SHARON L. ROBERTS, RN., Ph.D

California State University, Long Beach

Behavioral Concepts
and the
Critically Ill Patient

Second Edition

ACC APPLETON-CENTURY-CROFTS/Norwalk, Connecticut

UNIVERSITY OF ALASKA ANCHORAGE LIBRARY

ISBN 0-8385-0632-1 01

86 87 88 89 90/10 9 8 7 6 5 4 3 2 1

Prentice-Hall International (UK) Limited, *London*
Prentice-Hall of Australia Pty. Limited, *Sydney*
Prentice-Hall Canada Inc., *Toronto*
Prentice-Hall Hispanoamericana, S.A., *Mexico*
Prentice-Hall of India Private Limited, *New Delhi*
Prentice-Hall of Japan, Inc., *Tokyo*
Prentice-Hall of Southeast Asia Pte. Ltd., *Singapore*
Editora Prentice-Hall do Brasil, Ltda., *Rio de Janeiro*
Whitehall Books Limited, *Wellington, New Zealand*

Library of Congress Cataloging-in-Publication Data

ROBERTS, Sharon L., (date)
  Behavioral concepts and the critically ill patient.

  Includes bibliographies and index.
  1. Nurse and patient. 2. Critically ill—Psychology.
I. Title. [DNLM: 1. Critical Care—nurses' instruction.
2. Intensive Care Units—nurses' instruction. 3. Sick
Role—nurses' instruction. WY 154 R647b]
RT86.3.R625 1985   610.73'61   85-18657
ISBN 0-8385-0632-1

Editorial/production supervision and
  interior design: *Carol L. Atkins*
Cover design: *Edsal Enterprises*
Manufacturing buyer: *John Hall*

Printed in the United States of America

Contents

Chapter 3

HOPELESSNESS   95

Chapter 4

TERRITORIALITY AND SPACE   120

Chapter 5

HOSTILITY AND ANGER   144

Chapter 6

POWERLESSNESS   173

Chapter 7

AVOIDANCE AND DENIAL   197

Chapter 8

LONELINESS   223

Chapter 9

PSYCHOLOGICAL IMMOBILITY   252

Chapter 10

DEPERSONALIZATION   276

Chapter 11

TRANSFER ANXIETY   298

Chapter 15

STRESS   406

Chapter 16

FAMILY IN CRISIS   431

Chapter 17

DEPRESSION   457

Preface

The patient who enters a critical care unit is confronted with a multi-faceted setting that converges upon the patient in an attempt to maintain or strengthen his life system. Likewise, the nurse is confronted with a similar set of circumstances. While attempting to provide expert knowledge and quality patient care, the multiarticulating parts of the critical care environment, including the patient, can become lost. The critically ill patient's physiological parameters are constantly monitored by means of highly sophisticated technology. Unfortunately, technology has not been developed to monitor behavioral parameters. The second edition of *Behavioral Concepts and the Critically Ill Patient* is a consolidation of reference points from which the student and clinician can further investigate the behavioral world of critical care.

This edition has been organized around the nursing process: collection of data, assessment, diagnosis, implementation, and evaluation. The nursing assessment component of each chapter has been divided into regulatory behaviors and cognitive behaviors that will help the critical care nurse recognize overall behavioral problems. Furthermore, four chapters have been added to the revised text. These chapters cover the important topics of stress, loss, pain, and depression.

The first chapter, *BEEP*, has been expanded with additional physiological parameters and flow charts. The mnemonic BEEP provides a structure of behavioral, emotional, environmental, and physiological assessment which is applied to the patient and family. Most chapters contain case studies designed to assist the student in applying the particular behavioral concept being discussed. While this book's primary focus is on behavioral concepts, physiological concepts or problems are not to be minimized. For the student who would like to pursue specific physiological problems as they apply to the critically ill, *Physiological Concepts and the Critically Ill Patient*, written by this author and published by Prentice-Hall, Inc., is recommended.

While there are those who falsely believe nurses in critical care provide care for machines or that they simply are technicians, the informed person realizes that the nurses' responsibilities are enormous. Nurses are the ones who gather data, assess, diagnose, and determine whether or not a particular intervention will occur. As June Abbey pointed out in the preface of the first edition, "The nurses who courageously risk need to comprehend the phenomena which they meet, for they cannot encounter experience by escape, neither can they support, afford, or appreciate that which they do not understand. This book brings together the wired, monitored world of the critically ill with the lonely, frustrated internal world of fear."

Special thanks are extended to the book's production editor, Carol Atkins, for her effort and help on this project.

Sharon L. Roberts RN, PhD
Professor
Department of Nursing
California State University, Long Beach

1

BEEP: Behavior, Emotions, Environment, and Physiology Systematically Assessed in the Critically Ill Patient

BEHAVIORAL OBJECTIVES

1. List the four major levels of assessment according to the system.
2. State the four components of behavioral assessment.
3. Identify the twelve components of emotional assessment.
4. Discuss how three of the emotional components apply to the critically ill patient.
5. State the six components of environmental assessment.
6. Discuss how two of the environmental components apply to the critically ill patient.
7. Identify the nine components of physiological assessment.
8. Describe how each of the nine physiological components can be applied to the critically ill patient.

Psychological and physical assessment are significant components of the nursing process and are utilized by nurses working in various critical care units such as intensive care, coronary care, hemodialysis, respiratory care, and neurological care. Furthermore the critical care nurse draws upon knowledge of physical assessment skills to assist in the formulation of a nursing diagnosis of an individual suffering from physical dysfunction. The systematic assessment of a critically ill patient should be an orderly and precise method of collecting information about his* behavior, emotions, environment, and physiology. Of course, any systematic assessment should include observations on each of the factors that may influence the state of a critically ill patient's ability to cope with illness. "An individual's state of health and ability to cope with illness is influenced by his physiologic status, by his perception of and reaction to his social and physical environment, as well as by his understanding of what to expect and what he can do for himself. It is also influenced by stresses within the environment" (Giblin 1971, p. 113).

Today critical care nurses can, should, and do make observations and judgments about their patients. Nurses have become more knowledgeable in the contributing science and more competent in analytical thinking so that they are able to make decisions without waiting for medical direction. Critical care nurses are like computers with monitors themselves. They are filled with vital information designed to correlate with alterations in the patient's physiological status. Prepared with knowledge about how to care for the critically ill patient at his bedside, the nurse can produce valuable information and supply specific actions designed to assist the patient in recovering from illness or to provide supportive care in a pleasant manner. The nurse has the responsibility of assessing, intervening, and evaluating while simultaneously maintaining a warm, caring relationship with each of her patients. Such an approach necessitates continuous involvement between nurse and patient.

The critical care nurse needs a systems approach to making pertinent assessments, on the basis of which she formulates an overall diagnosis of the critically ill patient. A systems approach requires an understanding of how things work together in groups or classifications. If the nurse understands the overall pattern of a system, the significance and purpose of each part is clearer. The saying about not being able to see the forest for the trees implies that gaining a perception of the overall picture derived from assorted small facts is difficult if there is too much detail. I think of the trees as a series of assessments the nurse makes and of the forest as the overall diagnosis based on the assessments. It is difficult for the critical care nurse to assess details and to formulate a diagnosis equally well unless she has a systematic way of making her assessments. The critical care nurse has physiological knowledge regarding the normal functions of a particular system that enables her to observe deviations from the normal and to assess her critically ill patient's problem. The critical care nurse, as a human-to-human monitor, can collect,

---

*Of course critically ill patients as well as their nurses may be either male or female. For convenience, however, throughout this text the masculine pronoun is used to refer to the patient and the feminine pronoun is used to refer to the nurse.

record, transmit, and act upon data received only when she understands the normal; the nurse cannot be expected to recognize physiological dysfunction if she does not know what to look for normally. Frequently nurses in critical care units know what to do, when to do it, and how to do it, but fail to understand, even in a general way, the reasons behind their actions. A better understanding of these reasons gives nursing care its significance and allows the nurse to assess potential patient problems.

The critical care nurse serves as a human monitor with functions akin to those of the various pieces of cumbersome equipment in the critically ill patient's environment whose safety alarm systems signal when the patient is in trouble. The cardioscope alarm rings when the patient's heart rate rises or falls below a set number, indicating bradycardia, cardiac arrest, ventricular tachycardia, or ventricular fibrillation. Respirators that have a built-in alarm mechanism buzz when the patient's bronchus becomes obstructed with a mucous plug or when the patient and machine become separated from each other. The IVAC machine, responsible for delivering to the patient a preset number of drops of intravenous solution each minute, has an alarm that informs the nurse if her patient's IV is dry or if the soluset chamber is empty. The nurse as a human monitor also has a built-in alarm system that signals what I call a BEEP when potential danger threatens the patient.

BEEP represents *B*ehavioral, *E*motional, *E*nvironmental, and *P*hysiological assessment (see Figure 1.1). The BEEP concept helps the nurse to make quick and thorough assessments of any critically ill patient and to formulate her nursing diagnosis, which is frequently the same as the medical diagnosis for critical care patients. When a nurse approaches her patient, she must have a starting point determined by the nature and severity of her patient's illness. BEEP enables the nurse to begin at any of the four major levels, helping her to organize her assessments into categories and to conclude with an overall diagnosis. This concept provides a logical, sequential method of making observations for each major level.

The behavioral components of BEEP consist of patient consciousness, behavior consistency, the characteristics of a patient's background, and his movement control. Emotional assessment deals with components such as depersonalization, the frustration of helplessness, and patient despair. Environmental components include the effect of equipment, spatial relations, and sensory overload upon the patient. Physiological components include sclera color and condition of pupils; central venous pressure; systolic and diastolic arterial pressure; chest, cardiac, and bowel sounds; and the status of the pulmonary, cardiovascular, and renal systems. Flow charts in the following sections provide greater detail about each of these assessment levels. For example the nurse may begin her assessment by observing one part of the physiological system: she may observe that her patient's CVP is 24. After making additional assessments, she would formulate a nursing diagnosis of cardiac tamponade.

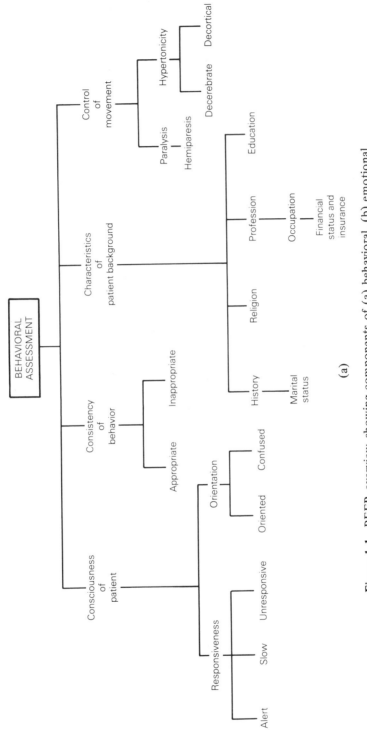

Figure 1.1 BEEP overview showing components of (a) behavioral, (b) emotional, (c) environmental, and (d) physiological assessment.

(a)

4

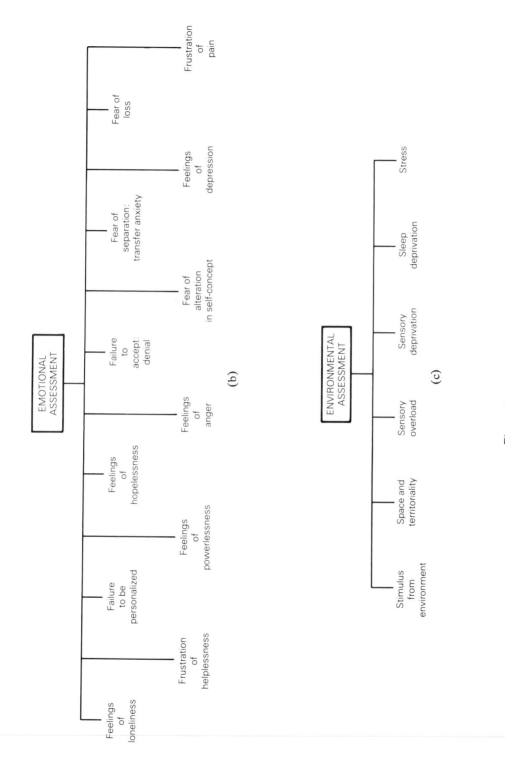

Figure 1.1 (continued)

5

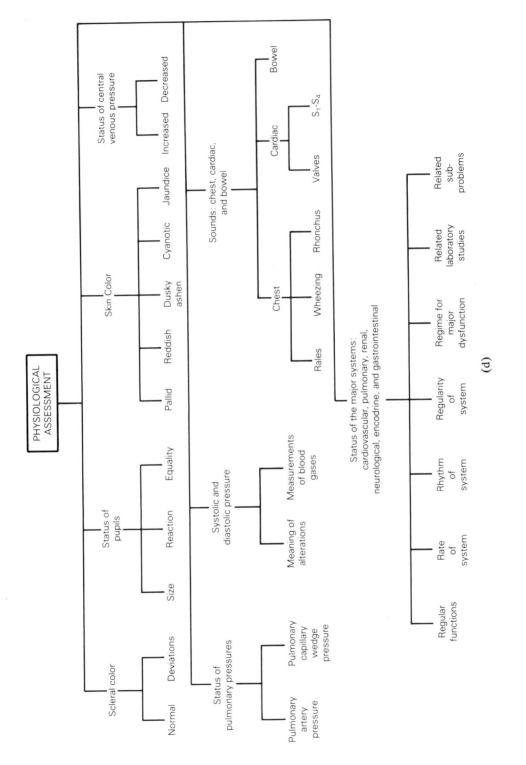

Figure 1.1 (continued)

BEHAVIOR ASSESSMENT

By extending her hand to her patient, squeezing his hand, and saying hello, the critical care nurse is able to make observations and assessments regarding his consciousness, consistency of behavior, and control of movement. By extending her hand, the nurse assesses whether her patient is able to extend his hand and find her hand. Usually when someone squeezes a hand the normal response is to squeeze back. When the nurse squeezes her patient's hand, she can assess his sensory-motor function and degree of hand grasp. Naturally the critically ill patient must be conscious in order to find his nurse's hand and then grasp it. When the nurse says hello, she is communicating a personal and warm interest in him. This entire process takes only a few seconds and yet provides the baseline information for making judgments about the patient's care or progress. If she observes a deviation, the nurse can begin gathering additional data in an attempt to formulate her nursing diagnosis and appropriate interventions.

Consciousness of Patient

The patient will be responsive or unresponsive, oriented or disoriented. Normally the patient will be reasonably alert and quick to respond to his environment. One frequently sees extremely alert behavior in patients who have survived a major physiological crisis. Excessive alertness may be attributed to initial hypoglycemia, anxiety, fear, impending hypovolemic shock, hyperthyroidism, or thyrotoxicosis. In addition some medications may cause the patient to become excessively alert. An excessively alert patient may be reacting to his environment. In questioning him, the nurse may discover that the patient is afraid of what is going on around him. For example, the patient may worry that the crisis confronting a patient next to him might happen to him, too, especially if both patients share similar physiological problems or surgeries. In this instance the nurse would assess that the particular problem is acute anxiety.

The nurse who observes that her patient is drowsy may note that he has received medication for pain. Therefore, she may assess that the drowsiness and slowness to respond is due to pain medication. If this is not the case, however, the nurse may infer that her patient's drowsiness or slowness to respond may be due to the following: electrolyte imbalance such as hyponatremia, hypochloremia, or hypokalemia; hypoxia or oxygen deficiency at the cellular level; ammonia intoxication where glutamine synthesis is interfered with, thereby altering cerebral metabolism; increased intracranial pressure; impending stroke; hypoxemia; CO_2 narcosis; or hypercarbia. The nurse can validate her inference by any of the following procedures: lumbar puncture, skull series, EEG, blood gases, electrolyte, or liver panel. Although the laboratory values may all be within normal limits, a lumbar puncture may reveal an elevated pressure, and an electroencephalogram may show a space-occupying lesion. The nurse then assesses that her critically ill patient has increased intracranial pressure, which compresses brain cells as the pressure builds up in the cranial cavity. The initial patient behavior may be confusion, disorientation, and delirium. However, this condition may deteriorate into deep coma.

The confused patient who does not have increased intracranial pressure may present an interesting assessment problem: the nurse may infer that her patient's confusion is due to hyponatremia (120 mEq/ℓ), hypokalemia (2.5 mEq/ℓ), increased BUN (7100 mg/dℓ), medications, sleep deprivation, hypercapnia, respiratory failure, or CHF causing decreased cardiac output and decreased cerebral perfusion. After finding the patient's electrolyte panel and blood gases normal, the nurse may listen to her patient's chest and take his vital signs. She discovers that he has bilateral rales, decreased blood pressure, and an increased heart rate. The nursing diagnosis becomes CHF with a decreased cardiac output. The decreased cardiac output results in decreased cerebral perfusion and anoxia, both capable of causing confusion.

Consistency of Behavior

The critical care nurse may assess appropriate changes in behavior such as a sudden withdrawal from environmental interaction due to depression; anger because of forced limitations or altered life-style; or denial of the physiological dysfunction for fear of further physiological loss. Furthermore, the patient behavior may be consistent with an anxiety response.

The nurse may observe degrees of anxiety in her critically ill patient. Initially the entire experience of acute illness may make him anxious. As his anxiety begins to subside, and as the reality of his illness with its potential threat to his being enters his consciousness, the patient may sleep much of the day, turn his back to the door, or avoid talking to staff. In presenting her observations to the patient, she discovers that this is his third major infarction in two years. He feels discouraged and fearful that he may not survive. The nurse then assesses his problem as depression. She should support him through the adaptive stage and offer realistic encouragement.

Inappropriate or sudden changes of behavior are also assessed by the nurse. Possible causes of inappropriate changes are cerebral metabolic disturbances attributed to cerebral insufficiency caused by reduced cardiac output and reduced cerebral perfusion pressure or hypoxia. Sudden changes in the patient's behavior should alert the nurse to possible metabolic disturbances that can be observed in conditions such as cerebral insufficiency with a reduced cardiac output. Neural cells are extremely sensitive to decreased oxygen supply. The first observation the nurse may make to support her assessment of anoxia is restlessness.

Characteristics of Patient Background

Characteristics of the critically ill patient include first of all a patient history. The patient history includes basic data such as diagnostic impression; biographical data and reliability of history; chief complaint; present illness; past medical history (chains), including childhood diseases, hospitalization, allergies, injury or other illness, narcotics, and surgeries; social history; and review of systems.

Other characteristics of the critically ill patient include his occupation, education, age, marital status, nationality, religion, number of children, insurance, and possibly financial status. Personal idiosyncrasies such as the time he wants his bath, his food likes and dislikes, and his previous patterns of coping with illness also merit consideration. The nurse may obtain this information by using a nursing history form. Learning personal characteristics about her patient enables the critical care nurse to participate in his world and to offer a more personal approach to his care. The patient's cultural background can be an influential factor in his care. For example, if the patient is a Gypsy and an influential leader within his clan, the nurse should understand the family's overwhelming concern for and protection of the patient, as well as the meaning of illness to his culture.

Control of Movement

It is especially important to observe the movements of patients who have suffered neurological injuries, who have fallen at home without apparent neurological trauma, or who have undergone neurological surgery. Nurses can also observe movements of patients who return from open heart surgery to assess possible cerebral embolism. Alteration in movement consists of paralysis, hemiparesis, and hypertonicity. Progressive hemiparesis can occur from compression either of a hemisphere or of the brainstem itself. The compression may be attributed to a lesion, injury, or clot. Furthermore, progressive hemiparesis can be a sign of impending stroke. Hypertonicity can be either decerebrate movement, whereby inhibiting signals from the basal ganglia and cerebral cortex to the retricular areas are removed, thus causing rigidity; or decortical movement, whereby cortex function is lost. Such abnormal movements are due to loss of higher inhibition upon brainstem and spinal reflex circuits.

EMOTIONAL ASSESSMENT

After the critical care nurse has assessed and diagnosed her patient's behavior, she can begin the assessment of his emotional status. Her patient may not experience all of the problems discussed here, but she must understand that such emotional conditions do exist.

Feelings of Loneliness

Loneliness can occur as existential or real loneliness and loneliness anxiety or fear of aloneness. In assessing existential loneliness, the nurse will note that it can result from two causes: the threat of illness and the psychological pain. Likewise loneliness anxiety is also assessed according to two causes: the fear of aloneness in the present environment and the fear of aloneness in the future. The nurse may observe that her patient is quiet, withdrawn, and tearful. She realizes that even though he is surrounded by hospital personnel, he still feels lonely. The people who take care of him in the early stages of his crisis have little significance in his normal life. The patient's behavior may be due to his presence in an unfamiliar environment, in which chairs, tables, bed, and curtains all belong to someone else. Some critical care units do not have television sets so patients cannot keep up with their favorite and familiar programs. The patient must submit to restrictions upon all the familiar activities of daily living, including contact with his family. This is particularly true for the aged patient in critical care, who lives in a constantly constricting environment. His aged friends may be unable to visit. His behavior and circumstances lead the nurse to diagnose his problem as loneliness.

Once the diagnosis is formulated the nurse intervenes to reduce existential loneliness by minimizing the threat of illness and minimizing psychological pain. Loneliness anxiety or fear of aloneness is reduced by fostering relatedness to the environment and fostering relatedness to the future.

Frustration of Helplessness

The critical care patient may feel that he has no control over his care or environment. The patient may say, "You treat me like a baby," or "Is diaper service part of my care?" Such statements stem from the situation in which someone else determines what he will eat, when he will be bathed, when his linen will be changed, and how he will defecate or urinate. As his treatment restricts all his normal activities, the patient finds himself dependent upon another person, his nurse. His problem is the frustration of helplessness.

Failure to Be Personalized

The nurse may assess depersonalization or dehumanization through the patient's detachment from the environment and himself. Depersonalization is a subjective mental phenomenon having as its central feature an altered awareness of the self.

The nurse may hear her patient say, "I am just another piece of equipment," or "You decided to talk to the old fossil." The nurse may discover that the patient heard himself being referred to as "the man in bed 7," "the acute myocardial infarction," "the man with the bleeding ulcer," "the foul-smelling patient with gangrene," or "the old fossil next to the window." The patient may feel lack of personalization when his nurse enters his room to check his cardioscope, IV tubing, and Foley; listen to his chest; take his vital signs; and *then* decide to say hello and introduce herself. By the time the nurse stops to say hello, the patient already feels like just another object to be manipulated. His problem is depersonalization.

Feelings of Powerlessness

Powerlessness can be assessed first as loss of control involving physiological loss of control, psychological loss of control, and environmental loss of control. Second, it is assessed as lack of knowledge. The nurse may observe a critically ill patient pulling out his IV tubing, refusing to wear his oxygen mask, or getting out of bed. He feels as if he has no power over his environment; therefore he assumes power by pulling tubes or defying orders. The nurses and doctors who make decisions regarding his well-being are total strangers to the patient. If he is an executive in charge of a company in which he makes major decisions each day, he may feel stripped of his decision-making power. The critical care nurse diagnoses his problem to be powerlessness.

Once the nurse makes her diagnosis, she intervenes to create feelings of powerfulness. First, to whatever extent is realistic, the nurse returns control in the form of physiological control, psychological control, and environmental control. Second, the nurse reinforces the patient's learning and knowledge level.

Feelings of Hopelessness

Hopelessness can be assessed according to two categories. First there are factors threatening the internal resources of the patient: his illness and his ability to cope accordingly. Second, there are his perceptions of the external resources such as the environment and persons within that environment who can help him. The nurse may assess that her patient seems depressed. Such is the case of the critically ill patient who experiences his third acute myocardial infarction in a relatively short period of time, or the patient who returns to the hospital for the third time in one year with CHF and pulmonary edema. Another example is the patient who transfers to the general floor and several days later extends his MI. This particular patient feels depressed regarding his progress. The patient's depressed behavior coupled with his current or previous illness leads the nurse to diagnose his problem as hopelessness. The nurse must then supply her patient with a realistic element of hope.

Once the nursing diagnosis of hopelessness has been made, the nurse's interventions are designed to foster hopefulness by helping the patient find reality in the current illness, motivating the patient through education towards a future, establishing meaningful goals, and encouraging the family to participate in the patient's care.

Feelings of Anger

There are two general characteristics of anger and hostility expression inhibited to be assessed: the perception of a threat and the location of the agent of harm. The critical care nurse observes that the patient is angry and hostile. He yells and screams at people who approach him. The patient's behavior may be his only defense against an unfamiliar environment. He may feel he has no control over the course of events that will eventually lead to his recovery. The patient may be angry at being ill because illness is not a part of his life-style.

The critically ill patient's display of anger may be the only energy output or control system he feels he has in a strange, unyielding environment. His behavioral output in the form of anger is the patient's way of handling and adapting to a very unpleasant situation. Instead of dismissing the patient as irascible, the nurse should accept and understand the patient and motivate his behavior toward acceptance of his situation.

Once the nursing diagnosis of anger and hostility is made, the nurse attempts to mobilize the patient's internal energies into appropriate external expressions of his feelings.

Failure to Accept: Denial

Avoidance and denial can be assessed first according to direct-action tendencies: directly expressed avoidance with fear, fear with avoidance expression inhibited, or avoidance without fear. Second, it is assessed according to defensive reappraisal: denial.

The nurse who observes that her patient is jovial and quite talkative about his family, animals, or business may mistakenly feel that he has accepted his current illness. She should assess the happy-go-lucky patient as being in the denial stage of adaptation. The patient discusses peripheral topics in order to keep the spotlight off himself and his feelings. The critical care nurse realizes that the patient's high level of anxiety makes him unable to assimilate his environment and to derive meaning from it. Once he has assimilated his surroundings, he will receive still more stimulus. As the pieces of his environment begin to fit together, and he realizes the implications of his illness, the patient may momentarily choose to deny. The nurse should diagnose his behavior as temporary denial.

Once the nursing diagnosis of avoidance and denial has been made, the nurse's interventions are twofold: protecting the patient's personal integrity and helping him to accept the illness or disfigurement.

Fear of Alteration in Body Image and Self-Concept

Responses to alteration in body image and self-concept can be assessed according to four phases: impact, retreat, acknowledgement, and reconstruction.

The male patient who has had a severe myocardial infarction with little myocardial reserve may be dependent upon his wife to be the breadwinner. The nurse may observe the patient showing hostility toward his wife. In talking to the nurse about her assessment, he may express that he is really hostile at himself for being ill and dependent. Virtually all acute illnesses, whether they leave internal or external scars, cause some changes in body image. The degree of change varies with each individual and depends upon his previous ability to cope with crisis. The nurse must assess the significance of illness for the individual and what changes, if any, will occur in his self-concept. In the case mentioned above, the nurse assesses that the patient and his wife have been forced suddenly to make role changes. In addition the patient has to change his self-concept. The patient's behavior is due to his fear of alteration of body image.

After the diagnosis of fear of alteration in body image or self-concept has been made, the nurse designs interventions around the four phases of impact, retreat, acknowledgement, and reconstruction.

Feelings of Anxiety: Transfer Anxiety

Transfer and the anxiety it generates occur in two different situations: when the individual is transferred from one critical care unit to another, and when the patient is moved from a critical care unit to a general floor. Transfer anxiety can be further assessed according to three components: primary anxiety, fright, or expectant anxiety.

When the critically ill patient is admitted into critical care, he is most anxious about the threats to his biological well-being. The critical care unit may represent biological security, but it does not represent emotional security. Everything around him, including the technical language used by the staff and the wires, tubes, and pieces of equipment, is foreign to him. However, as the days progress and the biological crisis subsides, the patient realizes that he and his nurse have built an emotional bond. Then the critical care unit takes on a new meaning to the patient. He feels a sense of emotional security. His nurse knows his needs, fears, and concerns. He feels secure knowing that either his own nurse or another one is visually present to care for him. Just when the nurse-patient bond is at its peak, the patient is transferred to a subacute unit or to the general floor. The transfer may be anticipated, or it may occur suddenly due to the need of space for a more critically ill patient. In either case the patient will experience transfer anxiety. The important factor is the degree to which he experiences this type of anxiety: a patient who is not prepared for his transfer may have an anxiety reaction that causes him to be readmitted into critical care.

In order to minimize transfer anxiety, the nurse can begin her work the moment a patient arrives in a critical care unit. After the diagnosis of transfer anxiety has been made, the nurse begins to reduce the conditions that lead to the three components of transfer anxiety: primary anxiety, fright, and expectant anxiety.

Feelings of Depression

The nurse can assess depression according to a general model of self-regulation involving three stages: self-monitoring, consisting of perception of the loss and perception of life stressors; self-evaluation, consisting of a negative view of self, a negative view of experiences, and a negative view of future; and self-reinforcement.

When the critically ill patient is confronted with an illness or injury, he experiences feelings of depression. Feelings of depression may not be an immediate behavioral response to illness. Instead the nurse may observe that the patient is jovial one day and withdrawn, silent, or fearful the next. When losses are noted and seen as related to the patient's emotional state, the depressed individual is likely to consider the loss as deserved or as punishment for some real or assumed transgression.

After the nurse diagnoses the patient's behavioral response as depression, nursing interventions are grouped into two categories: fostering cognitive reappraisal and facilitating realistic independence.

Fear of Loss

Loss or the threat of loss can be a new experience for the critically ill patient. In assessing depression in the critically ill patient, two factors are significant. First is the concern for physiological survival. Second is the competent behavior utilized as the patient copes or adapts to his physiological threat and which involves three degrees or orders of denial: first-order denial, second-order denial, and third-order denial.

Loss or the threat of loss can be a new experience for the patient. The loss can be the result of acute illness, injury, or disease. For some critically ill patients it is an adaptation to dying. For others it is the loss of health or the loss of a limb, a blow to their self-concept, or the sudden necessity to change their life-style. It should be noted that the type of physiological loss or injury has tremendous significance for some patients. Some critically ill patients use negation as a process through which they respond to something perceived as a threat. Negation behaviorally manifested as denial is a defense behind which the patient can retreat. If he denies the loss, then its meaning or future implication cannot be emotionally assessed.

Once the nurse has diagnosed the patient's behavioral response due to loss, interventions are organized around, first, internal variables of pathological processes, psychological processes such as self-esteem and personality variables, age and prior experiences, beliefs and values, and anxiety. Second, interventions are organized around external variables that encompass the critical care environment; social-cultural values and available support systems.

Frustration of Pain

Pain can be assessed according to two components: physiological and psychological. The physiological component includes pain threshold, pain tolerance, and pain reaction. The psychological component includes the perception of past experiences and the perception of pain as a threat to the patient's physical or emotional integrity.

Pain viewed as overwhelming by the critically ill patient demands his immediate attention because it disrupts ongoing behavior and thought. Pain serves as a motivating force that drives the person into activity aimed at stopping it. For the patient in coronary care, chest pain is a signal of potential physical loss. The chest pain reinforces the patient's perception of cardiac involvement. Serial EKGs and isoenzymes support the diagnosis of acute myocardial infarction. The pain tells the individual that a breach in the protective barrier has taken place.

After a diagnosis of pain has been made, the critical care nurse organizes nursing interventions around three categories: prepain experience, actual pain experience, and postpain experience.

ENVIRONMENT ASSESSMENT

The critical care nurse who makes assessments and diagnoses regarding the events that alter her patient's behavior must also look clearly at his environment. The environment can channel the critically ill patient's progress toward an affirmative or a destructive outcome.

Environmental assessment is an aspect of the patient's care that is frequently taken for granted. As we know, the environment contains sensory stimuli that affect the patient. The stimuli enter the patient through any one or all of his senses. Each stimulus can then play upon his battered senses. The critical care nurse may be so adapted to the environment that she fails to observe its effect on the patient.

Stimulus from Equipment

The nurse may assess that her patient is hallucinating. The critically ill patient will find himself surrounded by various pieces of unfamiliar equipment, each of which has its unique sound that creates a very noisy world. The stimulus produced by either the patient's equipment or that of someone else close to his bed can lead to sensory overload. Whether the patient is critically ill or heavily sedated, he is unable to judge what is normal around him. Therefore the sounds emanating from his environment become magnified to frightening levels. If the incoming stimulus from his environment is great, the nurse might consider it to be the origin of his behavior.

Space and Territoriality

The nurse assesses alteration in space and territoriality according to body factors, which include space around the individual, self-ego dimension, and illness necessitating intrusive procedures; environmental factors such as the physical setting and environmental props; antecedent factors that involve intrusion; and organism need states.

After repeated intrusions into the patient's personal territory, the nurse may observe that he is angry, hostile, and argumentative. The critically ill patient has a limited space no larger than his bed. This space may be only three or four feet wide. The territory around his bed contains various pieces of equipment: a cardioscope, an arterial line, a CVP manometer, chest tubes and bottles, a hypothermia machine, a respirator, an IVAC machine, or a hemodialysis machine. The equipment takes space and intrudes into the patient's already limited territory. The nurse may diagnose that her patient's behavior is due to territorial intrusion.

It is significant for critical care nurses to obtain information from the patient or family about territoriality needs when doing a nursing assessment. The critical care nurse uses proxemics when organizing various interventions. The four distance zones defined in proxemics are termed intimate, personal, social, and public.

Sensory Overload

All behavior is completely determined by, and pertinent to, the perceptual field of the behaving organism. The field of perception is responsible for the individual behavior. Sensory overload involving the phenomenal or perceptual field can be assessed according to four properties: fluidity, intensity, direction, and stability.

Sensory overload, also referred to as environmental overdose, can occur immediately after the patient is admitted into a critical care unit. The nurse may hear her patient say, "Can't they turn off the noise and let me rest? I am going out of my mind." After admission into critical care, the patient must submit to several diagnostic procedures. The procedures can be done in a relatively short period of time, overwhelming the patient. He begins to feel overloaded. In addition to activities that created the overload, the sounds within his environment create what the nurse should diagnose as sensory overload.

After the diagnosis of sensory overload has been made, the nurse designs her interventions according to the use of proxemics and the four distance zones—intimate, personal, social, and public.

Sensory Deprivation

Sensory deprivation is assessed according to its causes—reduction in stimulation of the senses, reduction in meaningfulness of stimulation, removal from familiar stimulation, and restrictions imposed on bodily movements—and the resulting behavior caused by deprivation.

Sensory deprivation in ICU can also be called emotional-touch deprivation. A patient may have been very critical for a period of three days. During this time the nurse has primarily observed his physiological condition. Because he was critical, he could not receive family visits. Now that the patient is physiologically stable, the nurse observes that he is quiet and withdrawn.

The nurse may give more time to the patient's equipment than to the patient himself, leaving him with very little tactile stimulation and causing emotional-touch deprivation. The nurse also realizes that while her patient was critical, he was unable to differentiate meaningless from meaningful stimuli, and therefore he blocked out all stimuli. The patient's current behavior leads the nurse to diagnose his problem as emotional-touch deprivation.

Once a diagnosis of sensory deprivation has been made, the critical care nurse can facilitate deprivation avoidance by being aware of the patient's physical environment. The nurse accomplishes her goals through management of the patient's environment and by maintaining meaningful stimulation.

Sleep Deprivation

Sleep deprivation is assessed by the nurse in two ways. She first looks at situations in the patient's environment that create increased sensory input. The increased input deprives the patient of his rest and sleep. Second, there are situations that require more sleep, such as illness. The once-quiet patient may become the angry man throwing objects in his room or becoming confused. In critical care units the nurse may have to awaken the patient every one to four hours to check his vital signs, measure his urine output, or suction him. The patient is unable to sleep, and even tranquilizers or sedatives fail to help. Sleep deprivation causes angry and confused behavior.

After the diagnosis of sleep deprivation has been made, the nurse's role is to create an environment conducive for sleep. Providing a conducive environment means that the nurse will attempt to minimize situations leading to increased stimulus input and to facilitate sleep required by illness.

Stress

Stress is assessed according to a stress framework. The stress framework consists of three components: degree and/or duration of stress, which is in turn divided into psychological categories (threat phase, danger impact phase, and postimpact victimization phase) and physiological categories; previous experiences involving stress tolerances and perception of stressful events; and available resources, which include external and internal resources.

Stress affects all critically ill patients. Hospitalization in critical care with a biophysiological illness can create both physiological and psychological stress. For such patients the stress they experience revolves around loss of significant others, loss of identity, loss of familiarity, and loss of function or purpose.

When the diagnosis of stress has been formulated, nursing interventions focus on the three phases within the stress framework. These include interventions based on the degree and/or duration of stress, the patient's previous experience with stress, and the resources available to alleviate stress.

PHYSIOLOGICAL ASSESSMENT

Having assessed the critically ill patient's behavioral, emotional, and environmental systems, the nurse begins the sometimes tedious task of making physiological assessments. The logical and sequential system of collecting data that is presented in this section can greatly reduce the tedium. It is beyond the scope of the chapter to include all physiological reasons behind the assessment process or physiological deviations. The physiological component is presented as an overview or comprehensive examination of possibilities.

The nurse can make physiological assessments and diagnoses by beginning with the sclera and continuing until the status of the major system has been examined. The status of the major systems—pulmonary, cardiovascular, and renal—will be discussed in detail because these are the systems most commonly affected by illness. The status of minor systems—endocrine, neurological, and gastrointestinal—will be discussed in less detail. Regardless of the systems involved, the nurse can make observations about each system's regular functions, rate, rhythm, regularity, and regime of major dysfunction, as well as about related problems and related nursing care. The assessment or diagnosing process remains constant, so that the critical care nurse may incorporate any illness or pathology into the data-collecting framework.

Sclera Color

Normally the sclera of the eyes are white. The nurse may observe that her patient's sclera is red or bloodshot. In talking with the patient, she learns that he had a painful night and feels discouraged about his progress. The nurse assesses her patient's problem to be a feeling of hopelessness and concludes that he needs additional emotional support. If the nurse observes that her patient's eyes are yellow, she may infer that the color is due to an increase in bilirubin. This in turn may be due to hepatic failure or biliary tract obstruction. To validate her inference, she will look in the patient's chart, where she might find that his bilirubin and alkaline phosphatase levels are both elevated. On the basis of the alkaline phosphatase level, the nurse assesses her patient's problem to be obstructive biliary disease. Figure 1.2 shows in more detail why the patient's sclera may be jaundiced.

Status of Pupils

To obtain accurate measurements of pupil size, the nurse should use a flashlight with good batteries and provide an environment in which the degree of darkness will be consistent. To keep the light source consistent, the nurse should use the same flashlight each time. The nurse checks the pupils for size, equality of size, and reaction to light (see Figure 1-3).

Problems associated with the optic nerve are characterized by (1) disturbance or loss of visual acuity, (2) pupillary abnormalities, (3) visual field defects, and (4) changes in the fundus oculi. Only the first two will be

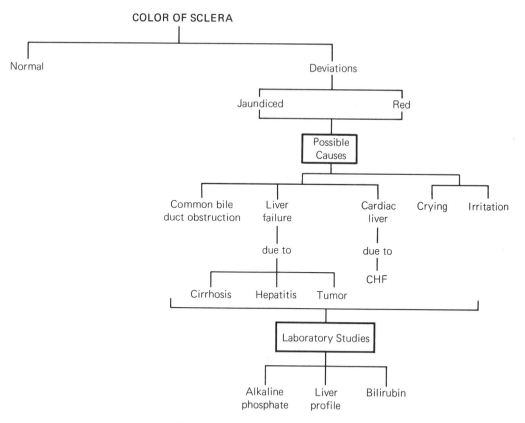

Figure 1.2 Assessment of sclera color.

briefly discussed. The optic nerve may be involved primarily by trauma and by a host of inflammatory and compressive lesions between the retina and the optic chiasm (Mancall 1981).

Disease of the optic nerve is associated with partial or complete loss of vision (amblyopia). Tumors that compress or infiltrate the optic nerves cause a slowly progressing impairment. In papilledema caused by increased intracranial pressure, the visual acuity is ordinarily preserved, but may deteriorate subsequently as secondary ("consecutive") optic atrophy ensues (Mancall 1981).

Pupillary abnormalities are common in the face of optic nerve disease and reflect interruption of the afferent portion of the light reflex arc. With acute changes of the optic nerve, the pupil is often dilated to at least some extent. The involved pupil fails to react to direct light, but the consensual response is preserved (Mancall 1981).

Diseases of the ocular nerve lead to changes in ocular motility and problems affecting the oculomotor nerve cause pupillary alterations. The normal pupil is round, centrally placed, regular in outline, equal in size to its fellow, and responds promptly to light, both direct and indirect (consensual),

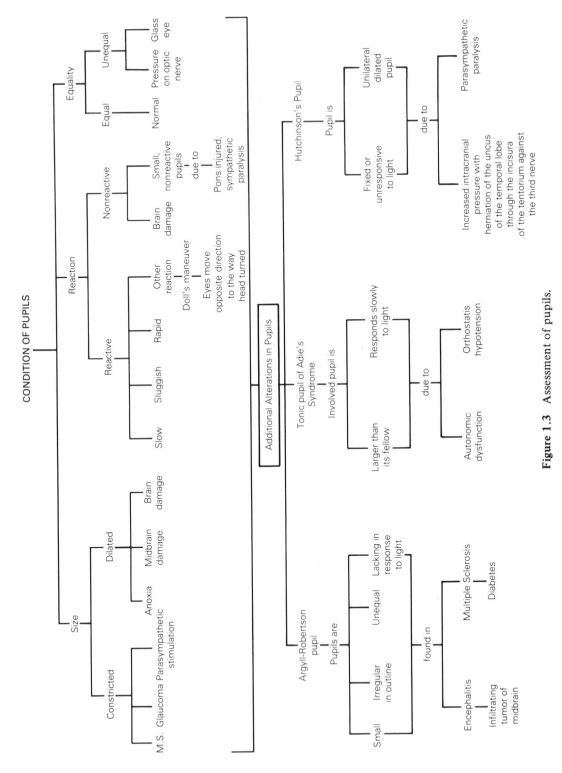

Figure 1.3 Assessment of pupils.

and to accommodation. Unequal pupils (anisocoria) may be observed in otherwise entirely normal individuals. A pupil is said to be slow or sluggish in its reaction when it contracts slowly or imperfectly to direct light, and over a less than anticipated range (Mancall 1981).

Alterations in the critically ill patient's pupils can reflect physiological changes other than neurological. In cases of respiratory or circulatory failure, excess carbon dioxide in the blood causes the pupil to be dilated. In checking reaction to light the nurse records the rapidity (e.g., slow, sluggish, or rapid) of the pupil. The equality of the pupils may be affected by things other than hematoma on the third cranial nerve. The patient may have a glass eye in which there is no reaction by the pupil. Another factor to consider is that the patient may have glaucoma necessitating eye drops that constrict the pupil. The nurse may observe that both her patient's pupils are constricted. She further observes that the patient is receiving morphine sulfate for pain. The nurse assesses that her patient's pinpoint pupils are due to morphine effect and observes him closely for respiratory depression. Figure 1.3 shows why the pupils may be unequal, nonreactive, or dilated.

Skin Color

The nurse can observe the skin color of the critically ill patient's lips, cheeks, chin, earlobes, and nails. The lips often show the most rapid color changes because they are very vascular and their blood vessels are superficial. The continuum of color changes ranges from pallor to reddish to dusky-ashen to cyanotic to jaundiced. For possible causes of color changes refer to Figures 1.4(a) to (d).

It should be noted that for the dark-skinned critically ill patient, the nurse may assess slightly different changes in skin color. For example, in pallor there is the absence of underlying red tones that give dark skin a flow. In brown skin there is a yellow-brown appearance, whereas black skin will manifest an ashen-gray appearance. Pallor assessed in dark-skinned patients implies shock and anemia. In assessing jaundice, the nurse should keep in mind that the sclera of darkly pigmented individuals have heavy deposits of subconjunctival fat that contains carotene to mimic jaundice. If the palate of the patient does not have heavy pigmentation, jaundice can be detected.

The critical care nurse can also observe warmth of the skin (see Figure 1.5). Temperature elevation may follow surgery, infection, dehydration, or acute myocardial infarction, in which there is tremendous cellular death. Neurologically a rise in temperature may be due to failure of the thermoregulatory mechanism (induced by compression). However, elevation more commonly indicates respiratory or urinary tract infection. A rise in temperature can increase myocardial activity, thus increasing the workload of the possibly damaged heart, or can increase metabolic rate, which in turn can increase the temperature.

While checking the temperature of her patient's skin, the nurse should also look for evidence of diaphoresis. She can observe the forehead, the

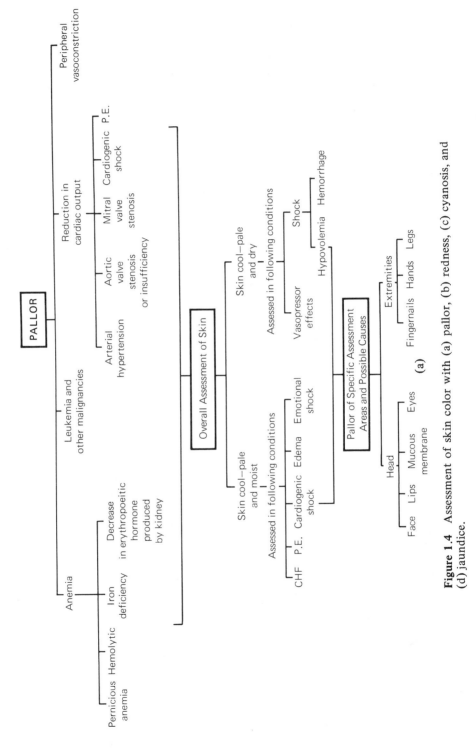

Figure 1.4 Assessment of skin color with (a) pallor, (b) redness, (c) cyanosis, and (d) jaundice.

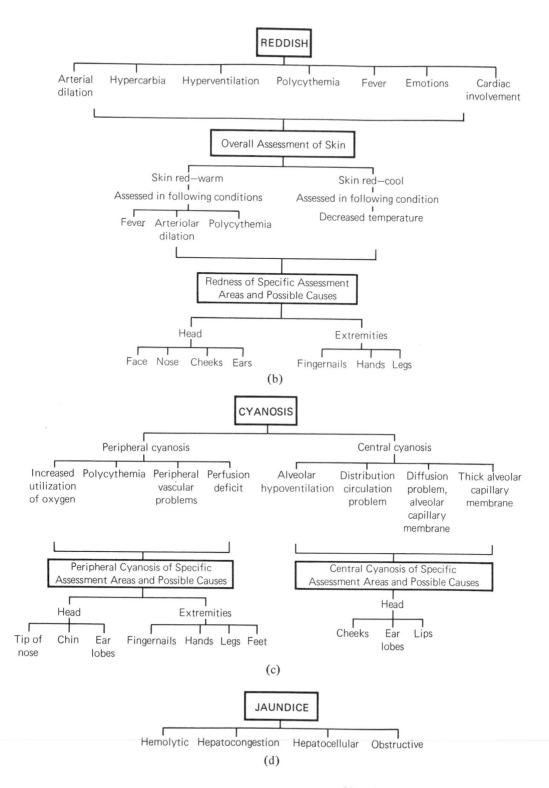

(b)

(c)

(d)

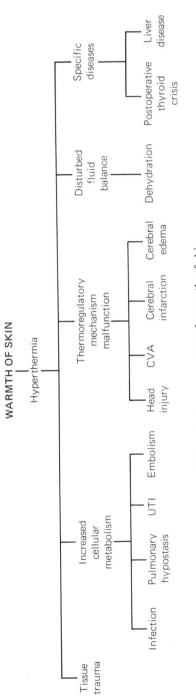

Figure 1.5 Assessment of warmth of skin.

palms, and the upper lip. A patient who is in acute pulmonary edema may be extremely diaphoretic from head to toe. Diaphoresis of the forehead and palm of the critically ill patient may signify impending shock. It is possible to discern the sometimes sudden fall of fluid pressure in shock other than by the more obvious changes in pallor and pulse pressure. The nurse may observe that patients inspire sharply, as though surprised, when their splenic and pulmonary reservoirs become mobilized. In addition, perspiration may spread from forehead to palm.

The nurse may observe that her patient's skin color is dusky-ashen. She further observes that his skin is cool and extremely diaphoretic to the touch. The nurse finds that her patient's blood pressure is 88/60, as compared to an earlier recording of 120/60, and she notes that his cardioscope pattern shows sinus tachycardia at a rate of 140; his central venous pressure is 18, with neck vein distention; his urine output for the last two hours has been 15 cc; and he has bilateral rales. On the basis of these observations, the nurse would formulate a diagnosis of congestive heart failure with impending pulmonary edema.

Status of Central Venous Pressure

Central venous pressure measures the mean right atrial pressure and also reflects the right ventricular end diastolic pressure. It is influenced by the preload, contractility, and afterload of the right ventricle. The preload for the right heart is the volume of blood in the right ventricle at the end of diastole, which is determined by the venous return. Preload changes will lead to changes in CVP. Poor contractility of the right ventricle causes an increase in the right ventricular end diastolic pressure. An increased LVEDP subsequently causes a rise in CVP and RLVEP. Afterload signifies the pressure the right ventricle must overcome in order to pump blood into the pulmonary system. An increased afterload causes an increased CVP. The mean right atrial pressure ranges from 1 to 6 mm Hg. Right ventricular systolic pressure is 15–25 mm Hg with diastolic pressure at 0–8 mm Hg. Therefore the normal patient when lying at a 45° angle in bed has flat cervical neck veins. Refer to Figure 1.6 for deviations in central venous pressure.

The nurse observing a patient who has just experienced open heart surgery for coronary artery bypass notes that his venous pressure is 28. After checking the catheter for patency, the nurse observes that her patient's blood pressure is 80/60, his urine output for two hours is 15 cc, his neck veins are distended, his color is cyanotic, the cardioscope pattern is sinus tachycardia (150), and he is restless. On the basis of these observations and the data collected by the nurse correlated to the type of surgery, the nurse infers that her patient's problem is cardiac tamponade. A chest X-ray may reveal a small heart validating the nurse's inference and confirming a nursing diagnosis of cardiac tamponade.

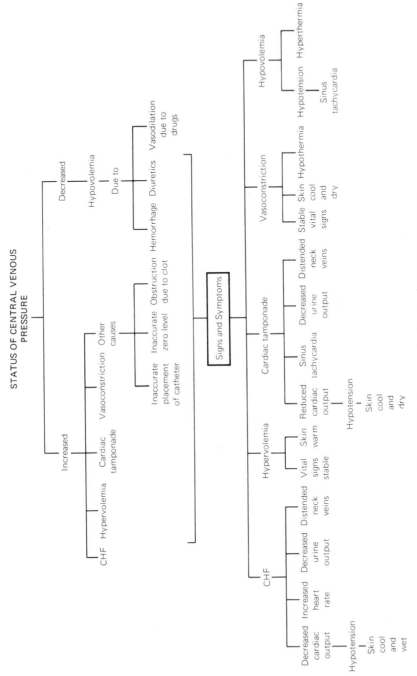

Figure 1.6 Assessment of central venous pressure.

Status of Pulmonary Pressures

The Swan-Ganz catheter allows the nurse to monitor pulmonary artery pressure (PAP) and pulmonary artery wedge pressure (PAWP). The pulmonary artery wave form is represented by two positive deflections. The first represents the systolic pressure generated from contraction of the right ventricle. The second positive deflection signifies the dicrotic wave following closure of the pulmonic valve. The normal pulmonary artery systolic pressure is 20–30 mm Hg with the diastolic pressure as <12 mmH. The pulmonary artery mean pressure, which determines the afterload for the right ventricle, is less than 15 mm Hg. Afterload is the amount of tension the ventricles must develop during contraction to eject blood. Arterial pressure and ventricular size or radius determine afterload. Therefore afterload is related to the resistance of blood ejected from the left ventricle into the aorta and is determined by peripheral vascular resistance.

A pulmonary capillary wedge pressure (PCWP) is obtained when the balloon in the Swan-Ganz is inflated. The inflated balloon blocks the high pressure generated by the right ventricle so that only pressure from the left atrium is recorded. The PCWP measures the left atrial mean pressure and left ventricular end-diastolic pressure. Preload is related to the volume of blood distending the ventricle at the end of diastole and is reflected in the left vetricular end diastolic pressure (LVEDP), which is estimated by PCWP. Ventricular compliance will determine the intraventricular pressures for any given volume. In other words, preload or myocardial fiber stretch increases the force of contraction to a certain point and subsequently increases the volume of blood ejected from the left ventricle. On the other hand, excessive preload produces a fall in contractility and ultimately cardiac output. For normal values and alterations in both PAP and PCWP see Figure 1.7.

Systolic and Diastolic Arterial Pressure

While arm cuff blood pressure accurately reflects the true intraarterial pressure in the well patient without complications, frequently it is difficult or impossible to measure in the critically ill patient with cardiopulmonary disease. Intraarterial pressure monitoring allows accurate measurement of systolic, diastolic, and mean pressures and is used increasingly for patient monitoring during cardiac surgery and in critical care units (Daily and Schroeder 1981).

Meaning of Arterial Blood Pressure. The maintenance of normal blood pressure requires an effective pump and cardiac output, moderate vascular tone, and an effective circulatory blood volume. During ventricular systole the aortic valve opens and blood is rapidly ejected into the arterial system, causing an increase in both arterial pressure and volume. The peak pressure reached is termed the systolic arterial pressure and reflects the maximum systolic LV pressure. The systolic pressure also reflects the compliance

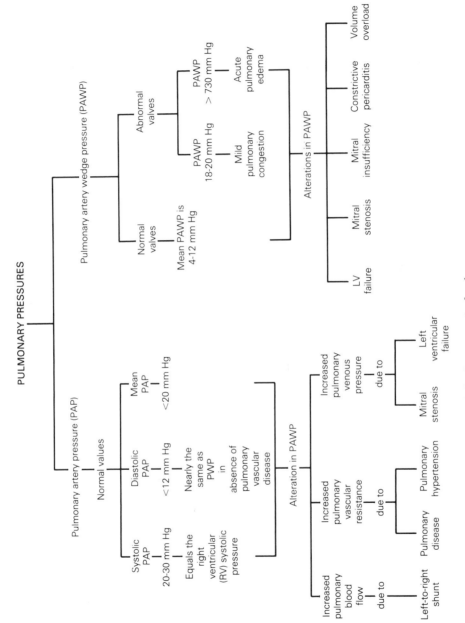

Figure 1.7 Assessment of pulmonary pressures.

of the large arteries and total peripheral resistance. After the phase of rapid ejection, runoff of blood from the proximal aorta to the peripheral vessels occurs, causing the aortic pressure to decline to minimum levels until the next ventricular ejection. The nadir of declining pressure is termed the diastolic arterial pressure and reflects both the velocity of runoff and the elasticity of the arterial system. The mean arterial pressure is represented by the formula

$$\frac{systolic - diastolic \times 2}{3} .$$

Cardiac output is a significant component in assessing arterial blood pressure. When the Swan-Ganz catheter with the thermodilution lumen is used, the external end of the thermistor portion of the catheter is connected to a bedside cardiac output computer. Cardiac output is the amount of blood ejected by the heart per unit of time and is reported as liters per minute. Therefore cardiac output is the product of heart rate and stroke volume ($CO = HR \times SV$). Cardiac output is affected not only by the factors within the heart but by resistance to ejection of the blood from the ventricle (afterload). The higher the systolic blood pressure, the higher the resistance to ejection of an adequate stroke volume. The normal resting cardiac output is 4–8 ℓ/min (Daily and Schroeder 1981). See Figure 1.8 for factors causing low cardiac output.

If the critically ill patient experiences a decrease in cardiac output, his heart will compensate by increasing its pumping ability, resulting in sinus tachycardia. The patient may be unable to compensate further and to handle adequately the sinus tachycardia (160–180), and he may go into congestive heart failure and pulmonary edema. The nurse will observe decreased blood pressure, increased size of cervical neck veins, and decreased urinary output. The nurse's observations will lead her to assess his problem as congestive heart failure.

Vascular tone depends on the sending of signals in the carotid sinus to the vasomotor centers. These centers control heart rate; thus, an increase in sympathetic stimulation causes tachycardia. Likewise, a decrease in vagal tone causes bradycardia.

The critical care nurse must be aware of the vagal effects caused by suctioning. This is particularly significant for the patient who has had a myocardial infarction and is having arrhythmias. Suctioning such a patient may cause bradycardia. If the patient is having frequent PVCs, the ectopic beats might take over as the primary pacemaker, causing ventricular tachycardia or ventricular fibrillation. Furthermore, bradycardia can lead to decreased cardiac output and pump failure. If the nurse, while suctioning or passing a nasal gastric tube, observes that her patient suddenly develops sinus bradycardia, she may then infer that the cause is from the vagal effect of her procedure.

An effectively circulating blood volume depends on a moderate level of arteriolar and venous tone and control of regional blood flow. When the critically ill patient is hypotensive due to myocardial infarction and an in-

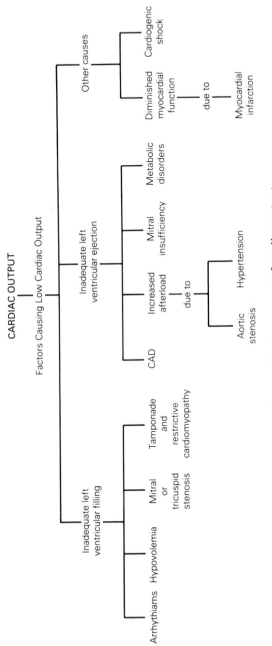

Figure 1.8 Assessment of cardiac output.

adequate pump, or in hypovolemic shock due to hemorrhage, sustained reflex vasoconstriction of the skin, muscle, and visceral arteries keeps blood flowing to priority organs. The nurse may observe that her patient, who has just returned from surgery for abdominal aortic aneurysm resection, is restless. If the observes decreased blood pressure, absence of urinary output, cool and dry skin, weak thready peripheral pulses, if the cardioscope pattern shows sinus tachycardia, and if there is a decrease in the central venous pressure, the nurse would assess that her critically ill patient is possibly in hypovolemic shock secondary to hemorrhage. There are three critical factors: (1) the patient has just returned from surgery, (2) he has a low venous pressure indicating hypovolemia, and (3) he has weak peripheral pulses. These factors lead to a nursing diagnosis of hemorrhagic shock.

There are other reasons besides shock that explain why a critically ill patient may be hypotensive. For example, he could have any one of the following problems: hypoxia, pain, cardiac tamponade, arrhythmias, hypovolemia, low cardiac output, metabolic acidosis, medication overload, anxiety, decreased ADH, or decreased aldosterone. On the other hand, the critically ill patient may be hypertensive because of any one of the following factors: pain, activity, CHF, carbon dioxide retention, renal disease, vasopressor drugs, increased ADH, or increased aldosterone.

Measurement of Blood Gases. The arterial line is an excellent source for arterial blood needed to assess the critically ill patient's blood gases. The patient need not experience frequent and often painful femoral punctures to make this assessment. Blood gases are helpful in assessing the patient with chronic obstructive pulmonary disease who is on a respirator or the patient who has recently experienced open heart surgery.

The critical care nurse may be the first person to receive her patient's blood gas report. She must know how to interpret the values and correlate them with observations made of the patient. Sometimes the patient looks more critical than his blood gases indicate. In correlating her observations and blood gases, the nurse can formulate an overall assessment of her patient's respiratory status. For example, a patient's blood gas may consist of the following: pH 7.24, pCO_2 55, HCO_3 28, and pO_2 70 mm Hg. The nurse observes that her critically ill patient's respirations are shallow, slow, and moist. She further notes that he is not receiving oxygen. On the basis of her observations and the blood gas report, the nurse would make a diagnosis of respiratory acidosis caused by hypoventilation. The nurse intervenes by first encouraging her patient to breath deeply while she simultaneously administers oxygen or ventilates the patient. Second, the nurse suctions the patient in an attempt to reduce secretions and to increase diffusion of oxygen across the alveolar-capillary membrane. Refer to Figure 1.9 for examples of blood gas deviations. It should be noted that a noncompensated acidosis or alkalosis will show the following changes in $PaCO_2$ and HCO_3: in metabolic acidosis $PaCO_2 > 40$; in metabolic alkalosis $PaCO_2 < 40$. Likewise in respiratory acidosis $HCO_3 < 24$; in respiratory alkalosis $HCO_3 > 24$.

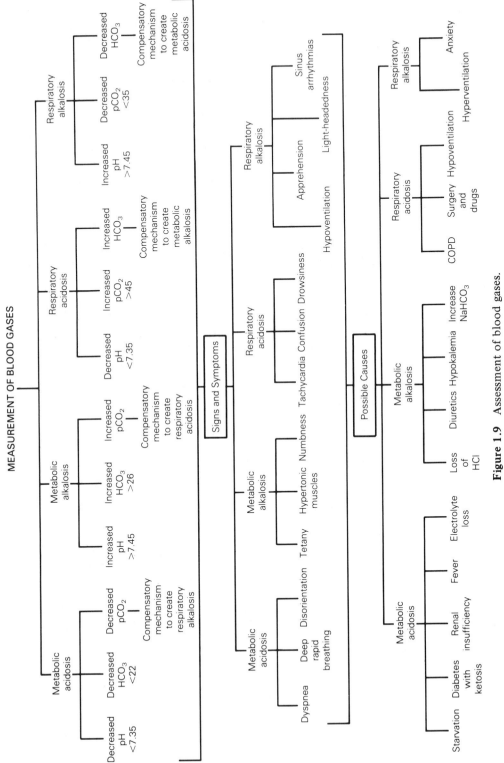

Figure 1.9 Assessment of blood gases.

Sounds: Chest, Cardiac, and Bowel

The critical care nurse uses auscultation skills in assessing chest, cardiac, and bowel sounds.

Chest Sounds. In assessing the chest the nurse will listen first with the diaphragm in the suprascapular area on the right, and next on the corresponding left side of the chest. The nurse makes her way down to the interscapular region on both sides in order, and finally to the right and left lower lobes.

In the normal lung, the sounds heard are threefold: vesicular, bronchial, and bronchovesicular. Vesicular breath sounds originate in the alveoli and have a soft, breezy quality of medium pitch. Inspiratory phase is longer (3:1) than the expiratory phase. Bronchial breath sounds are found in patients with significant atelectosis or consolidation in the lungs. The sounds are loud and high-pitched, expiration phase is longer than inspiratory phase, and there is a pause separating inspiration and expiration. Bronchovesicular breath sounds are heard where the trachea and the bronchi are closest to the chest wall, above the sternum and between the scapulae. These sounds have two characteristics: the inspiratory and expiratory phase are equal, and there is a blowing sound of medium to high pitch.

Abnormal or adventitious breath sounds consist of the following: laryngeal stridor, rhonchus, asthmatic breathing, bronchial breath sounds, rales, absent breath sounds, and pleural rub. Figure 1.10(a) categorizes the type of chest sounds, characteristics of each sound, and possible causes for their occurrence. A more detailed breakdown of rales is presented in Figure 1.10(b) (Delaney 1975a, 1975b).

In making her initial overall assessment of the patient, the critical care nurse must listen for both chest and cardiac sounds. While listening to her patient's breath sounds, she may note a decrease in sounds over the right side of his chest. The nurse might then observe that her patient's neck and face are slightly cyanotic, his respiratory rate is increasing, and he is becoming restless. Having collected these observations, the nurse would diagnose the problem as caused by obstruction of bronchus from a mucous plug or pneumothorax. The nurse may intervene by suctioning the patient in an attempt to relieve the obstruction. At the same time she should order a chest X-ray to document the presence of a pneumothorax.

Cardiac Sounds. Cardiac sounds are more difficult to assess. Each heart valve sound is reflected to a specific area of the chest wall. The aortic valve will often be heard best in the aortic area, which is located in the second intercostal space (2-ICS) next to the right sternal border. The pulmonic area is located opposite the aortic area in the 2-ICS near the left edge of the sternum. The tricuspid area is found lower down the left sternal edge at the fifth intercostal space. The mitral area is also in the 5-ICS of the cardiac apex (Thompson 1981).

When she cares for a patient who has had a valve replacement, it is imperative that the nurse listen to the newly implanted valve. She must estab-

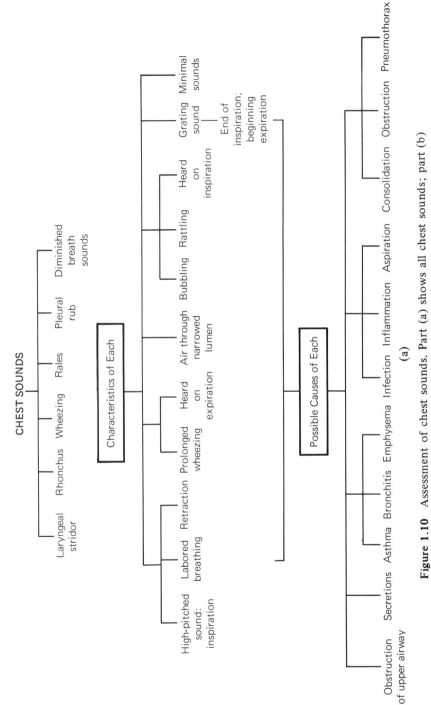

Figure 1.10 Assessment of chest sounds. Part (a) shows all chest sounds; part (b) gives a detailed breakdown of rales.

ADVENTITIOUS BREATH SOUND

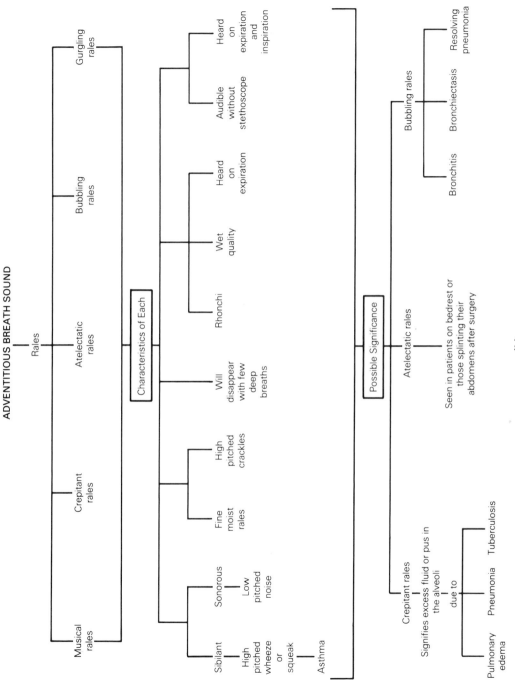

(b)

lish a normal baseline sound, so that if a suture ruptures she can note the change and immediately assess the problem. The nurse may be the first person to hear a pericardial friction rub. Figure 1.11 shows characteristics of heart sounds, various types of heart sounds, their origin, and the general abnormalities of each.

Bowel Sounds. Bowel sounds or absence of sounds should be included in the overall assessment of the critically ill patient. Of course, the significance of such data will depend on the type of surgery experienced. If a patient has had bowel surgery, the nurse may want to note the first instance of bowel sounds, which may return in three to five days.

Status of Major Systems

In assessing the critically ill patient's pulmonary, cardiac, renal, neurological, endocrine, and gastrointestinal systems, the nurse can observe important factors according to the eight R's: regular functions, rate of system, rhythm of system, regularity of system, regime, related laboratory studies, related subproblems associated with the system, and related nursing care. Only the first four will be briefly discussed.

The critical care nurse uses physical assessment skills in examining the major systems. The assessment process consists of inspection, palpation, percussion, and auscultation (Guzzetta and Kenner 1981). The last was discussed earlier under the section on sounds. Inspection refers to the visual examination of the patient in which normal and abnormal features are noted. The nurse inspects for size, appearance, symmetry, normalcy, anatomical landmarks, color, movement, temperature, and abnormalities.

Next the nurse utilizes palpation skills. In palpating the patient, the nurse assesses texture, temperature, moisture, elasticity, position, pulsations, vibrations, consistency, and shape. The nurse uses light pressure and with the fingertips identifies the presence of pain, tenderness, swelling, organ enlargement, muscle spasm, rigidity, or crepitus.

After palpation the nurse percusses the patient to determine size, density, organ boundaries, and location. The sound heard on percussion can be tympanic, resonant, dull, or flat. Tympanic sound is clear and hollow, has a higher pitch than a resonant sound, and a very high intensity. It is also of long duration and possesses a musical quality. A resonant sound, too, is a clear and hollow sound. However, a resonant sound is lower in pitch, more variable in intensity, and less musical in quality than a tympanical sound. It is heard when percussing a normal lung. A dull sound is high-pitched and thudding, similar to the sound heard over the heart. Finally a flat sound is low-pitched and abrupt. It is usually produced by percussing a solid mass.

Pulmonary System. The critical care nurse inspects the head and neck by observing for signs of respiratory distress such as airway difficulty, gasping, cyanosis, open mouth, flared nostrils, and/or use of accessory muscles.

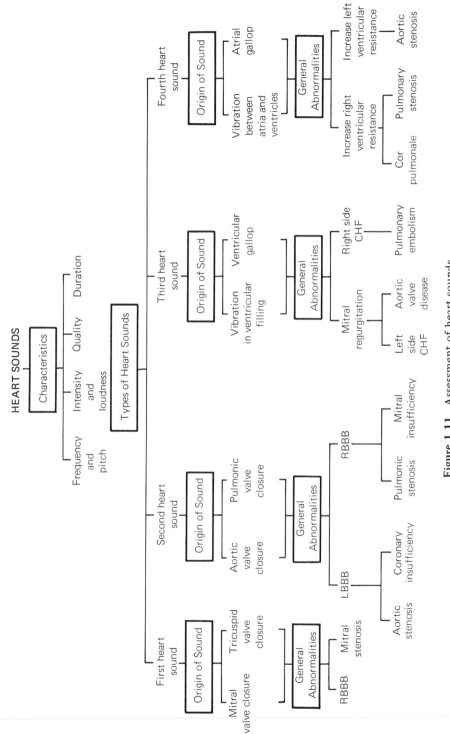

Figure 1.11 Assessment of heart sounds.

Next the nurse assesses bilateral jugular vein distention, inspiration–expiration ratio, sputum, and odor of the breath.

The nurse inspects the patient's rate and rhythm of respirations, noting whether the respiratory excursions are regular or irregular, easy or labored. The symmetry of the chest is inspected, together with color changes or paradoxical movements. The contour and size of the chest is inspected and its anteroposterior diameter is noted. Lastly the extremities are inspected for clubbing of the fingers or toes. Alterations in the angles of the nail from 160° to 180° can indicate the presence of pulmonary disease.

Palpation of the chest permits assessment of excursions, any unilateral asymmetry, tenderness of the chest wall, muscle tone, swelling, and tactile fremitus. Tactile fremitus is assessed when the nurse places her hand on the patient's chest and has the patient say 99. The phrase produces intense vibrations. Strong vibrations can be palpated over areas where there is consolidation of the underlying lung. Decreased tactile fremitus is associated with pleural effusion and pneumothorax.

Lastly, the nurse percusses the chest by tapping it with the finger. When she does this, the vibrations of the tissues, lung, and chest wall produce an audible sound wave. The vibrations are described according to their acoustic properties of frequency, intensity, duration, and quality. Frequency signifies the number of vibrations per second. Intensity refers to the amplitude of the sound wave. Duration refers to the length of time the sound is heard. Quality is the characteristic most difficult to describe; it involves pitch, intensity, and harmonies.

The vibrations produced in the chest are also assessed as resonant, dull, flat, or tympanic. A resonant chest sound has low pitch, variable intensity, long duration, and a nonmusical quality. A dull sound has a higher pitch, decreased intensity, short duration, and a nonmusical quality. A flat sound has a higher pitch, less intensity, short duration, and a nonmusical quality. A tympanic sound has a higher pitch, loud intensity, long duration, and a relatively rich (musical) quality.

The nurse begins percussion of the apices and proceeds to the bases, moving from the anterior areas to the lateral areas and then to the posterior areas. Any changes in the sound waves are produced by changes in the underlying structures. Patients with emphysema or air in the pleural cavity produce a hyperresonant or tympanic sound. Decreased air from consolidation in atelectasis or pneumonia produces a dull sound.

The critical care nurse who assesses her patient's respiratory status may discover that his respiratory rate is 32 per minute and very shallow. She also notes that the rhythm of his chest is unequal: rhythm is unilateral rather than bilateral. If the nurse also observes that her patient's skin color is becoming slightly cyanotic, she may infer that his problem is due to an obstruction. The nurse should obtain blood gases, use suction, or change the patient's position.

A chest X-ray and changes in blood gases may document that the unilateral chest movement was due to a pneumothorax. The regime for such a problem is the insertion of a chest tube, which restores a more normal intrapleural pressure. Besides continued observation of her patient's respiratory rate, rhythm, and regularity, the nurse must observe his chest tube. She should milk the tube every one to two hours to prevent stasis of drainage, which would result in clot formation. The nurse will also note the presence and/or amount of drainage, its color, and the presence or absence of bubbling in the water seal chamber. Figures 1.12(a) to (e) show the regular functions, rate, rhythm, and regularity of the pulmonary system, regime for pulmonary dysfunction, related laboratory and/or diagnostic studies, and related subproblems.

Cardiovascular System. Inspection and palpation of the cardiovascular system can be done simultaneously. The nurse inspects the external and internal jugular veins to estimate venous pressure, right atrial pressure, and right heart failure. The hepatojugular reflex (HJR) is also assessed. Firm pressure is placed over the right upper quadrant of the patient's abdomen for 30 to 40 seconds. An increase in jugular venous pressure of more than 1 cm during this period is abnormal. If present, this sign reveals that the right heart is unable to accommodate an increased blood flow without a corresponding rise in venous pressure and implies right heart failure. Jugular venous pulsations are inspected bilaterally and at the base of the neck. Next the arterial pulses are palpated for rate, rhythm, amplitude, and equality. Peripheral pulses including the brachial, radial, femoral, popliteal, posterior tibial, and dorsalis pedis pulses are assessed. While inspecting and palpating the extremities, the nurse notes alterations in color and temperature of the extremities, complaints of cramps, intermittent claudication, clubbing, edema, varicosities, and pain. Lastly, the nurse inspects the chest for distortion of the thoracic cage, bulges, lack of symmetry, scars, and petechiae. The apical impulse (PMI) is located with the percordium being assessed for other pulsations or thrills. The normal apical impulse is the size of a penny. If it is as large as a quarter, left ventricular enlargement is suspected. Pulsation or thrills are also assessed. Palpable pulsations in the second or third intercostal spaces to the left or right of the sternum suggests pulmonary hypertension, aortic aneurysm, or systematic hypertension. Palpation of a right ventricular lift along the left sternal edge is indicative of possible right ventricular hypertrophy (Guzzetta and Dossey 1981).

Finally, precordial percussion is done to define the cardiac borders. Percussion is done with the patient placed in a supine position. The left border of cardiac dullness (LBCD) is defined by percussing the third, fourth, and fifth left intercostal spaces. Percussion is begun over resonant lung tissue near the axilla and moves medially until relative cardiac dullness is heard.

To assess her patient's cardiovascular status, the critical care nurse must first know the regular functions of that system. Briefly the functions consist of the following: the systemic arteries serve as a pressure reservoir by means of the elastic properties of the walls; the capillaries control a major portion of pressure between the arteries and veins; the venous system acts as a con-

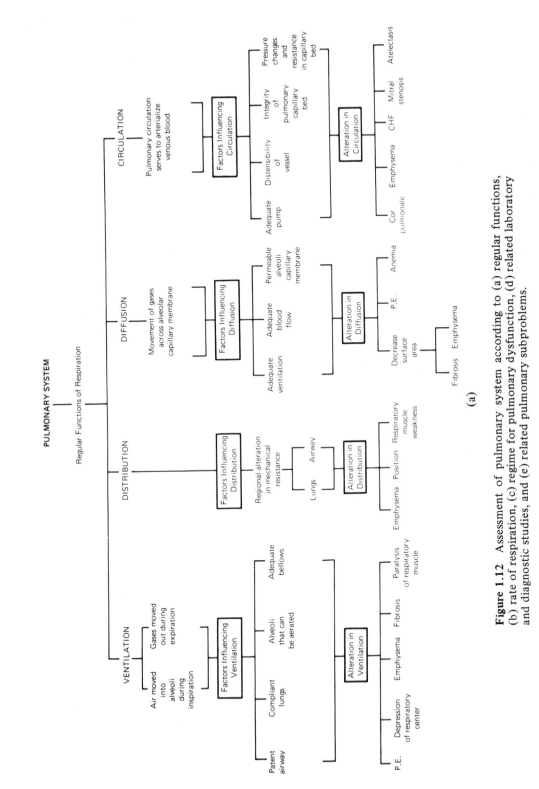

Figure 1.12 Assessment of pulmonary system according to (a) regular functions, (b) rate of respiration, (c) regime for pulmonary dysfunction, (d) related laboratory and diagnostic studies, and (e) related pulmonary subproblems.

40

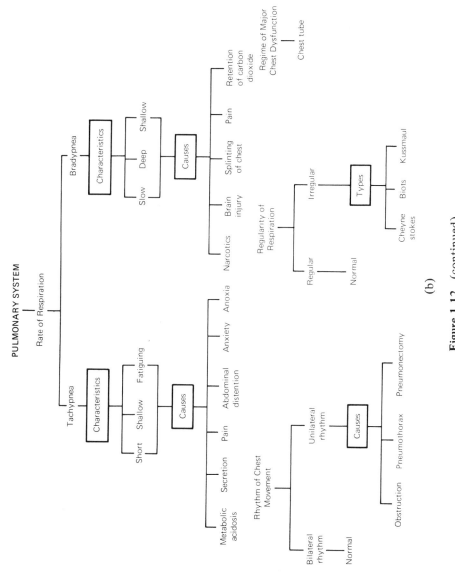

Figure 1.12 (continued)

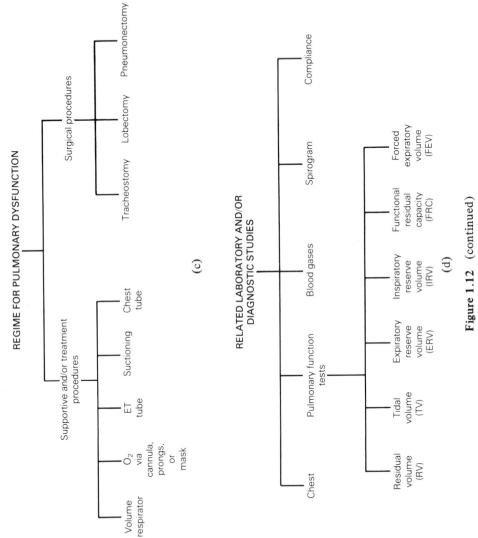

REGIME FOR PULMONARY DYSFUNCTION

Supportive and/or treatment procedures

- Volume respirator
- O₂ via cannula, prongs, or mask
- ET tube
- Suctioning
- Chest tube

Surgical procedures

- Tracheostomy
- Lobectomy
- Pneumonectomy

(c)

RELATED LABORATORY AND/OR DIAGNOSTIC STUDIES

- Chest
- Pulmonary function tests
  - Residual volume (RV)
  - Tidal volume (TV)
  - Expiratory reserve volume (ERV)
  - Inspiratory reserve volume (IRV)
  - Functional residual capacity (FRC)
  - Forced expiratory volume (FEV)
- Blood gases
- Spirogram
- Compliance

(d)

Figure 1.12 (continued)

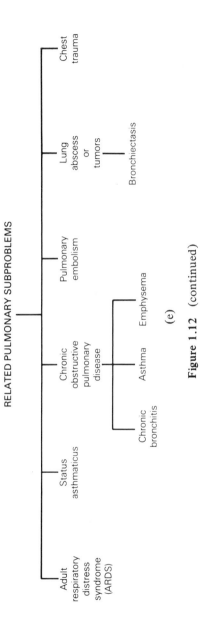

RELATED PULMONARY SUBPROBLEMS

Adult respiratory distress syndrome (ARDS)

Status asthmaticus

Chronic obstructive pulmonary disease

Chronic bronchitis

Asthma

Emphysema

Pulmonary embolism

Lung abscess or tumors

Bronchiectasis

Chest trauma

(e)

Figure 1.12 (continued)

duit to channel blood from the capillaries to the heart; the pulmonary vessels supply the alveolar membrane; and cardiac output represents effective volume of blood expelled by either ventricle of the heart in a unit of time (Rushmer 1961).

While taking her patient's apical heart rate, the nurse may observe that his heart rate is 48 per minute. Using a cardioscope to determine his rhythm, she observes that the P waves do not correspond regularly to her patient's QRS pattern. The atrium seems to be functioning independently from the ventricles. Furthermore, she observes that the patient's blood pressure and urinary output have decreased, and notes that the patient is complaining of dizziness. As a result of these observations, the nurse realizes that the patient cannot tolerate his rhythm. The nursing diagnosis of her patient's rhythm is A-V dissociation or complete heart block. The nurse realizes that regime for such heart dysfunction is either Isuprel or a pacemaker. It is important that the nurse know what observations to make (e.g., decreased blood pressure, decreased urine output, dizziness, and relationship of P waves to QRS complexes) in order to formulate the nursing diagnosis of complete heart block. Figures 1.13(a) to (f) show the rate, rhythm, and regularity of the cardiac and/or conductive system, regime for cardiovascular dysfunction, related laboratory and/or diagnostic studies, and related subproblems.

Renal System. In assessing the renal patient, the nurse inspects for the following: changes in level of consciousness such as lethargy or coma; skin color alterations such as grayish tinge indicating anemia, bruises indicating fragile skin capillaries, and skin turgor; edema; respiratory pattern indicating air hunger as found in severe acidosis; decreased urine volume; muscle tremors, weakness, and weight loss; tetany; and asterixis.

The nurse palpates the kidney to determine its size and shape. Further palpation will reveal the presence of tenderness, cysts, and masses. The bladder is palpated for the presence of urine assuming the patient does not have a Foley catheter. A grossly enlarged bladder can indicate bladder neck obstruction.

Next, percussion is performed at the costovertebral angles in an attempt to elicit pain or tenderness. Pain or tenderness can indicate conditions such as calculi, renal abscess or tumor, and glomerulonephritis.

Finally the nurse auscultates the aortic or renal artery for bruits. They are auscultated in flanks or intercostal regions of the anterior abdomen. The presence of a bruit can be indicative of hypertension, atherosclerosis and aneurysm (Stark 1981).

In assessing the critically ill patient's renal status, the nurse applies her knowledge of the regular functions of the renal system: glomerular filtration, tubular reabsorption, tubular secretion, acid-base balance, electrolyte balance, and hormone and enzyme synthesis (renin and erythropoietin). The nurse may assess that her patient's BUN (20–30 mg/100 mℓ/day) and creatinine (1–2 mg/100 mℓ/day) levels have increased while the patient's urinary volume has decreased to 400 mℓ/day. Based upon these findings the nurse may

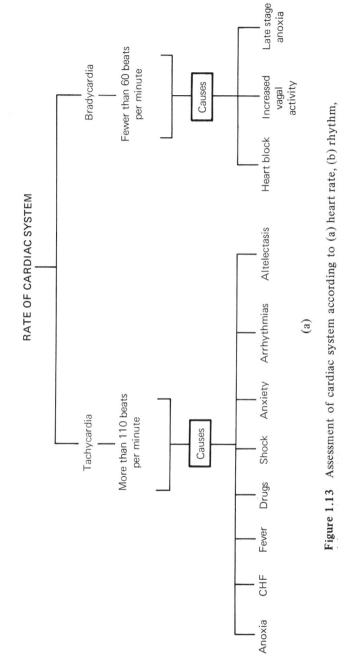

Figure 1.13 Assessment of cardiac system according to (a) heart rate, (b) rhythm, (c) regularity, (d) regime for cardiac dysfunction, (e) related laboratory and/or diagnostic studies, and (f) related subproblems.

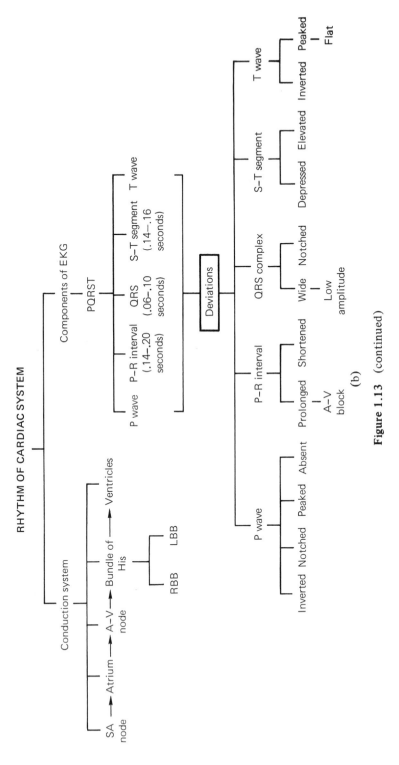

Figure 1.13 (continued)

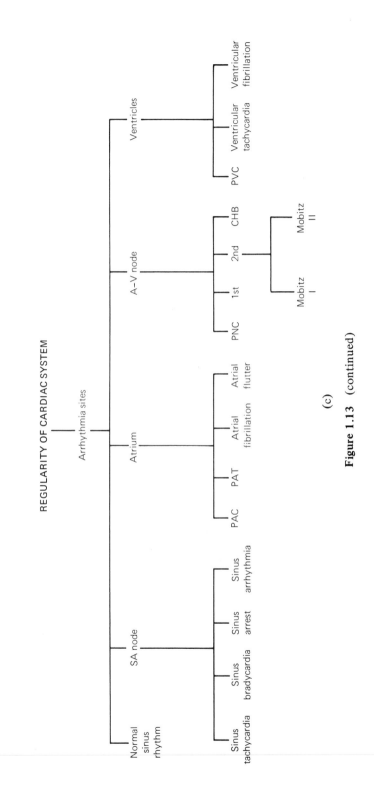

Figure 1.13 (continued)

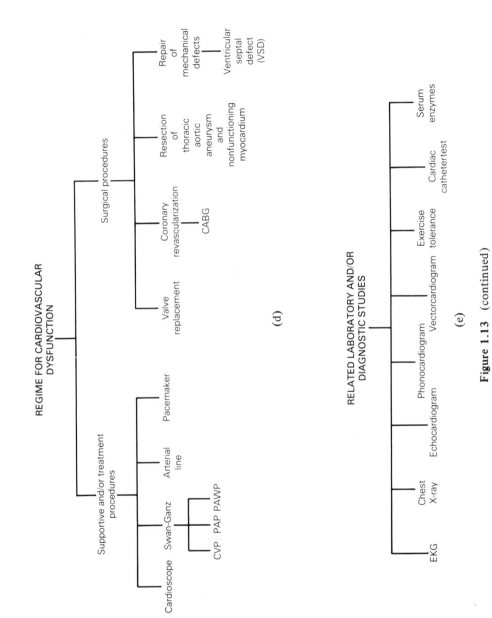

REGIME FOR CARDIOVASCULAR DYSFUNCTION

Supportive and/or treatment procedures

Cardioscope   Swan-Ganz   Arterial line   Pacemaker

CVP   PAP   PAWP

Surgical procedures

Valve replacement   Coronary revascularization   Resection of thoracic aortic aneurysm and nonfunctioning myocardium   Repair of mechanical defects

CABG

Ventricular septal defect (VSD)

(d)

RELATED LABORATORY AND/OR DIAGNOSTIC STUDIES

EKG   Chest X-ray   Echocardiogram   Phonocardiogram   Vectorcardiogram   Exercise tolerance   Cardiac cathetertest   Serum enzymes

(e)

Figure 1.13   (continued)

48

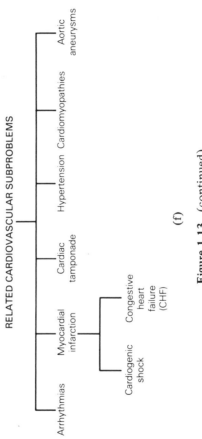

RELATED CARDIOVASCULAR SUBPROBLEMS

Arrhythmias Myocardial infarction Cardiac tamponade Hypertension Cardiomyopathies Aortic aneurysms

Cardiogenic shock Congestive heart failure (CHF)

(f)

Figure 1.13 (continued)

diagnose the problem as acute renal failure. Naturally the nurse will make observations regarding the renal system. These additional observations can be found in Figures 1.14(a) to (f).

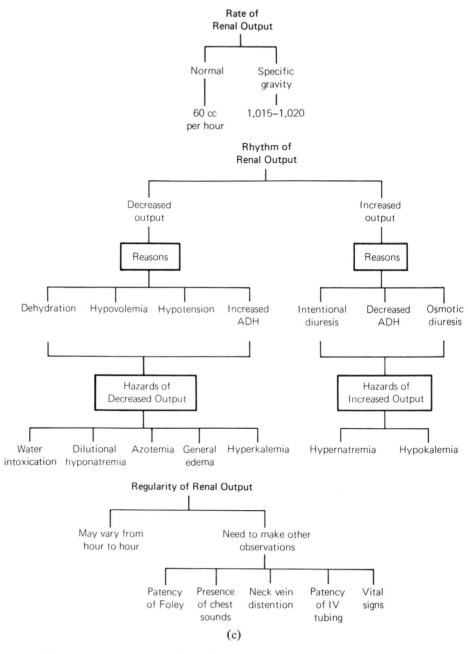

(c)

Figure 1.14 Assessment of renal system according to (a) rate of output, (b) rhythm of output, (c) regularity of output, (d) regime for renal dysfunction, (e) related laboratory and/or diagnostic studies, and (f) related renal subproblems.

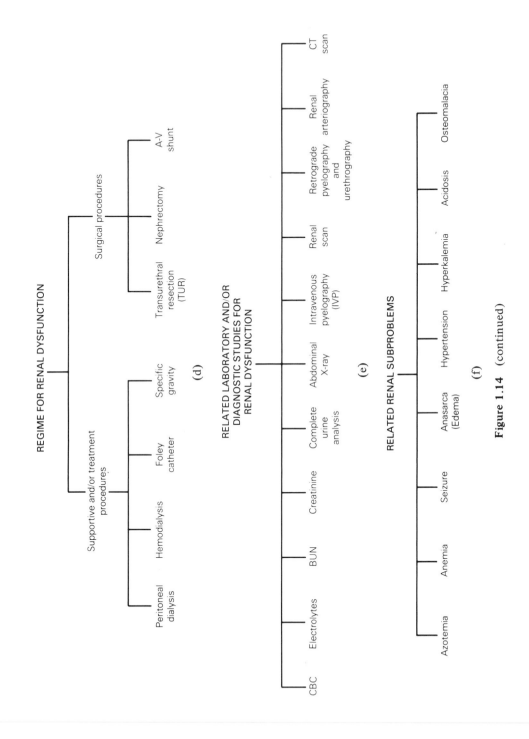

REGIME FOR RENAL DYSFUNCTION

Supportive and/or treatment procedures
- Peritoneal dialysis
- Hemodialysis
- Foley catheter
- Specific gravity

Surgical procedures
- Transurethral resection (TUR)
- Nephrectomy
- A-V shunt

(d)

RELATED LABORATORY AND/OR DIAGNOSTIC STUDIES FOR RENAL DYSFUNCTION

- CBC
- Electrolytes
- BUN
- Creatinine
- Complete urine analysis
- Abdominal X-ray
- Intravenous pyelography (IVP)
- Renal scan
- Retrograde pyelography and urethrography
- Renal arteriography
- CT scan

(e)

RELATED RENAL SUBPROBLEMS

- Azotemia
- Anemia
- Seizure
- Anasarca (Edema)
- Hypertension
- Hyperkalemia
- Acidosis
- Osteomalacia

(f)

Figure 1.14 (continued)

Neurological System.   The critical care nurse begins her assessment by inspecting the patient's level of consciousness and content of consciousness. Level of consciousness is controlled by the reticular activating system in the brainstem. The content of consciousness is controlled by the cerebral hemisphere located above the cerebellar tentorium. The patient's alertness, ability to cooperate, educational level, and handedness are evaluated. The mental status examination tests the patient's immediate recall, recent or short-term memory, remote sensory interpretation, and use of previously gained knowledge and behavior (Kenner 1981).

Next the nurse assesses the patient's respiratory pattern. Identification of respiratory patterns helps to identify the lesion site and to anticipate patient problems. Respiratory abnormalities consist of the following: posthyperventilation apnea, Cheyne-Stokes breathing, central neurogenic hyperventilation, apneustic and atoxic breathing. The pupillary response is assessed, including size, reaction to light, consensual light reflex, and equality. The nurse can also assess the 12 cranial nerves to determine whether or not any abnormalities exist.

Palpation is involved in assessing the motor system. The assessment includes determination of muscle bulk, tone, strength, and symmetry, and the presence of abnormal muscle movements. Any hypertrophy or atrophy of muscles is also noted. To assess any suspected asymmetry, the corresponding muscles on the opposite limb are measured. The patient's muscle tone is evaluated by passive range-of-motion exercises and active movements, noting any involuntary resistance, spasticity, flaccidity, or rigidity.

It is beyond the scope of this chapter to include all aspects of the neurological assessment. Other components include sensory movement, reflexes, and vital signs. The assessment process also includes knowledge of the regular functions (Nikas 1981). See Figures 1.15(a) to (e) for the regular functions of the brain.

Endocrine System.   The critical care nurse can inspect the patient's general appearance for distribution of subcutaneous fat relative to maturation level, appearance relative to age and sex, and facial expressions and body movement. Next, she inspects the distribution of hair, paying attention to the scalp and face. The patient's eyes are then assessed for periorbital edema and visual acuity. Any behavioral changes or alteration in level of consciousness should be noted. Finally the skin is inspected for turgor, pigmentation, lesions, vascularity, and texture. Palpation and pressure is done to determine the boundaries of the glands and the pressure of an enlarged gland. The thyroid gland can be auscultated for bruits.

Of the five glands comprising the endocrine system, only two will be briefly mentioned: the pancreas and adrenal glands. The regular functions of the pancreas consist of the secretion of insulin and glucagon. The regular functions of the adrenal gland are divided between the adrenal cortex and

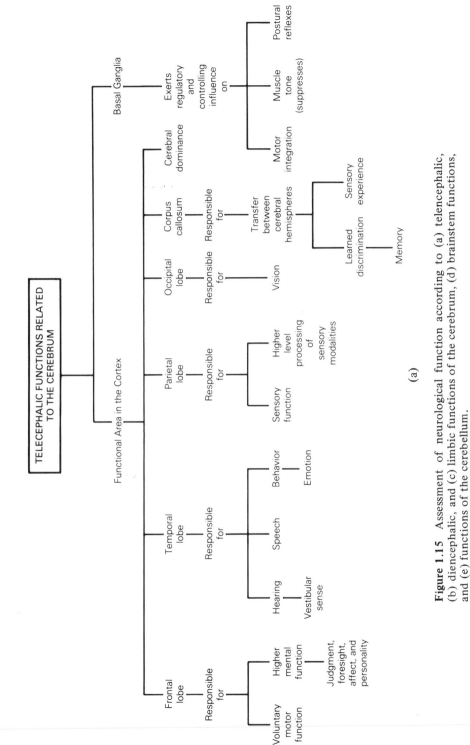

Figure 1.15 Assessment of neurological function according to (a) telencephalic, (b) diencephalic, and (c) limbic functions of the cerebrum, (d) brainstem functions, and (e) functions of the cerebellum.

(a)

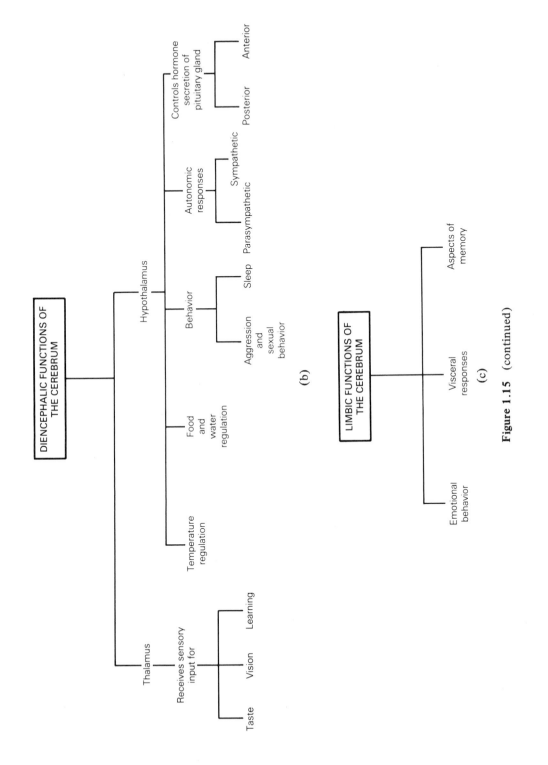

Figure 1.15 (continued)

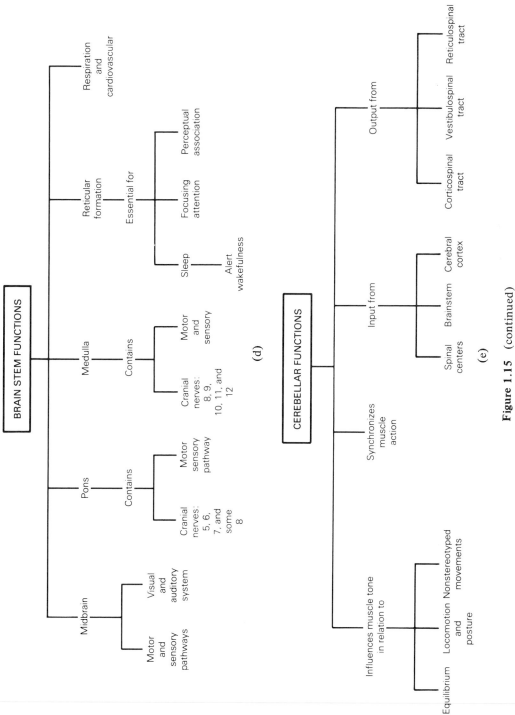

Figure 1.15 (continued)

adrenal medulla. The adrenal cortex produces the following hormones: glucocorticoids (cortisol), mineralocorticoids (aldosterone), and androgen. The adrenal medulla secretes the catecholamines epinephrine and norepinephrine. See Figures 1.16(a) to (c) for a brief discussion of rate, rhythm, and regularity of the pancreatic and adrenal glands.

Gastrointestinal System. The gastrointestinal system involves the upper gastrointestinal system including the oral cavity, pharynx, esophagus, and stomach; the lower gastrointestinal system including the small and large intestine; and accessory organs of digestion including the pancreas, gallbladder, and liver. Only the hepatic system will be discussed.

An abdominal assessment including inspection, auscultation, percussion, and palpation can be done at this time (Dossey 1981). The nurse inspects the patient's abdomen from the right side. Inspection includes examination of the abdominal surface, striae, old or new scars, rashes, lesions, dilated veins, shape, size, contour, and symmetry. Next the nurse systematically auscultates the abdomen by moving the stethoscope from quadrant to quadrant. The bowel sounds are auscultated for their frequency, quality, and pitch. Since most intestinal sounds originate in the small bowel, the nurse listens for high-pitched and gurgling sounds. Ausculation for bruits is performed in midepigastrium, where their presence could indicate stenosis of the renal arteries, and in the iliac region, where their presence could indicate iliofemoral artery stenosis. Finally if the critically ill patient has splenic infarction or liver tumor, peritoneal friction rubs are auscultated over the spleen and liver.

The abdomen is percussed to determine the degree of resonance, tympany, and dullness. The organs percussed consist of the liver for dullness, which can be obscured by gas in the colon, lung consolidation, or right pleural effusion; the stomach for tympany; and the spleen for tympany.

Lastly light and deep palpation are done to assess the presence of abdominal tenderness, muscular resistance, and masses. If masses are palpated, their size, shape, consistency, mobility, tenderness, and pulsation are determined and recorded. Masses in the abdominal wall remain palpable when the patient tightens his abdominal muscles. On the other hand, masses in the abdominal cavity are obscured when the patient tightens his abdominal muscles.

The liver is the largest organ in the body. The regular functions of the liver consist of the following: secretion of bile; metabolism of carbohydrates, fats, and proteins; synthesis of amino acids, albumin, globulins, prothrombin, and fibrinogen; deamination of amino acids for glucose availability; formation of urea to remove ammonia from blood; storage of vitamins; conversion of glucose to glycogen; formation of lipoprotein, cholesterol, and phospholipids; and detoxification of drugs, hormones, and toxic substances. See Figures 1.17(a) to (c) for additional information on the rate, rhythm, and regularity of the hepatic system.

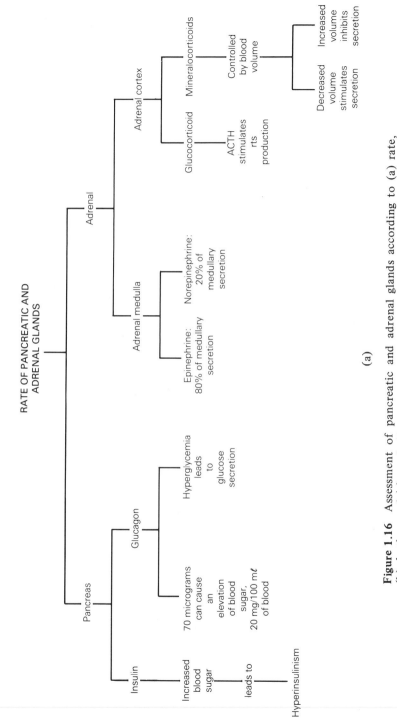

Figure 1.16 Assessment of pancreatic and adrenal glands according to (a) rate, (b) rhythm, and (c) regularity.

(a)

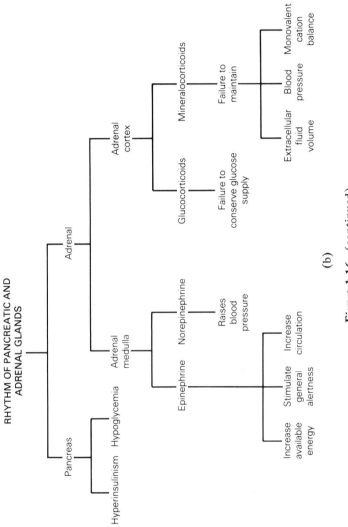

RHYTHM OF PANCREATIC AND
ADRENAL GLANDS

Figure 1.16 (continued)

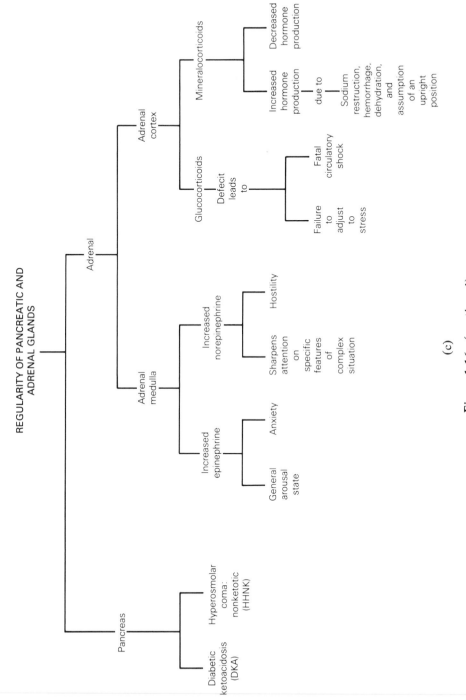

Figure 1.16 (continued)

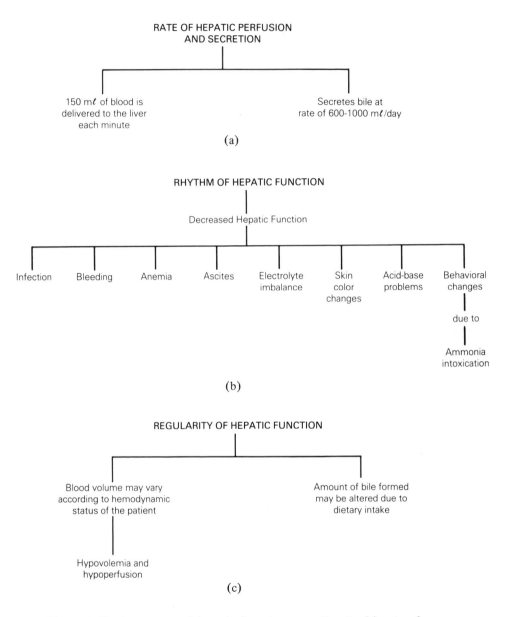

Figure 1.17 Assessment of hepatic function according to (a) rate of perfusion and secretion, (b) rhythm, and (c) regularity.

SUMMARY

To the nurse working in critical care units, the critically ill patient may simultaneously manifest many problems. As a result, the nurse will experience sensory overload. She may become unable to put the many pieces of data together systematically and formulate an overall picture of the patient. The BEEP concept permits the critical care nurse to observe her critically ill patient logically and, on the basis of her observations, to arrive at a nursing diagnosis of his problem. She will know what she should be observing regarding both behavior and physiology. With BEEP, the critical care nurse knows to start at the patient's head (e.g., consciousness) and continue to observe all facets of his inner feelings and outward appearance. Through systematic assessment of her critically ill patient's emotional status, the nurse can become aware of conceptual problems that may occur. For example, she sees how repeated illness can cause a feeling of hopelessness in her patient. She gains new appreciation for her patient's display of anger once she assesses its meaning to him. The BEEP concept also permits the critical care nurse to learn that the environment plays a significant role in her patient's well-being.

To provide successful nursing care in the various critical care units, the nurse must have a systematic means of observing and assessing her patient. It is possible that the nurse's assessment could mean the difference between life and death.

REFERENCES

ABBEY, JUNE, "Nursing Observations of Fluid Balance," *Nursing Clinics of North America*, 3, no. 1 (March 1968), 77.

ANDREOLI, KATHLEEN, *Comprehensive Cardiac Care*. St. Louis: C. V. Mosby, 1968.

BETSON, CAROL, "Blood Gases," *American Journal of Nursing*, 68, no. 5 (May 1968), 1010-1012.

―――, "Central Venous Pressure," *American Journal of Nursing*, 69, no. 7 (July 1969), 1467.

DAILY, ELAINE, and JOHN SCHROEDER, *Techniques in Bedside Hemodynamic Monitoring*. St. Louis: C. V. Mosby, 1981.

DELANEY, MARY, "Examination of the Chest, Part I: The Lungs," *Nursing '75*, (August 1975a), 12-14.

―――, "Examination of the Chest, Part II: The Heart," *Nursing '75*, (September 1975b), 41-46.

DOSSEY, BARBARA, "Abdominal Assessment," in *Critical Care Nursing: Body-Mind-Spirit*, ed. C. Kenner, C. Guzzetta, and B. Dossey, pp. 159-167. Boston: Little, Brown, 1981.

GIBLIN, ELIZABETH C., "Foreword to 'Symposium on Assessment as Part of the Nursing Process," *Nursing Clinics of North America*, 6, no. 1 (March 1971), 113.

GILBO, DONA, "Nursing Assessment of Circulatory Function," *Nursing Clinics of North America*, 3, no. 1 (March 1968), 54-55.

GUYTON, Arthur, *Textbook of Medical Physiology*. Philadelphia: Saunders, 1971.

GUZZETTA, C. and C. KENNER, "A Practical Approach to the Nursing Assessment," in *Critical Care Nursing: Body-Mind-Spirit*, ed. C. Kenner, C. Guzzetta, and B. Dossey, pp. 143-158. Boston: Little, Brown, 1981.

KELLY, LOWELL, *Assessment of Human Characteristics*. Monterey, Calif.: Brooks-Cole, 1967.

KENNER, CORNELIA, "Neurological Assessment," in *Critical Care Nursing: Body-Mind-Spirit*, ed. C. Kenner, C. Guzzetta, and B. Dossey, pp. 143-158. Boston: Little, Brown, 1981.

LEHMAN, JANET, "Auscultation of Heart Sounds," *American Journal of Nursing*, 72, no. 7 (July 1972), 1242-1246.

MANCALL, ELLIOTT, *Essentials of the Neurological Examination*. Philadelphia: F. A. Davis, 1981.

MARRIOTT, HENRY, *Practical Electrocardiography*. Baltimore: Williams and Wilkins, 1968.

NIKAS, DIANA, "The Nervous System," in *Core Curriculum for Critical Care Nursing*, ed. N. Borg, D. Nikas, J. Stark, and S. Williams, pp. 173-259. Philadelphia: Saunders, 1981.

RUSHMER, ROBERT, *Cardiovascular Dynamics*. Philadelphia: Saunders, 1961. (Reprint from Orange County Medical Center)

STARK, JUNE, "The Renal System," in *Core Curriculum for Critical Care Nursing*, ed. N. Borg, D. Nikas, J. Stark, and S. Williams, pp. 263-311. Philadelphia: Saunders, 1981.

THOMPSON, DONALD, *Cardiovascular Assessment*, St. Louis: C. V. Mosby Co., 1981.

YOUNG, JESSIE, "Recognition, Significance and Recording of the Signs of Increased Intracranial Pressure," *Nursing Clinics of North America*, 4, no. 2 (June 1969), 224-225.

2
Sleep Deprivation

BEHAVIORAL OBJECTIVES

1. Define *sleep.*
2. Compare and contrast the differences between REM and NREM sleep.
3. Define *sleep deprivation.*
4. State two situations in which the critically ill patient experiences increased input.
5. State two situations in which the critically ill patient needs more sleep.
6. Identify five NREM regulatory behaviors.
7. Identify six REM regulatory behaviors.
8. State eight cognitive behaviors associated with sleep deprivation.
9. Design a nursing care plan to promote sleep.

Sleep is something familiar and enjoyed by us all. At the end of a long and stressful working day, we look forward to a good night's sleep. Many television commercials focus on measures to help us sleep, such as the use of medications or the purchase of a firm mattress. Each is advertised as a means to obtain a safe and restful sleep. Sleep is such a vital part of our lives that one room in our home is entirely devoted to it. Large stores have departments devoted to beds, sleepware, and accessories. Sleep is so important that we even devote a portion of our wardrobe to it. Beds themselves come in all sizes and shapes, including water beds. All this attention is not unusual when one considers that we spend one-third of our lives asleep. According to Cohen (1979), sleep and wakefulness are characteristics of a fundamental circadian rhythm of activity-inactivity in human beings. The cycle of sleep and wakefulness is one of the most common phenomena in human life. It should be noted that a person who lives 70 years will spend 27 of them asleep, and approximately 5 to 7 of these will include vivid dreaming experiences.

Individuals are even categorized into good and bad sleepers. Good sleepers are those who fall immediately to sleep. They sleep for an appropriate period of time, six to eight hours, and awaken refreshed. Bad sleepers, on the other hand, have difficulty falling and remaining asleep. They toss and turn most of the night. When they finally fall asleep, it is early in the morning. They awaken just as tired as when they went to bed. No one really knows why one individual is a better sleeper than another, and no one really understands why one individual needs only four hours sleep a night whereas someone else may need eight hours.

Segal (1969) points out that "many centuries ago, sleep was regarded as a type of anemia of the brain. A Greek physiologist, Alemacon, believed that blood retreats into the veins, after which the partially starved brain goes to sleep. Plato, on the other hand, supported the idea that the soul leaves the body during sleep, wanders the world, and wakes up the body when it returns" (p. 48). It is a mystery why we allow ourselves to be set aside from the rest of the world in quiet sleep. Sleeps seems to replenish our body's depleted energy system and get it into a state of readiness for the coming day's event. The restorative theory holds that sleep is a period of recovery or restoration of physiological, neurological, and/or psychological states. This position implicitly underlies earlier toxin theories of sleep and is certainly the most widely held intuitive notion about sleep (Webb 1979).

Scientists and technicians are developing new ways to investigate the human mind during sleep. In time their findings will help nurses working in critical care units, for it is in such stimulus-oriented environments that sleep is frequently interrupted, thus causing deprivation. It is not the intent of the critical care nurse to create sleep deprivation, but the nature of the patient's illness, together with the intense surveillance required, frequently causes this problem. Before discussing sleep deprivation, we must first define the concept of sleep and examine its meaning and some of its purposes.

DEFINITION OF TERMS

Our bodies contain numerous interrelated energy systems. Each depends on the others for sending and receiving energy messages. The primary energy control center is the brain. Like a condensed computer, the brain controls the body's energy systems to maintain a relatively normal homeostatic state. Like any energy system, however, the primary controller needs its own source of energy, which can eventually become depleted unless recharged. We have all had the experience of starting our car in the morning only to find the battery dead. The battery must be recharged if the car is to take us to our destination. Sometimes the process takes three hours, other times it takes a totally new battery. Our bodies function on a similar principle. We cannot replace our brain as we can our battery. Instead we can recharge its depleted energy system through the mysterious world of sleep. Sleep involves many degrees of detachment from the existing world. While in a deep state, the individual drifts through various levels of consciousness as if on waves (Segal 1969). It is this detachment from the world that allows our mind and body to reorganize and regenerate themselves in preparation for the coming day. Sleep is not a freezing point in our existence. Even while we sleep, our mind is active. The action takes the form of dreaming.

Sleep: Meaning and Purpose

In behavioral theory sleep is described as a mode of behavioral adaptation to the environment which is characterized as a behavioral state of diminished responsivity. The amount, period length, and placement of sleep are species specific endogenously determined tendencies. The purpose of these episodes is to adapt effectively the organism for survival (Webb 1983).

Zelechowski (1979) notes that sleep is defined as a state of unconsciousness from which an individual can be aroused through use of sensory stimuli. The reticular activitating system (RAS) is involved in the process of keeping an individual awake. The stimuli that keep us awake accomplish this goal by activating the reticular factor. When a patient experiences hypoxia or hypoglycemia, the RAS is altered with the result being induced unconsciousness. It should be noted that sleep can occur in two ways. First, it can result from reduced stimulation in the RAS such as in NREM sleep. Second, it can occur from abnormal channeling of signals in the brain during REM sleep.

As we sleep we are not totally alienated from the outside world: we respond and react to incoming stimuli. Our response is determined by the depth of our sleep. The deeper the sleep, the more difficult it is to arouse us. We have all experienced the quiet and pleasant Sunday afternoon nap. Maybe we have attended church in the morning, eaten a large meal, and read the voluminous Sunday newspaper. All these circumstances force us into a sleep state. Suddenly we become aware of someone calling our name while shaking our shoulder. The person is trying to tell us that we are wanted on the telephone. In the process of awaking, we may become confused as to the time, date, or place. Once fully awake, we can intelligently answer the telephone. Given another 30 minutes of sleep, in all probability, we would have heard the telephone ringing. The phenomenon occurs because as we sleep we go through various stages. Each stage has its own unique characteristics.

Sleep can be divided into two major periods: synchronized (non-rapid eye movement or NREM state) and desynchronized (rapid eye movement or REM state). The synchronized NREM state is further divided into four stages. Stage I represents a transition between the awake state and the sleep state. During this stage the individual is still somewhat aware of his surroundings but is relaxed and dreamy. People in stage I jerk involuntarily and can awaken in the process. The sleeper may enjoy a floating sensation or drifting with idle thoughts and dreams. His muscles are relaxing and his heart rate is slowing down. He can be awakened easily and might insist that he had not been asleep at all. Stage II acts as a door between REM and NREM sleep. The individual in stage II experiences slow rolling of the eyes from side to side. If awakened, which can be done easily with a modest sound, the sleeper may still think he has been awake all along. At this point, he has been sleeping soundly for perhaps ten minutes. Stage III is associated with deeper sleep. In this stage a louder noise is required to awaken the individual, perhaps a calling of his name. His muscles are very relaxed and he breathes evenly. His heart rate slows, his temperature declines, and his blood pressure drops. Finally stage IV represents a period of profound sleep from which arousal is difficult. It is a time of relatively dreamless oblivion. Breathing is even and heart rate, blood pressure, and body temperature fall (Segal 1969; Hayter 1980; Wotring 1982; Rosenblatt, Hartmann, and Zwilling 1973).

The second major period of sleep is desynchronized or REM sleep. It is distinguished by rapid eye movements associated with a low voltage irregular EEG pattern. REM sleep is also called active or paradoxical sleep because of the high levels of neurological and general physiological activity demonstrated during these sleep periods. REM sleep is associated with general physiological activation. During this time the patient can experience increased oxygen consumption, increased ectopic beats, increased heart rate, increased cerebral metabolic rate, and decreased cerebral blood flow. In addition there exists a wide fluctuation in blood pressure. The respiratory pattern during REM sleep mimics Cheyne-Stokes. A gasping type of snoring may occur during REM due to a decreased tone of the oropharyngeal muscles. Furthermore REM sleep is a time of autonomic excitement, hormone release, and metabolic acceleration. The hormones are significant determinants in our vitality, metabolism, and ability to resist infection. REM sleep also seems to facilitate emotional adaptation to both the physical and psychological environment. When the patient is undergoing tremedous stress or new learning, REM sleep is required. During REM sleep the day's events are reviewed and significant information is categorized and integrated into the brain's storage system. Problems are often solved during REM sleep, or more perspective is gained about areas of concern. The REM state of the first stage is only a few minutes, but approximately 25 percent of total sleep time is REM sleep (Wotring 1982; Sebilia 1981; Hayter 1980; Rosenblatt, Hartmann, and Zwilling 1973).

NREM sleep restores one physically whereas REM sleep is significant for learning, memory, and psychological adaptation. The critically ill patient may vacillate between stages I, II, and III. If the normal sleep pattern is disrupted night after night, the overall effect can be devastating. This is especially significant because critical care patients are already sick and stressed. Critical care units are notoriously noisy places. Although nurses encourage their patients to sleep, the sounds of bedpans dropping, telephones ringing, charts falling into their racks, or machines humming, buzzing, and beeping make stages I to III difficult to achieve. Besides being awakened by strange or loud noises, the patient may be awakened for procedures or treatments.

According to Gaarder's (1966) model, sleep has two important functions. One is the destructuralization of neurological data storage stimuli that emerged during the course of the day. It is assumed that each day one stores a great deal of information. Most of this information is irrevelant to one's long-range goals and takes up needed space. Sleep functions to destructuralize stored data. It is not necessary that we remember what time we got out of bed, what was said during breakfast conversation, or how many cups of coffee were consumed. Gaarder believes that such data

> ... were stored by the establishment of reverberating circuits in neural tissue. This implies a given cell would maintain collateral interactions with other cells so that the spike firing of the cell occurred in a determined way rather than at random. The determinance of the firing pattern would be equivalent to the structure of the neural system imposed in the storage of data and there would be a limit to the capacity to store this structure. The destructuralizing aspect of the adaptive function would be the clearing out of this part of the storage area so that it would be empty during the next active waking part of the cycle for new storage.* (P. 254)

Such a function may not be achieved in critical care units, where sleep is continuously interrupted. The amount of incoming stimuli and data may be far greater than the amount of sleep and its subsequent destructuralizing. Not only is the patient placed in a noisy environment, but he is also forced to sleep without his customary nighttime equipment. He is placed in a narrow bed instead of a spacious one. The narrow bed, moreover, becomes his dining area, bathroom, living room, and bedroom. All his daily activity occurs in this one area. Furthermore, he is not permitted to wear his customary sleep uniform. Instead, he has to wear a traditional hospital gown. Other deviations from his normal nighttime routine make sleep and destructuralization of stored data difficult.

The second function attributed to sleep by Gaarder is the reinforcement of the structure of the organism's emergent character for the purpose of adapting: "The reinforcement of character function assumes that at any particular period of an individual's life it is advantageous for him to take from a given day certain things that occurred and additively structure them into his character in such a way as to be better prepared for the next day" (p. 254). If the individual is deprived of his sleep, the normal function of character reinforcement is also depressed. Illness threatens the individual's integrity, forcing him to lose confidence in his own being. It creates changes that he must assimilate. The waking hours are packed with numerous people and machines moving in and out of his environment. The critically ill patient must rely on the nighttime to integrate changes into this character. If his sleep continues to be interrupted at night, such integration may not take place; it may be delayed until after he leaves a critical care unit.

*Copyright 1966, American Medical Association.

According to Greenberg (1981), dreaming is a vital part of the sleep state that permits integration of changes into the individual's character. Dreams consist of images that include memories of experiences connected with important feelings of the dreamer. These images are ways of representing the feelings and experiences with which they are connected. In addition dreams become a way of organizing them so that they can be meaningfully integrated by the dreamer. Dreams are important to psychological function. They provide a mechanism for maintaining a continuity and meaningfulness in our life experiences, allowing us to draw on past experiences in our approach to the present and allowing us to make use of present experiences to modify old modes of behavior.

Sleep Deprivation

According to McFadden and Giblin (1971), "Sleep or dream deprivation is defined as lack of adequate sleep or dream time as related to prior or unusual sleep patterns" (p. 249). Human beings cannot tolerate going without sleep for very long. If forced to go without sleep they experience behavioral, psychological, and physiological changes. Sleep deprivation, especially of stage IV sleep, has been associated with decreased growth hormone secretion. Stage IV sleep is significant to the sick individual because it plays a vital role in tissue healing and physical restoration. Depriving a person of REM sleep will leave him continually fatigued and with poor powers of concentration. In addition, individuals deprived of REM sleep demonstrate increasing perceptual difficulties leading to behaviors such as confusion, paranoia, and hallucinations with increased anxiety and short-term memory impairment (Sebilia 1981; Klell 1974; Wotring 1982). Many studies have been made of prisoners of war who were deprived of sleep for prolonged periods of time. It was during such experiences that their character structure reached its lowest and weakest point, and it was easy to break a sleepless man emotionally. It would be unusual for a critically ill patient to go over 200 hours without sleep, but he may go 48 to 72 hours without adequate periods of sleep.

It is important to note that an individual who is deprived of REM sleep from frequent interruption of REM state will spend more time in REM when finally allowed uninterrupted sleep. This type of sleep is referred to as *REM rebound*. REM rebound can be problematical for the patient with coronary artery disease. The physiological demands of REM sleep can lead to arrhythmias. Furthermore cardiac patients seem to have more pain and experience heart failure most frequently between 4:00 A.M. and 6:00 A.M. This is one time when most people have the majority of their REM sleep (Hilton 1976; Hayter 1980; Wotring 1982).

Researchers do not really comprehend what lies behind an individual's need for sleep. They do know, however, that when an individual goes without sleep for an extended period of time, he experiences behavioral changes. This is particularly true in critical care units, where the nature and severity of the individual's illness requires repeated visual, tactile, and machine surveillance.

SLEEP DEPRIVATION IN CRITICAL CARE

Each of us maintains certain situations or habits. These habits become a part of our health pattern. Our response to the events of the coming day is influenced by the time at which we go to sleep and by how well we sleep. We all know people whose daily habits are so routine that they become predictable. Regular habits help to keep us organized. Sleep, as a necessity of life, is no exception to the rule. Luce (1971) believes that

> Regular hours of sleep keep us in tune with ourselves, and the hour we select for bedtime calibrates our day with twenty-four hour world of society. This unit of twenty-four hours is only one of the periods expressed in our behavior, but it is our most important social time unit. As the hours go around each day, we change visibly. Our mental acuity, the keenness of our senses, our vulnerability to stress or infection, even subtle displays of vitality and idiosyncrasy all show circadian rhythms.* (P. 119)

There may be a time such as during acute illness in which a regular rhythm of sleep cannot be achieved. A sudden disruption in the normal sleep pattern or even in the rituals or preparation for sleep can lead to sleep deprivation.

All human beings sleep. Some individuals sleep more than others. Sleep deprivation has tremendous significance for critical care patients. We know that REM sleep deprivation can lead to fatigue, irritability, and increased sensitivity to pain. A patient whose biological integrity is already severely weakened can grow worse. An aged patient deprived of sleep may complain of pain. His nurse may administer a medication to relieve the pain, but analgesics that serve temporarily to reduce the pain simultaneously make older patients confused. Confusion may further reduce the individual's sleep, thus creating further deprivation and emotional pain. Illness can reduce the total normal sleeping time, depriving the patient of some of the normal stages of sleep.

The concept of sensory deprivation can be applied to the critical care patient in two ways. The first way looks at situations in the patient's environment that create increased sensory input. The increased input deprives the patient of his rest and sleep. Second, there are situations that require more sleep, such as illness. However, we know that normal uninterrupted sleep is almost impossible in noisy and stimulus-oriented critical care environments. If the individual needs more sleep during his illness and is unable to attain it, he may experience sleep deprivation more quickly than patients in other areas of the hospital. We will discuss both situations—increased stimulus input and increased need of sleep—in accordance with the function of sleep identified by Gaarder.

*© 1971 by Pantheon Books, a Division of Random House, Inc.

Situations of Increased Input

According to the model of sleep and its functions proposed by Gaarder (1966), an increased input of stimuli would require an increased amount of sleep to destructuralize the overcrowded data storage. If this is the case, then our goal in caring for the critically ill patient would be to provide the necessary rest and sleep. The patient in acute crisis has already sustained an overwhelming amount of sensory input prior to his arrival in a critical care unit. He experienced the sudden impact of illness, the anxiety of getting into an ambulance, the hysterical outbursts of family members, the ambulance ride, the admitting process of the emergency room, the pain, the ride to his temporary home, and finally admission into a critical care unit. Once in the unit the incoming stimuli do not diminish; they increase.

Due to the severity of the patient's illness and the need for continuous monitoring and care, his normal sleep patterns and cycles are highly susceptible to interruption and changes. The patient in critical care is affected by pathophysiological alteration, necessary supportive devices, constant surveillance, lack of privacy, reduced meaningful stimuli, and personal reaction to illness or hospitalization. All of these variables influence the patient's reaction to stress and subsequently its effect upon sleep-inhibiting factors (Hilton 1976).

There are two general types of patient cases in which increased sensory input occurs. The first includes patients admitted as emergencies. The second includes patients admitted for elective surgery. The emergency may dictate an overwhelming amount of nursing surveillance and supportive devices. A patient may have had a routine operation only to sustain complications necessitating admission into critical care. Like the patient who has elective surgery, he is exposed to tremendous environmental stimulation. The following two patient cases depict examples of increased sensory input.

Case 1.   Mr. B. was a 38-year-old man, married, and the father of three children. He and his family had just returned from church when his children informed him that they wanted hamburgers for lunch. Mr. B. decided to get them the hamburgers. He took their orders and told them he would return in ten minutes. In the meantime Mrs. B. and the children changed clothes, set the table, and got ready to eat. On the way to a nearby drive-in, a car suddenly crossed the middle line and crashed into Mr. B.'s car. The impact was so great that it pushed Mr. B.'s car into the next lane, causing it to collide with another car. In the process of the collision, Mr. B.'s car burst into flames. Luckily a few bystanders risked their lives to save Mr. B. By the time they were able to free him, he had sustained burns. While he lay in the street waiting for the ambulance, he was aware of cars passing, horns beeping, people yelling or looking at him, and finally the distant sound of a siren. After what seemed like an eternity, the ambulance arrived. Mr. B. was painfully but gently placed on a stretcher and taken to the emergency room. Meanwhile his family had completed the prelunch preparation and were waiting for their father to return with their lunch. Then Mrs. B. received a phone call informing her of the accident and that her husband had been taken to the emergency room of a nearby hospital.

Burn patients in this particular hospital usually went directly to the burn unit. Patients went to the Hubbard tank, where burns could be cleaned, assessed, cultured, medicated, and dressed. Due to Mr. B.'s accident, it was decided to medicate the patient and take a series of X-rays in the emergency room before transporting him to the burn unit. By the time X-rays had been ordered and taken, other treatments and procedures were also begun. Once the X-rays were taken, Mr. B. was quickly whisked to the Hubbard tank. Here another series of intrusive and painful procedures began. Assessment of his burns revealed second- and third-degree burns over 40 percent of his body. The burns involved his arms, face, chest, and back. While in the Hubbard tank, many people poked and probed his body. Parts of his body ached with pain. Staff members took blood samples for routine laboratory work, electrolytes, and other procedures. Finally Mr. B. was moved directly into the burn unit.

Here another series of events occurred, creating additional increase in sensory input. Mr. B. was painfully lifted onto a narrow bed. Next, staff members applied various pieces of supportive devices. Each piece had its own unique function and characteristic noise. The patient barely had time to become familiar with his bed when nurses connected the supportive devices to strategic points of his body with wires and tubes. Intravenous therapy had already been initiated in the emergency room, and now the tubing was threaded into an IVAC machine. EKG leads were connected to his cardioscope, and nurses attached a nasal-gastric tube, a Foley catheter, an arterial line, and central venous pressure tubing to Mr. B. Because of heat loss, a heat cradle was placed on his bed. Nurses checked urine output, blood pressure, CVP, temperature, pulse, respirations, reflexes, and pupils each hour.

During the next twelve hours, Mr. B.'s blood gases revealed the beginning signs of respiratory insufficiency. Intermittent positive pressure breathing every two hours seemed to be ineffective. Mr. B.'s mouth and cheeks had been burned, making it difficult for him to hold a mouthpiece. His doctors decided they would have to perform a temporary tracheostomy so his breathing could be assisted by a volume respirator. All these treatments and procedures, with the exception of the tracheostomy, occurred in a relatively brief period of time. The patient hardly had a chance to incorporate one stimulus when another was instituted.

Throughout the next several days, Mr. B.'s condition remained critical. His condition required frequent surveillance by both nurses and doctors. It was necessary for the burn nurses to monitor his blood pressure, TPR, CVP, and urinary output hourly. In addition, he required frequent suctioning. All the interventions were necessary, but they kept Mr. B. awake. Furthermore, coughing stimulated through suctioning was painful to the burns on his chest. The number of concerned people in his environment, coupled with all the supportive devices, greatly limited Mr. B.'s normal sleep rhythm. It seemed that just as he fell into a relaxing sleep someone touched him, jarred his bed, or made a noise that awakened him. The nurses began noting a change in Mr. B.'s behavioral response to them. It seemed that as they approached his bed, he became hostile or irritable. On the fourth day after his arrival in the burn unit, Mr. B. began screaming at his nurse after he deflated his tracheostomy cuff.

MR. B.: What are you trying to do now?

NURSE: I am about to clean your tracheostomy tube and suction you.

MR. B.: Do you have to do that right now?

NURSE: What's wrong, Mr. B.?

MR. B.: What's wrong? You are what's wrong. Why can't all of you leave me alone?

NURSE: I just want to clean your tracheostomy inner cannula.

MR. B.: (Grabs the nurse's hand.) Get out of here and leave me alone! I don't want it cleaned now.

NURSE: Mr. B., you are hurting my hand.

MR. B.: Good. You have been hurting me. I'll let your hand go if you leave me alone.

NURSE: Let me reinflate your cuff, and I'll leave you alone.

MR. B.: Please get out of here. (His agitation increases to the point where medication is required.) All I want to do is sleep.

Even though the nurse acknowledged Mr. B.'s wishes and left him alone, other environmental stimuli continued. As Foulkes (1966) has pointed out,

> During sleep external stimuli are by no means eliminated. It may happen, for instance, that a housefly is captive in the bedroom. Not only does its buzzing provide a fluctuating auditory stimulus, but tactile stimulation will also be produced if it chooses to land on one's forehead. Nor are bodily sensations entirely absent during sleep. Digestive processes may continue to apply themselves to what was eaten and a host of other stimuli producing body processes persist during sleep. (P. 154)

Even while the critical care patient sleeps, sensory input from his environment continues. Unfortunately, nurses can never completely eliminate excess stimuli. Machines will continue to hum, buzz, and beep along as they perform their vital functions. Nurses, doctors, and other patients are human beings who will continue to make humanlike noises.

The psychological stress associated with critical care, together with the reality of facing new and potentially threatening experiences, cause a need for more REM sleep. Illness, disease, injury, and the need for hospitalization create psychological stress while simultaneously making it less likely that REM sleep will be obtained.

Many times we do not realize all the incoming stimuli the patient has endured prior to his arrival in critical care. Mr. B. had experienced tremendous sensory input. First, his car collided with two other cars. In the seconds that followed, he found himself threatened by fire. The next weeks added additional threats, all of which created their own stimuli. While Mr. B. awaited his ambulance, he experienced the stimulus of pain together with the environmental stimuli of cars and people. Once inside the ambulance, he experienced the sensory input of a siren sounding his journey through the city. Finally he arrived in the emergency room, where he was exposed to additional stimuli. He was poked, probed, and percussed. All these events were stored in his mind. Mr. B. needed time to sleep to destructuralize stored data.

The more incoming stimuli there are, the more time a patient needs to sleep so he can destructuralize the data. But when more sleep is needed, less seems to be available. As the patient remains critically ill, input of stimuli continues. Nurses, doctors, and machines continue their surveillance. The individual continues to store data until he reaches his input limit, and then he may react behaviorally, as did Mr. B. He becomes hostile and irritable. Mr. B.'s behavior was manifested in his statements, "Why can't all of you leave me alone," and "Get out of here."

Mr. B., like many patients in critical care units, experienced sleep deprivation. In attempting to monitor the patient's biological system so that any threats to its integrity can be anticipated, his nurses threatened his psychological integrity. We sometimes forget that this experience, especially to the severely burned patient, may be a totally new one. He is exposed to new faces, new procedures, new situations, and above all a new bed. Such new encounters affect both his biological and psychological integrity. Individuals in new situations all show the same quiet, intense orienting to their surroundings, with signs of tension.

According to Gaarder's model, sleep serves to reinforce the individual's character structure. Mr. B. may need to internalize changes in his self-concept. Included in his altered self-concept may be changes in his life-style. He needs quiet, uninterrupted time to think about these changes. Initially the changes may be too threatening for him to think about on a conscious level. Therefore, he pushes the thoughts to his unconscious. There the thoughts remain unless he can sleep and dream. It may only be through dreaming that a patient like Mr. B. is able to think about a painful situation. If he is not permitted periods of uninterrupted sleep, he may not experience reinforcement of his character structure.

Mr. B. represents one type of patient who experienced sleep deprivation due to tremendous sensory input. His admission to the hospital was an emergency. There are other patients who experience similar situations of sensory input. The individual who gets his hand caught in a machine may need to wait several hours while it is determined whether or not his hand can be freed. The woman who has a myocardial infarction while climbing in the mountains with friends may be forced to wait while a friend obtains help and returns to her side. The aged lady who lives alone and falls in the bathroom may wait for hours until a neighbor hears her screams. Each of these individuals has already experienced tremendous sensory input. Each should be quickly admitted and encouraged to sleep, in order to allow him to de-structuralize all the data taken in during the crisis and to reinforce his character structure. Furthermore, sleep can fortify the individual for the next series of situations leading to sensory input.

The elective patient presents a different problem than does the emergency patient. Elective patients enter critical care free of the sensory stress felt by emergency patients; they have chosen to submit to surgery necessitating a few days hospitalization in critical care. Their biological systems have been steadily deteriorating over the years, thus preparing them for eventual illness or surgical intervention. Mr. O. is an example of such a patient who had surgery and experienced both a complication and deprivation.

Case 2. Mr. O. was a 57-year-old man who for the past several years had experienced angina. His angina attacks had become more severe in recent months. He was hospitalized for cardiac catheterization in order to determine the severity of his coronary artery disease. The test revealed severe stenosis, or narrowing, of all three major coronary arteries. It became apparent that open heart surgery would be recommended. The cardiac surgical team decided to perform a triple bypass on Mr. O. Mr. O. did not like the idea of surgery in general, let alone surgery involving his heart. He feared being immobilized for a prolonged period of time, the incisional pain, and the possibility that something might go wrong. His wife, his doctor, and former cardiac surgical patients encouraged him to submit to the procedure. Finally Mr. O. agreed to have the surgery.

An intensive care nurse who would handle the postoperative care of Mr. O. went to his room, on another floor, and explained the surgical procedure, postoperative care, and the length of time he would be in intensive care. Next, she invited him to tour the intensive care unit and see for himself his new temporary home. This would give him the opportunity to see various pieces of supportive equipment used by other patients. The nurse attempted to explain each piece of equipment and each procedure.

Mr. O. toured the intensive care unit, had his preoperative teaching, and then returned to the quietness of his room. There he pondered, slept, and dreamed about the coming surgical event. The following morning, Mr. O. was taken to surgery. The surgical procedure was uneventful, and Mr. O. was admitted to intensive care. His bed was surrounded by pieces of equipment. The dresser top no longer contained pictures of his grandchildren, flowers and cards from friends, or his glasses and book; it held foreign-looking objects—bottles, tubes, tape, and gloves. Around his bed were a cardioscope and the assorted paraphernalia of cardiac treatment. While Mr. O. was still lethargic and unaware of his environment, nurses set the various pieces of silent equipment into motion, connecting them one by one to the newly arrived open heart patient. The nurse and the machines monitored all aspects of Mr. O.'s activities.

When the wires, tubes, and machines were all connected, the nurse pushed the buttons, turned the dials, and regulated the flow rates. In this postoperative phase, her job was to elicit information from the supportive devices and from her own assessment in order to provide a plan of care for Mr. O. The entire process involved soliciting information on an hourly basis, necessitating continual disturbance of the patient. For the next two days, the nurses maintained close surveillance of Mr. O. His cardioscope pattern showed occasional ectopic beats necessitating a lidocaine drip.

On the morning of his third postoperative day, Mr. O.'s nurse noted that his premature ectopic beats were increasing in frequency. The flow rate of his lidocaine was increased, but this did not seem to control the ectopic beats. At the same time, Mr. O.'s doctor was notified of the arrhythmias and minimal response to the medication. Before the doctor came, Mr. O.'s rhythm changed to ventricular fibrillation. A cardiac arrest was immediately initiated. The doctors decided to do direct cardiac massage. During the process Mr. O. remained unconscious. After several minutes of direct massage and defibrillation, the arrhythmias converted to a normal sinus rhythm. Mr. O. awakened to find his chest open and heart exposed. The look on his face was one of extreme fear. Sensing his obvious fright, the nurses and doctors attempted to explain what had happened. They tried to reassure him that he was all right and that they were waiting to return him to surgery. Mr. O. simply stared at the ceiling.

Mr. O. was taken to surgery where his newly transplanted coronary arteries were assessed for possible damage. None being found, the doctor resutured the patient's sternum and returned him to his bed in intensive care. He slept until early afternoon. This was to be his last sleep for several days. During the next three days, he was monitored even more closely than before his arrhythmia complication. Mr. O.'s sleep deprivation had two causes: environmental stimulus input and his own alertness. He observed everything going on around him, whether it pertained to him or not. He listened intently to what the nurses said about his care or progress. He continually asked the nurses what they were doing, what they were finding out, and how he was progressing. Reassurances did not seem to relax Mr. O. to the point of sleep. The result was that Mr. O. was unable to achieve a sleep state due to frequent surveillance. The significance of frequent interruption in critical care units focuses on the fact that the interruptions cause the patient to experience more waking time and stage I sleep. In patients with fixed myocardial oxygen supply, such interruptions of sleep increase myocardial oxygen consumption and may contribute to myocardial ischemia and increased PVC frequency (Sebilia 1981).

Even if uninterrupted periods of sleep had been provided, Mr. O. would not have utilized them. He would have interpreted this intervention as neglect or avoidance, and he would have become all the more alert and watchful. The patient was creating his own type of sleep deprivation. He seemed to be afraid to sleep. Medication did not help, and as a matter of fact, he tried to resist it. The nurses noted a change in Mr. O.'s behavior over the three-day period. Instead of asking his usual questions, he became noncommunicative. His fatigued and frightened eyes continued their surveillance of his environment.

Studies of open heart patients have found that these patients develop cardiac psychosis due to sleep deprivation. Sleep deprivation has obvious effects of behavior. Apart from tiredness, there is irritability, suspiciousness, and speech slurring which soon become evident; mild forms of paranoia are not uncommon. In addition time disorientation and visual misperceptions are encountered after one or two nights of sleep deprivation (Horne 1983). Mr. O. was no exception. After only three days of sleep deprivation, he experienced irritability, fatigue, and tiredness. The nurses began observing a change in his thinking and speech pattern. They observed him talking to himself. On the afternoon of the third day after his emergency, Mr. O. became extremely angry, combative, and paranoid. Mr. O.'s nurse was beginning to take a CVP reading when he began screaming.

MR. O.: Don't do that!
NURSE: What do you mean, Mr. O.?
MR. O.: You know what I said. Don't play games with me.
NURSE: I really didn't hear you.
MR. O.: I told you not to do that.
NURSE: What, Mr. O.?
MR. O.: You know. You all know none of this will do any good.
NURSE: I am not following you, Mr. O.
MR. O.: Yes, you are. You are all playing games around here.
NURSE: What kind of games?
MR. O.: The games of life and death. Who decides which one lives and which one dies? (*He laughs.*) I know what you are up to. (*He becomes increasingly more agitated*)
NURSE: Try and relax, Mr. O.
MR. O.: How can I relax when I have to see who tries to do me in?
NURSE: What do you mean?
MR. O.: You know, you all know! Not get these things off me. (*Reaches for his tubes and wires.*)
NURSE: (*Nurse grabs his hands.*) Please try to relax.
MR. O.: Don't tell me what to do. I'll do whatever I want. (*Continues to pull his tubes.*)
NURSE: Mr. O., don't do that!
MR. O.: I'll do what I want before you all kill me. Let me out of here. (*Now there are several nurses all holding the patient*).
NURSE: We are all trying to help you.
MR. O.: Sure, you are. I see you already have my casket ready. (*Points to a bed scale.*)
NURSE: That is a bed scale, Mr. O.

MR. O.:   Is that what they teach you to say?

NURSE: No, Mr. O., it is a bed scale.

MR. O.:   Get out of my way. (*Finally grabs the nurse's wrist and again pulls his tubes.*)

NURSE: Relax, Mr. O. (*The nurse calls his doctor, who orders a Valium to relax the patient.*)

The patient has finally reached his limit of both stimulus input and sleep deprivation. He spent two complete days prior to his complication without uninterrupted sleep. After his complication, he spent an additional three days in sleep deprivation. He could not match the normal pattern of sleep he had achieved on the general floor in intensive care. His critical condition necessitated intensive surveillance. Furthermore, his own fear of threat to his biological integrity made sleep impossible. Instead, he remained in a psychological state of readiness, alert to the possibility of complications. He seemed afraid to submit to the soothing world of sleep. He became increasingly more fatigued, irritable, confused, and finally paranoid. His perceptions of environmental objects were distorted. This became obvious when he perceived a bed scale as being a "casket." As Luby (1966) has reported,

> between forty-eight and seventy-two hours of sleep deprivation, subjects will start to lose conversational or perceptual sets and begin to respond to intrusive, internal cues. Bodily sensations of an unusual and frightening nature are reported by almost all subjects. Depersonalization experiences are quite common—feelings of floating, body deadness, or detached self-observation. (P. 191)

An important point worth mentioning is the patient's association of sleep with death. As the patient's perception is altered, he perceives sleep as death. He fears that if he should fall asleep, he may never again awaken. Therefore, the nurse may find her patient fighting the thing he needs most—sleep. If the patient is unable to sleep because he fears death, the nurse can help him verbalize these fears; then he can discover that his fears are normal and temporary.

Like Mr. B., Mr. O. could not achieve the two functions of sleep. First, he had difficulty destructuralizing stored data collected from tremendous stimulus input, in the form of intensive surveillance and his postoperative crisis. Surgical intervention, especially involving the heart, is traumatic even when it occurs in the operating room. To awaken and find one's heart exposed could shock the patient into avoiding sleep. This crisis occurred when he was asleep. Therefore, he will fight sleep for fear that another complication may occur. As Hume notes,

> The individual fails to realize that the occurrence of sleep is not determined exclusively by a punitive endogenous oscillator, whether the subject is under temporal isolation in an isolation chamber or in the world outside. The decision to attempt to sleep depends on the level of interest in what one is doing or what is happening in the environment and how much sleep one intuitively feels from experience one needs for their scheduled activity on the following day. (P. 22)

Impending surgery can lead to sleep deprivation. Some patients are sleep-deprived prior to surgery. Among the causes of preoperative sleep deprivation are anxiety, noise, and unfamiliar surroundings. Postoperative sleep can be affected by pain, frequent nursing observations, anesthetic agents, and the inability of a patient to lie comfortably due to incisional site and supportive devices. Ellis and Dudley (1976) point out three major changes in sleep after surgery. First there is a marked reduction in REM sleep. The severity of the surgery seems to influence the degree and duration of REM reduction. Second, there may be a reduction in stage III and stage IV sleep. The degree of alteration is dependent upon the severity of the surgery. Surgical trauma and drugs affect the patient's ability to achieve the slow wave of deep sleep. Third, a lack of inherent rhythmicity in sleep is often noted postoperatively. The postoperative variables that influence or determine the pattern of sleep consist of analgesic drugs and nursing observations.

The nurse may not be able to provide her patient with a normal sleep pattern, but she might be able to control the amount of stimulus input, which would obviously lessen the need for destructuralizing stored data. The amount of sleep needed by the patient is not as significant as the quality of sleep. Uninterrupted periods of sleep allow both destructuring of stored data and reinforcement of character structure, the second function of sleep.

Mr. O. and Mr. B. needed sleep to reinforce their threatened character structures. A patient may need to incorporate the chain of events that have occurred since his surgery. Mr. O. experienced all the routine postoperative surveillance, but he also underwent cardiac arrest and direct cardiac massage. Following his return from surgery, he became preoccupied with fear of additional biological threats. This became apparent when he continually asked his nurses what was happening and how he was progressing. He did not seem to find peace in the nurse's reassurances; instead, he continued his own watchful surveillance. He fought sleep.

Any patient who goes without sleep may not be able to accept or assimilate all the events into his changed character structure. The structure might change in a behaviorally bizarre manner. Postoperative confusion and bizarre behavior on the part of the open heart patient are not unusual. Some patients may experience them to a greater degree than others. Fass (1971) has noted that "after transfer from the intensive care unit, these patients usually return to reality quickly in a place where sleep is less interrupted. Definite causes of their hallucinations and strange behavior are not known but drastic reduction in allowing sleep and dreaming may play a significant role" (p. 2317).* The nurse may not be able to facilitate or provide a normal sleep pattern; the nature of critical care units makes this difficult. But she may control the amount of incoming stimuli so that what sleep becomes available is of a qualitatively good nature.

*Copyright, American Journal of Nursing Company. Reprinted, with permission, from *American Journal of Nursing.*

Situations in Which More Sleep is Needed

In some situations an individual requires more sleep than at other times. Physical illness is one of those situations. As Gaarder (1966) points out, an individual in biological crisis requires more sleep:

> Physical illness often leads to increased need to sleep. This would be because there is an increase in the amount of body image input that must be stored. Entero and exteroceptive input are probably stored in a common area, and enteroceptive stimuli are probably more imperative and less susceptible to inattention. Therefore, the enteroceptive input of disease would fill storage much faster, resulting in the need of sleep to erase the filled storage. (P. 259)

However, sleep may not always come when it is needed the most. This is frequently the case in critical care units. Although his nurse may tell the cardiac patient in coronary care to rest and sleep, the impact of cardiac illness creates emotional stress that makes rest difficult. Furthermore the patient must submit to frequent monitoring of his blood pressure, respiration, cardiac rhythm, intravenous flow rate, temperature, and urinary output. His nurse will tell a respiratory care patient who has severe emphysema to rest and sleep in an attempt to reduce his physical activity. Reduced activity would decrease the amount of oxygen needed. Just as the patient achieves rest or sleep, he is awakened by the sensation of being suctioned.

Most critical care patients can tolerate periods of sleep deprivation. Most patients can accept this because they are away from their normal sleeping environment. "We know that patients in hospitals, away from their usual sleeping environments and beset by the problems caused by illness, frequently have difficulty meeting one of their most basic physiologic needs—the need for sleep—at a time when they require it most" (Long 1969, p. 1896).* Some patients in critical care tolerate sleep deprivation because they realize that as their condition improves, the intense surveillance will subside. These patients are unusual; most patients react consciously and unconsciously to sleep loss. One behavioral response is hostility or irritability.

Some critical care patients go for long periods of time without uninterrupted sleep. In critical care, sleep is low on the priority scale. Nurses have to concentrate on getting their treatments and procedures completed, although the patient may not understand the nurse's goal. As sleep becomes less obtainable to the patient, it becomes one of his immediate priorities. The following example shows what happened to a critical care patient who experienced sleep deprivation.

Mrs. L., a 62-year-old woman, had experienced intermittent claudication for several years. At the onset of her peripheral pain, diagnostic tests

*Copyright, American Journal of Nursing Company. Reprinted, with permission, from *American Journal of Nursing.*

revealed an abdominal aortic aneurysm. Her doctors believed that as long as the aneurysm remained constant in size, surgery would not be necessary. In addition to the abdominal aneurysm, Mrs. L. also had a history of hypertension and had had one previous myocardial infarction. Since her myocardial infarction Mrs. L. has tried to walk a mile each morning. Much to her displeasure, her pain became more severe and she was hospitalized for additional X-rays and possible surgery. Diagnostic X-rays revealed an increase in the aneurysm's size; surgery would be necessary. Needless to say, Mrs. L.'s history of cardiac disease and hypertension became a preoperative concern. Mrs. L. did not look forward to the temporary immobility caused by surgery. Nevertheless, she felt more immobilized by the pain, so she submitted to the surgical procedure.

After Mrs. L.'s surgery, she was transferred to intensive care, where she could be closely observed for the next few days. Her blood pressure, respirations, peripheral pulses, temperature, cardiac rhythm, and urine output were monitored frequently. Mrs. L. was aware of her sensory-oriented environment, her nurse's surveillance, and incisional pain. Although medication could halt her pain, nothing could be done about the surveillance and environmental input. Over a four-day period, Mrs. L. experienced several biological crises. Each crisis required nursing and mechanical surveillance, and each contributed to the creation of additional problems. The patient's immediate environment became a beehive of activity. Mrs. L. continued to remain hypertensive, necessitating blood pressure readings every two hours. A chest X-ray revealed pneumonitis. This required coughing, positioning, suctioning, IPPB, blood gases analysis, and medication for incisional pain so that she could cough and deep-breathe. Next Mrs. L. developed shortness of breath, diaphoresis, cyanosis, bilateral rales, and some peripheral edema. Doctors ordered rotating tourniquets, additional IPPB treatments, intravenous medications, a chest X-ray, and central venous pressure readings.

The nurses also noted a reduction in Mrs. L.'s urinary output. Hourly urinary output and specific gravities were done to monitor her renal function. Laboratory studies revealed rising BUN and creatinine levels. The doctors diagnosed Mrs. L.'s renal problem as acute tubular necrosis resulting from perfusion deficit. From the time of Mrs. L.'s cardiac crisis until the reduction in her urinary output, her blood pressure had dropped. Since Mrs. L. was normally hypertensive, the sudden decrease became alarming. By the end of Mrs. L.'s fifth postoperative day, her cardiac output had improved, and her blood pressure returned to its higher level. It was hoped that once she was out of cardiac failure the patient's renal problem would also subside, but her renal problem continued to the point where peritoneal dialysis was necessary.

Throughout the five-day period since Mrs. L.'s surgery, she experienced pneumonitis, congestive heart failure, pulmonary edema, and acute tubular necrosis. As various pieces of equipment were wheeled into her environment and attached to her, she became aware of each new biological complication. She was also aware of being poked, pinched, stuck, palpated, or percussed.

Each additional complication reduced her ability to achieve uninterrupted sleep; she could only nap between the hourly parade of seemingly necessary activities. Finally Mrs. L. reached her limit. Like Mr. O., she became hostile, irritable, angered, and somewhat confused. The once-quiet and pleasant woman now became an angry person yelling at her nurse, "Leave me alone," "Stop bothering me," and "I just want to sleep."

Sleep at such a time is not always possible. Sleep and rest facilitate the patient's biological well-being, and sleep deprivation may serve to foster biological distintegration. Luce (1971) notes how important biological functions are tied to the sleep cycle:

> Hours of sleep and waking normally set the phase of kidney activity, for elimination function, for increases and decreases in metabolism, body temperature, and many other intermeshed functions. When we shift our hours of sleep these functions also shift. Unfortunately the parts of the body shift at varied speed, so that heart, kidneys, liver, and adrenal glands may adjust at different rates. (P. 75).

The patient who experiences a sequence of consecutive biological crises needs time to adapt physiologically to each crisis. Sleep and dreaming become one way in which the individual is able to restore the energy depleted by the crisis and mobilize himself for the next sequence of events. The individual who is not permitted periods of uninterrupted sleep may not be able to cope with current threats or adaptive changes. According to Greenberg (1972),

> When an individual meets a situation which is stressful for him, the stressfulness is due to the arousal of memories of prior difficulties with similar situations. The person's initial defense reaction is usually of an emergency or generalized type (such as global denial or repression). Then during the dream experience, these feelings from the past and the current stressful stimulus are integrated, and the individual's character defenses for that particular set of emotions and memories are used to deal with the current threat. (P. 260).

A patient like Mrs. L. defends herself against further sleep deprivation by pushing the people creating deprivation out of her environment. Such is the case when the patient finally reaches his stimulus input limit and yells that he wants to be left alone.

We do not know why we need sleep in illness. We do not know "why we have sleep to restore our well-being and efficiency, nor do we know whether, as one might surmise, some chemical substance may accumulate in the brain or elsewhere during wakefulness, to be removed by the sleep it promotes" (Oswald 1962, p. 178).

We do know that illness necessitating critical care leads to tremendous stimulus input. The stimulus input comes from the environment and from changes the individual must make as he adapts to an altered or new self-concept. It is through sleep, according to Gaarder's model, that the individual reinforces his character structure. The individual bombarded by threats to his biological integrity retreats into the world of sleep and dreaming to protect his psychological integrity. Foulkes (1966) addresses the importance of dreaming as a protection against such threats:

> The functions sometimes ascribed to mental activity during sleep are those mentioned by psychoanalysis: the protection of sleep and the maintenance of personality integrity. The dream is viewed as the means by which the continuance of the state of sleep is assured and by which potentially harmful thoughts and impulses find discharge without any interference in wakeful personality functioning. (P. 193).

Critical illness also creates alterations in the normal sleep rhythm. It is imperative for the critical care nurse to remember that "along with alterations of activity and sleep, a continuum of vital functions is intermeshed, leaving their gradually changing signs in the blood and urine, in our levels of hormones, and in the utilization of food" (Luce 1971, p. 145–146). Therefore, if biological function is closely interrelated with sleep, sleep should become one of the priority needs of the critical care patient.

Patients whose illnesses are serious enough to warrant critical care need to have a normal sleep rhythm. The length of time in sleep is not as imperative as the routine of uninterrupted sleep: a somewhat normal pattern of minisleep should be fostered. A patient like Mrs. L., who experienced several complications over a relatively short period of time, needs to sleep in order to destructuralize stored data from stimulus input and to reinforce her character structure. Originally she feared postoperative immobility from pain. As her postoperative complications grew, however, her fears extended beyond that of pain. Mrs. L.'s experience and need state are not unique. Other critical care patients need sleep to maintain and restore their threatened biological and psychological integrity. The patient who experiences his first myocardial infarction needs the vehicle of sleep to work through some of his fears or anxieties about his newly acquired sick-role status. Since this is his first admission to coronary care, he has no previous experience on which to draw. The cardiac patient experiencing his second myocardial infarction has memories of the past experience and an awareness of limitations or additional changes in his life-style that may take place in the future. A patient with chronic emphysema may enter a respiratory care unit for the third time in one year. This time his pulmonary system is decompensated to the point where he needs a permanent tracheostomy. In addition, the patient may realize that when he leaves the respiratory unit, he will be limited to minimal activity. He may be forced to spend his waking hours sitting in a chair. Contemplating such a physically limited future changes his self-concept. He therefore needs time to integrate these changes, including hostile feelings, into his character structure. Such integration takes place during sleep. The burn patient also needs to integrate character structure changes that may have occurred as a result of disfigurement. The sleep needs of the hemodialysis patient are considerably less. He is only hospitalized in hemodialysis unit for a period of six to eight hours. Many patients take time to sleep or rest. They have already experienced the original biological crisis that required hemodialysis. Now they must face the continual adaptation to limitations created by renal failure. They can sleep, whereas patients in other critical care units such as intensive care, burn, respiratory care, or coronary care units cannot as easily do so. Critical care nurses have a tremendous responsibility in intervening to facilitate a relatively normal sleep pattern, but it must be remembered that there will always exist situations in which sleep is somewhat difficult to achieve.

NURSING ASSESSMENT OF SLEEP DEPRIVATION

The nurse assesses sleep deprivation through the patient's behavioral response. The responses can be categorized into regulatory behaviors and cognitive behaviors. Regulatory behaviors result from REM deprivation leading to physical fatigue. Cognitive behaviors are due to REM deprivation causing psychological alterations.

Regulatory Behaviors

The regulator system involves inputs, processes, effectors, and feedback loops. It involves stimuli from the external environment and from changes in the internal state of dynamic equilibrium. The inputs are chemical in nature or have been transduced into neural information (Roy and Roberts 1981). The regulatory behaviors are physiological responses.

During NREM sleep the brain rests and the body is quiet. However, REM sleep is characterized by tremendous activity. Both sleep periods manifest themselves through specific regulatory behaviors. The NREM or synchronized period is characterized by the following regulatory behaviors (Fabijan and Gosselin 1982):

NREM Sleep Regulatory Behaviors

Decreased blood pressure
Decreased heart rate
Decreased respiratory rate
Decreased urine volume
Decreased plasma volume
Decreased metabolic rate
Decreased O_2 consumption
Decreased CO_2

The EEG waves of the patient in NREM sleep are slow and of high amplitude.

The REM or desynchronized state is a physiologically active period in which the following regulatory behaviors occur (Sebilia 1981):

REM Sleep Regulatory Behaviors

Increased heart rate
Increased respiratory rate
Increased blood pressure
Increased autonomic activity
Increased metabolic activity
Increased gastric secretions
Increased 17-hydrocortisone
Increased catacholamine level

During REM sleep the patient's cardiovascular demands may be suddenly and abruptly increased. Rosenblatt, Hartman, and Zwilling (1973) point out that, in an individual with a normal vascular system, the increased cardiac demands are met with no abnormal consequences. In patients with coronary artery disease, hypertension, or arrhythmias, however, a sudden outflow of sympathetic stimuli may result in increased arrhythmias, angina pectoris, and myocardial infarction. Therefore the REM stage of sleep is a vulnerable period for developing cardiac arrhythmias associated with sudden outflow of sympathetic activity and changes in blood pressure. When PVCs occur during slow heart rate as in stage IV, they may be due to irritable foci in damaged areas of myocardium that initiate arrhythmias. Attention to heart rate becomes significant for the cardiac patient since heart rate is a primary determinant of myocardial oxygen consumption.

Normally during sleep the cerebral blood flow in the cortex of the brainstem decreases. The exception is during REM sleep when the blood flow markedly increases in the brain and brainstem. An increased cerebral blood flow may have special significance to the acute head injury patient already experiencing increased intracranal pressure (Williams and Jackson 1982).

Gastric secretion is also increased during REM sleep. Critical care patients with peptic ulcers seems to have more pain during REM stage. Gastric secretion peaks between 1:00 A.M. and 3:00 A.M. It is characteristic of peptic ulcer disease that the person awakens at that time with pain (Hayter 1980).

Finally, convulsions are a regulatory behavior, that is more likely to occur during REM sleep. Because long periods of REM sleep occur shortly before the person awakens, it is during this time when nighttime convulsions occur (Hayter 1980).

In summary, NREM sleep is associated with reduced body activity while REM sleep is more active. Therefore when the critically ill patient is deprived of NREM sleep, he experiences physical fatigue.

Cognitive Behaviors

The cognator system involves inputs from internal and external stimuli which include psychological and social factors. The specific aspects of the cognator mechanism consist of perceptual/information processing, learning, judgment, and emotion (Roy and Roberts 1981). The cognitive behaviors are psychological responses.

During REM sleep the mental aspect is an extreme state of divergent thinking. Lewis and Glaubman (1975) hypothesize that the psychological effect of REM deprivation varies in a dimension of creativity versus rote learning. On the creativity pole, REM deprivation has a damaging effect, while on the rote learning pole, it has a beneficial effect. The cognitive behaviors associated with sleep deprivation consist of the following (Hayter 1980; Zelechowski 1979; Fabijan and Gosselin 1982):

REM Deprivation Cognitive Behaviors

Lassitude
Lethargy
Hallucinations
Disorientation
Confusion
Restlessness
Irritability
Apathy
Poor judgment
Memory disturbance
Delusions
Paranoid ideation
Hostility

If REM deprivation occurs repeatedly every night while the patient is in critical care, he is likely to become confused and disoriented and to experience hallucinations.

Furthermore REM deprivation also causes changes in the patient's dreaming pattern. Dreams play a role in psychologically helping an individual to adapt, problem solve, and integrate his daily activities. Another line of thought attributes to dreaming and REM sleep internal information processing. The information processing focuses on material not successfully handled during wakefulness (Lewis and Glaubman 1975; Sebilia 1981).

NURSING DIAGNOSIS OF SLEEP DEPRIVATION

The nursing diagnosis is a statement of the current problem. To make her diagnosis, the nurse takes into account regulatory and cognitive behaviors as well as the sources of stress causing the problem. The problem is sleep deprivation. Stressors contributing to sleep deprivation can be categorized as internal or external. Internal stressors involve fear; anxiety; age; illness; disease; or injury; and medical or chemical alterations. The environmental noises associated with a critical care unit are an important source of external stressors. Internal and external stressors can combine to cause NREM and REM deprivation.

NURSING INTERVENTIONS AND SLEEP DEPRIVATION

The critical care nurse's role is to provide an environment conducive for sleep, not sleep deprivation. Providing a conducive environment means that the nurse will attempt to minimize situations leading to increased stimulus input and to facilitate sleep when required by illness.

Minimizing Stimulus Input

In order for the critical care nurse to minimize situations of stimulus input leading to sleep deprivation, she must be aware of the situations in which excess stimulation occurs. The nurse has only to look as far as the critically ill patient's immediate environment. The stimuli creating sleep deprivation are there. According to Gaarder's (1966) model, patients require sleep to destructuralize stored data collected from the day's activity. By minimizing the degree or quality of stimulus input, the critical care nurse may also minimize the actual amount of sleep needed by the patient. Stored data come from both verbal and nonverbal input.

Verbal input comes from the patient's doctor or nurse. We have all experienced the situation in which a group of eager doctors gather around the patient's bed. Unfortunately their discussion may have no meaning to the individual, and instead of impressing him, it may serve to frighten him. Consider the example of Mrs. Q., a 45-year-old woman admitted to coronary care with a diagnosis of acute myocardial infarction. On the morning following her admission the doctors gathered around her bed to listen to the exciting new "case." A young intern, trying to impress his superior with a thorough review and discussion of the patient's problem, related her symptoms and proceeded to discuss her EKG, pointing out that the changes indicated an anteroseptal myocardial infarction. Naturally, everyone clamored to review her EKG tracing and to examine changes in the various leads. Next they discussed her serum enzyme levels. Finally they had a session of show and tell, in which they discussed the various articles they had read.

Mrs. Q. tried intently to follow the doctor's discussion. The more verbal input she received, the less secure she felt. The longer the doctors discussed her situation, the more she fantasized about her problems. Mrs. Q. believed her condition was most critical. Because she feared a potential threat to her biological integrity, she created her own sleep deprivation by watching her cardioscope. She wanted to be aware of any irregularities in order to alert the nurse. The coronary care nurses finally convinced Mrs. Q. that her cardiac rhythm was stable and normal, and they tried verbally to destructuralize all the stored data collected when the doctors were discussing her clinical picture. The nurses discovered that most of the data she collected were in error. Destructuralizing the data gave them a chance to provide realistic and understandable verbal input.

Most critical care units encourage the nurse to participate in patient rounds. The nurse can listen to what is being discussed and can observe the patient's reactions. She can then act in a leadership role to encourage the patient to ask questions or seek clarification; if the patient is not ready, then the nurse can share this data when the patient achieves his own readiness level. Usually critical care patients pick a time when they feel ready for some verbal input, but even then the nurse must minimize the amount of verbal input in order not to overload her patient. She should instead enhance his understanding of what led to his admission into a critical care unit, of the nursing care plan devised to meet his needs, and of future needs. She must do this teaching gradually. The patient needs time to integrate all these events and data into his character structure. If the amount of meaningless verbal input is minimized, it is quite possible that the quality of sleep can also be enhanced. Meaningful verbal input consists of information the patient is able to comprehend and use. All other data become useless and take valuable storage space in the individual's already troubled mind.

The patient's need for sleep, when appropriate, can be given priority over the checking of vital signs or other nursing activities. Prior to awakening the critically ill patient, the nurse observes him to determine whether or not he is in REM stage sleep. Because this stage lasts a short time, it may be beneficial to wait until it ends before awakening the patient (Hayter 1980). A major nursing intervention is to eliminate the unnecessary causes of sleep deprivation. Unnecessary activities should be eliminated while nursing care be planned to allow for adequate periods of sleep. Through an understanding of the 60 to 90-minute sleep cycle it may be possible to design nursing care on a more flexible basis (Sebilia 1981).

Nonverbal input involves stimuli emanating from the patient's environment: lights; noises from nurses, doctors, other patients, and mechanical devices; gestures and facial expressions; and touch. Many critical care units maintain some type of light surveillance through the entire 24 hours. The patient never really realizes when it is day or night. He may doze off and awaken to the continual glaring of lights. He may think it daytime when it is night. Luce (1971) has pointed out that "light is a synchronizer. Light is an important time giver for human beings. It has been conjectured that the intensity of illumination might influence the activity and physiological rhythms of man as it certainly influences birds" (p. 57). Continual light may make some people more secure than others. They may feel that while the lights are on they are being watched. Artificial illumination may take the place of sunlight coming through the patient's window. In some critical care units, windows are not available for each room. The critically ill patient in such an environment is disoriented to time. Continual artificial illumination may have unwanted effects on the patient's biological systems. "Light, particularly in certain parts of the spectrum, may have potent effects upon metabolism and well-being. It is an important synchronizer of waking and sleep, and thus circadian cycles. Without the daily light alteration, as studies of the blind give witness, metabolic functions may become irregular" (Luce 1971, p. 274). The critical care nurse can encourage the dimming or elimination of nighttime lights. Naturally some patients need continual light. In the future it may be possible to devote special areas in open critical care units to continual artificial illimination of the patient. Furthermore, hospitals should provide clocks for each patient that indicate A.M. and P.M. If at all possible digital clocks would even be more helpful.

A second source of nonverbal stimulus that leads to sleep deprivation is noise. Noise comes from both human and mechanical sources. Human sources include doctors or nurses chattering in the distance and other patients moaning, groaning, or snoring. Environmental noises consist of squeaky doors, oxygen, ventilators, suction tubing, footsteps, other patients, and sudden crashes. Noises from mechanical or supportive devices can create sleep deprivation. The machines hum, buzz, click, or beep along as they perform their function. The supportive devices can have two effects on the critically ill patient. Their presence can reassure the patient that technology is monitoring his biological being, and the patient may feel secure when he hears the equipment humming along, but the stimulus created by various alarms, lights flashing, or clicks may annoy the patient who is trying to sleep. He may just drift into sleep and suddenly be awakened by the buzzing of his cardioscope or volume respirator. One patient who has minimal supportive devices may lie next to a patient who has several pieces of supportive devices. The noises emanating from another patient's environment create sleep deprivation.

Patients in critical care, especially intensive care, become aware of each other's problems. Quite frequently, a less critically ill patient will conduct his own observation surveillance of a neighbor. He listens to the volume respirator in the event the machine or patient would cease to function. The critical care nurse, aware of the situation, needs to reassure the individual that although his neighbor may have more supportive devices, he is progressing satisfactorily. Critical care patients may indirectly seek to support one another because they are in such great need of support themselves. Maybe such behavior tells something about a need to provide more active-overt support. The buzzes and beeps cannot be completely eliminated. The nurse may minimize stimulus input created from these devices by giving the patient earplugs. A patient wearing a hearing aid may be encouraged to remove it at night or at specific times during the day in order to decrease stimulus input and increase sleep. The critical care nurse may find time during the day when environmental activity is reduced, she can encourage uninterrupted sleep periods.

A third source of stimulus input involves gestures and facial expressions.

Critical care nurses often provide stimulus input from their nonverbal behavior by frowning, for example, as they regulate equipment. The patient may misinterpret his nurse's nonverbal behavior; because she frowns, he surmises that something must be wrong. If the nurse frowned at the patient's nasal-gastric tube, then he will probably monitor his own tube closely. Critical care patients identify the object of concern and make it their own concern. This was the case with Mrs. Q., who continually watched her own cardiac rhythm dart across the cardioscope. The nurse's nonverbal behavior may have nothing to do with the patient, but the patient, being hypersensitive to environmental cues, will personalize her behavior. Critical care nurses must be aware of their own behavior and the effect it has on others. An individual in biological and psychological crisis needs support and reassurance. If such an atmosphere is provided, he feels confident that a crisis will not occur while he sleeps.

The fourth and last source of nonverbal stimulus is touch. Touch appropriately used can be meaningful, but when used inappropriately it can lead to excess stimulus input. Many of the treatments and procedures done to critically ill patients involve touch. The nurse touches her patient when she takes his blood pressure and temperature, milks his chest tubes, changes his dressings, replaces his EKG leads, bathes him, and makes his bed. There are times when the patient's illness demands intensive surveillance, but at other times, when the patient's condition improves, the intensive surveillance unnecessarily continues. Although such a patient may have stabilized to the point of achieving sleep, the surveillance routine continues. It is possible that during the night, the nurse can depend on other means of assessing her patient. She can utilize the various supportive devices connected to her patient. If the patient's cardioscope patter and respiration are normal, and his urine output is adequate, then he need not be awakened for vital signs.

The critical care nurse's goal is to minimize extraneous stimulus input. She can attempt to reduce stimuli from unnecessary light, from noises emanating from people or machines, from anxiety-provoking facial expressions, and from excessive touch. The nurse turns off the maximum number of lights, keep meaningless noise at a maximum, refrains from unexplained frowning, and assesses the necessity of hourly monitoring the patient. She may not be able to eliminate their presence totally, but she can minimize the quantity of the stimulus input. In addition, the nurse can foster sleep through use of relaxation measures, exercises, and possibly daytime naps. While minimizing the stimulus input, she can help the patient to maintain a relatively normal sleep pattern in situations that require more sleep.

Maintaining Sleep Rhythm

The schedule of each individual's night sleep is somewhat consistent. The sleep pattern may, however. change with age or illness. In the hospital, the normal sleep pattern is altered by anxieties aroused from illness, pain associated with illness, and situational changes disrupting sleep. Each individual enters the critical care unit with his own unique sleep pattern and ritual. The nurse's goal can be to formulate individualized planning for adequate sleep periods. As Fass (1971) points out, "Individualized planning for rest periods and sleep can be as therapeutically important to a patient's health as the medication and treatments the physician has prescribed" (p. 2316).* According to Cohen (1979), the effects of aging on sleep appear to be in the reduction of REM and delta (stage IV) sleep. Also, there is reduction of the latency to the first REM period due to loss of stage IV. There are certain characteristics in the sleep of the aged. They consist of more awakenings; poorer quality of spinales, and relatively similar duration of REM periods across the night. In addition there are similar sleep characteristics between the aged and depressed patient. Both tend to have short REM onset latencies, smaller amounts of delta sleep, and shortened or fragmented sleep. Furthermore both may involve dissociation of biological cycles, disturbance of catecholamine functioning, and defects in short- rather than long-term memory.

The nurse can create a sleep-oriented environment. She can gradually prepare her patient for sleep by learning his presleep ritual. If the patient normally begins his preparation by taking a shower, the nurse can provide him with water so he can at least wash his face and hands. If this is biologically impossible, the nurse can assume the responsibility. He may then brush his teeth and get into his sleep clothes, helped by the nurse if necessary. The last presleep activity the nurse can undertake is to minimize extraneous noises and dim artificial lights. All the preparatory stages get the patient into a sleeping mood, which must be continued throughout the night in order to facilitate a constant sleep state.

The mood of sleep is most disturbed at night. At a time when the patient is most in need of rallying all defenses to combat severe illness for trauma, sleep interruption can turn into sleep deprivation and thus deny the patient the restorative benefits of sleep (Fabijan and Gosselin 1982). Not only does sleep disruption lead to sleep deprivation, it also alters the individual's tolerance for sedatives and pain tolerance. Flurazepam (Dalmane) temporarily improves sleep patterns in insomniacs. Slow-wave sleep can be markedly suppressed with flurazepam 30 mg, but stage IV sleep can be recovered within two weeks after discontinuation of the drug; the 30 mg dose can act as a moderate REM suppressant as do many hypnotics. However REM rebound may not be observed during two weeks of drug withdrawal (Wotring 1982). REM rebound can occur following an abrupt withdrawal of many of these drugs and may also occur during the night when the patient sleeps beyond the pharmacological action of the drug. To reduce the response, the drug can be gradually discontinued by reducing the dose every five or six days (Wotring 1982).

Hypnotics are expected to promote sleep at nighttime, but their effect

*Copyright, American Journal of Nursing Company, reprinted, with permission, from *American Journal of Nursing.*

should not persist beyond waking. The daytime residual effects may give rise to hangover and impaired performance. It should also be noted that REM sleep is suppressed by barbiturates and enhanced after discontinuation of these drugs (Borbely 1983).

Sleep deprivation can make the individual less tolerant of pain. As Long (1969) points out, "In a situation where the patient is awakened frequently throughout the night, as in the intensive care unit, the nurse can be alert to the signs of sleep restriction. Perhaps especially important is her awareness that the patient will have an increased sensitivity to pain if he has not had enough sleep" (p. 1898).* Sleep lessens the need for pain medication. Sleep and dreaming also enable the individual time to reinforce his character structure.

Depending upon the severity of his illness, the patient may need more than his normal amount of sleep to integrate various changes into his new personality structure. The critical care nurse can listen to the patient's fears. The burn patient fears physical disfigurement and his altered body image. His dreams may become nightmares. He needs to have a supportive ear ready to listen to his fears and anxieties. Even when given the opportunity to talk about his nightmares, the patient may create his own sleep deprivation by refusing to discuss them. A patient may be afraid to sleep because he fears the reality of his dreams or he fears that a crisis will occur while he sleeps. In this way the individual himself can create deprivation.

NURSING EVALUATION

Evaluation of the patient's problem and nursing care is an ongoing process. The nurse assesses regulatory and cognitive behaviors supporting the diagnosis of sleep deprivation. Interventions designed to minimize sleep deprivation are evaluated for their effectiveness. Effectiveness is measured by the control, reduction, or elimination of sleep-disturbance behaviors after the patient has been permitted uninterrupted sleep. The cognitive behaviors may not totally disappear until the patient is removed from critical care.

The nurse evaluates how hospitalization interferes with usual sleep habits. Nurses are in a position to positively aid in restoration of healthy relationships by individualizing hospital routines and planning therapeutic nursing interventions (Leddy 1977).

SUMMARY

Sleep is something every critical care patient needs. It sometimes receives low priority, but as we learn about sleeping, dreaming, and waking, sleep will become a high-priority need. Sleep is necessary if the patient is to destruc-

*Copyright, American Journal of Nursing Company. Reprinted, with permission, from *American Journal of Nursing.*

turalize the stored data compiled from various environmental stimulus inputs. Too much stimulus input and too little time to destructuralize may only serve to confuse the patient. He also needs sleep to reinforce his threatened or changed character structure. It may be the process of dreaming that allows forbidden thoughts to enter the patient's consciousness. The patient retreats into the world of sleep to recharge his depleted battery and becomes ready for the next day's events. The critical care nurse can intervene to minimize meaningless stimulus input and to maintain a relatively normal sleep rhythm. It is not the quantity of sleep that is important; minisleep can have a beneficial effect. Sleep is a composite of various rhythms that travel through many levels of altered consciousness. The critical care patient who is deprived of this experience for a length of time becomes behaviorally disoriented, irritable, hostile, or fatigued. Such behavioral reactions commonly serve to threaten further the individual's already-threatened biological and psychological integrity.

REFERENCES

BURDICK, J. A., G. BRINGTON, L. GOLDSTEIN, and M. LASZIO, "Heart-Rate Variability in Sleep and Wakefulness," *Cardiology*, 55 (1970), 79-83.

BORBELY, ALEXANDER, "Pharmacological Approaches to Sleep Regulation," in *Sleep Mechanism and Functions*, ed. Andrew Mayes, pp. 232-261. Cambridge, Mass.: Van Nostrand Reinhold, 1983.

COHEN, DAVID, *Sleep and Dreaming: Origins, Nature and Functions.* New York: Pergamon Press, 1979.

DOHNO, SATOSHI, JAMES LYNCH, DAVID PASKEWITZ, KENNETH GIMBEL, and SUE THOMAS, "Sleepwalking Changes in Cardiac Arrhythmia in a Coronary Care Patient," *Psychosomatic Medicine*, 39, no. 1 (January-February 1977), 39-43.

DOHNO, SATOSHI, DAVID PASKEWITZ, JAMES LYNCH, KENNETH GIMBEL, and SUE THOMAS, "Some Aspects of Sleep Disturbance in Coronary Patients," *Perceptual and Motor Skills*, 48 (1979), 199-205.

ELLIS, B. W., and H. DUDLEY, "Some Aspects of Sleep Research in Surgical Stress," *Journal of Psychosomatic Research*, 20 (1976), 303-308.

FABIJAN, LUVA, and MARIE GOSSELIN, "How to Recognize Sleep Deprivation in Your ICU Patient and What to Do about It," *The Canadian Nurse*, April 1982, pp. 21-23.

FASS, GRACE, "Sleep, Drugs and Dreams," *American Journal of Nursing*, 71, no. 2 (December 1971), 2317.

FOULKES, DAVID, *The Psychology of Sleep.* New York: Scribner's, 1966.

GAARDER, KENNETH, "A Conceptual Model of Sleep," *Archives of General Psychiatry*, 14 (March 1966), 253-54.

GRANT, DONNA and CYNTHIA KLELL, "For Goodness Sake—Let Your Patients Sleep," *Nursing '74*, October 1974, pp. 55-57.

GREENBERG, ROMAN, "Dreams and REM Sleep—An Integrative Approach," in *Sleep, Dreams and Memory*, ed. William Fishbein, pp. 125-133. New York: S P Medical and Scientific Books, 1981.

HARTMANN, ERNEST, "The Functions of Sleep and Memory Processing," in *Sleep, Dreams and Memory*, ed. William Fishbein, pp. 111-124. New York: S P Medical and Scientific Books, 1981.

HAYTER, JEAN, "The Rhythm of Sleep," *American Journal of Nursing*, March 1980, pp. 457-461.

HELTON, MARY, SUSAN GORDAN, and SUSAN NUNNERY, "The Correlation between Sleep Deprivation and the Intensive Care Unit Syndrome," *Heart and Lung*, 9, no. 2 (May-June 1980), 464-468.

HILTON, ANN, "Quantity and Quality of Patient's Sleep and Sleep-Disturbing Factors in a Respiratory Intensive Care Unit," *Journal of Advanced Nursing*, I (1976), 453-468.

HORNE, J. A., "Mammalian Sleep Function with Parheular Reference to Man," in *Sleep Mechanism and Function*, ed. Andrew Mayes, pp. 262-312. Cambridge, Mass.: Van Nostrand Reinhold, 1983.

HUME, KENNETH, "The Rhythmical Nature of Sleep," in *Sleep Mechanisms and Functions*, ed. Andrew Mayes, pp. 18-56. Cambridge, Mass.: Van Nostrand Reinhold, 1983.

KLELL, GRANT, *Nursing 1974*, November 1974, 56-57.

LEDDY, SUSAN, "Sleep and Phase Shifting of Biological Rhythms," *International Journal of Nursing Studies*, 14 (1977), 137-150.

LEWIS, ISAAC, and HANANIA GLAUBMAN, "The Effect of REM Deprivation: Is It Detrimental, Beneficial or Neutral? *The Society for Psychophysiological Research*, 2, no. 3 (1975), 349-353.

LONG, BARBARA, "Sleep," *American Journal of Nursing*, 69, no. 9 (September 1969), 1896.

LUCE, GAER GAY, *Body Time*. New York: Pantheon, 1971.

LUBY, ELLIOT, "Sleep Deprivation: Effects on Behavior, Thinking, Motor Performance and Biological Energy Transfer Systems," *Psychosomatic Medicine*, 22 (1969), 406-419.

LUKAS, JEROME, "Noise and Sleep: A Literature Review and a Prepared Criterion for Assessing Effect," *Journal Acoustical Society of America*, 58, no. 6 (December 1975), 1232-1241.

McFADDEN, EILEEN, and ELIZABETH GIBLIN, "Sleep Deprivation in Patients Having Open-Heart Surgery," *Nursing Research*, 20, no. 3 (May-June 1971), 249-253.

MILNE, BARBARA, "Sleep-Wake Disorders and What We Do about Them," *The Cardiac Nurse*, April 1982, pp. 24-26.

MORRIS, GRAY, Misperception and Disorientation during Sleep Deprivation," *Archives of General Psychiatry*, 2 (March 1960), 247-254.

MOSES, J. M.; L. C. JOHNSON, and A. LUBIN, "Sleep Stage Deprivation and Total Sleep Loss: Effects on Sleep Behavior," *The Society for Psychophysiological Research*, 2, no. 2 (1975), 141-146.

OSWALD, JAN, *Sleeping and Waking*. New York: Elsevier Division, ASP Biological and Medical Press, 1962.

——, *Sleep*. Baltimore: Penguin Books, 1968.

ROSENBLATT, GERALD, ERNEST HARTMANN, and GEORGE ZWILLING, "Cardiac Irritability during Sleep and Dreaming," *Journal of Psychosomatic Research*, 17 (1973), 129-134.

ROY, SISTER CALLISTA, and SHARON ROBERTS, *Theory Construction in Nursing: An Adaptation Model*. Englewood Cliffs, N.J.: Prentice-Hall, Inc., 1981.

SEBILIA, ALBERT, "Sleep Deprivation and Biological Rhythms in the Critical Care Unit," *Critical Care Nursing*, May-June 1981, pp. 19-23.

SEGAL, JULIUS, "To Sleep: Perchance to Dream," *Today's Health*, 47, no. 10 (October 1969), 48-50, 54, 86-87.

SMITH, RICHARD, LAVERNE JOHNSON, DONALD ROTHFIELD, LEONARD ZIR, and BARRY THARP, "Sleep and Cardiac Arrhythmias," *Archives of Internal Medicine*, 130 (November 1972), 751-753.

WEBB, WILSE, "Theories of Sleep Functions and Some Clinical Implications," in *Function of Sleep*, ed. René Drucker-Colon, Mario Shkurovich, and M. B. Sterman, pp. 19-35. New York: Academic Press, 1979.

———, "Theories in Modern Sleep Research," in *Sleep Mechanism and Functions*, ed. Andrew Mayes, pp. 1-17. Cambridge, Mass.: Van Nostrand Reinhold, 1983.

WILLIAMS, ROBERT, and DANIEL JACKSON, "Problems with Sleep," *Heart and Lung*, 11, no. 3 (May-June 1982), 262-267.

WOTRING, KATHLEEN, "Using Research in Practice," *Focus*, October-November 1982, pp. 34-36.

ZELECHOWSKI, GINA, "Sleep and the Critically Ill Patient," *Critical Care Update*, February 1979, pp. 5-13.

3

Hopelessness

BEHAVIORAL OBJECTIVES

1. Define the terms, *hope, helplessness,* and *hopelessness.*
2. Identify the possible threats to the patient's internal resources.
3. Identify the factors that can affect the patient's perception of his external resources.
4. State three regulatory behaviors associated with hopelessness.
5. State five cognitive behaviors associated with hopelessness.
6. Design a nursing care plan that fosters hopefulness.

An individual's most valued, private, and strongest resource is hope. Hope is an intrinsic component of life. It provides dynamism for the spirit thereby saving people from apathetic inaction (Miller 1983). Although we, as human beings, need hope in our lives, very little has been written about the concept. Every day the hopeless in life bombards our senses in news reports, in the books we read, in the movies we see, and in the daily invasion of our homes by television. Pleasant or positive news does not rate much coverage. The mass media seem less interested in reporting how a child's life was saved or how the families experiencing a natural disaster supported one another, because these events do not sell newspapers.

"Good news" stories often provide a source of hope to others, and the idea that hope has sources implies that it is an attribute of some open system, which depends upon input, which consumes what it takes in, and which generates activity while doing so. Hope is a mental state that has something to do with the maintenance of cyclical processes involving intake and feedback. Hope refers to some general characteristic of living organisms which they continue to possess as long as they live and without which they cease to do so (Rycroft 1979).

In fact, one of the most remarkable characteristics of human beings is that no matter how hopeless things may be, they still maintain an element of internal hope. This is probably the motivating force that enables prisoners of war and their families to survive during their separation from one another. Each has hope that the other exists. The prisoners have hope that the war will end and that they will be returned to their families. Each family has hope that their loved one is still alive. In spite of the great physical separation and the dismal condition of prisoner camps, hope still prevails. But hope cannot be achieved alone. Hope must be an act of the community, an organization, or two people struggling together. People develop hope in each other, hope that they will receive help from the other.

Not only is it related to other persons, but hope relates to things outside of us in a futuristic way. Hope is an attitude toward the future. It is a feeling that consists of two components: we desire something we do not yet have and we desire something we believe we could or may gain. Hope occupies a key position between the present and the future. Hope is therefore a present attitude towards a future known to be intrinsically contingent and uncertain (Rycroft 1979).

While a person has hope, he also wishes. He hopes for a response; this may involve wishing. The two go hand in hand. If we do not wish for something, of no matter what significance, then we have no hope in the thing we want. We are then playing games with ourselves, and at times we become apathetic about achieving the thing we originally hoped for. This is particularly true of mental illness. More has been written about mental illness and its relationship to hopelessness than any other illness, except perhaps for the hopeless feelings of a patient's experiences while dying. Death and dying have gained prominence in nursing literature throughout the last decade. Kübler-Ross (1971) noted in her studies of dying patients that hope was the only thing that persisted throughout the stages of dying. Hope provided these people with strength at a time when they desperately needed it. Nursing can look at other patient groups and take note of the void regarding explanation of their feelings of hopelessness.

The patient's degree of hopelessness can be better understood by determining the patient's perceived sense of powerlessness, duration of powerlessness, and the severity of losses suffered (Miller 1983). Unfortunately little has been written about the hopeless and helpless feelings of the patient in a critical care unit. Needless to say, when his body becomes ill, he experiences the frustration of hopelessness and helplessness. Both frustrations do not necessarily go hand in hand; they can occur separately. The critically ill patient can feel helpless about his illness, but he may not lose hope in his body's ability to restore itself. There are times, however, when the critically ill patient does feel helpless because his physical condition may seem so very hopeless. It then becomes the critical care nurse's role to foster a realistic sense of hopefullness. She can try to make her patient responsible for his own care.

It is ironic that even with modern technology our bodies still become sick. The only saving factor is that technology allows us to live longer. We now face a dilemma: with all our technology, will we increasingly prolong death rather than life? Regardless of the outcome, human beings have hope because they know science has progressed and is progressing to unmeasurable limits. They realize that humans can accomplish virtually anything they choose. If this is true, then why does the patient still experience hopelessness? What causes his feeling of hopelessness? These are a few of the issues that should be examined from the viewpoint of the critically ill patient.

DEFINITION OF TERMS

The greatest hope of all individuals is that there is nothing wrong, physiologically, with them. This becomes the individual's hope, and he might suffocate from it if he builds too high a psychological wall between the well and the ill. The more people push illness out of their minds, the greater the distance to hope. The individual subjects himself to his own sense of hopelessness. Hope is a sense of the possible, and hopelessness means to be ruled by a sense of the impossible.

Hope

The purpose of hope is to ward off feelings of despair. Despair leads to disorganization, helplessness, and hopelessness. Hope, on the other hand, is an essential concomitant of life and growth. Hope is made up of affective and cognitive components. Both occur in varying patterns and degrees to maintain psychological equilibrium. The affective components signify the emotional element of hope, namely, faith, trust, confidence in self and others, and fortitude. These emotional elements are behaviorally manifested as determination, motivation, inspiration, and encouragement. The cognitive component of hope is the way in individual perceives and processes reality. It is made up of selected information that will support the desired hope (Lange 1978).

Lynch (1965) defines hope as the fundamental knowledge and feeling that there is a way out of difficulty, that things can work out, that we as humans can somehow handle and manage internal and external reality, that there are solutions in the most ordinary biological and psychological senses of that word, that, above all, there are ways out of illness. Hope gives the individual a sense of security in the knowledge that there are solutions to problems. It may seem to the patient that the solutions are a long time in coming, but the individual with hope feels that a solution is possible. His doctors may be deciding which drug would be of greatest benefit in treating his illness, and many patients trust that their physicians will pick the best one. If the individual did not feel this way about himself and others, he would have nothing. He would have no energy. Wishing and hoping generate energy. Energy creates within the individual a desire or motivation to achieve a goal. The goal for a critically ill patient may be simple (e.g., to dangle for the first time) or more complex (e.g., to ambulate). Regardless, the individual has hope that he will accomplish the goal. Without energy the patient has no sense of motivation. He is dominated by his feelings of the impossible. He has no direction. "Hope, therefore, is energized by belief in the possibility of getting somewhere, in the possibility of reaching goals. The somewhere, the goals, can be as many as the wishes and things we propose to ourselves" (Lynch 1965, p. 34).

According to Schneider (1980) hope is not normally present in an individual's conscious awareness. Instead it is as an underlying sensation and belief that hope functions as a foundation for dealing with the process of living. Hope is a requirement for an evolving life under normal circumstances. Therefore during periods of crisis such as illness, hope becomes essential for one's biological and psychological existence.

Each of us moves into the future as long as we have hope. This means that we would not brush our teeth after eating unless we had hope of avoiding tooth decay. Apparently hope is something halfway between knowing and willing, for none of us can know the future or know what will happen if we do not participate in that future. We know from past experience that brushing our teeth limits tooth decay. Our action rests upon our knowledge of the past. Hope is opposed to despair. The individual who despairs essentially gives up. He separates himself from his selfness and from his peers.

The individual who hopes can transcend a difficult situation. He has the inner strength to overcome the difficulty, thus liberating himself from the darkness. His sense of hope is that there is a way out. On the other hand, the individual who has a sense of hopelessness believes there is no way out. According to Lynch (1965), "Hope is truly on the inside of us, but hope is an interior sense that there is help on the outside of us. . . . The act of taking help from the outside is an inward act, an inward appropriation, which in no way depersonalizes the taker or makes him feel less a man" (p. 31–32). Hope and help are closely related. There are times when we realize that our own internal resources are not sufficient to handle or cope with the situation. These strengths must be added to from the outside. This need of help is a continuing fact for every human being. Many difficulties make us increasingly more aware of it.

Therefore hope becomes a basic need to all individuals. Hope implies a desire and trust in the future. Without hope, the patient and his family will be unable to cope with the current illness, injury, or disease.

Helplessness

The term *helplessness* refers to a complex syndrome of emotions, thoughts, and behavior. Helplessness occurs in situations such as illness where events are uncontrollable. It is the sense of being overwhelmed by the loss of control over the outside world. The syndrome of helplessness may occur at any time during life that an individual experiences a threatened loss of something or someone who is a source of direct gratification. For many critically ill patients the experience of illness and treatment bring about feelings of helplessness (Lange 1978).

Each of us has experienced a moment when we had a helpless feeling. There may have been a time when we have watched a child run, trip, and fall. Maybe we were only an arm's length away but were helpless to break her fall. When an individual becomes sick, he feels helpless. His body has lost control and can no longer rely on its own physiological adaptation or homeostatic mechanisms. The body needs external help. Nurses also experience helpless feelings, especially when they watch a patient die and realize that they have done everything possible to make the patient comfortable.

Lange (1978) has proposed a theory of learned helplessness resulting from situations in which the outcome is independent of the individual's responses. The result is a reduction of motivation to try to control the outcome; interference with new learning or alternate responses that might control the outcome; and feelings of anxiety as long as the controllability is uncertain and feelings of depression when the events are predictable but still not controllable.

Schneider (1980) points out that helplessness is being in a situation in which responses occur not as a result of actions by the person in the situation, but appear to be uncontrollable from his perception. Helplessness involves the mental state of a person when he blames his failures and frustrations on the environment where he looks for a solution. An ill person realizes that he is unable to help himself. He finds himself confronted, at a critical moment, with a medical problem that cries out for help. Although he may be able to help himself, serious illness or injury obliges him to seek external help. Sometimes individuals feel both a sense of helplessness and hopelessness; the individual accepts the fact that the disease process is progressive and irreversible and that all efforts to intervene are of no use to either the people in the helping relationship or to the patient. Hopelessness, more so than helplessness, is one of the most difficult areas in which the critical care nurse works, for she must try to feel hopeful, no matter how grave the situation.

Hopelessness

According to Siomopoulos and Inamdar (1979), a hopeful existence entails a positive feeling state, and a dimension of future time involving two factors: a projection of the past into the future or a restructuring of a potential future. Hopelessness becomes then an all-pervasive affect state with an unpleasant quality.

Hopelessness is always entering our lives. It can be used in either a creative and positive way or negative way. If allowed to take control, it is capable of immobilizing the individual. Feelings of hopelessness become manifest at certain times in our lives. At these times, we learn about ourselves and try to channel hopelessness toward a positive outcome. If not channeled in a positive manner, hopelessness can block any effort to change a situation constructively.

Schneider (1980) notes that hopelessness is an emotional state implying a sense of impossibility with the feeling that life is too much to handle. Hopelessness therefore is an individual's state when he is unable to cope and feels that no change in the immediate environment is possible. According to Lynch (1965), "Hopelessness is rooted in structures of thought, feeling, and action that are rigid and inflexible. They are absolutized and repetitious structures that have become so many traps. If, therefore, one of the central qualities of the hopeless is the feeling of entrapment, a central quality of hope is freedom" (p. 63). Hopelessness involves a number of powerful human feelings. It arouses a sense of the impossible: what a person wants to do or accomplish is beyond his reach. He comes to a wall that he cannot climb. The individual may also experience the feeling of futility. He senses that there is no goal, no reason, and he therefore has no hope or wish. Hope allows the individual to imagine a future. Hopelessness, on the other hand, lacks this central vision, or image, of what could be.

Lange (1978) defines hopelessness as a state of acute or prolonged desperation that signifies the feeling of being beyond hope. It reflects the sense of overwhelming defeat or loss of control over one's self. The person feels unworthy of help and may refuse it when offered.

According to Lynch (1965),

> Hopelessness does not imagine and it does not wish. Hope does, but hopelessness does not. It is characteristic of the latter that it does not have the energy for either imagining or wishing. It is deeply passive, not in any of the good senses of the word, but in its most unhappy sense. Its only fundamental wish is the wish to give up. In particular situations it cannot imagine anything that can be done or that is worth doing. It does not imagine beyond the limits of what is presently happening. (P. 50).

It has been proposed that an individual's hopelessness can be objectified by defining it in terms of a system of negative expectancies concerning himself and his future life (Lester and Trexler 1974).

There are times in life when everything seems to collapse on us at once. For example, the water heater breaks and floods the house, ruining a newly laid carpet. Next the dishwasher and stove break at the same time. Finally one car is accidently driven into the side of the garage while the fan belt on the other car breaks. At this point, the victim will say, "I feel like just giving up," or "What's the use, nothing seems to go right anymore." Most persons have enough inner strength to handle each crisis even if they occur simultaneously. They maintain a sense of hopefulness that the storm will pass. The hopeless individual not only feels like "giving up," but he actually does. He decides that, even if he has resources and even if help is available, there is no use, no good, no sense in action or in life. The feeling of hopefulness is a major concern of the critical care nurse. She needs to foster hopefulness, but before doing this she must be aware of how the patient comes to feel hopelessness in the first instance.

THE CONCEPT OF HOPELESSNESS APPLIED
TO THE CRITICALLY ILL PATIENT

Persons respond to stimuli from many sources: emotions, physiological state, attitudes, beliefs, perceptions of others, and environment. Illness itself can be a stimulus. The factors influencing the patient's hopelessness fall into two categories. First, there are factors threatening the internal resources of the patient: his illness and his ability to cope accordingly. Next are his perceptions of the external resources such as the environment and persons within that environment who can help him.

Threats to the Patient's
Internal Resources

Threats to the patient's internal resources involve threats to his sense of autonomy, self-esteem, independence, strength, and integrity. The patient may feel an internal hopelessness if his ability to function is impaired, if the goal of his existence is frustrated, or if those he loves are separated from him. The individual may despair when his function is impaired or lost. He may feel that he will never be whole again. He fears that he will be forced to give up those things vital to his internal being. He loses hope in himself and in his own internal resources. Normally the patient who hopes refuses to give up before the inevitable. He accepts the situation, he realizes his inability to rise above and beyond it by his own will, but he knows that assistance will be coming and that he will be helped according to his own hope.

Schneider (1980) points out that an individual is helpless when an outcome occurs independent of his voluntary responses. This occurs when he experiences response independence. In learned helplessness, the person has learned that he is helpless. On the locus of control scale, individuals who are externally oriented learn helplessness much more readily than do internal oriented individuals.

The patient who despairs will submit to the imminent loss of his integrity and being. For example, a CCU patient who enters the unit for the second time in one year may give up completely. This admission is more severe, and his physician tells him he has had another myocardial infarction superimposed on his old infarction. Shortly after his admission, the patient begins to show signs of congestive heart failure and arrhythmias. The patient begins to despair because this time "things seem worse." He has hope because he lived through the previous experience, but he knows his condition is critical. In time he develops complete heart block, and his doctor implants a temporary pacemaker. As other complications develop, the patient may lose his sense of hope and submit to hopelessness.

Another example of hopelessness involves a patient who had no previous experience with surgery. This man in ICU had intense pain in his legs, especially when he was active. His pain increased in intensity over a period of several weeks. He also complained of color and temperature changes in both his legs. Always active, he had never been ill before, nor had he experienced surgery. His doctors diagnosed the problem as an abdominal aortic aneurysm with intermittent claudication and agreed that they should perform an aneurysm resection with a dacron graft replacement. The patient consented to this relatively simple surgical intervention. Since this was the patient's first experience with a surgical procedure, he did not know what to expect. The word *surgery* conjured up negative internal feelings. He saw it as his last chance before death. As a result, he despaired at the thought of an operation and submitted to hopelessness.

The burn patient who has second- and third-degree burns over 50 percent of his body will obviously despair. He feels a tremendous loss. He realizes that even with the most successful grafts, he will never be the same again. He fails to realize that even though he may not be the same in the future, he might become something more than he was in the past. He needs this hope. Naturally the despair overshadows all other feelings, and as time passes from days to weeks, he will feel a sense of hopelessness.

Like the burn patient, the hemodialysis patient and the isolation patient also experience despair. Their despair is related to both loss and time. Burn patients and hemodialysis patients have lost a vital part of themselves, but grafts restore the skin and hemodialysis aids renal function. In time they can attain a sense of hopefulness. But to all three patients, time is their biggest enemy. The isolation patient experiences the time-oriented days waiting for his culture to return negative. The hemodialysis patient's time revolves around the days he is on the dialysis machine and the length of time his dialysis exchange takes. The burn patient must wait for the grafting process to heal.

Lange (1978) notes that when the patient experiences loss of hope, it can have a deleterious effect leading to giving-up behavior. Giving-up behavior can further contribute to physical and psychological disequilibrium. It should be noted that hopelessness and helplessness may occur together indicating an actual, threatened, or unresolved loss for which nothing can be done. An acute biological injury or illness represents a threatening experience to the patient's internal resources and the family. In many instances, the critically ill patient requires dramatic nursing care.

Regardless of the patient's reasons for being in a critical care unit, there is a time when his own internal resources become threatened or even totally drained. It is during this traumatic time of realizing his own emptiness and seeking external help that the patient may experience his most overwhelming period of hopelessness. Illness may evoke within the critically ill patient a lifelong dread of the vulnerability of his body. He may feel his wholeness destroyed. His body is in essence quite vulnerable and helpless. Naturally the patient despairs when he realizes the vulnerability of his own body. But if he submits to desperation, he loses an important internal resource, his motivation.

Motivation plays a significant role in the recovery process. According to Stotland (1969), "Motivation is a positive function of the perceived probability of goal attainment and of the importance of the goal. Motivation is indicated by the organism's acting, either overtly or cognitively, toward the attainment of goals. These actions include attending to and thinking about those aspects of the environment that are perceived as relevant to goal attainment" (p. 14). Learned helplessness can have an effect upon motivation and cognitive functions. The individual's motivation to initiate responses to control other events become decreased. Furthermore the cognitive function involved in learning that a response has succeeded in producing the desired outcome may also be impaired (Schneider 1980).

The patient's goal is a major determinant of his motivation. He must believe that his actions will bring about a result. His goal may be good health, although he is realistic enough to know that due to his particular illness, he can never be restored to the same previous level of wellness. Nevertheless he makes this his goal. The patient might be highly motivated to achieve a goal with low expectation of actually achieving it. The goal still has great significance to him. As long as his illness remains essentially stable, the patient continues to be motivated. The hope for goal attainment becomes his internal resource. With each positive day or test result, his goal becomes increasingly more realistic. The patient is more receptive to things within his environment that will facilitate attainment of the goal. He may become preoccupied with how to obtain his goal. There are, however, other patients who do not have this same internal positive motivation. Their illness pushes them into the darkened world of hopelessness. Hopelessness in critical care units becomes most apparent in patients with multiproblems, those who are burned, or those who have an infection superimposed on a loss.

Mr. T., a 55-year-old man, is an example of a multiproblem patient. He had been relatively healthy until a few weeks prior to his hospitalization, when he complained of pruritis, discomfort after eating, and stool color changes. A gallbladder series revealed cholelithiasis and the need for a cholecystectomy. Mr. T. did very well before and during surgery. After his operation, he developed an episode of hypotension. The episode lasted for one hour and was attributed to his anesthetic agent. His blood pressure was maintained by means of a vasopressor. After two hours, the medication was stopped. To ensure his well-being, he was transferred to ICU. His vital signs remained within the normal range. Within the next 48 hours, Mr. T.'s urinary output decreased. Diuretics did not seem to alter the situation. Several times Mr. T. asked his doctors and nurses what was wrong, and several times he received the answer, "Nothing serious; things will improve." The other answers were too technical for his comprehension. The doctor decided that the problem might be attributed to volume deficit. He also noted that Mr. T.'s hemoglobin and hematocrit were low. Two units of blood were ordered to be given simultaneously over a two-hour period. After one hour, the nurse noted that Mr. T. had marked chest sounds, diaphoresis, shortness of breath, hypotension, and slight cyanosis. The diagnosis of congestive heart failure with impending pulmonary edema was made. Rotating tourniquets, diuretics, and IPPB were initiated. Throughout the episode, Mr. T. remained alert and aware of what was happening. Even though he was aware of the seriousness of his condition he remained quiet. Everyone around him focused on his immediate crisis to the exclusion of his questions. Naturally the crisis was of top priority; even as the crisis subsided, he was told to rest and not to talk. Mr. T. followed orders and closed his eyes.

Over the next two days, Mr. T.'s condition rapidly deteriorated. His BUN and creatinine levels increased. His doctors decided to begin peritoneal dialysis in order to assist his failing kidneys and reduce his hypervolemia. Meanwhile Mr. T. became jaundiced. Doctors thought that his jaundice was due to hepatomegaly caused by CHF. Furthermore he developed arrhythmias, multifocal premature ventricular contractions, and atrial fibrillation. The diagnosis on Mr. T.'s card index were cholecystectomy, acute tubular necrosis, CHF, pulmonary edema, hepatomegaly, and arrhythmias. The peritoneal dialysis had very little success. The only alternative remaining was hemodialysis. Mr. T. was less alert, and he seemed to spend most of his time sleeping. The nurses believed the situation to be hopeless. Everything attempted seemed to fail. They realized that his prognosis was poor, and it seemed to become increasingly more so each day. One day as his nurse was working around his bed, Mr. T. began to talk with her. Usually his conversations were only one word or one sentence. This time it was different.

MR. T.: Nurse, why are they doing these things to me?
NURSE: What things, Mr. T.?
MR. T.: You know. All these tubes and procedures. They really don't know what they are doing, do they? It is all just guesswork.
NURSE: Who are "they"?
MR. T.: My doctors, of course. What's the use. We know I'll never pull through this.
NURSE: What do you mean?
MR. T.: I know I am going to die. Why don't they. . . . (*He then shuts his eyes and turns his head away from the nurse.*)
NURSE: (*Leaves the patient's bed.*)

Within the next 48 hours, Mr. T.'s condition became more critical. Without warning he had a respiratory arrest necessitating a tracheostomy and volume respirator. While his intermittent suction bottle clicked, his volume respirator sighed, and the hemodialysis machine hummed, Mr. T. lapsed into the noncommunicative world of the unconscious.

Initially Mr. T. had hoped that his original symptoms would be rectified through surgical intervention. He realized that with any surgery there is always the possibility of complications. He did not perceive them to be a threat to his being. Besides, complications happened to other people. He maintained the hope that shortly after surgery he would awake, maybe in pain, but that his problems would be over. This was the goal that motivated him. Instead, he awakened to find himself not in the quiet environment of the recovery room but in the somewhat noisy and busy ICU. Further groggy investigation revealed that he had developed a postoperative complication— one that "occurs in some patients" and one that "can be reversed." Therefore, even with the knowledge of a complication, he was assured that it was reversible. This assumption enabled him to maintain his hope and his motivation. His goal was still in sight; it was just further away.

Up to this point, it never occurred to Mr. T. that the goal might not be attained. As the complications continued, his motivation began to falter. He began to lose hope in himself. His internal resources were suddenly threatened; consequently, he mobilized his energy toward defending his resources rather than toward motivation. When Mr. T. looked around him, he sensed the impossibility and futility of hoping to be whole again. His perceptions of the staff were reflected in his comment, "We know I'll never pull through this." He was simply validating the hopeless expressions he had come to see around him. Finally, as his body tried desperately to adapt to each physiological complication, he lapsed into unconsciousness. He lost the hope of ever getting well and submitted to the monster despair.

At a time when the critically ill patient's sense of biological security is threatened, he becomes sensitive to events in his environmental surroundings. If additional mechanical devices enter his immediate environment, he immediately feels that his condition has become more critical. At the same time, he learns to assess his nurse's nonverbal expression for feedback regarding his progress. The patient may see and hear his nurse talking with another patient about his transfer out of critical care and ultimately his transfer home, but her discussions with him focus on the here and now. Consequently, the patient begins to assume that he no longer has a future. If he cannot hope in a future, he may find little security hoping in the present. What we learn from Mr. T.'s experience is that nurses should be extremely careful of their nonverbal and verbal expressions in order not to create a hopeless environment.

Another patient, Mr. C., was admitted to a burn unit with second- and third-degree burns over 40 percent of his body. The burns were on his chest, arms, hands, and upper thighs. He was 30 years old and single. He had sustained the burns when he fell asleep while smoking a cigar in bed. Mr. C. had the usual admission procedures: assessment and treatment of his burns, laboratory work, and cultures. His burns made Mr. C. virtually dependent upon his nurse for everything. Every day he was taken to the Hubbard tank, where his nurse cleaned, treated, and dressed his burns. Each day he asked his nurse, "How much longer will I be this way?" Burn patients sometimes show evidence of marked concern over their injuries during the acute phase. Mr. C.'s nurse tried to reassure him that he was "progressing adequately." She realized that "hope is important for the burned patients who escaped from fires but were burned. The recovery mechanism in these cases may be broadly defined as mobilization of hope of recovering, followed by the restoration of interpersonal relationships and self-esteem, including transaction from enforced passivity to constructive activity" (Stotland 1969, p. 5).

According to Lange (1981), individuals strive to cope with the impact of serious illness in a variety of ways. When the critical care nurse has knowledge regarding stressors affecting the patient or family's ability to cope, she is better able to support, maintain, or restore hope. The critically ill patient may deny or minimize the seriousness of the biological crisis. In so doing, the patient maintains hope by not facing the crisis. It provides time for other coping mechanisms or styles to be developed. Another coping style is to seek information that will relieve anxiety contributing to a threat to the patient's internal resources. Providing information about treatments and risk factors decreases helplessness. The feeling of helplessness is decreased because the patient has a time dimension whereby specific treatments and/or emotions can be anticipated.

The nurse can try to foster hope in her patient. Another source of hope are the patients around Mr. C. He sees other patients in the unit who have similar burns. Each one is in a different stage of recovery. He tries to maintain his internal sense of hope that as they progress, so will he. As the days progressed, Mr. C. became increasingly more concerned about the future. Prior to the injury, his future consisted of his job as a mechanic and his other life goals. As a mechanic, he realized, his hands were extremely important to him. He saw his burns as ruining his future. He feared that his current girl friend would be repulsed by his burns. He further despaired that he would never again work as a mechanic. He felt several losses: his sex appeal, his job, and his self-esteem. With burn patients the realistic problems regarding the effect of their injury on future plans often merge imperceptibly into the patient's personal interpretation of his injury. This was the case with Mr. C.

Mr. C. had been in the burn unit for three weeks. During the next few days, he seemed to become less active verbally and more depressed. He refused to eat and resisted turning or going to his daily therapy. When his nurse insisted upon his participation, he became angry. He finally screamed at his nurse, "I am sick of everyone telling me what to do. I am tired of having people wait on me. Just leave me alone. I am not getting anywhere anyway!" To the patient, dependency had become a problem. If the burn patient has previously had some unresolved conflicts in regard to dependent relationships, it becomes apparent in the initial treatment period. The entire situation may be difficult to accept. The patient may not understand the unavoidable dependency the burns require.

Despite the fact that Mr. C. was free of complications, he still felt hopelessness. As previously mentioned, time becomes the burn patient's enemy. The burn patient has difficulty seeing the subtle changes in his burns. This is part of the recovery phase in which time literally stands still. It is no wonder that burn patients become depressed, angry, or hostile. Mr. C.'s goals were women and work. Now he felt these goals were beyond his reach. This fear caused him to reject the individual who became his external source of motivation, his nurse.

It is not unusual for the burn patient to experience feelings of resentment. The resentment may narrow the patient's perception of others including the care received. It is possible he may not appreciate his care because he does not feel appreciated. Like the patient with multiproblems, the burn patient can become hopeless about his internal strengths and the recovery process. Hopelessness for the burn patient centers primarily around the illness or injury and its effects upon his future goals.

Mrs. G. experienced organ loss. A 40-year-old mother of three, she had a history of severe renal disease. For several months, Mrs. G. had noted frequent and intense headaches, energy loss, weight gain, and blurred vision. She avoided going to the hospital because of her family. She felt that she had caused her husband to be away from work too frequently. Because of their financial instability due to her frequent hospitalizations, she feared that he might lose his job. She felt guilty about leaving her three daughters, who ranged from age 14 to 16. Regardless of her reasons, Mr. G. insisted that she be hospitalized for diagnostic work. Neither realized the seriousness of the situation. Diagnostic work revealed that Mrs. G. was in renal failure. Her doctors informed the G. family that bilateral nephrectomy must be performed to avoid further increase in toxic products. They further informed the family that Mrs. G. would have to be on hemodialysis the rest of her life.

Naturally Mrs. G. was shocked at the news. All she could remember was that her kidneys must be removed and that she would be on a machine the rest of her life. The information had come too fast and was overwhelming. A hopeless feeling immediately flooded her. She thought of her children who would have to assume more of the domestic responsibilities. She felt hopeless about becoming a financial and psychological burden on her family. As her concerns and questions mounted, she became more depressed. Her feelings of hopelessness removed any sense of motivation she had prior to the news that she would lose her kidneys. It was a situation beyond her immediate understanding.

Mrs. G., like other patients experiencing loss of function or of a part, felt a sense of hopelessness. Such patients have no previous knowledge that might give them hope for the future. Initially the words "must be removed" or "hemodialysis" are so overwhelming that the patient may be unable to transcend the situation. In time Mrs. G. might realize that before the days of hemodialysis, she might have died, never seeing her daughters grow to be women. If the individual is unable to transcend the crisis, he despairs to the point of hopelessness.

The Patient's Perception
of His External Resources

External resources consist of the environment and other people. Hope is directly related to help from others. As Rycroft (1979) reminds us, individuals are social beings and as such put their faith in others. The sources of hope in an individual reside in his past, present, and imagined future relationships with others, from whom he acquires hope and to whom he may give hope. Hope is a social, cultural quality which is engendered within a social, historical matrix and transmitted from one generation to another. The individual senses that there is help outside himself. People who are stressed, sick, and feeling hopeless can be assisted by others who guide and plan the patient's care, namely, his nurse and physician, and his family members and friends. However, the patient's perception of his external resources may be as he wants to perceive it. The critically ill patient who is in a state of learned helplessness is reluctant to initiate voluntary responses because he sees his future as bleak. He fails to seek assistance from people in the environment. The patient believes that he has lost control of his illness and the treatment designed to alleviate his biological crisis.

The patient in a critical care unit may perceive the unit to be a frightening place. The environment around the patient is noisy and busy. He must lie in bed connected to various pieces of equipment such as IVs, a chest tube, an O_2 mask, or cardioscope leads. He realizes that each piece of equipment serves a special purpose. Some of the equipment, such as the cardioscope, reassures the patient that he is being observed, but most of the equipment serves to make him aware of how really helpless he has become. It also forces him to realize how vulnerable his body is. Now he depends upon objects to record, monitor, or maintain body function. Each new piece of equipment makes him feel even more helpless and hopeless. He feels that death must be the inevitable outcome. The patient's doctor, for example, may hear adventitious breath sounds and order IPPB treatments. The patient remembers that prior to his aunt's death she also had IPPB treatments. He correlates IPPB with his aunt's death, and he assumes his condition has deteriorated to her level. Another patient may be told he will need a temporary pacemaker. His frame of reference is a TV program in which a patient had difficulty with his pacemaker. The patient fails to realize that the actor's problems were written into the script to make the program more dramatic, but his only association with pacemakers is those problems. The nurse must be sensitive to her patient's perception of treatments in his environment.

The patient normally assimilates the original treatment or piece of equipment into his being because he perceives it to be part of the recovery process. The IVs, oxygen mask, Foley, CVP, and cardioscope leads all gain acceptance. The patient hopes these things will be discontinued when his condition stabilizes; at least this is what the people in his environment tell him. But if additional pieces are added while none are removed, the patient may despair of his situation. He believes that his body is steadily losing control, necessitating more external environmental help.

A patient who always accepted his IPPB treatment may suddenly refuse it. He may have been taking the treatment for three consecutive days. Since the doctors have not informed him that his chest film shows marked improvement, he feels the treatments are not accomplishing their goal. Had he been kept informed, the X-ray results would have motivated him toward further use of the machine. He would then have had the hope that his lungs would clear and the use of the machine would be discontinued. This communication breakdown frequently occurs. Each member of the health team assumes the other has informed the patient of his progress. It is only later that they discover that he was not informed, did not hear the results of his test, or did not understand the results.

The patient also has perceptions of his nurse and the other members of his health team. These persons play a vital role in determining his hopes—or hopelessness. Obviously there are times when it becomes difficult for the nurse to be anything else but hopeless, as the case of Mr. T. illustrated. Mr. T. seemed to deteriorate with each passing day. The nurse could see no improvement, even though the health team tried new treatments and procedures. A nurse's feelings of hopelessness may be manifest when the doctors order a new procedure. The nurse may inadvertently groan and say such things as, "What is he trying to do?" or "What good do they hope the treatment will accomplish?"

The nurse conveys her personal attitude to the patient and his family. She must remember that "when the patient becomes the object of the hopeless and helpless feelings of the staff, his hopelessness and helpless feelings about himself become intensified" (Shea 1970, p. 33). The hopelessness of the patient's illness or injury may render his nurse helpless. There will be times when the critically ill patient's condition does seem hopeless, and the nurse may feel justified in her own internal feelings of hopelessness; but if such feelings are communicated, the patient may reach a premature level of emotional standstill. He would succumb to a sense of hopelessness in his own biological integrity, underscored by his perception of hopelessness in the health team guiding his therapy. He views events internal and external to his being as "waste of time." If the health team seems hopeful, on the other hand, the patient will also feel hopeful. He will continue to strive emotionally toward a higher level of wellness, because he will have hope in his biological integrity. The nurse must be careful not to express her feelings of hopelessness verbally or nonverbally to the patient or his family.

Shea (1970) points out how hopelessness can be used as a protective mechanism by staff members:

> The fusion of helplessness and hopelessness into an entity results from the fact that when staff members feel helpless about intervening in a patient's illness, they utilize hopelessness as a defense for protecting them from feelings of failure. This response is frequently rationalized by the use of stereotypes and diagnostic labels that enable the staff to feel comfortable about ceasing to interact effectively with the patient (P. 32)

Therefore the nurse could use her feelings of hopelessness as a defense. She assumes that the critically ill patient with multiple complications will die. The defense of hopelessness serves to protect her from becoming too emotionally involved with the patient. This is a normal expression of feelings. The nurse may fear that if she invests too much energy in the patient's care or becomes too close, she will be left with an empty feeling if the patient dies.

The critical care nurse may need help in channeling her energy toward both the patient and his family. The nurse should keep in mind that she and other members of the health team are making the critically ill patient as comfortable as possible. There are times when the patient's illness will reach stability; however, the mechanical devices decorating his immediate environment give the impression of instability. His nurse realizes the equipment is alienating her from providing the human contact so desperately needed by her patient. To get close to her patient, she may literally need to crawl over chest tubes, IV tubing, suction bottles, respirator, peritoneal dialysis bottles, or cardioscope wires. This alone makes her feel hopeless. No wonder the nurse is discouraged from making personal close contacts on a frequent basis.

Modern technology, moreover, takes away some of her technical responsibility. Blood pressure is now monitored by an arterial line. Eventually, other technical procedures will be done by computers. This may only serve to make the patient feel more helpless; after all, the equipment and machines cannot motivate him and give him hope for continuing. They cannot talk to him, listen to his concerns, answer his many questions, give him positive reinforcement, laugh or cry with him, or tell him how he is progressing. All the machines can do is hum, beep, and buzz as they go about their technical business. The tragedy is that the equipment cannot always save the patient's life—it may only prolong his dying. The patient may finally put his hope in the machines. The nurse must help her patient seek other ways of maintaining hope, a hope that comes from within and is reinforced by people who help from the outside.

In summary, institutional systems including critical care have a tendency to be insensitive to the patient's need for control over events. Patients are not permitted to participate in their own care or make decisions. For some patients it is beneficial to relinquish control and independence as it might threaten their biological stability. Other patients desire a greater degree of control. Loss of control over simple things leads to efficiency but may not promote health (Seligman 1975).

NURSING ASSESSMENT OF HOPE AND HOPELESSNESS

Prior to looking at any behavior, it is important to remember that all people are unique and have their own constellation of psychosocial and personality characteristics which produce behavior (Dubree and Vogelpohl 1980). The nurse assesses hopelessness through the patient's behavioral response. The responses can be categorized into regulatory behaviors and cognitive behaviors.

Regulatory Behaviors

The regulatory system involves stimuli from the external environment and from changes in the internal state of dynamic equilibrium. The regulatory behavior or physiological responses associated with hopelessness may be few in comparison to the cognitive behaviors. Nevertheless the critically ill patient experiencing hopelessness may manifest the following regulatory behaviors:

Regulatory Behaviors
Weight loss
Appetite loss
Weakness
Sleep disorder

Cognitive Behaviors

The cognator system involves inputs from internal and external stimuli which include psychological and social factors. The specific aspects of the cognator mechanism consists of perceptual/information processing, learning, judgment, and emotion. The cognitive behaviors are psychological responses.

Before discussing specific cognitive behaviors, it may be useful to examine three major behavioral responses to the shattering of hope. First, some individuals resign themselves to fate. They have an average optimism and hope for the best but may then lose the capacity to dream. Second, some individuals who lose hope tend to isolate themselves from others. They withdraw in order to avoid being hurt by more unfulfilled hope. Third, a result of shattered hope may be destructiveness. Frustration due to unreached goals can cause the individual to direct destructive drives toward the self. This behavior results because the drive is no longer subordinated to other goals (Dubree and Vogelpohl 1980).

While there are numerous behaviors associated with hopelessness and/or despair, the following is a partial list of cognitive behaviors (Lange 1978; Miller 1983):

Cognitive Behaviors
Reduced activity
Passivity
Saddened expression
Lack of motivation
Interference with learning
Diminished interest in external objects
Muteness
Motionlessness

The hopeless individual experiences a lack of future orientation. The primary wish of the person who feels hopeless is to give up. Such a hopeless individual may manifest apathy, marked by a negative attitude, noninvolvement, withdrawal, boredom, and absence of feeling and concern (Lange 1978). Research by Schneider (1980) found that hopelessness characterized by indifference, apathy, and emotional deadness as a continuous state was rare, but as an intermittent state it was a frequent occurrence.

NURSING DIAGNOSIS OF HOPELESSNESS

The nursing diagnosis is a statement of the patient's problem. The patient's internal resources may be threatened due to illness, injury, or disease. Likewise the patient may perceive his external resources to be limited. Both factors are stressors. The stressors can lead to regulatory behaviors and/or cognitive behaviors. Behavioral manifestation coupled with an assessment of the patient's biological crisis help the critical care nurse formulate the nursing diagnosis of hopelessness.

NURSING INTERVENTIONS TO FOSTER HOPEFULNESS

Following the initial crisis, the patient should begin to feel elements of hope and hopefulness in encounters with people around him. These encounters have two dimensions: they involve other patients in the unit and they involve members of the health team.

Quite frequently, a patient will say to his nurse, "How is Mr. J. today? You know he had surgery the same time I did." This becomes a reference point for the patient. He is indirectly asking his nurse, "Am I doing as well or better?" Contact with other patients in a critical care unit is probably most evident in burn and hemodialysis units. In these units, patients seem to develop an early realization that there are other people experiencing the same kind of injury. When the burn patient sees visual evidence of another patient's progress, his own sense of hopefulness increases. Nurses in burn units can encourage hopefulness by taking frequent pictures of the patient's burns. As a patient becomes depressed and hopeless about his future, his nurse shows him pictures of another recovered patient who had similar burns. The fact that someone else survived the crisis serves as a motivating force to attain the same goal. In ICU it is quite possible, depending upon the patients, to place two people side by side who have had the same surgery. For example, two patients who have had coronary artery bypass could become unit mates. On the other hand, if there were preoperative indications of complications, it might not be possible to place the patient beside another patient who has had similar or same type of surgery. This might serve to discourage or alarm the patient rather than motivate him. If the patient's condition is stable, however, he can be placed beside another patient with the same surgery. The two patients can evaluate each other's progress. If one patient dangles earlier than the other, it may serve to motivate the patient who has not reached this goal. He sees that another person has accomplished the goal and survived to attempt more taxing goals. He has realistic hopes that he can accomplish the same goal.

The nurse helps the patient to find reality in the current illness situation. According to Miller (1983), reality surveillance is a cognitive task in which the individual searches for clues that confirm that maintaining hope is feasible. Another component of reality is phenomenal grounding, which refers to what the person in the situation believes provides ground for hope. It is this phenomenal grounding that provides reassurance to the individual.

Another approach in utilizing patient-peer contact is to involve a postoperative patient in the teaching of a preoperative patient. The nurse can certainly instruct the patient from a theoretical level, but it is the other patient who has actually experienced the surgery. This can be a useful technique for open heart surgery patients. Naturally, the one helping must have had a positive experience. Patients can help and support each other on a very practical level.

The nurse can serve as a tremendous motivating force in her patient's environment. Patients in crisis are able to perceive the attitude of hopelessness or hopefulness of those providing their care. The patient begins to believe that his nurse has power and ability to help him. He derives comfort in knowing that she must want to help him. He has trust in this stranger who is steadily becoming a very important friend. Before the patient can truly hope in his nurse, he must sense that she hopes that her interventions will be effective and that the crisis will be resolved. He can then transcend the crisis. Mr. T. sensed a feeling of hopelessness in his nurse. He realized that she did not have faith in her own intervention, nor did she have faith in his external resources. Since she already had more knowledge and experience than he, her feelings, thought Mr. T., must be correct. He reconciled himself to hopelessness. Unfortunately, and too often, nurses have a tendency to give up prematurely on a particular patient. We prematurely reach a level of hopelessness when not all avenues of care have been explored. We give up because we feel the situation is hopeless. And then the patient quite miraculously responds to therapy and gets well, much to our amazement.

Hope becomes a real entity when it contains elements that the individual can control and personally affect. When the patient acts or becomes involved in his care more options present themselves and hope grows (Dubree and Vogelpohl 1980). Therefore permitting a patient to control as many events as his energy level and/or restrictions permit prevents feelings of hopelessness. The patient with chronic pulmonary or renal disease may lack the energy necessary for controlling more than minute aspects of his care. Lange (1978) points out that the nurse who is knowledgeable about the normal progression of an illness, injury, or disease encourages the patient to exercise his controls over specific aspects of care.

Nursing's aim is to encourage people to live a full life. It is not always possible to reverse a disease process, yet biological science is often capable of replacing a diseased organ or restoring its integrity. Nursing does not return the patient to his previous physiological level. Instead, it helps the patient to live as abundantly as possible.

The goal of the critical care nurse is to help the patient reach out to others for support regardless of the helplessness of a situation. The question that immediately comes to mind is how does the nurse help her patient reach a higher level of being? The nurse accomplishes her task by motivating him and by channeling his internal energies toward a goal he can attain—one that is realistic for his level of illness. She motivates him by influencing his internal and external resources.

Motivation refers to action, to doing something rather than doing nothing. That something can be overt or covert; it can entail skeletal, perceptual, or cognitive behavior. Moreover, as Stotland (1969) points out, "Motivation refers to the directed quality of the action taken; the organism will choose acts that seem more likely to lead to goal attainment over acts that seem less likely to do so, and it will attend to those aspects of the environment that are relevant either in an instrumental or in a consummatory way" (p. 8). Dubree and Vogelpohl (1980) believe that a major nursing intervention for hopelessness is to motivate the patient. The nurse identifies the patient's strong points and provides the strength to see positive alternatives and to move ahead. She attempts to reduce the threats he feels against his internal resources. She simultaneously reinforces the realistic perceptions he has of his environment and the people in it. According to Monaco (1969), the nurse accomplishes this by becoming a "catalyst, helping to mobilize the positive forces that will activate his progress toward an improved standard of being. In this way, she enables or stimulates the patient to take his own steps—even faltering ones—toward a goal" (p. 1719).*

The alleviation of hopelessness is a significant nursing concern because it contributes to the patient's sense of power and prevents other harmful consequences of illness and therapy. Hopelessness can have an effect upon the critically ill patient's response to therapeutic measures. If the patient does not believe that the therapeutic measures will have a significant or positive effect upon his current illness, he experiences hopelessness and depression. Some patients measure therapeutic measures according to a time dimension. In other words the patient expects to have his pulmonary, renal, or cardiac problem resolved immediately. Naturally when this does not occur he becomes hopeless. Therefore the nurse points out stages of progress towards biological stability. This, together with continued supportive encouragement, sustains hopefulness.

The key word in helping the critically ill patient overcome his feelings of hopefulness is *goal*. The nurse might devise a plan involving degrees of goal attainment from simple to increasing complexity. She realizes that a patient could be highly motivated for a goal of minor significance but of high probable attainment. For example, the second-day postinfarction patient

*Copyright, American Journal of Nursing Company. Reprinted, with permission, from *American Journal of Nursing.*

may be allowed to brush his teeth and wash his face. These are relatively simple tasks that are taken for granted until they are restricted. When the responsibility for such tasks returns to the patient, he senses that he is improving and feels hopeful. The next day he might be given another goal: shaving with an electric razor. The nurse can start on a safe level, one that she knows her patient can attain. After evaluating the positive or negative effects of the activity, she can create another goal. The critical care nurse realizes that "hope of attaining a goal and the importance of that goal also influences the organism's affective state. The higher an organism's perceived probability of attaining a goal and the greater the importance of that goal, the greater will be the positive affect experienced by the organism" (Stotland 1969, p. 8).

The nurse keeps in mind that the strategies for reversing hopelessness in the patient require a tremendous amount of patience and commitment. When the patient is in a psychological state of hopelessness, he experiences feelings of impossibility and entrapment. Therefore the nurse attempts to focus on the possibility of attaining various goals. This may require establishing learning activities that will help the patient master his current crisis and learn. For example the nurse can establish learning goals when she works with the hemodialysis patient who is learning home dialysis. She starts with the basic procedure of cleaning the A-V shunt, caring for equipment, and maintaining a proper diet, and she then might demonstrate how to set up the machine and how he will eventually connect himself to the machine. She works with the patient and motivates him through each phase of his learning. The nurse in the burn unit works in a similar fashion with her burn patient, first establishing short-term goals and then progressing toward long-term ones. A burn patient like Mr. C., whose hands were burned, needs daily range-of-motion exercises. Each day his nurse can establish goals that serve to restore and maintain function of his hands. The first may involve reducing contractures, and the ultimate goal might be squeezing a ball. Another patient who has had a mitral valve replacement may be moving toward the goal of ambulation. His nurse starts the patient at the simple level of turning, progresses toward dangling, standing at the bedside, walking around the bed, and finally ambulating further. As the patient achieves each small goal the nurse encourages him to reach for the next one.

As all three patients move closer toward their ultimate goal, they become increasingly more motivated. However, if the patient feels he has to accomplish too many intermediate goals before he achieves the big one, his motivation will diminish. Therefore, nurses should establish a reasonable number of intermediate goals, each of which builds on the patient's prior accomplishment. An initial goal should be close to the patient's starting point and it should have a high probability of attainment.

As the patient moves towards his goal, the nurse evaluates the positive or negative outcome. If the patient's movement is in a positive direction, then the nurse's intervention has been successful. The patient may be ready for more complex goals. The nurse then fosters goal-directedness in her patient by deciding upon a goal that can be achieved together. For example, the postoperative cardiac surgical patient and his nurse would work together toward the long-term goal of ambulation. The two people plan for the goal in the following manner:

NURSE: Mr. L., I imagine you are tired of lying in bed.

MR. L.: Yes. My back is sore.

NURSE: Since you are doing so well, we can increase your activity. It might take the soreness out.

MR. L.: That would be great. How can I get out of bed with all these tubes?

NURSE: You won't be getting completely out of bed the first time. Have you ever heard the word *dangle*?

MR. L.: Yes. That's where you hang your legs over the side of the bed.

NURSE: Right. The tubes will all follow you with no problem. We start with dangling and see how well you do.

MR. L.: What happens if I don't do well?

NURSE: We will try again this afternoon. Remember your body has been through some extensive surgery, so it can't be expected to perform as it did before surgery.

MR. L.: What happens if I do well?

NURSE: This afternoon I'll have you stand at your bedside.

Mr. L.: It sounds like I am getting better.

NURSE: Yes, you are. Ready to try dangling?

MR. L.: Yes, let's go.

In this situation the nurse provided Mr. L. with an attainable goal. His condition was stable, and it seemed as though he could be successful. She gave him positive reinforcement that his progress was normal. She presented the goal of dangling in a positive manner. Motivation, we should note, is like an accumulating pressure; it seeks discharge or diffuse motor activity. Mr. L.'s motivational need was position, to facilitate better pulmonary ventilation, to stimulate circulation, and to prepare for more complex activity. The more complex activity would be standing beside his bed. The patient had hope of satisfaction, based upon the opportunity to relieve the tension in his back and eventually to ambulate. He realized that increasing activity meant his condition was improving, and he was hopeful of leaving the ICU in a relatively short period of time.

The nurse can be careful to establish a number of small goal-directed interventions that instill a sense of hopeful satisfaction. As the patient becomes more hopeful about his internal resources, his original feelings of threat will lessen. He realizes that his internal resources can be stimulated toward execution of a plan. The nurse creates an atmosphere conducive to goal attainment and goal satisfaction. The goal must have a high probability of attainment; it must have meaning to the patient; and it should build toward attainment of more complex goals. The nurse can accomplish such a plan only by maintaining the proper personal attitude.

The nurse can maintain an attitude of hopefulness with each patient and family, no matter how grave the situation is. Hopefulness is a necessary condition for action, for without this positive attitude, very little can be accomplished. The hopeful nurse is enthusiastic, active, and energetic about the care she provides. As the patient draws upon her energy in an attempt to replenish his curative powers, she becomes more involved with the patient. As mentioned previously, hopelessness can be a defense utilized by the critical care nurse to avoid closeness or involvement. The hopeful nurse enters the situation with this awareness, but she will usually believe that it is far better to have actively touched another's life in an attempt to meet his needs than to turn away from him in a fatalistic manner. The latter approach only fosters guilt feelings and perpetuates a sense of failure. If the patient should die, the nurse feels guilty. Frequently she might say, "I wonder if I could have done more?" The activist approach fulfills the nurse, the patient, and the family. The nurse should continue to work in a positive manner. This does not imply she denies a possible outcome of death in her patient; such a concern is constantly present in her mind. It does imply that she realizes the alternatives and chooses to work in an affirmative direction.

NURSING EVALUATION

The critical care nurse assesses various regulatory and cognitive behaviors that support the diagnosis of hopelessness. Interventions designed to facilitate hopefulness and minimize hopelessness are evaluated for their effectiveness. When the patient is able to gain control over aspects of his care, to become involved in learning activities that help him cope with the immediate situation, and to develop meaningful goals, then the nurse's interventions have been effective. Some of the cognitive behaviors may not be eliminated until the patient is transferred out of critical care. The transfer is viewed as a positive step towards wellness and eventual discharge.

SUMMARY

The nurse can trust her patient's will to live. In all instances, she must help the patient to look forward to some worthwhile life goal. The patient who hopes does not stop at the momentary crisis. Instead, he extends himself— he reaches out to being. In reaching out, he must reach toward someone. That someone must share a similar hope. When he finds this hope shared by the critical care nurse, he can be restored to being.

REFERENCES

BECK, ARRON, and ARLENE WAISMAN, "The Measurement of Pessimism: The Hopelessness Scale," *Journal of Consulting and Clinical Psychology*, 42, no. 6 (1974), 861-865.

BROWN, BRENDA, "An Innovative Approach to Health Care for the Elderly: An Approach of Hope," *JPN and Mental Health Services*, 15, no. 10 (October 1977), 27-35.

DAVIES, A. F., "Varieties of Hope," in *The Sources of Hope*, ed. Ross Fitzgerald, pp. 24-35. Australia: Pergamon Press, 1979.

DUBREE, MARILYN, and RUTH VOGELPOHL, "When Hope Dies So Might the Patient," *American Journal of Nursing*, November 1980, pp. 2046-2049.

FITZGERALD, ROSS, "Hope, Meaning and Transcedence of Self," in *The Source of Hope*, pp. 244-254. Australia: Pergamon Press, 1979.

FULLER, JOHN, *Motivation*. New York: Random House, 1968.

HAMBURG, DAVID A., BEATRIX HAMBURG, and SYDNEY DE GOZA, "Adaptive Problems and Mechanisms in Severely Burned Patients," *Psychiatry*, 16, no. 1 (February 1953), 1-20.

HENRI, DESROCHE, *The Sociology of Hope*. London: Routledge and Kegan Paul, 1979.

HIROTO, DONALD, "Locus of Control and Learned Helplessness, *Journal of Experimental Psychology*, 102, no. 2 (February 1974), 187-193.

KRANTZ, DAVID, DAVID GLASS, and MELVIN SNYDER, "Helplessness, Stress Level, and the Coronary-Prone Behavior Pattern," *Journal of Experimental Social Psychology*, 10 (1974), 284-300.

KÜBLER-ROSS, ELIZABETH, *On Death and Dying*. New York: Macmillan, 1971.

——— , "Hope and the Dying Patient," *Nursing Digest*, 5 (Summer 1977), 82-84.

LANGE, SILVIA, "Hope," in *Behavioral Concepts and Nursing Interventions*, ed. Carolyn E. Carlson and Betty Blackwell, pp. 171-190. Philadelphia: Lippincott, 1978.

LESTER, D. and L. TREXLER, "The Measurement of Pessimism: The Hopeless Scale," *Journal of Consulting and Clinical Psychology*, 42, no. 6 (1974), 861-865.

LYNCH, WILLIAM F., *Images of Hope*. Baltimore: Helicon Press, 1965.

MILLER, JUDITH FITZGERALD, *Coping with Chronic Illness: Overcoming Powerlessness*. Philadelphia: F. A. Davis, 1983.

MINKOFF, KENNETH, ERIC BERGMAN, ARRON BECK, and ROY BECK, "Hopelessness, Depression and Attempted Suicide," *American Journal of Psychiatry*, 130, no. 4 (April 1973), 455-459.

MONACO, JUDY, "Motivation by Whom and towards What?" *American Journal of Nursing*, 69, no. 8 (August 1969), 1719.

NOVAK, MICHAEL, *The Experience of Nothingness*. New York: Harper & Row, 1971.

NOWOTNY, JOAN, "Despair and the Object of Hope," in *The Source of Hope*, ed. Ross Fitzgerald, pp. 44-66. Australia: Pergaman Press, 1979.

RYCROFT, CHARLES, "Steps to an Ecology of Hope," in *The Sources of Hope*, ed. Ross Fitzgerald, pp. 3-23. Australia: Pergamon Press, 1979.

SCHNEIDER, JUDITH, "Hopelessness and Helplessness," *JPN and Mental Health Services*, 18, no. 3 (March 1980), 12-21.

SELIGMANN, MARTIN, *Helplessness*, San Francisco: W. H. Freeman & Co., 1975.

——— , *Helplessness on Depression, Development, and Death*. San Francisco: W. H. Freeman & Co., 1979.

SHEA, FRANK, "Hopelessness and Helplessness," *Perspectives in Psychiatric Nursing*, 2, no. 1 (1970), 32-38.

SIOMOPOULOS, GREGORY, and SUBHASH INAMDAR, "Developmental Aspects of Hopelessness," *Adolescence*, 14, no. 53 (Spring 1979), 233–239.

STOTLAND, EZRA, *The Psychology of Hope*. San Francisco: Jossey-Bass, 1969.

VAILLOT, SISTER MADELEINE CLEMENCE, "Hope: The Restoration of Being," *American Journal of Nursing*, 70, no. 2 (February 1970), 268–273.

VERNON, M. D., *Human Motivation*. Cambridge: Cambridge University Press, 1969.

4

Territoriality and Space

BEHAVIORAL OBJECTIVES

1. Define the terms *territoriality, space,* and *privacy*.
2. State the functions of territoriality.
3. Identify the four components of territoriality.
4. Describe the functions of privacy.
5. Compare and contrast body factors, environmental factors, antecedent factors, and organism need states as they apply to the critically ill patient.
6. State four regulatory behaviors associated with territoriality.
7. State how cognitive behaviors can influence the patient's perception of his critical care environment.
8. Design a plan of care that utilizes proxemics.

The need for a territory of one's own is universal. People providing health care can contribute a great deal to the patient's well-being by assisting him to meet his territorial or spatial needs. Many institutions such as hospitals have usually limited their interest and concern with space to closet or drawer space for personal belongings and storage space for linen, equipment, and supplies. Increasing attention is being given to the patient's feelings regarding personal space, territory, or privacy. Members of the health team seem to focus little attention upon the effect of physical and physiological intrusion into the patient's space or territorial bubble. With the rapid development of critical care units, hospital personnel direct more interest toward the use of space in these areas. More space is needed not only to house the critically

120

ill patient, but to contain the various pieces of equipment that might be needed. If there is adequate space for each patient, none need experience territorial invasion by his neighbor's supportive devices. Nurses should examine how territory and space are utilized for the patient's benefit and also how the concept of privacy relates to territory and space—both physical and psychological space.

When examining human territorial behavior, it is desirable to view it according to three categories, namely, the individual, the small group, and the large group. Individual territory begins in a person's home. Each family member within the home has his or her own bedroom, bed, or particular side of the bed; Furthermore each individual has his own closet and drawer space as well as a specific place to hand his tooth brush.

It has been noted by Dubos (1965) that most animal species develop a complex social organization based on territoriality and a social hierarchy comprising subordinate and dominant members, the so-called pecking order. The place of each animal in the hierarchy is probably determined in part by anatomical and physiological endowments and in part by history of the group. The same principle applies to humans. In Western culture, a relationship between physical and social territoriality is frequently evident. As Pluckhan (1968) notes, the "amount of space a person has rights to often is related to his personal significance or financial status. For example, a large home on a double lot is generally symbolic of high income and status" (p. 393).

Both in regular units and in critical care units, patient status depends upon having a private room, a private duty nurse, a room full of flowers or cards, and frequent incoming phone calls. A high-status patient's nurse will place him high on her priority list or high in the pecking order. The less wealthy patient may be placed in a four-bed ward in the windowless corner of a critical care unit. The wealthy patient may have more social prominence than the poorer patient. The more socially prominent the patient, the more access he has to physical territory, in terms of both quality and quantity. In addition, his personal territory may extend throughout the hospital via connections with the significant people within hospital hierarchy.

Most members of our culture encounter unnecessary and extensive conflict in their day-to-day interaction with artificial environments. Critical care units are artificial environments. As designed environments, they are under the control of an environmental designer, or architect, who is inclined to see his or her efforts as directed toward the satisfaction of human needs, although architects may design critical care units with the financial need of the administration, not the psychological needs of the critically ill patient, in mind. The design should be environmentally conducive to the patient's well-being. While artificial environments are often monotonous and unstimulating, they may simultaneously be viewed as chaotic and overstimulating (Struder, 1970, p. 113). The routines in critical care may be monotonous to the patient, but the environment may be noisy and overstimulating. Current designs use soft and relaxing colors. Curtains and carpets can be and in many instances have been added to many coronary care units. They can provide pleasant visual stimulation and help to reduce noise. The patient's territory in critical care units should be designed to allow both openness and privacy. Partitions should be placed around each patient's bed in order to promote his privacy and reduce the transmission of meaningless stimuli to other patients. Ideally, the partition should be made out of material that absorbs most sounds.

DEFINITION OF TERMS

Researchers who have investigated territory seem to conceptualize it in two ways. It is conceptualized, first, as a spatial or geographic phenomenon and, second, as a behavioral phenomenon. To apply territorial and spatial concepts to the care of the critically ill, it would seem advantageous to view territoriality primarily as a behavioral system expressed in a spatial-temporal frame of reference. According to Carpenter (1968), "the drives and incentives or motives, and the sensory-response and learning process are all different aspects of the behavioral systems or territoriality" (pp. 228–229). Before seeing how territoriality, space, and privacy apply to various patients in critical care units, we will define these terms.

Territory and Territoriality

Territory refers to a specific place or area within which the satisfaction of important needs or drives take place. *Territoriality* is that conscious or unconscious behavior that is characteristically developed in the individual's tendency to indicate possession or ownership (Johnson 1979). Territories are fixed geographical areas that members of various species maintain and defend against intrusive behavior by others. Stea (1970) further states than in the case of humans, "territorial behavior reflects the desire to possess and occupy portions of space, and, when necessary, to defend it against intrusion by others. A distinction also needs to be made between territorial units of individuals, territorial clusters, and territorial complexes involving multiple people, as well as stationary and moving territories" (p. 3). Pastalan, who has done much research in the area of territoriality, believes that a territory is a delimited space that an individual or group uses and defends as an exclusive preserve. It involves psychological identification with the place, symbolized by an attitude of possessiveness and arrangements of objects in the area (1970, p. 4). Edward Hall (1966), an anthropologist, defines territoriality as behavior by which an organism characteristically lays claim to an area and defends it against members of its own species.

Territoriality is one aspect of the dynamic flow in the individual-environment relationship, namely, the sense of controlling an area of space (Bullock-Loughran 1982). Conceptually territoriality has to do with a specific place within which one's needs are met. The possession of a territory satisfies three basic needs in all species: identity, stimulation, and security. Identity is the powerful among all species (Holl 1981). Finally it is believed that territories frequently have peripheral or fringe areas that are neither territory which cannot be invaded without permission nor public space (Hayter 1981).

Functions of Territories and Territoriality. Territories function as places where one can spend time in privacy thereby allowing sustained or protracted action and thought (Johnson 1979). Territoriality offers protection from predators and also exposes to predation the unfit who are too weak to establish and defend a territory. One most important function of territoriality is proper spacing, which protects against overexploitation of that part of the environment upon which a species depends for its living. Territoriality is also associated with status. Humans exhibit territoriality and have invented many ways of defending what they consider their own land (Hall 1966, pp. 9-10).

Territoriality also serves four functions: security, privacy, autonomy, and self-identity (Hayter 1981). *Security* consists of safety from harm together with a feeling of safety. If an individual is in a place he controls, he feels safer, less threatened, and less anxious. The person may be safer in his own territory because it is organized for his specific needs. Therefore, the individual may be able to function better and more safely than in any other place. *Privacy* is the second function of territoriality. Personal territory provides privacy and protected communication. While in his own home, a person can be himself. Furthermore the privacy provided by territoriality facilitates emotional release. The individual controls space to the point that he can refuse entry to others or not. *Autonomy*, the third function of territoriality, implies that the person is in control of himself and what happens to him. While in his own territory, a person may feel free to ask questions or resist a course of action. However when placed in a foreign territory such as critical care, the patient may submit to a treatment or agree to a regimen. He passively submits to others because he does not feel sufficiently in control to refuse or raise questions. The fourth function of territoriality is *self-identity*. The person who has a space of his own promotes self-identity and self-expression. Territoriality provides an opportunity to express one's individuality. It should be noted that the space a person has jurisdiction over can become an extension of himself including his own values, beliefs, and interests.

Components of Territoriality. Territoriality can be viewed from several perspectives at once. Territoriality has a multifocal meaning involving four components: body factors, environmental factors, antecedent factors, and organism need states. These component parts of territoriality will be applied to the critically ill patients.

No matter what theory we use, as we "stand in line for coffee, in a tow line on the ski slopes, or in the supermarket checkout line, we realize that the recognition of territorial rights is one of the most significant attributes of our civilization. We may even become concerned when someone's cigar or cigarette smoke floats into our air" (Pluckhan 1968, p. 390). Territoriality has direct applications in open critical care units, and all critical care nurses who want to understand the silent language of space should pay heed to it.

Space

Personal space and individual territory are thought to be equal. Personal space is the space that we carry around with us. Some personal space is so related to one's self-identity that it has many behavioral implications in terms of understanding or foreseeing both one's own spatial relations and one's relationship with others (Trierwailer 1979). Territory, relatively stationary, is usually much larger in area. According to Pastalan (1970) an individual, whether he is hospitalized or at home, will "delineate the boundaries of his territory with a variety of environmental props both fixed and mobile so that they are visible to others, while the boundaries of personal space are invisible though they may sometimes be inferred from self-markers such as facial expressions, body movements, gestures, olfaction, visual contact, and voice intonation" (p. 212).

The concept *space* has been defined as "room to move about in" and "room to put our bodies in." In and of itself, it is a nonentity. It is essentially the nothingness that exists between "self" as the point of departure and some object or person perceived in the world "out there" (Pluckhan 1968, p. 390). Some regard an internal concept of the spatial organization of the world to be part of the body image. Thus, the immediate buffer zone around the body is considered as a separate facet of the body image, which comprises not only an internalized projection of the body's boundary and position but also a sensitized projection of the immediate area around the body.

Another aspect of space is preferred personal space. It is the amount of distance an individual prefers between himself and another for comfortable conversation. The amount of space preferred or selected by an individual is related to several variables such as culture, eye contact, sex, state of anxiety, and self-esteem. Self-esteem seems to correlate with preferred personal space. Individuals with a low self-esteem or whose self-esteem is threatened by a situation prefer greater distance between themselves and others (Giorella 1978).

According to Sonnenfeld (1970), space, then, is sensible space: it has significance according to the purpose for which it is sought and the conditions under which it is experienced. Space is adequate if it allows for privacy. The determinants of spatial adequacy, both in its isolation and difference dimension, lie in part in the nature of the space and in part in the individual and the constraints on his activities.

Privacy

Privacy in whole or in part represents the control of transactions between persons and others, the ultimate aim of which is to enhance autonomy and minimize vulnerability (Margulis 1977). Privacy and the invasion of privacy involves a balancing of normative and individual interests. It seems that control and choice are involved in privacy. For example, psychological privacy serves to maximize freedom of choice or the ability to control what goes on in defined areas of space (Johnson 1979). According to Pastalan, privacy, because of its unique human behavioral states, may constitute a basic form of human territoriality. Privacy may be defined as the right of the individual to decide what information about himself should be communicated to others and under what conditions (Pastalan 1970, p. 89). From this basic definition Westin (1967, p. 7) elaborates on the relation of the individual to a social group, stating that privacy is the temporary and voluntary withdrawal of an individual by physical or psychological measures.

Margulis (1977) has defined privacy according to the selective control of access to oneself, which involves six properties. First, it involves the dialectic process involving differential accessibility of the self to others over time and with changing circumstances. Second, privacy is an interpersonal boundary control process that regulates and controls social interaction. Third, in privacy there is an optimum level of interaction that equals the ideal balance between forces to be open versus closed. In other words, the open individual may have too little privacy whereas the closed person will have too much privacy. Fourth, desired privacy versus actual privacy are distinguished. When achieved and desired privacy are equal, optimal privacy exists. When desired levels exceed achieved levels, crowding occurs. Likewise when achieved levels exceed desired levels, social isolation occurs. The fifth property of privacy is that it is a bidirectional process. Input includes incoming social stimulation from others and output includes interaction from self to others. Sixth, privacy applies to various social units.

Functions of Privacy. Margulis (1977) has identified three functions or purposes of privacy regulation processes. The higher functions build upon, integrate, and are more controlled than the lower functions. The initial or least controlled function of privacy is management of self-other boundaries. The next highest function focuses on how people use the information drawn from social interaction to both define self-other roles and to interpret oneself in relationship to others. The third and ultimate function of privacy is self-identity. Self-identity includes self-understanding, knowledge of where one begins and where one ends.

Proshansky, Ittelson, and Rivilson (1970) have identified four functions of privacy: autonomy, emotional release, self-evaluation, and limited or protected communication. In this scheme, a basic function of privacy is to protect and maintain the individual's need for personal autonomy, which is a sense of individuality and conscious choice in which the individual controls his environment, including his ability to have privacy when he desires it. Psychologists and sociologists have linked the development and maintenance of this sense of individuality to the human need for autonomy—the desire to avoid being manipulated or dominated wholly by others. Autonomy is threatened by those who are not discreet in their intrusion and either do not recognize or choose to ignore the importance of privacy or feel that the casual and uninvited help may be sufficient compensation for the violation. The critically ill patient faces continual manipulation, intrusion, and external control over his very life. His personal sense of autonomy may feel threatened.

The second function of privacy is to provide emotional release, the safety-valve effect. Privacy, whether through solitude, intimacy, or anonymity, may serve the function of emotional release. Social and biological factors create tension so that people need periods of privacy for various types of emotional release. Because life in critical care units imposes stress on the patients, they need opportunity for privacy in order to find emotional release. With the door shut the patient may tell the nurses what he thinks of his doctor, his food, or his care.

The third function of privacy is self-evaluation. In a state of solitude or withdrawal during reserve, the individual not only processes information but also makes plans by interpreting it, recasting it, and anticipating his subsequent behaviors. According to Pastalan (1970), "Every individual needs to integrate his experience into a meaningful pattern and to exert his individuality on events. To carry on such self-evaluation, privacy is essential. At the intellectual level, individuals need to process the information that is constantly bombarding them, information that cannot be processed while they are still on the go" (p. 91). Privacy also allows a person to decide when to inject his private reflections into public conversation.

The last function of privacy is limited and protected communication. First, it meets the individual's need to share confidences and intimacies with people he trusts such as his spouse, minister, or physician. Second, it establishes a psychological distance in all types of interpersonal situations when the individual desires such distance or when it is required by normative role relationship. Withdrawal into privacy also provides psychological distance. A person can communicate his need for privacy nonverbally, through facial expressions and bodily gestures, or verbally, by changing the subject of a conversation (Pastalan 1970, p. 92).

Degree of Privacy.   The four degrees of privacy are solitude, intimacy, anonymity, and reserve. All but anonymity actually apply to patients in critical care units. *Solitude* is a state in which an individual is separated from the group and freed from the observations of other persons. The patient in isolation may experience solitude. So do many patients in intensive care units who are subjected to jarring physical stimuli of equipment noises. The burn patient's peace of mind may continue to be disturbed by physical sensation of heat, cold, itching, and pain, yet he may still experience solitude, which is the most complete state of visual privacy that individuals can achieve.

Privacy also provides *intimacy*. Typical units of intimacy are husband and wife, the family, a friendship cycle, or a work clique. Whether close contact brings relaxed relations or abrasive hostility depends on the personal interaction of the members, but intimacy does provide a basic need of human contact.

Reserve, the final degree of privacy that we shall discuss, is the creation of a psychological barrier against unwanted intrusion. This occurs when the individual's need to limit communication about himself is protected by the willing discretion of those surrounding him. The manner in which individuals claim reserve and the extent to which it is respected or disregarded by others is at the heart of securing meaningful privacy (Pastalan 1970, p. 90).

As the definitions of territoriality, space, and privacy indicate, every living thing has a physical boundary that separates it from its external environment. There is also a nonphysical boundary that exists outside the physical one. This new boundary is harder to delimit than the first, but it is just as real. No matter how crowded the area in which the patient temporarily lives, he will try to maintain a zone or territory around himself. No one knows exactly how much space is necessary for any individual, but what is significant is what happens to the critically ill patient when his territory is threatened or breached.

With these definitions in mind, we will apply the concepts of territoriality, space, and privacy to the critically ill patient in critical care units, examining the critically ill patient according to Pastalan's (1970) definition of the four component functions of territory.

THE CONCEPT OF TERRITORIALITY APPLIED TO THE CRITICALLY ILL PATIENT

Territoriality as it applies to various critically ill patients will be examined according to the following: body factors, environmental factors, antecedent factors, and organism need states.

Body Factors

Body factors include space around the individual, self-ego dimension, and illness necessitating intrusive procedures. Lyman and Scott (1967) point out that "there are body territories, which include the space encompassed by the human body and the anatomical space of the body. The latter is, at least theoretically, the most private and inviolate of territories belonging to an individual. The rights to view and touch the body are of a sacred nature, subject to great restriction" (p. 241). The patient, however, regardless of age or severity of illness, relinquishes the privacy of his or her own body. Shortly after admission into critical care, the patient's body is explored, manipulated, or intruded upon. Granted, the adult patient can maintain a degree of control through refusal to sign consents for intrusive procedures, but since failure to compromise and submit could greatly hinder the patient's progress, the patient usually complies.

Self-ego dimension refers to a developmental process that, in our society, focuses on autonomy and, by implication, personal dignity. There is another sense in which the self is critical to the understanding of privacy. Any array of reasons given by individuals for seeking and maintaining their privacy reveals an attempt to protect, nurture, extend, and enhance the self (Laufer and Wolfe 1977).

Illness or admission to a critical care unit almost always creates a threat to the territory of expertise or role because it temporarily interferes with the individual's perception about his own expertise or role function. Therefore illness is a threat to the individual's security. During illness a person is less able to defend his territory against invasion, yet he is also less likely to tolerate invasion of it (Hayter 1981). The critical care patient's anxiety level can increase when he experiences an intrusion into his body territory. Intrusion or manipulation is more likely to involve the critically ill patient.

Intrusive procedures or supportive devices connected to the affected body part make the individual more aware of its temporary or permanent loss. As Lyman and Scott (1967) state, "Body space is . . . subject to creative innovation, idiosyncrasy, and destruction. First, the body may be marked or marred by scars, cuts, burns, and tattoos. In addition, certain of its parts may be inhibited or removed without its complete loss of function" (p. 250). Body territories can be altered due to illness or extended through various pieces of equipment which support the affected body part. Intrusion into the individual's body territory can be a threatening experience in and of itself.

Depending upon the severity of the patient's illness, the intrusive procedures happen quickly. The patient already feels anxious and threatened by virtue of being ill, and the loss of or invasion of his territory adds to his anxiety. If the patient uses psychic energy to defend his territory, he may be depleting the energy reserves needed for recovery. At a time when the critically ill patient's need for his own territory is increased, he is more likely to have it invaded (Hayter 1981).

Environmental Factors

Environmental elements influence the patient's ability to perceive, have, and use available options. The environmental dimension is composed of a series of elements that act as boundaries of meaning and experience. The elements of the environmental dimension involve the physical setting and its environmental props (Laufer and Wolfe 1977). Since critical care units are designed for high-priority patients who require continuous, intensive nursing observations and interventions, they should be large enough to accommodate the various pieces of equipment needed. This is not always the case. In many units, the territory and space around the patient's bed is too small, and when equipment is needed the space becomes even smaller. There are two formats for critical care units: (1) an open space, in which each patient unit is usually separated by four or five feet and an imaginary territorial boundary or curtain; and (2) a closed space, in which each patient has a private room. Figures 4.1(a) and (b) are schematic drawings of open and closed ICU units.

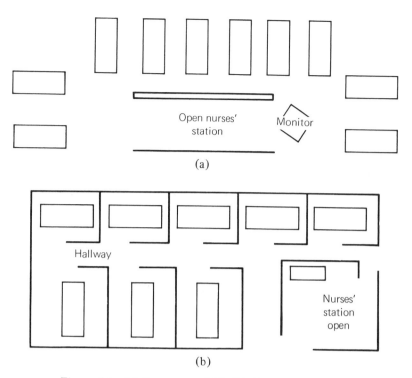

Figure 4.1 (a) Open space ICU. (b) Closed space ICU.

Open spaces or open units are less costly, and the nurse can see her patients at all times. The majority of critical care units, with the exception of isolation units, are organized as open units. Because each bed is separated by only an artificial boundary or curtain, environmental stimuli carry easily from patient to patient. When patient A's curtains are pulled, he knows exactly what territory is his—the distance from his bed to the curtains. If his curtains are opened, he loses his territorial boundaries. Patient A no longer feels a personal sense of territorial ownership or privacy. His territory now flows into that of patient B, lying in the adjacent bed. The only personal physical space of which patient A is certain is the space in which he is lying—his bed.

If the condition of patient A requires various pieces of equipment, these new elements may extend into the territory of the patient lying on either side of him. Patients B and C may feel they have lost a portion of their territorial ownership. Instead of owning a territory four feet wide, they may now find their space reduced to an area less than three feet wide. The equipment serves to decrease patient A's sense of privacy, because the curtains or artificial boundaries may not be easily pulled around the equipment. Moreover, curtains might obstruct the vision of the nurse if she should happen to be in another area of the unit. Patient A would probably say, "Please pull my curtain partially around me." The curtain becomes a private possession for both A and B. Patient B may not want to see patient A and all his equipment; consequently, he also would want the curtains pulled.

Just as the curtain can serve to provide privacy and a territorial boundary, it can also serve to isolate another patient. For example, the nurse may decide to pull a curtain along both sides of a critically ill patient in order to protect the two patients in adjacent beds from becoming frightened. One of the patients, however, may resent this intervention because the curtain serves to cut him off from his environment. The curtain may make it impossible for him to see his nurse or other nurses. He may become fearful that no one will watch him or that he will not be able to get his nurse's attention.

The second type of artificial environment is the closed unit. Some critical care units still have private rooms for critically ill patients. In the closed unit or private room setting, walls separate the rooms. In each room there is a closet, sink, table, chair, and nightstand. The patient shares his bathroom with another patient. The walls provide some protection against the environmental stimuli of other critically ill patients. The critically ill patient's territory may be his territory in name only, because the nature of his illness may immobilize him, restricting his ability to ambulate and to lay territorial claim to his surroundings. The only real spatial orientation the critically ill patient has is his bed; he can touch his side rails—if it does not create electrical interference—or the sides of his mattress and realize that his body occupies the space. Although he sees a closet, chair, nightstand, bathroom, and cardioscope in the territory around his bed, he may not always see these objects as belonging to him. He may ask the nurse, "Whose machine is that?" "Who uses the bathroom?" or "Where did they put my clothes?"

By symbolically pacing off territory through placement of his belongings in their appropriate place, the patient can gain a sense of spatial orientation regarding the territorial boundaries of his living quarters. People in general are very possessive about their objects, ideas, and geographical places. The critically ill patient arriving in ICU or CCU cannot lay territorial claims by hanging up his clothes in his closet, finding his bathroom or urinal, or placing his belongings in a nightstand. Because of the seriousness of his situation, a patient enters the ICU and CCU on a stretcher that may be three feet wide, his hands folded across his chest or tightly clenched at his sides. Wheeled into either an open space, referred to as a "slot," or a closed space, referred to as a private room, the critically ill patient's stretcher is maneuvered to his new, temporary home—a bed about four feet wide—and two or three nurses move him to his bed. He is not able to get a spatial feel for his new environment, not even the width of his bed.

Once the patient is lying in bed, his nurses raise the side rails to ensure his safety. Most patients are connected to a cardioscope in order to evaluate cardiac pattern for rate, rhythm, and regularity. Nurses instruct these patients not to touch the side rails or the leads because such contact creates interferences, which could trigger the alarm mechanism. The various tubes or wires that are inserted or connected to the patient may further limit his mobility in bed, thus restricting him to one portion of his total spatial claim of four feet.

The critically ill patient is also connected to other environmental props that underscore his illness: the arterial line, a central venous pressure line, oxygen tubing, IV tubing, a Foley catheter, or a nasal-gastric tube. These props may be connected as separate units, or the venous and arterial pressure readings can be connected to one large piece of equipment called a crash cart. In either case, the critically ill patient finds himself spatially and territorially surrounded by a shroud of equipment, a nest in which all his care and treatments occur. Nurses usually discourage patients in open CCU or ICU units from arranging environmental props like pictures, cards, or flowers on the nightstand because they take up space in an already spatially limited environment. More space is available in the closed space units, and nurses allow environmental props to accumulate on the nightstand.

The burn patient presents a unique territorial challenge to the nurse. She usually first sees him in a room designed as a Hubbard tank. It is within this territory that the patient's burns are assessed, cleaned, cultured, medicated, and dressed. Nurses then transport the patient on a stretcher to his new home in the burn unit. Unlike the ICU or CCU patient, the burn patient's home or bed may not be temporary. Depending on the severity of his burns, the burn patient may remain in the unit from two to three months. His limited bed space takes on a permanent quality. If the burned patient's face is involved, he will not have visual orientation of the space or territory around him. This factor is significant because, as Hall (1966) points out, "man's sense of space is closely related to this sense of self. It is an intimate transaction with his environment. Man can be viewed as having visual, kinesthetic, tactile, and thermal aspects of his self which may be either inhibited or encouraged to develop by his environment (p. 63).

If the burn patient's eyes are swollen shut due to facial burns or edema, he cannot see what is his territory. Physically, his body is surrounded not only by the usual boundaries of skin but also by the boundaries of dressings. Like the CCU and ICU patient, the burn patient has environmental props, which may include a heat cradle attached to a frame over his bed. This may obstruct his view; he may only be able to see objects within his peripheral vision. If the cradle is placed over his chest and lower extremities, he may still be able to look up at the ceiling. Turning his head from side to side for peripheral orientation may be painful. Furthermore, the dressings, wires, tubes, and pain prevent him from assessing the size of his bed by feeling the edges of his mattress. Consequently, he cannot adapt spatially and territorially as well as the ICU or CCU patient. Because the burn patient must remain in the open burn unit for a prolonged period of time, his nurse should place significant personal possessions like family pictures in his immediate territory, where he can easily see them.

Unlike the ICU or CCU patient, who builds a single territorial nest and then receives his care in that nest, the burn patient has two territorial nests. One, the Hubbard tank, in which the patient's burns are cleaned, exercised, and re-dressed, may be a source of pain. The second territorial nest is the burn patient's bed, the space in which he spends all of his day either sleeping, eating, or watching television. Hopefully, he associates his bed more with pleasure than with pain. The burn patient's ability to make territorial claims will come slowly. He may even be able to ambulate around his bed.

The patient in the hemodialysis unit walks into the unit, gets a bed, submits to blood work, and then is connected to a hemodialysis machine, which has been maneuvered next to his bed. He has a nurse who will spend the next six to eight hours supervising him and his machine. He can see the entire unit and knows where the other beds and the nurse's station are located. Since he will only be in the unit for a relatively short period of time, he needs only a few personal environmental props—a magazine, a book, or his glasses. The only environmental prop within the immediate territory is the hemodialysis machine. Once the dialysis has been completed, the patient is free to return home.

The patient in isolation will be in a closed space. His territorial adaptation may be very similar to the critically ill patient in ICU and CCU. Depending on the severity of the patient's illness, he may be able to walk around and can lay territorial claim to his room. However, if he is on complete bed rest, he will have only visual spatial orientation. Like the critically ill patient in ICU and CCU, the isolation patient may also be surrounded by equipment or environmental props.

Antecedent Factors

Body factors involve intrusion into the individual's intimate territory. Intrusion also applies to antecedent factors. Antecedent factors of territoriality and space refer specifically to intrusion by others into the patient's personal territory and space. Most critical care patients are likely to experience feelings of intrusion, which begin the moment they arrive in one of these units. The patient has very little time to recover between tests and examinations. Subjected to intrusive procedures by one health worker after another, many patients become angry. As Minckley (1968) has pointed out, "in every individual the readiness to fight is greatest in the middle of his own territory; it is there he has the greatest chance of winning" (p. 511).* This may expain why some patients become angry with repeated questions upon admission to ICU or CCU. Most patients react by quietly submitting to the intrusion, perhaps because "when a man's territorial defenses are weakened or intruded upon, his self-assurance tends to grow weaker" (Fast 1970, p. 53).

The patient feels intruded upon by procedures and by pieces of equipment. If a patient in an open-area unit has several pieces of equipment around his bed, the equipment is likely to infringe upon neighboring territories. The patient intruded upon in this manner may react by closing his eyes, moving to the edge of his bed away from the equipment, or curling up on his side while turned away from the equipment. The patient who turns away or

*Copyright, American Journal of Nursing Company. Reprinted, with permission, from *American Journal of Nursing.*

moves closer to the side rail opposite the equipment is attempting to increase his territorial or spatial distance. This is nonverbal protection from territorial intrusion. A verbal defense might be anger and yelling directed at his nurse: "Get that junk away from my bed!"

The burn patient, like the CCU or ICU patient, feels intruded upon immediately after his arrival in the hospital, but he will have only one or two "intruders." In addition to people intrusion, patients in CCU, ICU, or burn units are also exposed to numerous procedural intrusions. Their personal territories are intruded upon by needles, wires, tubes, or pieces of diagnostic equipment. Even various necessary diagnostic tests, such as X-rays, EKG, and EEG, may be looked upon as intrusive.

The patients in hemodialysis and isolation possibly feel less territorial intrusion than patients in other critical care units. A hemodialysis patient is connected to the dialysis machine, which becomes the object of intrusion. Instead of drawing blood specimens from the patient, his nurse obtains them from the machine. The isolation patient has his own personal territory, a private room. Depending on his reason for being in isolation, the patient may wish to be intruded upon. Since it takes time to gown, the nurse may choose to talk to her patient from the doorway or not at all. Therefore, the patient may want someone to enter his room simply to talk.

Both the dialysis and isolation patients have little opportunity for privacy. Privacy and freedom from frequent territorial intrusions provide the patient with a feeling of autonomy. According to Pastalan (1970), without privacy there is no individuality. Who can know what he thinks and feels if he never has the opportunity to be alone with his thoughts and feelings.

Organism Need States

If a patient is out of his own personal territory, he has additional territorial needs. Institutions or hospitals interfere with all four functions of territoriality. There may be little or no privacy and the patient may feel insecure. The critical care patient has little control over the environment, intrusive procedures, or unit policies. All of these factors work against the individual's self-identity. The patient's needs in all critical care units are psychological and physiological in nature. The needs for protection, dominance, status, affection, and touch are all associated with the use of space and with territorial phenomena. The boundaries of the territories remain reasonably constant, as do the locations for specific activities within the territory, such as sleeping, eating, and nesting. Humans have created material extensions of territory as well as visible and territorial markers. Objects such as the radio, television, and telephone become an extension of the patient, but in open critical care units, where space is a problem, these extensions are not always available. The exception might be in isolation or burn units, where diversional activity is vital to the patient's psychological well-being.

Although the critically ill patient may need privacy, it is not always obtainable. Nursing and medical staff frequently intrude into the patient's personal territory in order to meet his need for protection; in meeting one need, they may be violating another need.

Personal space is another aspect of territoriality and organism need state. As stated earlier, personal space is the space a person carries around with him and does not want invaded. People differ in the size of the personal space "bubble" that is comfortable for them. Some patients tolerate and like the closeness of health care members whereas others do not. The patient's particular reaction is dependent upon who is coming close and for what purpose.

The patient also needs his family and friends at his time of crisis. In critical care units, visiting hours are limited, and only the immediate family is allowed to see the patient. By limiting the number of people visiting and the time spent with each visitation, the staff protects the patient from additional fatigue and stress. The patient may sleep through his wife's visitation and awaken to wonder why she has not visited. On the other hand, the patient may realize that his wife is sitting in the visitor's lounge. Because he cannot see her, nor she him, they quietly worry about each other. Therefore, the two need to be kept informed as to how each other is doing.

NURSING ASSESSMENT OF TERRITORIALITY PROBLEMS

The critical care nurse assesses territorial and spatial problems through the patient's behavioral response. The responses are manifested as regulatory behaviors and/or cognitive behaviors.

Regulatory Behaviors

The regulator system involves stimuli from the external environment and from changes in the internal state of dynamic equilibrium. The regulatory behaviors are physiological responses. In assessing territorial and spatial behavior, the nurse should keep in mind that physiological responses may be limited to behaviors associated with those occurring when one feels threatened or intruded upon.

Regulatory Behaviors
Increased heart rate
Increased blood pressure
Increased respiratory rate
Diaphoresis
Muscle tension

Cognitive Behaviors

Most of the behaviors associated with territoriality and spatial problems involve the cognator system. The cognator system involves input from both the internal and external stimuli. The stimuli include both psychological and social factors. As stated before, the specific aspects of the cognator mechanisms consists of perceptual/information processing, learning, judgment, and emotion.

Hayter (1981) notes that the greater the degree of an individual's psychological competence, the less his behavior will be affected by change in the immediate environment. Likewise, the less psychologically competent he is, the more vulnerable he is to his environment. There is increased stress and anxiety when the person's territory is threatened, thereby decreasing the individual's tolerance for stress. Because the patient's personal space is invisible, the nurse must make inferences about his cognitive response by such behaviors as facial expressions, body language, gestures, tone of voice, and visual contact.

The patient who is unable to tolerate repeated territorial intrusions can hallucinate. Hallucination and passivity phenomena probably signify the residual and the failure of the organism's attempt to externalize its problem in order to better control them.

Patients may use environmental props—objects and arrangements of objects in space. We have earlier referred to environmental props as various pieces of equipment around the patient's bed that give the impression of acute illness. The patient may bring his own environmental props in order to mark off his territory. Patients may exhibit a broad range of response to territorial intrusion, but usually they seem to emphasize verbal, communicative, and reactive mechanisms: argument, discussion, pleas, anger, and other forms of verbal behavior. The person who is ill reacts to crowded territory differently from the way he reacts when he is well. Two patients who have had the same type of operation may be lying side by side in the critical care unit. One of the patients suddenly develops a complication. The other patient may then fear that the same complication, which he does not understand in the first place, may happen to him. Therefore he reacts by demanding close attention and additional nursing care time. Such a patient is often labeled as demanding. He may simply be asking for someone to be with him because his own personal fear of being alone may suddenly have intensified.

Patients in critical care units may also use gestures, facial expressions, and other forms of nonverbal behavior. When their personal territory is intruded upon, patients also use weapon props for reactive purposes. Occasionally patients have thrown their flowers against the wall or floor out of anger. The patient who is intruded upon while reading his book may slam it shut out of frustration.

NURSING DIAGNOSIS
OF TERRITORIALITY PROBLEMS

The nursing diagnosis is a statement of the specific problem affecting the critically ill patient. It is based upon the regulatory and cognitive behaviors observed by the nurse. In this instance, the nurse assesses the patient's immediate environment for evidence of territorial or spatial intrusion and regulator or cognitive behaviors. Based upon the data collected, the nurse can diagnose territorial or spatial behavioral alteration. Furthermore the nurse can identify stress in the patient's environment which contributes to feelings of intrusion.

NURSING INTERVENTIONS AND USE OF PROXEMICS

It is important for nurses in critical care to obtain information from the patient or family about territoriality needs when doing a nursing assessment. The nursing history may contain a few questions that provide general information regarding territoriality needs. It is important to learn how the patient responds to territorial intrusion. Patients have feelings of anxiety when intrusions in their territories occur. Their reactions can result in active defense or flight.

The relationship between space and a feeling of freedom has potential therapeutic significance. As Hall (1959) notes, "Spatial changes give a tone to communication, accent it, and at times even override the spoken word. The flow and shift of distance between people as they interact with each other is part and parcel of the communicative process" (p. 160). Horowirtz (1965) points out a less dramatic although more significant therapeutic possibility in "the nurse's everyday use of space as a message system to convey her attitudes and intentions to the patient. For example, support may be given to a patient who is feeling isolated and estranged by moving closer. On the other hand, the patient's personal space must be respected and no unwanted intrusion made" (p. 27).

A willingness to be somewhat close in space conveys the message of a desire to be close in other human-to-human transactions. Such a message may serve to quiet the restless and agitated patient as well as to support one who seems to be withdrawn.

A person's sense of space has a bearing on his ability to relate to other people, to sense them as being close or far away. Hall (1966) has coined the word *proxemics* to explain this sense and has identified four distance zones commonly used by people: intimate, personal, social, and public. The nurse working in critical care units can use all but public distances.

Intimate Distance

At intimate distance, the presence of the other person is unmistakable and may at times be overwhelming because of the greatly stepped-up sensory inputs. Sight, olfaction, heat from the other person's body, sound, and feel of breath all combine to signal unmistakable involvement with another body.

There is a close and far phase of intimate distance, and the nurse working in critical care units moves between them. Because the nurse does technical procedures to her patient, she enters into close-phase intimate distance. The nurse has become accustomed to forcing her presence on the patient at those times that best suit her own schedule. For example, it is traditional to bathe a patient in the morning. The patient, however, may normally take his bath in the evening. The nurse should be flexible and decide with the patient upon a time that meets his needs, not hers. Also, the patient may have had a difficult or sleepless night in which he suffered many intrusions into his territory. Consequently, he wants to sleep rather than be further intruded upon with a bath. The nurse may choose to give her patient a relaxing backrub to help reduce his tension so that he can sleep.

The close phase involves touch and manipulation of the patient's skin. This can be reassuring and pleasurable to some patients. Again, the bath is a good example. If the nurse is unhurried in her approach, she can use this time to talk with her patient, get to know him as a person, and attempt to relax him. Usually this particular time of the day is utterly chaotic. Nurses seem to compete with one another to see how many patients can be bathed before the 8:30 A.M. breakfast trays arrive. Needless to say, nurses usually end up with more water and soap on them, the beds, and the floor than on their patients.

When the patient makes a vigorous resistance to invasion of territory, it means that his territoriality is threatened. Patients, including those in critical care, resist invasion of their personal space by looks, moving away, pretending to be asleep, or merely by not answering when spoken to. The nurse needs to become sensitive to nonverbal and verbal clues that a person's personal space is being invaded against his wishes. On the other hand, the nurse is also sensitive to clues that a particular patient desires closeness (Hayter 1981).

If the nurse makes frequent intrusions upon the patient's intimate territory, he may react with hostility or anger. For example, a nurse may take her patient's CVP and leave him in order to check another patient. In ten minutes, she returns to take his blood pressure; having completed this task, she leaves him to answer the phone or to answer a doctor's question. Ten minutes later, she reenters his territory to take his TPR. Each time she enters into her patient's intimate territory, she disturbs him. The patient may just begin to relax and fall asleep when his nurse returns to perform another technical procedure. Such repeated and disorganized intrusion can make patients angry and nervous.

Unnecessary intrusion into the individual's territory can be avoided by showing respect for a person's claim. The nurse assesses factors in the patient's environment that lead to a positive adaptation. Simple gestures such as introducing one's self, addressing the patient by name, asking preferences, not leaving the patient physically exposed, minimizing time spent in body contact, and explaining treatments all help to establish territory and reduce intrusion (Bullock-Loughran 1982).

Instead of moving in and out of the patient's intimate territory frequently, the nurse can enter once and thoroughly accomplish her nursing goals. This means the nurse's actions should be organized and purposeful. Once the nurse has made her overall intimate-level assessment, she can observe and assess changes in the patient's status from a distance. Observing and assessing from a distance takes a greater degree of nursing skill. Too frequent intrusions into the critically ill patient's intimate territory cause stress and fatigue.

Nurses sometimes follow the doctor's orders without exerting their own professional judgment. For example, the doctor may order vital signs to be checked every hour. In doing so, the critical care nurse observes that the patient's vital signs are stable and have been consistently stable for the past several hours. She can independently decide to observe the patient closely and depend upon her eyes and judgment rather than unnecessarily intruding upon her patient. The nurse must assess the appropriateness of frequent intrusions into her patient's intimate territory and must prepare the patient before intruding uninvited. All too often, we feel that our uniform gives us the right to intrude into a patient's environment. We forget to ask permission to intrude on our patient's intimate territory.

Immediately after the patient's arrival in critical care, he needs time to adjust to his new territory. At this time, the nurse should use intimate far-phase distance, a distance of 6 to 16 inches. At this distance, the patient can see, touch, and hear his nurse. She does not touch him, because in all probability he has just come from the emergency room or Hubbard tank, where much intrusive touch has taken place. Instead, she can use this initial time to orientate the patient verbally to his spatial and territorial surroundings. If the patient appears to be relatively stable, the nurse can talk to him. She can attempt to give him an opportunity to recover psychologically before proceeding with her intrusive tasks. Furthermore, a personalized nursing care plan developed in collaboration with the patient makes him feel in control of the situation.

The nurse may include the patient's family in the orientation process. By orientating the family and the patient simultaneously, the nurse saves herself time that could be better spent with the patient. In addition, family inclusion gives the nurse a chance to assess the family relationships, to find out what further teaching they may need, and to judge their level of anxiety. Family members will have much more positive feelings toward a critical care unit if they are briefed about staff expectations of them. While the family and patient are together, the nurse may spend time taking a brief nursing history. She should discuss the patient's personal habits and find out whether he has had previous hospitalization. She can also ask if her patient has insurance in order to cut back, if need be, on unnecessary laboratory expenses. While obtaining the history, she can take the time to explain some of the routines and together the family, patient, and nurse can decide where the patient fits into that routine. Once the nurse observes that her patient has relaxed, she can explain his cardioscope's purpose and safety alarm device. After the explanation, she can ask permission to connect his cardioscope leads, moving now from intimate far-phase to close-phase distance. When she has applied the leads, the nurse can return to intimate far-phase distance. The nurse can continue in the same manner until all the necessary intrusive procedures have been accomplished, and she can coordinate the intrusion of any auxiliary people.

Intimate far-phase distance can be used when working with aged patients in critical care units. If the aged patient has visual and hearing failure, communication at intimate far-phase distance is usually effective. It permits the patient to see the provider of his care, and it is conducive to the use of first names, if such is the preference of the patient. A nurse can ask permission to call her patient by his first name, in order to avoid intruding.

According to Trierwailer (1979), when an individual has no private time or space, there is no opportunity to get in touch with the self in order to maintain that sense of identity. When privacy is lacking, the personality tends to become diffused and disorganized.

Personal Distance

Hospitalization in critical care may result in losses of personal identity and autonomy and in a feeling of social isolation which leads to depersonalization. Depersonalization is conceptualized as the depreciation of self-concept or the loss of personal identity (Johnson 1979). The ability to exercise choice is experienced in any privacy situation as the ability to choose how and in what circumstances and degree the individual is to relate to others (Laufer and Wolfe 1977).

Personal distance is the distance that consistently separates the members of noncontact species. It might be thought of as a small protective sphere or bubble that an organism maintains between itself and others. Close-phase personal distance is 1½ to 2½ feet. At this distance, one can hold or grasp another person. Where people stand in relation to each other signals the nature of their relationship, how they feel toward each other, or both. For example, the nurse working in isolation may choose to stand in the doorway and talk to her patient rather than putting on a gown in order to move into personal close distance. By standing in the doorway, she nonverbally communicates that she either does not have the time or the interest to enter into his territory.

At personal close distance the patient can reach the environmental props located on his nightstand. However, he may not be allowed to reach his nightstand if, for example, this activity would increase his need for oxygen, which in turn would cause an increase in the workload of his already injured myocardium. The activity could also potentiate gastrointestinal bleeding or dyspnea in the pulmonary patient. The patient's environmental props should be arranged on top of his nightstand, so that he can see his glasses, pictures of his family, cards, flowers, and his watch. The environmental props may be his only reminder of home. Nurses can encourage the family to bring environmental props, such as drawings from the patient's children or grandchildren, that can be taped to the wall. This reassures the patient that he is not being forgotten. The nurse can give the patient's wife something from the hospital for the children or grandchildren, so that communication continues. In addition, the nurse can remember to keep the patient's nightstand close to him rather than out of reach in an unobservable corner. If the patient cannot reach his nightstand due to the seriousness of his illness, he may request that his environmental props be placed in bed. This is particularly true of the aged patient. Nurses may find tissues, books, dentures, and food in bed, wrapped in a tissue, and they can respect this quest for security.

Personal close distance involves two components, namely, visual access and visual exposure. *Visual access* is the ability to monitor one's immediate spatial surroundings by sight. A person's visual access in the critical care unit establishes the range of opportunities available for synchronizing his own behavior with the behavior of others who share the same environment. The amount of information he incorporates from the immediate surroundings can determine the number of potential interpersonal relationships from which he can choose and the number of cues available for anticipating changes in those relationships. Enabling the patient to maintain visual surveillance of the physical surroundings provides him with the means for identifying the range of behaviors which are acceptable. Depending upon where the patient's bed is located, the amount of information acquired through visual surveillance may be limited. *Visual exposure*, the second component of personal close distance, is the probability that one's behavior can be monitored by sight from one's immediate physical surroundings. It is a function of visual barriers such as equipment, bottles, curtains, or people; space; and, illumination levels relative to one's own position (Archea 1977).

It is at close-phase personal distance that the nurse can sit beside her patient and talk. Either the patient or the nurse can touch the other. By sitting within the patient's personal territory, the nurse communicates an interest or desire to be there. It is at this time that the patient may choose to blow off emotional release from his problems. When the nurse sits, she gives her patient her undivided attention. She communicates that she has the time and wants to share it with him. If the nurse were to stand over the patient, she might communicate a domineering effect. To assure her patient further of a genuine interest in listening to him, she may pull the curtains or shut the door, telling other staff members that the two want to be alone.

Far-phase personal distance is a distance of 2½ to 4 feet. Four feet is sometimes the distance between patient beds in an open critical care unit. The distance may become smaller if equipment fills the space. Keeping someone at arm's length is one way of expressing the far phase of personal distance. "Arm's length" in an open unit may only be accomplished by pulling the artificial boundaries or curtains. Curtains can be pulled along each patient so that all maintain a sense of personal distance or privacy. The nurse can make sure that equipment does not intrude into the territory of other patients. Again, if possible, curtains can be pulled around the critically ill patient to encompass all of his equipment. If the patient is at the end of an open ward against a wall, the majority of equipment can be placed against that wall to protect the other patient from intrusion.

Social Distance

The social distance ranges from 4 to 12 feet. In most open CCU, ICU, or burn units, there is a glass barrier or screen separating the nurses' station from the patient. In some open units, the nurses' station can be closed off from the patients. Patients and nurses can still see each other, but they are unable to hear what is being said. When there is a lull in the pace, the nurse may want to retreat into the heart of her own territory, the nurses' station. The distance between both patient and nurse then becomes far-phase social. By remaining in the glassed-off nurses' station, the nurse can peek into the patient's personal territory. The patient may view this as a type of intrusion, but he will certainly prefer it to constant physical intrusion.

People are social beings and can give their best only when the social part of their being is balanced with privacy. People must have the opportunity to acquire time and space that is under their own control in order to renew their sense of identity (Trierwailer 1979).

As mentioned earlier, one of the functions of territory is proper spacing. Ideally, there can be a social distance of 7 to 12 feet between each patient's bed in an open unit. This is approximately the space available in a closed unit. The nurse is usually the best person to decide where a patient belongs in the critical care unit. It stands to reason that one would not assign a critically ill patient with several pieces of equipment next to a less critical and more alert patient. The latter patient would most certainly feel territorial intrusion. One can place the more critically ill patients next to each other. The space around their beds will be crowded, but they will be less aware of territorial intrusion by each other.

At close-phase social distance, the nurse can remember to knock before entering. If the patient asks for his curtain to be pulled around him and and then asks his nurse to leave, she can treat that territory as she would his home. Before opening his curtains, the nurse can seek permission to enter.

Another way of strengthening the patient's social territory is through development of territorial expertise. Strengthening territory of expertise is accomplished by giving the patient a feeling of achievement, for example, by encouraging him to teach another patient with a similar problem. A patient who recently experienced coronary bypass surgery is able to share positive experiences with patients about to have the same surgery. Experimental knowledge is many times more valuable to patients than theoretical material obtained through a preoperative teaching program.

NURSING EVALUATION

The critical care nurse assesses regulatory and cognitive behaviors supporting the diagnosis of territorial or spatial problems. The nurse knows that people who come together in the bounded setting of hospital units experience a common set of problems, among the most significant being the assignment of space to the occupants. Nursing interventions are designed to reduce territorial or spatial intrusion and facilitate feelings of privacy.

The nurse evaluates how hospitalization interferes with feelings of territorial or spatial control. Nurses are in a position to reduce territorial intrusion and increase territorial control.

SUMMARY

The concepts of territoriality, space, and privacy are gaining more recognition in critical care units. Patients frequently voice complaints about intrusion into their personal territory either be equipment or by hospital staff. Because the nurse works daily in the critical care unit, she may feel possessive about the total territory, including the space in which her patient is located. She may temporarily forget to knock on the patient's door or to announce herself outside the curtains before entering his territory. The patient needs to feel that his bed or private room is his territory.

It is our opinion that all critical care units should be closed units. In a private room, a patient has the feeling of dominance, status, and privacy. The territory and space around his bed is his; he does not share it with another patient. He may feel a sense of protection from intrusion. Closed critical care units can be monitored by closed-circuit television. The patient knows he is being observed, and he may feel that it is a form of intrusion, but he will prefer the decrease in the frequency of physical intrusion. After all, if he were sick at home, he would spend the time sleeping and resting.

REFERENCES

ARCHEA, JOHN, "The Place of Architectual Factors in Behavioral Theories of Privacy," *Journal of Social Issues*, 33, no. 3 (1977), 116-137.

BLOCH, DOROTHY, "Privacy," in *Behavioral Concepts and Nursing Interventions*, ed. Carolyn Carlson and Betty Blackwell, pp. 226-239. Philadelphia: Lippincott, 1978.

BULLOCK-LOUGHRAN, PATRICIA, "Territoriality in Critical Care," *Focus*, October-November 1982, pp. 19-21.

CARPENTER, C. R., "Territoriality: A Review of Concepts and Problems," in *Behavior and Evolution*, ed. Anne Ross and George Gaylord Simpson, pp. 224-249. New Haven, Conn.: Yale University Press, 1968.

DAVIS, ANNE, "Micro-Ecology: Interactional Dimension of Space," *JPN and Mental Health Services*, 10, no. 1 (January-February 1972), 19-21.

DUBOS, RENE, *Man Adapting*. New Haven, Conn.: Yale University Press, 1965.

FAST, JULIUS, *Body Language*. New York: M. Evans, 1970.

GIOIELLA, EVELYNN, "The Relationships between Slowness of Response, State Anxiety, Social Isolation and Self-Esteem, and Preferred Personal Space in the Elderly," *Journal of Gerontological Nursing*, 4, no. 1 (January-February 1978), 40-43.

_____ , "Give the Older Person Space," *American Journal of Nursing*, May 1980, pp. 898-899.

HALL, EDWARD, *The Silent Language*. New York: Doubleday, 1959.

_____ , *The Hidden Dimension*. New York: Doubleday, 1966.

HAYTER, JEAN, "Territoriality as a Universal Need," *Journal of Advanced Nursing*, 6 (1981), 79-85.

HOLL, R., "Identities in Nursing: A Territorial Issue," *Supervisor Nurse*, August 1980, pp. 25-29.

HOROWITZ, MARDI, "Human Spatial Behavior," *American Journal of Psychotherapy*, 19, no. 1 (January 1965), 20-28.

JOHNSON, FREDDIE, "Response to Territorial Intrusion by Nursing Home Residents," *Advances in Nursing Science*, 1, no. 4 (July 1979), 21-34.

KLOPFER, PETER, and DANIEL RUBENSTEIN, "The Concept Privacy and its Biological Basis," *Journal of Social Issues*, 33, no. 3 (1977), 52-65.

LAUFER, ROBERT, and MAXINE WOLFE, "Privacy as a Concept and a Social Issue: A Multidimensional Developmental Theory," *Journal of Social Issues*, 33, no. 3 (1977), 22-42.

LYMAN, S., and M. SCOTT, "Territoriality: A Neglected Sociological Dimension," *Social Problems*, 15 (1967), 236-249.

MARGULIS, STEPHEN, "Conceptions of Privacy: Current Status and Next Steps," *Journal of Social Issues*, 33, no. 3 (1977), 5-61.

MAXWELL, ROBERT, JEANNE BADER, and WILBUR WATSON, "Territory and Self in a Geriatric Setting," *The Gerontologist*, 12, no. 14 (Winter 1972), 413-417.

MINCKLEY, BARBARA, "Space and Place in Patient Care," *American Journal of Nursing*, 68, no. 3 (March 1968), 510-576.

PASTALAN, LEON A. and DANIEL H. CARSON, *Spatial Behavior of Older People*. Ann Arbor, Mich.: University of Michigan Press, 1970.

PLUCKHAN, MARGARET, "Space: The Silent Language," *Nursing Forum*, 7, no. 4, (1968), 386-397.

PROSHANSKY, HAROLD, WILLIAM ITTELSON, and LEANNE RIVLON, "Freedom of Choice and Behavior in a Physical Setting," in *Environmental Psychology: Man and His Physical Setting*, p. 173-183. New York: Holt, Rinehart and Winston, 1970.

RAWNSLEY, MARILYN, "The Concept of Privacy," *Advances of Nursing Science*, 2, no. 2 (January 1980), 25-31.

REID, THEODORE, "Space, Territory and Psychiatry," *Mental Health Sociology*, 3 (1976), 77-91.

SONNENFELD, JOSEPH, "Variable Values in Space and Landscape: An Inquiry into the Nature of Environmental Necessity," *Journal of Social Issues*, 22, no. 4 (1966), 74.

STEA, DAVID, "Home Range and Use of Space," in *Spatial Behavior of Older People*, ed. Leon A. Pastalan and Daniel H. Carson, pp. 138-147. Ann Arbor, Mich.: University of Michigan Press, 1970.

STRUDER, RAYMOND, "The Organization of Spatial Stimuli," in *Spatial Behavior of Older People*, ed. Leon A. Pastalan and Daniel H. Carson, pp. 102-123. Ann Arbor, Mich.: University of Michigan Press, 1970.

TRIERWAILER, ROSEMARY, "Personal Space and its Effects on an Elderly Individual in a Long-Term Care Institution," *Journal of Gerontological Nursing*, 4, no. 5 (September-October 1979), 21-23.

WESTIN, A. F., *Privacy and Freedom*. New York: Atheneum, 1967.

5

Hostility and Anger

BEHAVIORAL OBJECTIVES

1. Define the terms *hostility* and *anger*.
2. State the two components of anger and hostility expression inhibited.
3. Identify the two components of anger and hostility directly expressed.
4. State five regulatory behaviors associated with hostility and anger.
5. Identify four cognitive behaviors associated with hostility and anger.
6. Design a nursing care plan that fosters energy mobilization.

Although all individuals feel anger, each has a different way of experiencing it. Some people yell and throw things while others use blame. Some people turn their anger inward and convert it into depression or transfer it into a body symptom or illness. Finally some people suppress the feelings of resentment and frustration that might threaten their self-esteem (Knowles 1981).

We have all watched a small child constructing a building out of blocks. Once she has finished, she takes tremendous pleasure in its destruction. After deliberately destroying the building by kicking the blocks, the child jumps up and down with great excitement and enthusiasm. The excitement diminishes and the child, once again, gathers her scattered blocks and begins a new building, repeating the cycle several times until she gets tired or bored. To the adult observing this phenomenon, the entire episode seems strange. To the child, the experience has been an acceptable way of displaying her anger.

If an adult were to enter into play activity with the child, he might discourage the child from destroying the creation. Adults want to preserve their energetic and creative endeavors. An adult's gratification comes in construction, whereas the child's gratification comes in destruction. If a child holds her gratification in control, she becomes further angered or frustrated. Her frustration may be directed towards the adult who unintentionally interrupted her normal play activity. The child may hit her adult construction partner, beginning a battle that might end with an angry adult and a crying child. The whole incident seems ridiculous, since both people entered the game with different goals and needs.

Madow (1972) has identified several historical ways in which man has created acceptable social outlets for anger. Often such social outlets have taken the form of sports. In ancient Roman times, gladiators fought for their lives while the spectators cheered. The bloodier the assault, the more excited became the crowd. People enjoyed seeing a human ripped apart by a lion or speared to death by another human. In more recent times, man turned his aggressive hostility toward another socially accepted outlet, sport hunting. The aggression was turned from a human to an animal. In all probability, the hunt was more exciting than the actual kill. Rodeo is another sport in which the beast becomes the focus of attention. It is more a game of skill and endurance than anything else. The cowboy tries to rope a steer or ride a bucking horse for as long as he can. Both are acts of aggression that have become acceptable vehicles for displaying anger.

Finally man turned to other sports such as football, basketball, boxing, wrestling, and baseball. In contact sports, it is one man's body against the other man's. Madow observed that after an aggressive game of football, the hostile impulses of the spectators are unleashed on the football field. The crowd rushes to the goal posts in a destructive attempt to get a souvenir. Spectators at contact sports yell and scream. The more physical the action, the more excited the crowd. Spectators actively yell at referees or umpires. In these sports it is socially acceptable for people to funnel their aggressive energies into hostile screams directed toward an authority figure, the umpire or referee. These authority figures may symbolize a boss, friend, or spouse. The spectator cannot yell, "You dirty bum," at his wife or boss, but he can yell it at the referee or umpire.

In adulthood sports become an acceptable outlet through which man channels his energies. Anger should be converted into something useful or acceptable. The individual who has difficulty finding an acceptable way of directing his energies become more angry and frustrated. Eventually he reaches his limits and explodes. What results is violent behavior. Our newspapers give daily accounts of rapes, beatings, and murders. The individual through anger or aggressive acts inflicts pain on others. Anger becomes the subjective experience that accompanies certain forms of aggression, as a state of physiological arousal that enhances the probability of aggression, or as an intervening (drive) variable that mediates the effects of frustration, on aggression. Anger is the name of an emotional syndrome; aggression—a response intended to inflict pain or discomfort upon another—is a way anger is experienced (Averill 1982).

Maynard and Chitty (1979) note that anger is one of the most universally troublesome feelings experienced by individuals. Due to its powerful nature, anger is difficult for some people to express effectively. The expression of anger can be frightening both to the angry individual and to the patient. The critically ill patient is not immune to the feeling of anger. He resents being sick, limited, disabled, or disfigured. The illness has prevented him from doing all the things he wants to do. A critically ill patient experiences anger in two ways: first, he expresses anger at his illness; second, the illness creates additional hostile or angry feelings within him. The patient may cope with his feelings in one or two ways. He may turn the anger and hostility inwards on himself, or he may externalize it by displacing it onto agents within his environment.

DEFINITION OF TERMS

It is well understood that human beings are very complex individuals. They can experience love and hate for the same object at the same time. A man may love his wife dearly, but he dislikes it when she tells him, "Pick up your shoes!" He responds negatively, not to her, but to her behavior. Children quite frequently enter into love-hate emotions with their parents. Any emotion can be considered potentially destructive. The significant point is in the degree of emotional response. We will define hostility and anger and then apply these emotional responses to the critically ill patient.

Hostility

According to Stearns (1972), hostility is generally a long-lasting affective phenomenon which may persist, once established, without repeated stimuli. This is one essential difference between hostility and anger. Another is that hostility is always directed against a person or persons. Hostility is not directed against a material object and nor against oneself. One can be angry with a nonfunctioning object and with oneself in the sense of frustration. Hostility is often related to aggression although aggression can have constructive significance rather than being purely hostile, just as hostility may be passively rather than aggressively expressed (Kiening 1978). One of the best definitions of hostility is that of Kiening, who defines it "as a feeling of antagonism, accompanied by a wish to hurt or humiliate others, which may produce subsequent feelings of inadequacy and self-rejection owing to loss of self-esteem. This feeling may be repressed or dissociated, or it may be expressed in various kinds of covert and overt behavior" (1978, p. 129).

Hostility as an energy concept can be a motivating force that takes the form of an impulse, reaction, or urge. The energy may be directed in a negative way towards injury or destruction. Furthermore it can be directed towards an object perceived to be threatening. The behavioral response of hostility and anger can be experienced on a conscious or unconscious level. In many instances, individuals do not realize that they are hostile or angry. The behavior of one individual may initiate hostility or angry feelings in another person. The individual initiating the feeling may be totally unaware of his or her own behavior. This is because each individual displays hostility in a unique way. One person may say, "I am upset," whereas another may react more intently by saying, "I am so mad I could kick down the door." The first individual may be controlling his hostility, minimizing the expression of his feeling to a simple statement. The second individual expresses more intensity by expressing her hostility in terms of actions. Both people may have a similar level of hostility, but each expresses it differently.

According to Kiening (1978), "It is seldom possible to assess the degree of hostility present by the directness or the intensity of its expression. Behavior indicative of hostility varies considerably with the individual. Even the ways in which the person acts out his hostility may differ according to the circumstances in which he finds himself and the degree of stress that he is undergoing" (p. 133). An individual who has enjoyed health all his life experiences tremendous stress when he is confronted with illness, especially illness that leads to limitation, disability, or disfigurement. A critically ill patient who becomes burned while starting a barbecue with liquid lighter fluid may feel hostility toward himself for having been so careless. He experiences not only the hostility of illness but also the hostility of self-humiliation.

Kiening (1978) has identified four factors that lead to the development of hostility. First, a person may experience frustration, loss of self-esteem, or unmet needs for status and prestige. The patient experiences frustration in the restriction of illness. His self-esteem becomes threatened as he is thrust into a forced dependency role. If he was a socially prestigious individual who enjoyed self-achieved status, he has difficulty accepting dependent relationships with his doctor and nurse. He may continually inform his nurse of his social significance and become hostile when she does not respond with awe. To the critical care nurse, the patient is no more or less significant than all other patients on the unit. The patient may try to overcompensate for his dependency by frequently informing all concerned who and what he is. His behavior is simply a way to reassure himself and strengthen his bruised or threatened self-concept. The second factor in the development of hostility involves the expectations which the patient has of himself or others. A critically ill patient may place tremendous hope in those providing his care. Because of irreversible pathology, however, they may be unable to restore him to his previous level of wellness. Consequently he will be disappointed that his expectations are unmet. He may also hold certain expectations of himself that cannot be fulfilled. Third, the patient may feel inadequate, hurt, or humiliated. As a result, he experiences hostility. Fourth, he can experience anxiety, which takes the form of anger. Kiening (1978) has identified three different ways in which a patient can respond on an action level, regardless of the factors that have led to his feelings of hostility: (1) repression and withdrawal, (2) disowning the feeling and overreacting by being extremely polite and compliant, or (3) engaging in some type of overtly hostile behavior, either verbal or nonverbal.

Anger

Anger is an emotional defense that occurs in an attempt to protect the individual's integrity and does not involve a destructive element. Aggression, on the other hand, is a negative implementation of anger which is shaped by experiential learning quite distinct from the individual's integrity (Daneish 1977). Anger can be viewed as a derivative of anxiety. Incorporated in the feeling of anxiety is a sense of powerlessness.

Averill (1982) points out that anger has biological, psychological, and sociological functions:

> Anger is defined as a conflictive emotion that, on the biological level, is related to aggressive systems and, even more important, to the capacities for cooperative social living, symbolization, and reflective self-awareness; that, on the psychological level is aimed at the correction of some appraised wrong; and that, on the socio-cultural level, functions to uphold accepted standards of conduct. (P. 317)

Knowles (1981) points out that anger is a relatively automatic response which occurs when the individual is threatened. When the person's hopes, values, safety, or self-esteem are threatened, the response may be anger. As an individual is able to identify his anger, it can be more effectively handled. Patients who automatically react to anger respond with customary thoughts, feelings, words, and in some instances violent acting-out behavior.

Like avoidance and denial, which will be discussed in Chapter 7, hostility and anger can be viewed as normal behaviors within the adaptive process. The critically ill patient ideally moves from shock and disbelief to developing awareness. It is within the developing awareness phase that the patient realizes what has happened. Furthermore, all the anxiety accumulated prior to this time converts to energy. The amount of energy accumulated depends on the degree of anxiety experienced by the patient in the initial crisis. It also depends on the amount of energy output permitted by the patient himself. In other words, if he actively denied his illness for fear of confronting the threat, he may not have realized energy was accumulating.

Any individual under stress situations can accumulate only so much energy before it must be channeled to an output action level. At the output level, the energy can be channeled constructively or destructively. The excess energy can take the form of hostility or anger. Both behavioral outputs result from a series of events in addition to accumulation of energy that begins with an unfulfilled goal. Individuals subjected to severe trauma or psychological stress have reacted in a violent rage. The stressfulness of a situation depends on two sets of factors—the nature of the threat and the resources of the individual to cope with the threat (Averill 1982).

Anger has advantages and disadvantages. Anger that is turned inward can force the critically ill patient into depression. This may serve to impede temporarily the patient's movement toward resolving the loss phase of adaptation. Anger that is turned outward may serve to motivate the critically ill patient. It is as if the patient maintains the idea, "I'll get better in spite of you." Both anger and hostility, within limits, are normal human responses. The fundamental and dynamic force behind hostility is frustration. Likewise, anger reveals a sense of frustration in attempting to achieve a goal that has been obstructed. We have all experienced the normal frustration of driving on the freeway. Imagine yourself in the fast lane of a freeway. You are trying to attend an important meeting that begins in 20 minutes. As far as you can determine, you have at least 20 more miles to go. You feel confident because you are progressing at a safe pace and seemingly will reach your destination and thus your goal on time. At this point of confidence you might begin to whistle or even hum along with the radio. Then suddenly another car pulls in ahead of you. The driver is moving at a less aggressive pace, much slower than your own. This forces you to slow down. His action annoys and frustrates you, so you decide to pass him. As you check the next lane you note a car to your immediate right and one immediately behind you. Now there is no place to go. Time seems to be fleeting, and your frustration level increases. The car ahead to you is obstructing the fulfillment of a desired goal—attending the meeting. The more frustrated you feel, the more anxious you become. As the anxiety increases, you also begin to feel hostile and angry at the individual driving ahead of you. You can cope on an action level on one of several ways: screaming at the driver while waving your fist; honking your horn; tailgating; or cutting ahead of the car to your right. The last two choices could lead to an accident. Possibly the best choice would be to turn on your headlights or honk your horn. But the hostile or angry person is too preoccupied worrying about the obstructed goal to think of safe alternative ways for achieving it. The critically ill patient is no exception. He daily experiences similar frustrations, which lead to hostility and anger.

THE CONCEPTS OF ANGER AND HOSTILITY APPLIED TO THE CRITICALLY ILL PATIENT

Once a threat is felt, the individual utilizes defense mechanisms of fear or anger. These innate defenses are immediate and automatic. Depending on the individual's prior life experiences and endowments, one of the two defenses takes a more predominant position. It should be noted that the two defense mechanisms consist of the following three stages (Daneish 1977):

1. Alert signal, which informs the individual of the potential threat
2. Condition of anxiety, which mobilizes the individual's needed defensive energy

3. Urge for escape or withdrawal and/or desire to attack and thereby eliminate the source of threat

Hostility and anger can be viewed as psychological defense mechanisms. According to Levy (1972) they involve "an unconscious process employed by an individual in order to obtain relief from the anxiety produced by a sense of danger" (p. 401). Both types of behavior can be found within the developing awareness or accepting illness phase of adaptation. This is the time when an individual who has been defined as ill assumes the sick role. In all probability, he has relinquished his attempts at avoidance or denial, and he recognizes his dependency role. The dependency role arouses feelings of regression and powerlessness that create, sometimes unconsciously, additional feelings of hostility and anger. Besides dependency and powerlessness, the critically ill patient realizes the reality of loss. The degree of loss may determine the degree of hostility or anger. The patient may have the feeling that he has lost something of tremendous value.

Loss takes the form of loss of function or of a bodily part. We take our health for granted until a crisis occurs, and we lose a portion of it. Suddenly what we have taken for granted gains preeminence in our minds. A patient who is admitted to a critical care unit for the first time may experience loss of function. The coronary care patient who enters the unit for his third myocardial infarction experiences a partial loss of function. The hemodialysis or burn patient experiences loss of an organ. One has lost his kidneys, necessitating hemodialysis, and the other has lost his protective membrane, his skin. Regardless of the situation, the critically ill patient focuses on the loss and new role created by the loss.

The loss in terms of illness, disability, or disfigurement creates anxiety within the individual. The patient experiencing illness for the first time is subjected to anxieties associated with the unknown. He may not understand what is happening, nor does he know what is expected sick-role behavior. A patient whose illness dictates frequent admissions to critical care units, on the other hand, experiences anxiety of the known. Such a patient may be predisposed toward tension and worry. He may have a need of acceptable channels for dependence on others. His repeated illnesses leave him confused and uncertain about himself in relation to other people and to his life goals. Unfortunately, he may interpret the frequency of admissions as diminishing his chances of ever getting well.

Whether the patient is new to a critical care unit or a repeater, he will experience the feeling of hostility or anger at some point in his hospitalization. This is likely to occur because the patient's integrity has been threatened. Hostility and anger are psychological defense mechanisms that serve to mask the vagueness and powerlessness of anxiety. It is imperative that the critical care nurse identify when a patient is experiencing some degree of anger. This behavior may be difficult to recognize. The patient may make verbal and nonverbal attempts to control, attack, or even injure himself. He may have learned ways of coping that camouflage his true feelings of anger. After all, society forces people to suppress their anger, and they may never learn acceptable ways of handling it. According to research studies, angry behavior is frequently inhibited. Some form of aggressive impulse such as verbal denial, or benefit, and physical aggression is almost universal during anger. Alternately, nonaggressive responses are very common during anger. When provoked impulses toward verbal aggression are experienced about twice as often as impulses toward physical aggression (Averill 1982).

In our discussion of applications to the critically ill patient we will deal with both inhibited and open expression of hostility and anger. A patient who inhibits his anger internalizes, it, and he may express it by indirect means. Open expression of anger appears as an externalized outburst.

Anger and Hostility Expression Inhibited: Internalization

There are two general characteristics of anger and hostility expression inhibited. Both characteristics are similar to those which will be discussed in the chapter on avoidance and denial. The first characteristic is perception of a threat, and the second is location of the agent of harm.

Perceived Threat. Anger results from several major sources. When personal progress toward a goal is blocked, the result is frustration and anger. Anger may also result when a highly valued individual such as the nurse or family member fail to live up to the patient's expectations. The feeling of anger is expressed as disappointment due to difficulty in directly expressing anger toward a significant person (Maynard and Chitty 1979). In this instance a perceived threat exists. The threat perceived consists of a blow to the individual's view of himself. A blow to the self-view may also take the form of illness, disability, or disfigurement. The critically ill patient may perceive the crisis to be more or less threatening than it really is. Thomas (1970) has addressed the role of perception of threat in generating anger:

> A person's perception of a situation directly determines his response to that situation. If the situation is perceived as threatening, anxiety will result. When personal security is disrupted through anxiety, energy is created and transformed into various types of behavior. Manifestations of anger may be the resultant behavior if the person perceives the anxiety-producing threat as one that can or should be managed through overpowering actions or thoughts. (P. 2586)*

Internalization of anger and hostility means that the critically ill patient turns his excess energies inward, because it is socially unacceptable to display anger overtly. He then creates indirect means of coping with anger and hostility. If such defense or adaptive mechanisms are unacceptable to him, he may react by escaping. He avoids his own feelings and withdraws. Accord-

*Copyright, American Journal of Nursing Company. Reprinted, with permission, from *American Journal of Nursing.*

ing to Kiening (1978), the patient's situation may activate threatening memories of childhood dependency:

> Regardless of the types of illness for which the person seeks medical help, the circumstances surrounding the event are usually sufficient in themselves to call forth a high degree of anxiety and/or hostility. He is placed in much the same situation as he was when early childhood experiences first evoked a hostile response. His is again weak and inadequate in a world of powerful authority figures upon whom he must depend to ward off danger or threat; he is painfully aware of his dependent status; his needs for love and approval are intensified by stress; and his very self-identity is threatened by the alien, impersonal world of the hospital. (P. 132)

Mr. E. was a 32-year old sales representative. He had worked in that capacity for six years and had been quite successful in his company. People in his company described him as a handsome, aggressive, dynamic, and pleasant man. His work required that he travel a great deal of the time. His manner and physical appearance, besides his abounding energy, made him successful. Because of his success, he was going to be promoted to head the sales department. This was a promotion that meant less time traveling and more time at home. It also meant he would need to spend extra time training someone to replace himself on the road. A young representative, Mr. F., had been picked for the job. Mr. E. had been supervising Mr. F.'s career and job responsibilities for the past two years. Mr. E. was looking forward to spending more time with his pregnant wife and two sons.

Both men shared a room in an older hotel. Mr. E. and Mr. F. were extremely exhausted from their two-week trip of negotiating and becoming familiar with various executives. Their work involved long hours of preparing summaries of meetings held and issues to be discussed in the next day's meeting. On one such night, both men had worked until 2:00 A.M. Out of physical exhaustion, they decided to go to sleep. At 3:30 A.M., without warning, an explosion and fire occured in the hotel. Mr. E. awakened to find his bed and pajamas in flames. He screamed and yelled for help. People came to his rescue and smothered the flames. The immediate threat he experienced was potential loss of life. He later revealed that before he lost consciousness he feared he would never again see his wife, his unborn child, or his two sons. When he finally regained consciousness, he painfully found himself in a strange location, a burn unit. In the process of awakening, he discovered that not only his surroundings had changed, but also his body had changed. His entire body burned and ached with pain. His eyes were swollen shut, and when he tried to open them he had difficulty focusing on objects. His arms and hands were wrapped with cumbersome dressings, so he could not feel the boundaries of his territory. When he did try to move his hands, the pain immediately curtailed further exploration. His chest ached with each respiration. Lastly, he discovered he no longer could speak. Assessment of his burns revealed second- and third-degree burns of his face, chest, arms, hands, and a portion of his back. Because of smoke inhalation, doctors performed a tracheostomy. Furthermore, his vision was partially impaired due to edema and medication. Besides discovering what portions of his body were burned, the severity of loss caused by the burns, and the possible consequences of the burns, he learned the painful news that Mr. F. had died in the fire.

The nurses noticed that Mr. E. seemed quiet during the next three days. When his wife, who had flown to be with him, visited, they hardly spoke to one another. In between dressing changes and other aspects of care, Mr. E. seemed to sleep or keep his eyes closed. As his nurse was preparing for dressing changes, they had the following dialogue:

NURSE: Mr. E., I am going to change your dressings.
MR. E.: So go ahead, no one is stopping you.
NURSE: Would you like to stop me?
MR. E.: Just go ahead, and get it over with.
NURSE: Okay. If you feel uncomfortable, tell me and we will stop for a while.
MR. E.: Just hurry up. I doubt they do any good, anyway.
NURSE: It is too early to see the progress.
MR. E.: What good will the treatments do? My career is finished. I don't want to talk anymore. (*He closes his eyes in silence.*)

Initially, Mr. E. experienced the threat of death. He consciously and realistically felt the threat. His anxieties revolved around the prospect of never seeing his family again. However, as his hospitalization continued, his anxieties increased, and the threats he felt become less recognizable and more diffuse. An anxious patient, like Mr. E., may realize that his apprehension is illogical, but he usually is unable to identify the source of the threat. The person feels attacked but is unable to act definitely because of the felt diffuseness of the causations.

Anger, as a patient behavior, serves as a mask. When the anxiety is converted into anger, the latter hides the powerlessness, and the tormenting vagueness. Anger may give the patient a sense of power. The burn patient has adaptive responses that are unique to him, but the behavioral adaptation response of a burn patient like Mr. E. to extreme stress or trauma is not unlike that experienced by other critically ill patients. Most patients in a critical care environment do experience feelings of powerlessness, regression, and dependency. Those feelings stem from anxieties caused by threat to self. The patient may be totally unaware that such feelings are causing him to react with anger and hostility.

Mr. Y., for example, was a 62-year-old Japanese admitted into intensive care for the third time in two years with congestive heart failure and pulmonary edema. His condition had steadily deteriorated since his previous admission. Even though he was warned about reducing his work schedule and advised to allow his sons to assume responsibility, he nevertheless could not relinquish control. He had bought a small travel business at an early age and developed it into a large chain of travel businesses. He derived great pleasure from watching the success of his creative endeavors. He was afraid that someone else would not care as deeply as he did for the business. Therefore he worked long hours.

He noticed that each day he became more fatigued and short of breath. Finally, one day the inevitable happened, and once again he found himself in a forced dependency role, a role he obviously disliked and attempted to avoid. The nursing staff remembered Mr. Y. as a very independent, self-directed, and stoic man. He never complained, even though he seemed to have difficulty accepting his forced dependency and limitations. Mr. Y. had a diagnosis of pulmonary edema when he was admitted, but he continued to maintain independence. As he was being admitted to the unit, he took the patient gown out of the nurse's hand and struggled to put it on. When his nurse intervened to help, he pushed her hands away. A day later, the biological crisis had subsided. Mr. Y.'s independence continued to the point of becoming a nursing care problem. If he needed a bedpan, he would not call his nurse. Instead he would reach for his nightstand, move the pan from its drawer, and struggle to place himself on the pan. All of this activity left him short of breath, diaphoretic, and in sinus tachycardia. At this point, he would call his nurse. The nursing staff repeatedly tried to teach Mr. Y. about his immediate or temporary limitations and about his dependency.

In addition to the dependency imposed by the nurse and doctor, the patient's family unknowingly imposed their own type of dependency upon the patient. When they came to visit Mr. Y., they shaved him, washed his face, combed his hair, straightened his blanket, and encouraged him to rest. All the family's concern and attention served to magnify Mr. Y.'s feeling of dependency and thrust him into the adaptive coping response of withdrawal. Like Mr. E., Mr. Y. seemed to sleep when his family visited. The staff also noted that Mr. Y. was becoming more noncommunicative. Here is an exchange that occurred when Mr. Y.'s nurse entered his room carrying a lunch tray:

NURSE: Good afternoon, Mr. Y.
MR. Y.: Hello.
NURSE: Are you hungry?
MR. Y.: No, but put it down, and I'll see what I can do.
NURSE: Here, I'll cut the meat for you.
Mr. Y.: I can do that, just put the tray down.
NURSE: (*The nurse puts his tray down and begins to cut Mr. Y.'s meat.*)
MR. Y.: (*Closes his eyes.*)
NURSE: There, Mr. Y. Have a nice lunch.
MR. Y.: (*Mr. Y. picks at his food and pushes the tray aside. He then turns on his side and goes to sleep.*)

Mr. Y.'s behavioral response was normal for a patient experiencing the threat of dependency. His statement, "I can do that, just put it down," was an attempt to regain control and independence. Instead, his nurse continued to cut his meat. The patient's behavioral response was one of anger. His anger was controlled to the point where it was manifested subtly, by pushing aside his tray.

Both Mr. E. and Mr. Y. reacted with their own type of hostility and anger. Each had their own unique reasons for reacting the way they did. In most instances, all critically ill patients perceive a threat of loss. The threats consist of loss of biological, psychological, and social integrity. Loss of biological integrity consists of those alterations in the homeostatic process that result from illness, irreversible pathology, or trauma.

The encroachment upon an individual's integrity involves a threat to self-image or loss of control and is anxiety-producing. Because of the relative discomfort and vagueness inherent in anxiety, anger emerges as a defense against it. Anger becomes an assertive protection against helplessness and serves as an alternative to anxiety (Moritz 1978). The patient can also experience a threat to psychological integrity revolving around the loss of independence and self-respect. Statements such as, "Go ahead, no one is stopping you," or "I doubt they will do any good," or "My career is finished," or "I can do that, just put the tray down," are frequently heard from critical care patients. Indirectly they signify feelings of bitterness, hostility, anger, hopelessness, and powerlessness. Threats to the patient's psychological integrity suddenly become overwhelming. Such awareness enhances his already existing feelings of anxiety. The anxiety makes any critically ill patient respond in abnormal ways. In the case of Mr. E., the nurse had to realize how devastated her patient felt. Davidson (1973) points out what an important role her response can play in Mr. E.'s recovery:

> To be burned is to suffer one of the most devastating, demoralizing and dehumanizing experiences a human being can survive. The challenge for health care workers is to assist the patient and family to cope with suffering, and to help them find meaning in the experience. There is a person in every burned body, and how this person is treated as he reacts to his injury determines the extent to which he will heal both physically and emotionally, and the adjustments he will make to his crisis. (P. 370)

Mr. E. must also go through the psychological pain of disfigurement or adaptive changes, long hours of agonizing grafting and procedures related to dressing changes, and disappointment over grafting failure.

Any individual in a critical care unit is exposed to enforced illness, which arouses feelings of anger and hostility. According to Kiening (1978), "most adults experience some degree of hostility during a period of enforced illness and hospitalization. The initial reaction to any illness is anxiety, which may be expressed as hostility. The dependency feelings that accompany acceptance of the illness may lead to feelings of hostility if this is the pattern that the patient usually follows in his attempt to cope with the stress" (p. 132).

A patient's cultural background can influence how he reacts to illness, specifically his own. He may withdraw or overreact to illness, its limitations, and the need to be placed in a critical care unit. Culturally, the patient would rather depend upon his family than strangers. Dependence on familiar people is acceptable, but dependence on strangers may be embarrassing. Normally the patient and his family members know their reactions to a crisis such as illness. In addition, the family knows what makes the patient angry or hostile. The nurse, on the other hand, does not. For example, Mr. Y. may be ashamed to depend on his nurse for even the simplest act of eating. Anger as a behavioral response may not be culturally permitted. Therefore, his behavioral response was more subtle. He did not verbalize his anger by saying, "Put that tray down, and get out of here." Instead he nonverbally pushed aside the tray and withdrew into sleep. In this case, the patient turned his anger inward and withdrew. In the Japanese society that constitutes Mr. Y.'s ethnic background, anger or verbal demonstration of disappointment or anger is not acceptable. This is one example of many cultural situations in which there may be a conflict between social and psychological systems of behavior. Anger is often motivated by a desire for personal gain or aggrandizement. This alone may be regarded as sinful. The major conflict with respect to anger would seem to lie within the social system itself. One indication of this is the fact that the failure to become angry upon adequate provocation has often been considered as sinful as the tendency to become angry for selfish ends (Averill 1982).

Illness and the possibility of disfigurement temporarily lead to unfulfillment or obstruction of a goal. Mr. E. believed that because of potential physical disfigurement, his career as a sales representative was finished. Therefore, his goal of achieving higher business and social prominence would be unfulfilled. The obstructed goal and threat to his own self-respect led to frustration, which in turn led to feelings of anger and hostility. Mr. Y. wanted to continue directly managing and supervising his travel business. To do less would mean obstructed or unfulfilled goal attainment. Most independent patients with goals and dreams become frustrated when unable to obtain their goal. Consequently, they react against the enforced illness and dependence.

Janus (1958) has pointed out that exposure to a threat of illness or body damage "tends to sensitize the individual to unacceptable hostile and destructive tendencies in his own aggressive behavior, so that even relatively minor aggressive actions, which are normally tolerated without affective involvement, are consciously or unconsciously felt to be violations of inner superego standards" (p. 54). Patients may continue to speak of being disappointed. "My career is finished," or "I doubt they [dressings] do any good, anyway." The patient may also speak of being frustrated: "So go ahead, no one is stopping you," or "I can do that [cut the meat], just put the tray down." The critically ill patient may be unaware that such expressions represent repressed anger. In terms of continuing affective reactions, the consequences of anger are largely negative. People tend to feel irritable, depressed, and/or anxious after an angry episode. Also, the angry person tends to view the reactions of the target in a negative light. However, the eventual outcome of a typical angry episode is often more beneficial than harmful. There may be changes in the behavior or attitude of the target, to an increase in mutual understanding, or to an increased self-awareness on the part of the angry person of his or her own strengths and weaknesses (Averill 1982).

The nurse can facilitate expression of her patient's feelings by helping him to realize that they are normal. The patient needs to know it is normal to feel angry or hostile that he is not progressing as quickly as desired, or that he must remain dependent on other people. By helping him to see his behavior as normal, she also helps him to see it as acceptable. The nurse should give her patient permission to react to his situation even if the reaction is directed toward the only person in his immediate environment, the nurse herself. Once his anger is expressed, he must be helped not to feel guilt or embarrassment. There are three ways in which the nurse can facilitate expression: she gives him permission to feel the way he does, she explains his behavior in terms of its normalcy, and she alleviates any feelings of guilt. The critically ill patient feels relief in knowing that his nurse is aware of how he feels and actually encourages its expression.

It must also be remembered that in illness the patient seems to regress. Regression can be directly related to the meaning and length of the illness. As previously mentioned, illness is a threat to psychological integrity. In critical care units, illness is sometimes magnified. Nurses move quickly, as if each step is to thwart a disaster. Equipment and strange noises around the patient make him very aware of his illness. In such an environment regression can, as Martin (1962) points out, serve a very useful purpose:

> Regression in itself is neither good nor bad; in illness it is simply inevitable. It often serves a useful function, but at times it can become an obstacle to recovery. If a busy executive has a heart attack and must go to bed, it should be obvious that he cannot, for the time being, carry on at his previous position. This circumstance is beneficial; it allows for rest and the process of healing. (P. 168)

While it may be physically beneficial to the patient, he may not, in time, continue to accept the forced dependency. He may instead express anger or hostility in a verbal or a nonverbal manner.

Threat to social integrity can take several forms. For Mr. E., it took the form of physical disfigurement. He feared that the adaptive alterations resulting from his burns could lead to unpleasant scars. He felt that this would not only change his career potential but that it would also alter his relationship with his wife. Since he was a handsome man, he might have fantasized that she would not love him. He felt the threat of social repulsion by his wife and business associates. Besides feeling his own personal social loss, he may have felt guilty over the death of Mr. F., whom he had picked for the job.

Mr. Y., on the other hand, may have experienced the threat to his social integrity through relinquishing control of his business. Within the Japanese tradition, Mr. Y. felt the social responsibility of maintaining absolute leadership, but his cardiac condition restricted what he could do socially. He could no longer be as independent and self-assertive as before; instead, he had to begin to learn areas of appropriate dependency. This would be true of any critically ill patient with a disability.

Agent of Harm Located. Anger may result when one's sense of authority is threatened. This is a common occurrence in critical care. The critically ill patient may locate what he believes to be the harmful agent; in fact, he may believe that *he* is the harmful agent. Such awareness is enhanced when he looks into the eyes of those he loves. He may feel that he is a burden to his family and to those providing his care. Critical care nurses frequently hear patients say, "My family would be better off without me," "I have been such a burden to my wife," or "I hope my husband remarries when I die." In such instances, the patient internalizes his anger and hostility toward himself. He may be fearful of exhibiting anger to the staff, on whom he depends for his care. The critically ill patient's internalization of anger may be the result of guilt feelings; he may feel guilty for temporarily abandoning his spouse and responsibilities. In addition to internal anxieties, the patient may not be able to cope with external restrictions imposed on him by his illness. He may struggle for independence. Such patients find that becoming dependent upon the hospital staff or family is too threatening.

Mr. T. was 58 years old, married, and the father of three. He was a construction worker. Less than one year previously, he had surgery for a partial bowel obstruction. Postoperatively he did quite well until he developed acute tubular necrosis. The doctors speculated that the complication, prerenal in nature, was caused by perfusion deficit. It was thought that temporary hemodialysis would alter the clinical picture. However, as the weeks progressed it became apparent that Mr. T. had renal failure; consequently, doctors implanted an A-V shunt. After Mr. T.'s discharge, it became necessary for him to enter the hemodialysis unit three times a week. Since Mr. T. was no longer able to work, his wife assumed the financial responsibilities for the family. Mr. T. had tremendous difficulty accepting the various role changes. Mrs. T. described her husband as withdrawn and depressed. She informed his nurses that Mr. T. failed to eat or follow the doctor's orders. The hemodialysis nurses described Mr. T. as passive-aggressive. The following exchange took place between Mr. T. and his nurse:

NURSE: Mr. T., how is everything going at home?
MR. T.: Okay. (*Closes his eyes.*)
NURSE: You seem quiet today. Is there anything you would like to discuss?
MR. T.: Talk. Talk. Talk. Hook me up to that thing so I can get out of here!
NURSE: Do you think that what we have to say is empty talk?
MR. T.: No. What difference does it make? I am just another one of the machines.
NURSE: Is that how you feel?
Mr. T.: What difference does it make how I feel? Let's get this over with! (*He closes his eyes and turns his head.*)

Mr. T.'s depression and withdrawal behavior demonstrated internalized anger and hostility. His comments, "Talk. Talk. Talk," "Hook me up to that thing so I can get out of here," "I am just another one of the machines," and "What difference does it make how I feel?" indicate feelings of powerlessness, anger, hostility, and bitterness.

Maynard and Chitty (1979) believe there are several major hindrances to the uninhibited expression of anger. The patient may fear reprisal, fear of loss, or fear alteration in a relationship. Critical care patients are prone to fear since their well-being rests in maintaining a positive relationship with the nursing staff. Such patients experience concern about what might happen if they antagonize members of the health team. The overall result is internalized anger. When anger is not expressed it becomes internalized. Internalization of anger contributes to stress.

Illness and disability serve to frustrate the individual. He is no longer able to be the principal provider for his family. Besides the restriction of his illness, the role changes serve to further damage his already bruised self-concept. According to Hays (1963), "A blow to the self-view occurs when a person suddenly sees himself more fully, when he grasps the meaning of some dissociated or selectively unattended aspects of experience that are threatening his self-respect" (p. 111). Mr. T. saw himself as dependent on his wife, his nurse, and the machine itself. All these factors forced him to see himself as less significant and as a detriment to his family. His failure to eat, communicate, or follow the doctor's orders demonstrated his lowered self-concept. He may have unconsciously felt that he had minimal social value, so that there was no reason to take care of himself. His own human feelings had been reduced to the level of a machine.

It is apparent that Mr. T. had needs that were temporarily unfulfilled. A patient may feel that no one really cares or wants to understand, and that there is no help within either the self-system or the interpersonal system. Mr. T. experienced an overwhelming sense of disappointment in himself, and like many critically ill patients, he turned his energies inward. It is too threatening to turn them overtly outward; instead, the patient disguises his anger. He may become negative: "What difference does it make how I feel?" The critically ill patient may not choose to strike out verbally but may refuse to eat or follow the doctor's orders, showing passive resistance. Then there are critically ill patients who can directly express their anger. Such expression may be both appropriate and inappropriate.

Anger and Hostility
Directly Expressed: Externalization

If the critically ill patient cannot force the threat away, or if guilt feelings reinforce his anxiety, he may express his anger overtly toward people in his environment. Nurses, doctors, or even family members can become scapegoats of the patient's anger. The external expression of anger and hostility follows a pattern similar to the internal expression of these behavioral responses: first, one perceives a threat; then, one locates an agent of harm.

Perceived Threat. Society often disapproves of outright behavioral expression of anger. Therefore the patient may channel his anger through what one might call demanding or uncooperative behaviors. These behaviors may be a normal attempt to maintain the dignity as a human being in a highly technical impersonal setting. Before a person expresses anger directly, he must perceive a threat. According to Lazarus (1966), "Anger does not occur unless there is threat. The full reaction of anger and attack with all its motor, affective, and physiological concomitants, requires the presence of threat appraisal. The reaction is then regarded as a process of coping with threat" (p. 298).

Anger plays a role in passive-aggressive behavior. The patient's anger may be expressed covertly by obstructionism or ineffective action. Some patients may subtly provoke others to their own disadvantage. This is accomplished through passive and sullen behavior. In many instances, the individuals are unaware of their own aggressive action (Murphy and Schultz 1978).

The threat perceived may revolve around an unfulfilled or obstructed goal. Depending on the significance of the goal to the individual, his behavioral reaction may be slight or extreme. He may express sarcasm, verbal attack, or rudeness. The patient's behavior, according to Kiening (1978), "is usually motivated by fear and a distorted perception of a threat to the self or the self-image" (p. 134). A critically ill patient may be very angry or only slightly angry. Lazarus (1966) has pointed out that "high degrees of threat will be associated with tremendous anger, and the intensity of the behavioral and physiological reaction will reflect the degree of threat. A person may be very frightened or only slightly frightened, and the motor and physiological indicators will also reflect this variation in degree of threat" (p. 298).

Mrs. L. was a 49-year-old patient who had been admitted into critical care units several times in recent years. Three years before, she was diagnosed as having emphysema. Since that time, her prognosis had deteriorated. With each admission, it became increasingly more difficult to wean her off the respirator. Mrs. L. was totally aware of the consequences of her pulmonary pathology. She realized that in time she would be dependent upon a respirator. Furthermore, she realized her husband or oldest daughter could continue to assume major responsibilities for her care and the house. Her energy level and ability to function physically continued to diminish. The threat of dependency on a respirator coupled with visions of a limited future created overwhelming anxiety within the patient. She desperately wanted to watch her children grow and develop into young adults. She realized that this goal would eventually be unfulfilled. Her frustrations and anxiety grew to the point of anger.

Upon Mrs. L.'s arrival in the critical care unit, she was extremely short of breath, confused, restless, and cyanotic. Because of Mrs. L.'s history and the current threat to her physiological integrity, the doctors decided to perform a tracheostomy and place her on a volume respirator. Several hours after the intervention was performed, Mrs. L. fought both her respirator and the tracheostomy. Even though she depended on them both for survival, she continued to fight the nurses for their removal. She frequently banged on the side rails or rang her bell. When the nurses attempted to make her comfortable, she would hit, poke, pinch, or try to bite them. In the process, she would become extremely agitated and angry. The critical care nurses became concerned because they feared a threat to her physiological integrity. Dudley, Wermuth, and Hauge (1973) describe the dangers of anger in the emphysemic patient as follows:

> [The critically ill patient] with severe clinical emphysema who becomes angry may experience severe dyspnea and have a measurable decrease in arterial oxygen tension (PaO_2) and an increase in arterial carbon dioxide tension ($PaCO_2$). These changes are secondary to the increased work of breathing, the increased skeletal muscle tension, and the increased cardiac output which are normal accomplishments of anger and of the pulmonary system's failing ability to supply the air exchange necessary to meet the metabolic demands of this increased energy expenditure. (P. 390)

The nurses were perplexed about Mrs. L.'s status. Biologically, her blood gases had stabilized. When the nurses attempted to wean her off the respirator, Mrs. L. became very agitated, short of breath, and cyanotic. One day, while Mrs. L.'s nurse was cleaning her tracheostomy, the two individuals had the following conversation:

NURSE: Mrs. L., I am going to clean your tracheostomy tube.

MRS. L.: (*Nods her head in agreement.*)

NURSE: I'll deflate the cuff around your tracheostomy tube so you can talk. (*She suctions the patient, gives her oxygen, and deflates the cuff.*)

MRS. L.: (*With her finger over the tracheostomy tube*) Why don't you nurses stop torturing me?

NURSE: Is that what you think?

MRS. L.: Well, aren't you?

NURSE: No, but apparently you think we are.

MRS. L.: (*Screaming*) You can help me by getting rid of all this equipment and let me go home.

NURSE: You are not ready to go home. Do you miss your family?

MRS. L.: Yes. (*She screams the answer, and tears begin forming in her eyes.*) I am a financial burden to my family. I can't stand to watch my husband suffer for me. (*She begins to cry and becomes short of breath.*)

NURSE: (*Reinflating the cuff and placing her on the respirator*) Your husband loves you very much. Naturally he suffers because you suffer. You would do the same. Try and relax. We will talk again later.

MRS. L.: (*Whispers and mouths the words*) Just get me out of here.

As stated earlier, a person perceives threat when a goal is obstructed. An obstructed goal leads to frustration, anxiety, and ultimately anger. Mrs. L.'s goal was to get rid of her dependency on the equipment and return to the safety of her home. She wanted to "get rid of" those pieces of equipment that served to remind her of her illness and her limited future. She, like many other critically ill patients with a physiological disability, is imprisoned by her illness, her fear of the future, and her concern about being a financial burden to her family. Anger, in Mrs. L.'s case, was triggered not only by frustration but also by disappointment, fear, and loneliness. Instead of internalizing her anger and withdrawing into depression, she openly expressed some of her feelings.

Critically ill patients, regardless of the threats to their biological integrity, reach a point where they can no longer internalize their actions. They convert excess anxieties into energy, and the energy must be dissipated externally. When a person internalizes anger, he feels powerless against threats to his biological, psychological, and social integrity. Anger projected externally gives the patient a sense of power. This kind of anger has significance, according to Hays (1963), because it "serves a very useful purpose, if it can be felt and expressed freely, because it usually promotes a pleasant, powerful feeling, which is quite the opposite of the feeling of anxiety for which it is substituted. But it also veils the original threat which gives rise to the anxiety" (p. 110). For some patients, the anger provides a sense of power that enhances the lowered self-respect and motivates the individual to fight the obstacle interfering with his goal achievement. Dudley, Wermuth, and Hauge (1973) point out that when critically ill patients encounter the severe threats associated with their incapacitating illnesses, disabilities, or disfigurement, "they cannot face their feelings or deal with their interpersonal conflicts without endangering their lives. Their rigid avoidance of changes in their emotional state and conflict tends to perpetuate their emotional and interpersonal problems and increase their frustrations, anger and despair with which, in turn, they cannot manage adequately" (p. 392).

Agent of Harm Located. According to Daneish (1977), threats can be either actual or assumed. Furthermore, threats can originate from the external environment as either physical or social threats. The individual can either meet the threatening stimulus and deal with it or disguise it. Some patients use manipulation to control others. In so doing, the passive-aggressive individual can manipulate members of the health team or family by triggering guilt and/or anger.

In order for a person to express or externalize his anger directly, he must identify an agent of harm. It must be kept in mind that the anger or hostility expressed may be displaced onto what the patient believes to be the harmful agent. The agent who is perceived as harmful may only symbolize the true threat. Frequently nurses, doctors, and family members become the scapegoats or displaced objects for the patient's anger or hostility. The patient may either attack or avoid the harmful agent identified. Lazarus (1966) proposes that the perceived strength of the threatening agent will determine which kind of response will occur:

> The location of such an agent does not permit us to tell whether the coping impulse will be attack or avoidance, since both forms of coping require the specification of an object to attack or to avoid. The kind of harmful agent, on the other hand, is crucial. To the extent that the power of the agent to retaliate against attack is great (when the balance of power strongly favors the harmful agent), avoidance and fear will occur. To the extent the harmful agent is comparatively weak against direct attack, attack will more likely be viewed as a viable coping process. It should be pointed out that overcoming the harmful agent does not necessarily eliminate its capacity for harm; otherwise, if it can be easily overwhelmed, there would be no appraisal of threat in the first place. (P. 300)

Anger comes in a variety of forms, such as physical or verbal attack. The direct release of anger requires a strong sense of self-worth for it is usually taboo to focus the anger towards the nurse or physician. However, there are times when the critically ill patient does respond through verbal attack. When verbal communication is not specific to solving the threat, a more aggressive approach occurs. In addition, when physical activity does not remove the threatening stimuli, the patient sometimes turns to verbal attack. Both physical and verbal attack are avoided as long as possible because of external or internal restraints (Moritz 1978; Rothenberg 1971).

In the critically ill patient's mind, the doctor and the nurse may come to symbolize the illness itself. This behavioral response may help to lessen some of the personal disappointment consequent to having an acute illness, severe disability, or serious disfigurement. The individual may feel justified in his anger or hostility, but he may not be able to demonstrate his anger overtly toward the staff. He may fear that if he expresses outward anger toward his nurse or doctor, they may retaliate by not providing him with care. They may symbolize an agent of harm too powerful to overcome, but a family member, one perceived to be comparatively weak as a retaliator, may be next in line to accept the patient's display of anger. The patient may feel safe verbally attacking his spouse, because her role is "to love me no matter what I do or say." Critical care nurses quite frequently overhear a patient making sarcastic or derogatory remarks to his spouse. The spouse leaves the room and tearfully seeks reassurance and explanation from the nurse. The family member should understand that the patient's behavioral response is an attempt to drive the anger-provoking object away. In this case, the object is illness and its obstruction to goal attainment. The patient may feel relief after his energy outburst of anger; however, he may simultaneously feel guilty for having sent his spouse out of the room in tears.

The patient may choose to attack the agent of harm—his nurse—because she is the most dominant individual in the patient's environment. She may not be too accepting of his outbursts. The nurse will probably feel she has done nothing to warrant such a behavioral response. If the nurse fails to recognize the meaning behind her patient's anger, she may feel hurt. Furthermore, she may become equally as angry as the patient, only she may not express it overtly or verbally. Instead she may express her anger nonverbally through avoidance behavior by reducing the time spent with her patient. If she responds with overt anger, the patient's anger may increase to the point of threatening his biological integrity. The nurse who reacts overtly or covertly to her patient's angry or hostile response may reinforce the patient's displacement of the origin of his problem toward the health team.

NURSING ASSESSMENT OF ANGER AND HOSTILITY

The nurse assesses anger-hostility through the patient's behavioral response. Anger-hostility responses can be categorized into regulatory and cognitive behaviors. Regulatory behaviors are the result of physiological changes associated with anger, hostility, or aggression. Cognitive behaviors involve psychosocial changes accompanying anger and hostility.

Regulatory Behaviors

The regulatory system involves stimuli from the external environment and from changes in the internal state of dynamic equilibrium. Regulatory behaviors associated with anger can turn to acts of aggression. The following are anger-related physiological responses or regulatory behaviors:

REGULATORY BEHAVIORS

Increased blood pressure
Increased pulse rate
Increased respiration
Muscle tension
Perspiration
Flushed skin
Nausea
Dry mouth

Other physiological responses involve gastrointestinal, respiratory, skin, genitourinary, arthritic, central nervous system, and circulatory disorders (Madow 1972). Anger turned inward can lead to gastric ulcer or ulcerative colitis. The gastric hyperfunction associated with anger is manifested by increased blood flow, motility, and acid secretion. Another area of the gastrointestinal tract affected by anger is the lower bowel or colon. The individual, who because of internalized anger experiences tremendous stress, may have a lowered resistance to respiratory infection such as colds or asthma.

Repressed anger can also affect the patient's skin. A common dermatological condition is pruritus or itching. A chronic itch causes scratching, which may break down the skin thereby resulting in a secondary infection known as neurodermatitis or dermatitis factitia (Madow 1972).

There are many causes of arthritis with repressed anger being a contributing factor. Some scientists have reported observing rheumatoid arthritis related to emotional disturbance such as hostility. Central nervous system and cardiovascular disorders are also associated with anger. Neurologically the angry individual can experience headache and backaches. Finally circulatory disorders such as hypertension and anger may result from repressed anger. In an individual with coronary artery disease, angina episodes may be precipitated by anger (Madow 1972).

Cognitive Behaviors

The cognator system involves inputs from internal and external stimuli which include psychological and social factors. The specific aspects of the cognator mechanism consists of perceptual/information processing, learning, judgment, and emotion. The cognitive behaviors are psychological responses.

According to Rothenberg (1971) the angry individual experiences an involuntary increase in muscle tension at the same time he perceives a threat. Rather than discharge the energy or tension through flight or fight, the angry individual can utilize verbal attack to remove the threat. The following cognitive behaviors are associated with anger and hostility (Maynard and Chitty 1979):

COGNITIVE BEHAVIORS	
NONVERBAL BEHAVIORS	VERBAL BEHAVIORS
Clenching of muscles or fists	Sarcasm
Turning away	Insulting remarks
Avoiding eye contact	Verbal abuse
Tardiness	Argumentativeness
Silence	Demanding

Physical attack can also occur. The cause of the patient's combative behavior needs to be assessed. Critical care patients who physically or verbally attack the nurse or family do so out of fear. Therefore anger needs to be dissipated regularly through cognitive and behavioral processes in order to avoid accumulation of negative feelings. Releasing anger's energy in socially acceptable ways helps to preserve self-image and reduce angry feelings (Knowles 1981; Averill 1982).

NURSING DIAGNOSIS OF ANGER AND HOSTILITY

The nursing diagnosis is a statement of the current problem. The nurse is able to diagnose anger and hostility through an assessment of various regulatory and cognitive behaviors presented by the critically ill patient. Stressors contributing to feelings of anger and hostility originate from internal and external stimuli. The patient may be angry at himself for becoming ill. External stressors identified by the patient consist of the critical care unit, nurse, family, or even supportive devices. The various stressors combine to cause feelings of anger and hostility.

NURSING INTERVENTIONS: ENERGY MOBILIZATION

The nurse acknowledges that there are numerous ways of expressing anger which on the surface may not appear to be expressions of anger. In order to facilitate effective expression of anger, the nurse must first be able to identify clues to the patient's feelings (Maynard and Chitty 1979). The critical care nurse must be able to recognize anger or hostility and explain its meaning to the patient. She must be able to identify overt and/or covert signs of angry or hostile behavioral responses. What the patient says may covertly camouflage his real feelings. What he overtly says may serve to make the nurse defensive, thus forcing her away from the individual she seeks to help. In facilitating her patient's movement toward resolving the loss phase of adaptation, the nurse must remember two significant factors. First, all behavior is meaningful and goal-directed. Second, anxiety converts into energy, which is subsequently expressed as anger. The anger felt by the individual can serve as a motivator.

Nursing responsibilities consist of helping the critically ill patient channel his internal energies into appropriate external expressions of his feelings. As previously mentioned, the patient can be given permission to feel and express anger. The nurse helps him to identify when he feels anger and the possible reasons why he feels as he does. Talking together can be one constructive way of appropriately channeling energy that might otherwise be converted into anger. When he finds appropriate channels for direct expression of anger or hostility, the patient no longer needs to feel guilty for having such behavioral reactions to the stress of illness.

We have looked at various case studies in which the individual either internalized or externalized his anger or hostility. In each instance the patient directed his anger toward a perceived threat: illness, disability, or disfigurement. The problem, whether it be acute tubular necrosis, congestive heart failure, second- and third-degree burns, coronary artery disease, abdominal aneurysm, or occipital tumor, threatens the patient's sense of biological, psychological, and social integrity. The basic nursing intervention is to recognize the patient's behavioral response. For example, a patient may say, "I am disappointed," "I am frustrated," or, as in the case of Mr. E., "So go ahead, no one is stopping you." Such statements are covert examples of a patient's anger or hostility. Because he may be unable to express his anger overtly, he represses it. Repressed anger can seriously aggravate already-existing threats to biological integrity. The nurse must acknowledge that the patient appears troubled. This conveys the nurse's concern and willingness to help. Regardless of the result, the nurse must be prepared to accept the patient. Furthermore the nurse continues to meet his nursing needs in every way possible (Kiening 1978).

The critical care nurse's goal consists of identification, acceptance-acknowledgment, exploration, and constructive channeling of anger (Self and Viau 1980). The patient's anger is identified by recognizing of verbal and nonverbal cues. Nonverbal expressions of anger such as muscle tension, stiff body position, scowl, fatigue, apathy, depression, and throwing things need to be pointed out. These behaviors can impede the patient's cooperation and constructive involvement in his own care. Therefore his overall recovery is altered. Once the patient is able to identify and verbalize his anger, he will need help to identify realistic goals to handle future anger and hostility. Helping the patient focus on the future tends to reduce tension and facilitate feelings of hope. The patient's involvement in his care needs to be directed toward using his strengths, resources, and potentials. Furthermore the patient can learn to manage any deficiences (Moritz 1978; Self and Viau 1980). The significant point is that the critical care nurse recognize that a particular problem exists. The patient may be unable to express his problem because it concerns personal fears known only to him. Mr. E., for example, may have realistic fears about goal attainment within his company. He may have relied heavily on his physical appearance to sell merchandise. Now that he has been severely burned, he fears disfigurement that cannot be helped through grafting. Mr. Y., already financially established, fears threats to his autonomy. He has difficulty accepting loss of control, power, or independence. Physically, he has become more disabled and limited in his activites. To be dependent upon others both frustrates and threatens his psychological integrity. Mr. T. fears threats to his manliness. His dependency on a hemodialysis machine and his inability to work have made him resent the fact that his wife has to assume financial responsibility. Each patient has reacted to the stress of illness, disability, or disfigurement by withdrawing. In each case, the critical care nurse can provide stimuli to help the patient externalize his ideas or feelings. Just as the nurse recognizes the need to give her patient relief from his physical pain, she also can acknowledge "the need for allowing the patient to ventilate his feelings in order to help him come to grips with the meaning of emotional pain. This assists him to focus on himself as a 'person' rather than a 'victim' who must survive both his crisis and the strange world of a hospital" (Davidson 1973, p. 371).

Next the nurse helps the patient accept his own angry or hostile feelings. The patient needs to know that his anger is normal. Furthermore he may be concerned about feeling angry because he lacks knowledge of effective ways to express the anger. In so doing the nurse recognizes the meaning of her patient's behavior and helps him understand its meaning. Beyond assessing the meaning behind anger or hostility, she must assess her patient's readiness to look more closely at a threatening situation. Her goal becomes that of reducing threats perceived by the patient. She can both reduce perceived threats and help her patient to look realistically at threats of loss. The nurse can help him identify alternative ways of coping with the stress of illness and of fulfilling his goals. Mr. E., for instance, needs honest reassurance that grafting could greatly reduce disfigurement. He also has to identify his own internal strengths and assets. His nurse can point out that it was his enthusiasm, initiative, knowledge, and ability to work with others, rather than his good looks, that made him successful. These attributes still exist. With support and positive reinforcement, Mr. E. can come to the realization that he can still pursue his personal and professional goals.

Mr. Y. needs support in looking at alternative ways of coping with loss of control, power, or independence. Instead of withdrawing into depression, he should see the positive consequences of relinquishing some control over his business. He can shift primary responsibility from himself to his sons, who are already familiar with the business. He can still assist them in decision-making responsibilities and thus maintain a sense of control and powerfulness. The nurse can help him accept a degree of physical dependence on his family. The patient may recoil from the fear of total dependence, but his fear may be unrealistic in the light of what he is still able to do. Therefore, the nurse and his family can identify those areas in which the patient will be taking a less active role. As the patient begins to understand the meaning of his illness and the consequences of future crises, he may recognize these same areas of reduced participation. This does not negate the significance of what he still can do, nor his leadership role within the family. It simply implies that responsibility has shifted.

A hemodialysis nurse can help patients like Mr. T. to maintain a realistic sense of manliness. The patient feels less a man because he is no longer the primary bread winner. The nurse can also help the family identify ways to foster his manly self-concept. Like Mr. Y., he needs to feel significant and needed by others. If his nurse and family allow him to remain withdrawn and depressed, his feeling of lowered self-esteem will increase. Avoidance by the nurse will reinforce his feelings that no one cares or that he is just another one of the machines to be manipulated. The nurse can try to get him actively involved with his own dialysis by teaching him about the hemodialysis machine and his relationship to it. She can encourage him to do as much of the work as possible, while his family can reinforce a manly self-concept by support and attitude at home.

Once the behavior has been identified and accepted, the nurse explores its origin. The nurse helps the patient identify a reality-based source of anger. Knowing the cause assists the patient to understand and to gain some control over the situation. The patient identifies threatening events in the critical care setting and, together with the nurse, alternative ways of reducing the threat are explored (Maynard and Chitty 1979; Self and Viau 1980).

The nurse helps the critically ill patient constructively channel the anger or hostility. The patient becomes involved in actions that will help him release his feelings and give him a sense of managing his situation. The nurse allows the patient to assume as much responsibility as possible in his own care. The overall nursing goal is to reduce aggressive tendencies by cognitive restructuring of the provocative situation. In addition the nurse encourages the anger to be externalized thereby preventing massive internalization and ultimate depression (Maynard and Chitty 1979; Self and Viau 1980).

The critical care nurse must remember that, unlike the above examples, not all behavior can be changed. A patient who recently sustained a severe myocardial infarction realizes the consequences of his illness and the medical restrictions imposed upon him. Nevertheless, he might continue to enjoy heavy smoking, eating, or strenuous work. These decisions become his and his alone. The nurse can serve as a catalyst or motivator toward meaningful change. She must also remember that restorative solutions to the problem may not exist. In other words, a patient may be so biologically decompensated that he will never achieve stability or a level of wellness. She will not be able to help him look at role changes or dependency-independency behavior. Her responsibility may be to help him accept the terminal aspects of his illness. In doing so, she listens to what he verbalizes. The critical care nurse must be prepared to accept direct anger and hostility generated by introspection.

It is not unusual to hear a nurse say, "I don't understand that man. I spent hours talking with him, and all he does is yell at me." The nurse may feel disappointed and frustrated. Like the patient, she can become angry and hostile. Her own reaction may not allow her to understand the meaning of his behavior and why he displaced his feelings on her. Hopefully, the nurse will not become defensive, because if she does so, she renders herself powerless. Instead, she can take the patient's behavioral reaction as a compliment to her nursing care. She has successfully motivated him to change from a withdrawn, passive individual into an active, verbally aggressive person. She has helped him channel his internal energies into outward expression. Once the behavior is externalized, her responsibility is even greater. We should repeat that behavioral responses of anger or hostility may be normal. According to Kiening (1978), appropriate expression of anger is a sign of maturity:

> A person whose needs for growth and self-realization are really threatened is acting in a mature way when he takes a stand for himself. The nurse needs to be perceptive in order to assess what is healthy and necessary for this person. Social pressures within the system still operate all too effectively in silencing the adult who feels aggrieved and angry at his unwelcome—and often unforeseen—situation. (P. 131)

The nurse assumes the responsibility of constructively channeling the patient's externalized energies.

Anxiety, as we pointed out above, converts into energy. An individual can only accumulate a certain amount of potential energy. It must be released at some time and in some direction, and the release may create problems. Overt expressions of anger may create biological problems for the patient. The patient with a decompensated pulmonary or cardiac system cannot tolerate prolonged expression of anger. The potential depletion of stored energy may compromise the individual's ability to perform limited functions, as was illustrated in the example of Mrs. L., who had severe pulmonary involvement. Dudley (1973) describes the special problems of anger in the pulmonary patient:

> Patients severely ill with pulmonary crisis are rarely able to tolerate emotional stress of even a routine nature. . . . Since the muscular system is usually not impaired, feelings of anger, anxiety, and fear which activate the skeletal muscles and places an increased demand on the pulmonary system will drive the arterial PaO_2 lower and the $PaCO_2$ higher. These cannot be compensated by the patient with severe pulmonary disease. (P. 392)

The nurse must therefore establish limits for externalized anger or hostility.

Critically ill patients unable to externalize their anger verbally may do so nonverbally. There are critically ill patients who skillfully remove their wires, tubes, and machines. A patient with an external pacemaker may take out his hostility on the little box sitting on his arm or chest. The hemodialysis patient may attempt to disconnect his A-V shunt, an effort that can even be viewed as suicidal. A patient with severe pulmonary pathology may remove the volume respirator from his tracheostomy tube, and he may even try to extubate himself. Naturally, the critical care nurse cannot accept such behavioral responses. She can acknowledge the nonverbal behavior for what it represents—possible attempts to regain control, power, or independence—and provide care accordingly. The patient discovers that by disconnecting his wires, tubes, or machines, he elicits a response from his nurse. He discovers that such behavior causes her to appear at his bedside immediately in an attempt to prevent a disaster. This gives the patient a feeling of control or power. Such thinking, in all probability, is unconscious, but he does control his nurse in this respect. He may also enjoy all the additional attention and care shown him while he nonverbally externalizes his anger and hostility. Here again the critical care nurse can help her patient look at other ways of coping with the illness and of gaining her attention. The individual has to learn ways that are acceptable to others while simultaneously meeting his own needs. Consequently, a nurse cannot ignore any behavior expressed by the patient. She can examine what this behavior might mean. If both the nurse and the patient share the goal of wellness and stability, then they will direct their energies toward a meaningful outcome.

The critically ill patient needs help in recognizing that his energy outbursts are really expressions of anger and hostility. The first step toward understanding and mastering this behavior is for the patient to admit that he is angry. Next, the nurse can assist him to identify why he is angry. Then she can help him identify the target of his anger. It may be threatening for the patient to admit he has lost behavioral control in becoming angry or hostile.

He may feel guilty or embarrassed. At this point, he needs reassurance that to be angry or hostile is a normal adaptive response to illness. If the patient's anger or hostility was displaced on his family, he will have to explore reasons why such displacement occurred. This is most important, because a family relationship can become badly damaged. A family member may have become defensive and said things that served to hurt the patient. It is conceivable that a fatal complication could occur, thus leaving the family member with memories of that last angry encounter. Such behavior leads to overwhelming guilt. Therefore, the family needs help in understanding the patient's needs. The nurse turns both her own energies and those of the family toward motivating the patient.

NURSING EVALUATION

The nurse assesses regulatory and cognitive behaviors supporting the diagnosis of anger and hostility. Interventions designed to minimize or reduce angry or hostile feelings are evaluated for their effectiveness. Evaluation is measured by the patient's ability to avoid internalizing all feelings of anger or hostility. Furthermore overall effectiveness is measured by the patient's ability to verbally express his feeling of anger, identify the source of his anger, and seek alternative ways of handling the anger.

SUMMARY

The critical care nurse is in a unique position to assist both her patient and his family. She can learn the reasons behind his behavioral responses. She assesses his behavior, helps him to assess its meaning, and motivates him to find appropriate ways of channeling his energy. The nurse must keep in mind that a patient in a critical care unit may not reward his nurse by becoming symptom-free; he may continue to complain of discomfort after all the staff has done. These patients, especially the disabled, may lack warmth and the capacity to relate. Occasionally one finds a patient who relates only on a hostile or angry level. He may never move beyond this level because he has successfully coped, using such behavioral responses, in the past. The nurse can support and reinforce the patient's positive attributes. Regardless of his behavior, she can acknowledge, understand, and try to motivate him toward the affirmative.

REFERENCES

AVERILL, JAMES, *Anger and Aggression: An Essay on Emotion*. New York: Springer-Verlag, 1982.
BROOKS, BEATRICE, "Aggression," *American Journal of Nursing*, 67, no. 12 (December 1967), 2519-2522.

DANEISH, HOSSAIN, "Anger and Fear," *American Journal of Psychiatry*, 134, no. 10 (October 1977), 1109-1112.

DAVIDSON, S. P., "Nursing Management of Emotional Reactions of Severely Burned Patients During the Acute Phase," *Heart and Lung*, 2, no. 3 (May–June 1973), 370.

DUDLEY, D. L., C. WERMUTH, and W. HAUGE, "Psychosocial Aspects of Care in the Chronic Obstructive Pulmonary Disease Patient," *Heart and Lung*, 2, no. 3, (May-June 1973), 390.

JANIS, IRVING, *Psychological Stress*. New York: John Wiley, 1958.

KARSHMER, JUDITH, "The Application of Social Learning Theory to Aggression," *Perspectives in Psychiatric Care*, 16, nos. 5-6 (1978), 223-227.

KIENING, SISTER MARY, "Hostility," in *Behavioral Concepts and Nursing Intervention*, ed. Carolyn E. Carlson and Betty Blackwell, pp. 128-140. Philadelphia: Lippincott, 1978.

KNOWLES, RUTH, "Handling Anger: Responding vs Reaching," *American Journal of Nursing*, 81, no. 2 (December 1981), 2196.

KRAMES, LESTER, PATRICIA PLINER, and THOMAS ALLOWAY, *Aggression, Dominance and Individual Spacing*. New York: Plenum Press, 1978.

LAZARUS, RICHARD, *Psychological Stress and the Coping Process*. New York: McGraw-Hill, 1966.

LEVY, N. B., "The Psychology and Care of the Maintenance Hemodialysis Patient," *Heart and Lung*, 2, no. 3 (May-June 1973), 401.

MACINNES, WILLIAM, "Internal Consistency of the Threat Index," *Death Education*, 4 (Summer 1980), 193-194.

MADOW, LEE, *Anger*. New York: Scribner's, 1972.

MAYNARD, CAROLYN, and KAY CHITTY, "Dealing with Anger: Guidelines for Nursing Intervention," *JPN and Mental Health Services*, 17, no. 6 (June 1979), 36-41.

MORITZ, DERRY ANN, "Understanding Anger, *American Journal of Nursing*," 78, no. 1 (January 1978), 81-83.

MURPHY, PATRICIA, and ELLEN SCHULTZ, "Passive-Aggressive Behavior in Patient and Staff," *JPN and Mental Health Services*, 16, no. 3 (March 1978), 43-45.

PILOWSKY, I., and N. D. SPENCE, "Pain, Anger and Illness Behavior," *Journal of Psychosomatic Research*, 20 (1976), 411-416.

ROTHENBERG, ALBERT, "On Anger," *American Journal of Psychiatry*, 128, no. 4 (October 1971), 454-460.

SAUL, JOSEPH, *The Hostile Mind*. New York: Random House, 1956.

SELF, PAMELA and JEFFERY VIAU, "Four Steps for Helping a Patient Alleviate Anger," *Nursing 80* December 1980, p. 66.

SLATER, P. J. B., *Psychopharmacology of Aggression*, New York: Raven Press, 1979.

STEARNS, FREDERIC, *Anger: Psychology, Physiology and Pathology*. Springfield, Ill.: Charles C. Thomas, 1972.

SUGGS, KATHRYN, "Coping and Adaptive Behavioral in the Stroke Syndrome," *Nursing Forum*, 10, no. 1 (1971), 101-111.

SVARE, BRUCE, *Hormones and Aggressive Behavior*. New York: Plenum Press, 1983.

THOMAS, MARY DURAND, "Anger in Nurse-Patient Interactions," *Nursing Clinics of North America*, 2, no. 4 (December 1967), 738.

_____ , "Anger: A Tool for Developing Self-Awareness," *American Journal of Nursing*, 70, no. 12 (December 1970), 2586-2587.

WHITEHEAD, WILLIAM, BARRY BLACKWELL, HIMASIRI DESILVA, and ANN ROBINSON, "Anxiety and Anger in Hypertension," *Journal of Psychosomatic Research*, 21 (1977), 383-389.

6

Powerlessness

BEHAVIORAL OBJECTIVES

1. Define the terms *alienation* and *powerlessness.*
2. Discuss how physiological, psychological, and environmental loss of control contribute to feelings of powerlessness.
3. Describe how lack of knowledge contributes to feelings of powerlessness.
4. State three regulatory behaviors associated with powerlessness.
5. Identify six cognitive behaviors associated with powerlessness.
6. Design a nursing care plan that fosters powerfulness.

All individuals experience some feelings of power. The manner and frequency with which one arrives at the feeling depends on various factors such as the quality of interpersonal relationships, exposure to adequate role models, learned patterns of how to exercise power and which type to use, and the degree of success achieved in the lower levels. Each individual consciously or unconsciously confronts the issue of power in determining who will define the relationship with another (Wilkinson 1979).

Human beings in the modern world are essentially alone. Put on our own feet, we are expected to stand by ourselves. We can achieve a sense of identity only by developing a unique and particular self to a point where each of us can truly sense "I am I." This accomplishment is possible only if we develop our active powers to such an extent that we can relate to the world without having to drown in it—if we can achieve a productive orientation. Alienated individuals, however, try to relate to the world in a different way: by conforming. They feel secure in being as similar as possible to others. Their paramount aim is to be approved of by others; their central fear is that they may not be approved of (Fromm 1967). Rogers (1948) has stated that the basis of incorporating an event into the self may be the person's awareness of a feeling of control over some of his or her world experience. An individual who has power over objects and persons may make them part of her self-picture. With an extension of the self to include objects and persons comes a feeling of increased self-potency (Rogers 1948). Maslow (1968) has addressed the relationship of persons to their environment as follows:

> The authentic or healthy person may be defined not in his own right, not in his autonomy, not by his own intra-physic and non-environmental law, not as different from the environment, independent of it or opposed to it, but rather in environment-centered terms, e.g., of ability to master the environment, to be capable, adequate, effective, competent in relation to it, to do a good job, to perceive it well, to be in good relations, to be successful in its terms. (P. 168)

Since a generalized expectancy of low control is thought to represent a more or less permanent personality trait in adults, it is obvious that one cannot easily or rapidly reduce a high degree of powerlessness. According to Johnson (1967), comparatively little empirical work has been done on the sources of powerlessness, although a link has been established between social structure and alienation. Hospitalization in critical care involves diminished contacts with significant others and decreased meaningful sensory input. The patient's world shrinks to the point where he feels he is no longer able to make decisions or judgments without distortion. Patients feel forced to relinquish personal views, knowledge, and expertise (Kritek 1981). In this chapter we will examine some of the possible causes of powerlessness, possible behavioral manifestations by the patient as he experiences powerlessness, and possible ways that the critical care nurse might foster a feeling of powerfulness in critical care units. Before discussing the etiology of powerlessness, the term *powerlessness* and other synonymous concepts will be defined.

DEFINITION OF TERMS

In 1959 Seeman pointed out that the term *alienation*, a pervasive theme in classical sociological theory, appears in a number of ways in the literature. His analysis led him to present research definitions for five basic variants: (1) powerlessness, (2) meaninglessness, (3) normlessness, (4) value isolation, and (5) self-estrangement. We will define only three terms—alienation, powerlessness, and meaninglessness—and will use only the first two terms in our presentation.

Alienation

Alienation is a complex, impairing process whereby the individual experiences a loss of awareness and a blurring of the inner emotions as a result of the sum total of his life experiences (Yoder 1977). Alienation involves feelings of estrangement or a sense of basic fragility of human life. There is the threat of nothingness and the solitary condition the individual experiences before a threat (Carser and Doona 1978).

In the last century, Hegel and Marx used the word alienation to refer not to a state of insanity but to a less drastic form of self-estrangement, one that permits a person to act reasonably in practical matters, even though he or she is marked by one of the most severe socially patterned defects. Marx called alienation the condition of man in which his own act becomes an alien power, standing over and against him, instead of being ruled by him. Fromm (1967) similarly defines alienation as a "mode of experience in which the person experiences himself as an alien. He has become, one might say, estranged from himself. He does not experience himself as the center of his world, as the creation of his own acts—but his acts and their consequences have become his masters whom he obeys" (pp. 111–112). According to Goffman (1961), the alienated person is out of touch with himself as he is out of touch with any other person. He, like the others, experiences himself as things are experienced, with the senses and with common sense, but he is not related to himself nor to the world outside in a productive manner.

A developmental perspective implies that alienation, or the lack of ego identity, can be avoided as an enduring personality trait through experiences and relationships designed to assist the person in accomplishing psychosocial maturation. Individuals who have fewer resources, including fewer relationship and fewer options, may experience more alienation (Bloch 1978). When such individuals enter critical care they may be confronted with even greater feelings of alienation.

The patient as an alienated person feels inferior whenever he suspects himself of not being in line. Since his sense of worth is based on approval as the reward for conformity, he feels naturally threatened in his sense of self and in his self-esteem by any feeling, thought, or action that could be suspected of being a deviation. The alienated person or patient experiences himself as a thing or an investment to be manipulated by himself and by others. He lacks a sense of self (Fromm 1967). He does not experience himself as the active bearer of his own powers and richness, but as an impoverished "thing" dependent on power outside of himself. As Dean (1961) suggests, "It may very well be that alienation is not a unitary phenomenon, but a syndrome" (p. 758).

According to Seeman (1959), one type of alienation refers to the individual's sense of understanding the events in which he is engaged. Seeman speaks of "high alienation," a form of meaninglessness in which the individual is unclear as to what he ought to believe—when the individual's minimal standards for clarity in decision making are not met. The individual cannot predict with confidence the consequences of acting on a given belief (Seeman 1959, p. 786).

Power

Power is the potential or actual ability of an individual to influence, cause, or prevent changes in cognition, attitude, behavior, or emotions of another individual in interpersonal relationships. Two areas of potential power consist of aggression and violence. In aggression, the individual reacts when self-assertion is blocked by moving into positions of power or prestige. Violence may occur when efforts toward aggression are ineffective. The individual verbally or nonverbally explodes (Wilkinson 1979).

Powerlessness

Powerlessness refers to the feeling of being separated from or external to one's endeavors rather than being a creator of one's endeavors. The individual feels powerless or unable to control the outcomes of his or her own behavior. In powerlessness, the individual has the expectation that the outcomes of his behaviors are not determined by what he does (internal control) but rather by the influence of outside forces caused by chance or luck (external control). Patients with an external orientation feel powerless to determine the consequences of their behavior (Bloch 1978).

Seeman (1959) defines *powerlessness* as the expectancy or the probability held by the individual that his own behavior cannot determine the outcome of reinforcements he seeks. The use of powerlessness as an expectancy means that this version of alienation is very closely related to the notion of internal versus external control of reinforcements. The latter construct refers to the difference between the individual's sense that he has personal control over the reinforcement situation, as contrasted with his view that the occurrence of reinforcements depends upon external conditions, such as chance, luck, or the manipulation of others (Seeman 1959). Therefore, powerlessness is a perceived lack of personal or internal control of certain events in certain situations.

According to Johnson (1967), powerlessness focuses on the social-psychological aspects of individual personality and may be considered a personality variable. But in the context of her definition, that is, the context of alienated man in mass society, the term indicates clearly a perceived relationship between the structural feature of social life in modern society and particular aspects of individual psychological structure and functioning.

The key to examining powerlessness is to examine it as a feeling on the part of the individual rather than in terms of one's own attitudes. How one analyzes powerlessness is not significant. The significant fact is whether or not the individual feels powerless. Stephenson (1979) identifies two kinds of powerlessness: trait powerlessness and situational powerlessness. *Trait powerlessness* is a person's usual affect or attitude toward life. The individual with trait or personality powerlessness may feel even more powerless in the situation of illness. *Situational powerlessness* is the lack of control thrust upon a coping or powerful person by a specific situation or series of events. Situational powerlessness is equally as significant as trait powerlessness and possibly can be better controlled by the nurse.

Johnson (1967) addresses the relationship of powerlessness and expectancy as follows:

> Powerlessness is equated with the perceived external control of events in the learning variable, expectancy. Operating as this learning variable, it could be expected to influence learning, either in the sense of the acquisition of knowledge or of developing effective, goal-directed behavior. The direction of this influence would be negative since knowledge or goal-directed behavior is simply irrelevant or unnecessary when the individual does not perceive that future events can be controlled by his own actions. (P. 40)

Each individual, whether he is well or ill, has a desire for power. This desire is described as *power want*. Kretch (1962) defines power want as the desire to control other persons or objects, to obtain their obedience, to compel their action, to determine their fate. The concept has enormous significance for the working of a society. Power want may have its origin in self-defense and self-enhancement. The objects that someone incorporates into his extended self are, according to several authors, objects within the control, or power, of that person.

Powerlessness can also be described in terms of whether a person sees himself as being in control of what happens to him or whether he feels events are due to chance. For example, did the patient's cardiac condition improve because he complied by taking his medications and followed his diet? On the other hand, he is faced with the notion that maybe his cardiac condition would have improved anyway (Stephenson 1979).

As mentioned previously, everyone wants to maintain an element of power and control over his being and his environment. When illness forces the individual to relinquish that control to a stranger, he may feel an overwhelming sense of powerlessness. It may be safe to state that the more acute the situation or the patient's illness, the less power the patient feels he has. Therefore, it is essential to discuss some of the causes of powerlessness in critical care units. We will use the concepts of alienation and powerlessness interchangeably.

THE CONCEPT OF POWERLESSNESS
APPLIED TO THE CRITICALLY ILL PATIENT

It is an obligation of the sick person to do everything possible to get well as soon as possible. On the other hand, he is encouraged by the hospital environment to be passive. When a person becomes a hospital patient he finds others doing things to and for him whether he wants them to or not. He experiences a lack of participation and a loss of his usual control over his environment.

There are essentially two potential causes of powerlessness: loss of control and lack of knowledge. Loss of control implies loss over oneself, one's behavior, and one's environment. Lack of knowledge implies insufficient knowledge regarding one's illness and the implications it has over one's being, one's family, and one's future.

Loss of Control

When the critical care nurse is looking for factors contributing to powerlessness, she looks for the stimulus most immediately confronting the client, namely, the physiological or biological crisis. The nurse also assesses the values, attitudes, traits, and past experiences affecting the patient's psychological well-being. Lastly, she assesses factors in the environment that influence behavior. Thus, the factors contributing to loss of control can be thought of as occurring in three categories: the physical, the psychological, and the environmental being of the patient.

Physiological Loss of Control. Physiological loss of control begins when the patient develops an acute illness. Prior to his illness, the patient had what he viewed as power over his body. He told his body what he wanted it to do, where he wanted it to go, and how he wanted it to perform. He had control and power over its mobility through space and time. He may have been the type of individual who took pride in his physical accomplishments. In acute illness, however, his physical being is in charge of the control panel. It now pushes the buttons that control the individual physiologically, and it forces him to curtail his activities or respond to pain: the patient has no physical control or power over the pain, bleeding, or respiratory distress that he experiences. Instead, these and other symptoms, over which he has no power, have brought him into a critical care unit. It is during the initial powerlessness episode that the patient may feel he is losing a part of his body. Smith (1964) points out that in acute illness, "It is the fear of loss of the whole or a part of the body that appears to be the focus of psychological concern. While the anxiety is conscious, the idea of loss may not be conscious at all; such an idea may be so grave a threat to the ego that the whole matter is repressed" (p. 36). The patient may not understand what caused his body to become critically ill. He may be experiencing guilt feelings over his current illness, and he may simultaneously feel a threat to his sense of physical integrity. According to Smith, it seems likely that every illness contains some degree of threat to body integrity. Serious illness especially arouses a fear of loss of function, a loss of capacity for understanding daily routines, or the sudden awareness of loss of control over one's own physical activities.

In illness the critical care patient is not expected to fulfill the normal role responsibilities that gives the individual some control over his life and which fulfill his self-ideal. When the breadwinner of the family becomes ill, however, he may feel that he should continue to influence certain family decisions and may also try to live up to the ideal of being a good provider by attempting to fulfill the work role despite his illness. Illness itself is an influencing factor leading to feelings of powerlessness (Roy 1976).

Physical illness may totally control the patient's consciousness and render him powerless to do or think about anything else. Illness, by its very nature, "tends to preoccupy its victim. Discomfort or pain in the body results in a withdrawal of whatever psychic investments one has made in the outside world" (Smith 1964, p. 38). During illness, the patient relinquishes physical and psychological control over his body. The patient may, on an unconscious level, feel that he is relinquishing ego control; to him this becomes synonymous with relinquishing life. In other words, to give up a type of ownership of his body in acute illness is to give up his claim to life itself. In illness, therefore, the patient physiologically feels loss of control or a sense of powerlessness. The physiological processes that undergo disequilibrium (e.g., loss of myocardium, conducive tissue, renal function, or pulmonary function of skin) render the patient powerless. It is the powerlessness over his body that brings the patient to the hospital, where a chain of events occurs that may further render him psychologically and environmentally powerless.

Psychological Loss of Control. Psychologically the patient becomes powerless or loses control the moment he arrives in the hospital. The alienated individual feels that his acts rule him, and that he is an inferior object to be manipulated by others, with no power of his own. Powerlessness is related to Engel's concept of giving-up/given-up. Giving-up due to a biological crisis is viewed as a transitional ego state in which coping devices are not yet evolved. This may or may not progress to a given-up state when a biological loss is viewed as final with little or no possible source of help. The giving-up period of illness may be preceded by a period of being unable to cope for some reason. Such a feeling may reduce the individual's ability to cope with other problems. When help is offered it may be rejected because the person feels nothing is able to alter the situation (Stephenson 1979).

The critically ill patient may be admitted into the hospital in one of two ways: he may be received in the emergency room or he may be directly admitted to one of the critical care units. Most patients admitted to either the emergency room or a critical care unit already have a personal physician. If the patient manifested symptoms at home or work, either his family or colleagues notified the appropriate physician. The patient who arrives alone in the emergency room may have the admitting intern or resident notify his physician. On the other hand, some patients have no personal physicians. They may be individuals who have been relatively healthy, or who are visiting the town on business. To facilitate these patients, some hospitals have what is called a physician of the month. He or she is on call in the emergency room, and becomes the personal or temporary physician of those patients who have none. The patient is thus powerless over who becomes his doctor.

Most patients quietly accept the doctor, realizing that they need someone to carry them through the critical stages of the illness. Once successfully through the crisis stage, such a patient may feel free to choose another physician. Initially, however, the choices of both doctor and nurse are made by someone else. The patient must quickly submit to these strangers and let them worry about his physical being. He may be in such a state of psychological shock that he fails to realize how critically ill he really is. According to Peplau (1952), the feeling of powerlessness "that is connected with putting oneself in the hands of a doctor or nurse is reinforced when the patient cannot find out what his real worries are. It is not a simple matter to consent psychologically to manipulation or partial destruction of one's own body and yet integrate the events as one experience in life among many from which something valuable has been learned" (p. 67).

If the patient comes first to the emergency room, he must submit to various diagnostic procedures. Someone from the admissions office may interview him, if his health permits, so he can properly be labeled and numbered. If a family member is present, the admission procedure can occur without the patient's presence. During the admission and history-taking processes, hospital personnel elicit personal information from the patient, who is again powerless to influence the type of information recorded. As Goffman (1961) points out, this process is a "violation of one's informational preserve regarding self" (p. 24). The patient realizes that if he is to get well, he must answer the personal and sometimes tedious questions. If he refuses to answer questions, he may fear he will not receive adequate therapeutic care. Outside the hospital, the patient could withhold objects of self-feeling such as his body, his immediate action, his thoughts, and some of his possessions from contact with alien and contaminating things. In the hospital, however, he soon discovers that hospital circumstances violate the territories of self, invade the boundary that he places between his being and the environment, and profane his embodiment of self (Goffman 1961). The patient has relatively little power over what goes into his chart and who reads it. Once in the chart rack, it becomes open territory for one and all. Needless to say, it is no wonder that patients begin to feel transparent. Everyone seems to know what is going on with the individual, but the patient may be kept in the dark as to what is happening around and within himself.

As the patient moves deeper into the admitting web, he may discover that the nursing staff has confiscated some of his personal belongings, such as his money, valuable jewelry, or important papers. Naturally the nursing personnel do not want to assume responsibility for such valuables. Again, the patient is powerless to determine which valuables remain with him and which are confiscated. Furthermore, the nurse may give the patient's family his clothes because there is no place for them in a critical care unit.

Just as personal valuables may be removed from him, he will have to submit to valuable information-gathering procedures needed to support or confirm the doctor's diagnosis. Most critical care units have essentially standard admission procedures. It is the severity of the patient's illness that determines any differences. In the emergency room, the staff performs only basic procedures like blood work (e.g., enzymes, electrolytes, CBC, blood gases, or type and cross-match), intravenous therapy, or administration of stat medication. Life-sustaining procedures (e.g., to counteract shock, cardiac arrest, arrhythmias, or bleeding) also begin in the emergency room. Exceptions to admission procedure depend upon the type of illness and the advice of the patient's doctor. A burn patient may go directly to the Hubbard tank for immediate assessment and treatment. Occasionally, the emergency room is filled, and consequently the doctors order the patients to be admitted directly to a critical care unit. The patient in any circumstances is basically powerless over the type of diagnostic procedures done or the admission procedure followed. The patient realizes he must submit to the siege of technicians parading into and out of his immediate territory. The number of unfamiliar people entering his environment will probably serve to intensify his feelings of powerlessness.

Once the patient is in a critical care unit, he must submit to additional necessary procedures. If the patient is still wearing his clothes, the nurse will remove them and give the patient a hospital gown. The nurse may begin to shave her patient's chest in order to facilitate EKG lead conduction, she may insert a Foley catheter to monitor renal function, or she might place an oxygen mask on her patient's face. If for some reason no one has started an IV, she will also begin this procedure. Furthermore, it is the nurse who orders an EKG, additional blood work, or a chest X-ray. Unless the patient's situation is most critical, the nurse may not spend all of her time with him. She may be preoccupied with carrying out her technical responsibilities. She therefore becomes a transient fixture within her patient's environment.

There may be more than one nurse participating in the admission-diagnostic procedures, and the atmosphere around the critically ill patient may be tense. The patient is powerless to determine the number of times his nurse or nurses enter and leave his environment. Although he realizes that they have their "duties" to perform, the tense and hurried atmosphere creates anxiety within the patient. The circumstances of acute injury and "the atmosphere in which treatment is usually given are conducive to the development of high levels of anxiety in all concerned" (O'Connor 1970, p. 210). Anxiety alone can serve to make the patient immobilized and powerless. The patient may be too anxious regarding his immediate prognosis to exhibit control over his environment. He worries that what he might do would interfere with his long-term prognosis.

Stephenson (1979) notes that a sense of power occurs when the patient believes an event or reinforcement is due to his own behavior or characteristics. On the other hand feelings of powerlessness reflect the patient's belief that whatever happens to him is due to forces outside himself such as fate, luck, or chance. The patient's opinion has a major effect on his compliance with the therapeutic regimen. The patient may feel his opinions are neither requested or respected if he is not sought out as a participating member of the decision-making team.

Another source of psychological powerlessness is loss of control in decision-making matters. The critically ill patient relinquishes the ability he normally has of deciding and choosing what he wants or does not want to do. Now someone else, usually a stranger, makes the decisions and choices for him. A dietitian, acting on the doctor's orders, decides the type of food he will eat. The hospital decides when he shall eat. His dinner may arrive at 5:00 P.M. although he usually dines at 7:00 P.M. The nurse even decides how the patient shall eat. If the patient has had an acute myocardial infarction, the nurse may choose to feed the patient. Another patient may have his activity restricted to the point that he voids and defecates in bed. The patient soon discovers that his daily activities are tightly scheduled and monitored by other people. All phases of the day's activities are tightly scheduled, "with one activity leading at a prearranged time into the next, the whole sequence of activities being imposed from above by a system of explicit formal rulings and a body of officials" (Goffman 1961, p. 6).

The patient is powerless to control the treatments he receives and the observations made of him. He may fail to comprehend the significance of frequent vital sign checks, CVP readings, hourly output readings, chest tube milking, or cough–turn–deep-breathing exercises. As previously mentioned, the patient feels transparent when his chart is exposed for all to read, and he also feels transparent when nurses continually monitor his cardiac, respiratory, renal, or physical activity. He may feel that his nurse is flying around his bed on frequent reconnaissance missions. He feels powerless to curtail the frequency of her visits. During the initial crisis, the critically ill patient may not recognize the significance of her data-collecting missions, but on the basis of the data, doctors and nurses make choices for the patient. Besides deciding what the patient will eat, they decide when he will sleep or be bathed. It is the nurse who determines the degree to which the critically ill patient will participate in his own care, based upon her ability to interpret his prognosis into nursing care terms. The nurse has the power to decide when the family members shall see the patient. Furthermore, she has the ability to restrict, discourage, or encourage visits by friends.

Patients may have one of two reactions to loss of control. First, the patient may feel guilty over his loss of control. Take for example the executive, whose daily life consists of controls in the form of policy and decision making. Suddenly and unexpectedly, he finds himself in a foreign environment in which he must psychologically adjust to loss of control. He loses his independence, and control now falls to other people—a nurse, a doctor, or his family. As a result, he may feel guilty for having other people, including strangers, assume his responsibilities. Second, the patient may actually enjoy being helpless. He may want to relinquish control to other people in his environment. It is possible that the physiological crisis takes all his attention. Therefore, he does not want the additional worry of making choices and decisions. Psychological feelings of powerlessness are caused by loss of control over admission procedures, the choice of doctor, decision-making ability, schedules, and routines.

Environmental Loss of Control.   Besides physiological and psychological loss of control, the patient also experiences environmental loss of control. Normally we choose where we want to live. We take many things into consideration before making the ultimate decision. In a hospital, this is not the case. Environmentally the patient experiences powerlessness the moment he arrives in his critical care "home." The powerlessness is demonstrated by the patient's inability to explore and choose where he wants to go within that unit. He is too critically ill to explore the unit, so someone else must make the decision, usually either the admissions office or the nurse receiving the initial call. The nurse assumes the patient's responsibility in considering all the reasons for choosing a certain bed, slot, or room. In time, the patient may wish to choose another area of the critical care unit. Depending upon his physical problems, his wish may be acknowledged.

The patient may feel powerlessness within his own personal territory. The territory around the patient's bed may be filled with environmental props such as a nightstand, curtain, bedside table, chair, sink, or call light. Other hospital environmental props within his immediate environment may include an IV pole, a Foley bag, chest tubes, a CVP manometer, an arterial line, a Swan-Ganz line, an oxygen unit, a volume respirator, or a cardioscope. The patient may have personal environmental props such as a watch or clock, glasses, cards, flowers, books, toilet articles, tissues, or a urinal placed on his nightstand. Usually these objects are kept within reach of the patient, so that if he should need any of them, they are accessible. With so much equipment around the patient's bed, however, his bedside table becomes a place for the nurse to put her own props—dressings, catheters, and bottles. If the critical patient does not have equipment around his bed, the bedside table and its personal props can be moved closer. Frequently, after nurses have bathed their patients, they unintentionally forget to return the bedside table to its original position near the patient. Consequently, he is powerless to reach his personal props. He may be unable to reach his glasses so that he can find the call light. If he needs the urinal, he is powerless to obtain it. The patient who is encouraged to force fluids may be unable to do so because they are out of reach.

Another environmental source of powerlessness is the call light. In lowering her patient's side rail to make his bed, the nurse may untie it and inadvertently forget to replace it when she completes her tasks. If the patient needs to call his nurse for the urinal, bedpan, or pain medications, he will be without means to get her attention visually. He may attempt to call his nurse, but if the unit is particularly noisy, his feeble voice may go unheard. Loss of visual communication with the nurse is especially traumatic for the tracheostomy patient. He depends entirely upon his call light for communication. The critically ill patient who is already in an anxiety crisis may depend heavily upon the security of visual and verbal contact with his nurse. Without such contact, he may feel overwhelming powerlessness and alienation.

Lastly the health team can become an influencing factor contributing to environmental loss of control. The critical care team exercises expert power over the individual especially when they demonstrate that they possess information that the patient does not have. Furthermore the same power applies in the application of skilled services. The health team has the skills necessary to assist the patient toward recovery. As an environmental stimulus, the nurse can positively influence the patient's sense of control.

Lack of Knowledge

Just as loss of control creates feelings of alienation and powerlessness, lack of knowledge can have the same or similar effects. A source of personal power is a knowledge base. Fragmented information, collections of data, and unsorted ideas do not provide a knowledge base. Rather, the individual's knowledge base needs to be an interrelated cohesive body of knowledge that is in a process of continuous growth (Field 1980). When the patient's knowledge base is limited regarding his condition, medication, and expected course of treatments, he has increased feelings of powerlessness (Bloch 1978).

We keep the patient powerless if we do not provide him with knowledge about what is happening within and around him. This is quite unintentional on the nurse's or physician's part. The acuteness of the situation simply dictates actions that do not necessarily include exploration or teaching. Such input has a low priority. Hopefully, it will be postponed only until a more opportune time. Most patients have never before been critically ill, nor have they experienced the powerlessness of illness. Therefore, they feel frightened when placed in a highly specialized and technical environment. If the patient does not understand what is happening, he may choose to deny the seriousness of the entire event. He denies what is happening because his illness, his environment, or his equipment has no meaning to him. He can understand nothing except the fact that he is ill. Therefore, some knowledge input is imperative. It need take only a few minutes or seconds to begin the process of knowledge input.

It is natural that the patient, who has answered questions about his previous illnesses and/or current symptoms, may want some simple explanations in return, not the usual medical terminology or professional jargon. If the patient receives only highly technical explanations for his current illness, he will still be without knowledge. He does not understand the complicated language that may have become second nature to the medical-nursing team. If the patient has to seek further explanation of the professional jargon, he may believe the staff will think he is stupid. Therefore, he remains essentially less informed and more confused or frightened. After all, he knows if anyone has fancy problems such as myocardial infarction, acute tubular necrosis, hyperkalemia, or deficient alveolar-capillary exchange, that person must be dying. According to Smith (1964), when one leaves the patient in ignorance about what is going to happen to him, one provides a fertile field for the activation of fantasy. All kinds of distortion, many of a fearful nature, may creep into the patient's thinking.

Stephenson (1979) notes that powerlessness has been shown to have a negative influence on learning. This is due to the fact that the individual who feels powerless does not believe that his actions can influence events. Consequently learning about his physiological problem is both irrelevant and unnecessary. The patient seeks knowledge about his illness as it relates to his care, treatments, family, and future prognosis. Someone who is to receive an A-V shunt, a permanent pacemaker implanation, a chest tube insertion, a peritoneal dialysis infusion, or skin grafts obviously needs explanations and time to assimilate the explanations adequately. Even simple procedures such as CVP readings and EKG rhythm recordings can be explained. As Smith (1964) points out, if the patient's "emotions are properly dealt with . . . that is, if in preparation for a treatment he is given some understanding of, and help in coping with his feelings . . . much can be done to reduce the emotional complications of illness" (p. 43). Each time the nurse performs a treatment, she can explain its significance, so that the patient sees meaning in her actions. As previously stated, the patient may see his nurse as someone on frequent reconnaissance missions. He may feel that she takes knowledge from his biological systems, but relatively little information is being put back into his system. Frequently, the health team reinforces powerless feelings by giving minimal if any information and by conveying the expectation that their interventions will be accepted without question. The patient may be treated as though he could not understand the information if it were offered (Stephenson 1979). If the patient is able to derive meaning from the nurse's interventions, then he can realize that her interventions are purposeful and goal-directed.

A patient who lacks knowledge about his illness may not realize how it will affect his role in his family. He may not realize that a role shift or alteration may be necessary. The family may be informed, but often the patient is not informed. This is not intentional on the part of nurses or physicians: they, with the family, may believe they are protecting the patient. They do not realize that the patient may be fantasizing about all types of unrealistic complications and limitations. In such circumstances the patient experiences intellectual powerlessness. He may need to know how much his family knows and what his prognosis will be so he can make both short- and long-term plans, mainly financial plans.

When the nurse provides her patient with knowledge, she is actually facilitating his progress through the stages of illness. One must remember that there are times when the nurse must be sensitive to the degree, type, and readiness of the patient for knowledge. If the patient has knowledge about himself, he is able to ask his physician or nurse additional questions that will further expand his knowledge. The end result of this process is a reestablishment of the patient's intellectual power.

NURSING ASSESSMENT OF POWERLESSNESS

The nurse assesses powerlessness through the patient's behavioral response. The behaviors produced by various forms of alienation have been a subject of interest and research. The specific responses are categorized into regulatory behaviors and cognitive behaviors. The regulatory behaviors, which are less well researched, result in physiological responses. Cognitive behaviors, which will be our primary concern, focus on psychological responses.

Regulatory Behaviors

The regulatory behaviors occur in response to stimuli from the external environment and from changes in the internal state of dynamic equilibrium. When emotions are blocked they find some other way to emerge. The critically ill patient experiencing powerlessness may manifest the following symptoms:

REGULATORY BEHAVIORS

Tiredness
Dizziness
Headache
Gastrointestinal disturbance

The patient may be too tired or dizzy to ambulate or participate in his care. His fatigue and lack of participation only further contribute to feelings of powerlessness or loss of control. In addition, the patient's headaches may interfere with his listening and learning attention span. Diarrhea can be a symptom of many emotional problems. Therefore its presence needs to be assessed in relationship to other treatments or therapy that could cause diarrhea. Once other physiological causes have been ruled out, external and internal stressful stimuli contributing to a feeling of powerlessness by the patient must be controlled.

Other regulatory behaviors can occur simultaneously with cognitive behaviors. When the powerless patient experiences anger, aggression, or hostility, he will manifest regulatory responses. The regulatory responses consist of increased heart rate, increased respiratory rate, and increased blood pressure. There seems to be more information available regarding the cognitive behavioral responses of powerlessness.

Cognitive Behaviors

The cognitive system involves the inputs from external and internal stimuli, including psychosocial factors. Powerlessness alters the cognitive mechanism by reducing the individual's ability to process information, learn, make decisions, and utilize judgment. The patient who feels powerless seems to have no interest in life. Because he is not sure who he is or what he wants, the alienated person feels empty. Life holds nothing because he looks for nothing, and he looks for nothing because he does not know what to look for (Yoder 1977).

The critically ill patient who has a low sense of control or feels powerless will manifest the following cognitive behaviors (Roy 1976; Stephenson 1979):

COGNITIVE BEHAVIORS

Apathy
Withdrawal
Resignation
Fatalism
Malleability
Low knowledge of illness
Statements of low control
Anxiety
Restlessness
Sleeplessness
Wandering
Aimlessness
Lack of decision making
Aggression
Anger

Some of these behaviors may be due to fear of loss of self-control or they may be due to projection or fears and suspicions secondary to alenation. The powerless patient feels anxious and uneasy. The patient restricted to complete bedrest is restless and sleepless. Feelings of victimization, aimlessness, and powerlessness cause the patient to be uncertain in determining his future. He may feel depressed and think that the hospitalization is unnecessary. His feelings of helplessness may lead him to leave the hospital against medical advice. The patient's apathy makes him unable to see choices of existence that are available to him. Finally the patient is without direction and lacks decision (Roy 1976; Stephenson 1979). Ideally, whatever emotional changes occur in the critically ill patient should be transient and reversible; unfortunately, this is not always the case. The critically ill patient is particularly vulnerable from the psychological point of view. Denied his ability to function in a self-help capacity, he must accept a position of enforced passivity and reluctant dependency. Most often those responsible for his care are strangers, yet he must place his hopes for survival in their hands. Finding himself in strange surroundings and plagued with various worries about the future, the critically ill patient is prone to psychological complications (O'Connor 1970, p. 210).

As the critically ill patient reaches his limit of physical, psychological, and environmental loss of control, he may experience the frustration of powerlessness. He was powerless to choose his own doctor or his location in a critical care unit, and now he is powerless to choose how props will be organized around his bed, what diagnostic work and treatments will be done, or how the day's tightly scheduled routines will be accomplished. The individual may be frustrated "as a consequence of the discrepancy between the control he may expect and the degree of control that he desires—that is, power takes no direct account of the value of control to the person" (Seeman 1959, p. 784). A patient's experiences in a critical care unit are controlled by other people; the patient becomes another person's experience. This may eventually become alarming to the patient. As Fromm (1967) points out, "the sense of self stems from the experience of myself as the subject of my experience, my thought, my feeling, my decision, my judgment, my actions. It presupposes that my experience is my own, and not an alienated one. Things have no self and men who have become things have no self" (p. 130). An acutely ill patient must relinquish his "my" aspect.

Physical illness and the immobility that results create an emotional intolerance that may complicate the patient's recovery. He may no longer be able to tolerate not having choices or decision-making responsibilities. He no longer has the power to guide his daily activities. It is no wonder that the patient may have nothing to do but "concentrate upon his own misery to the exclusion of whatever is happening around him. Most illness and its accompanying pain are likely to be transitory, but for the period of time an illness dominates its victim's consciousness, there is a shift of psychic energies to the self that results in an enlarged egocentricity" (Smith 1964, p. 38).

As the patient reaches a level where he cannot tolerate further powerlessness, he may exhibit temporary behavioral responses. For example, a patient with a massive MI who is told to remain immobilized may become angry if his bedside table is pushed out of reach. The burn patient who is encouraged to force fluids may become angry when his water pitcher is either empty or out of reach. The tracheostomy patient may become angry when his call light is accidently placed out of reach. Patients can express themselves in a variety of ways such as anger, hostility, withdrawal, or depression. When the patient's feeling of powerlessness has reached an intolerable level, he may not be able to recognize that people in his environment are concerned with his well-being and restoration of power. The patient becomes increasingly more alienated. As David (1955) has noted, subjects who are high on the syndrome of alienation will be less accurate in their perceptions than subjects who are low on the syndrome of alienation.

NURSING DIAGNOSIS OF POWERLESSNESS

The nursing diagnosis is a statement of the problem, namely, powerlessness. From her assessment of regulatory and cognitive behaviors, the critical care nurse is able to formulate her nursing diagnosis of powerlessness. While the patient is hospitalized in critical care, the nurse assesses numerous internal and external stressors causing him to experience loss of control.

NURSING INTERVENTIONS AND POWERLESSNESS

The patient's experience with nursing care may discourage him from taking any initiative in his own care or progress. His contacts with nurses may have been nurse-active, patient-passive, nurse-guided, or patient-obedient. The critical care nurse often unintentionally carries her activities beyond the necessary point. She may do things for the patient when he is quite capable of doing them, with guidance, for himself. As the patient's condition stabilizes, the nurse returns power to her patient. The critical care nurse accomplishes this in two basic ways: she restores control to the patient, and she reinforces his new knowledge.

Restoration of Control

During illness, the nurse can aim to remove the specific aspects that lead to powerlessness, namely, the low expectancy of control and the constant discrepancy between the patient's condition and his ideal self (Roy 1976). The nurse may restore physiological, psychological, and environmental control to the patient. By restoring control, the nurse may alleviate unnecessary or debilitating behavioral responses.

Physiological Control. As mentioned earlier, a patient feels acute illness as a threat to his security. The insecurity that results relates to his fears of death. Physiologically, this fear can become a reality. No matter what the precipitating crisis may have been (e.g., MI, pulmonary edema, third-degree burns, open heart surgery, drug overdose, or bilateral nephrectomy), the patient's physiological systems go through adaptive changes in response to the insult. These changes may necessitate temporary disequilibrium and reorganization on the part of certain bodily systems. For example, through the process of peritoneal dialysis, the patient with acute tubular necrosis may be utilizing his peritoneal cavity as an exchange site. The myocardial tissue of a MI patient whose heart experiences tissue loss may have to redistribute the workload in order to ensure that the remaining tissue can be effectively utilized. Furthermore, if this patient's pacemaker or sinoatrial node is altered, the next pacemaker site (atrial-ventricular node) must assume the responsibility. The patient who has lost 50 percent of his skin due to burns experiences tremendous fluid and electrolyte shifts.

It is during such reorganizations or adaptive processes that additional complications can occur. As the nurse carries out her surveillance of the patient she will note that his fears are either reduced or intensified. Regardless of what the patient's primary problem was, he needs reassurance as to how his physiological systems are regaining control and, hopefully, reaching stability. The nurse can point out to her MI patient, for example, that his

EKG pattern shows less S-T elevation or no arrhythmias, or that his serum enzymes may be decreasing from their previous high levels. The patient with acute tubular necrosis will be reassured when he learns that his kidneys are diuresing and his BUN and/or creatinine levels are decreasing. The burn patient feels less insecure when he begins to see his skin grafts take control. The pulmonary patient feels hopeful when he learns that his blood gases are stable and that he is being successfully weaned off the volume respirator.

To point out that the body is regaining control means that the nurse must know the expected physiological changes that accompany an insult. She must be able to differentiate expected responses from the positive changes in her patient's condition. As the positive changes occur, the patient will feel a sense of physiological powerfulness. This feeling can occur only when his physician and nurse inform him of his body's daily restoration of control. One must keep in mind, however, that there will be patients whose condition vacillates and who may never reach total control.

For example, some critically ill patients may not regain normal physiological control as quickly as desired. It may become more difficult for the nurse to identify areas in which she can return power to such patients. Her most important intervention in this instance is to point out to the patient that his progress has reached a slow stage of physiological adaptation. A positive factor is that his condition is not regressing. In other words, a physiological plateau is more desirable than physiological regression. In this respect, the nurse helps to maintain the level of power she has previously given the patient before he reached a plateau.

Psychological Control. Each patient has potential power. Kaplowitz (1978) points out that to have the capacity to exercise power is to have potential power whether the capacity results from the possession of such tangible, extrinsic resources as wealth, authority, or force. Furthermore, potential power can result from intrinsic intangible resources as dedication, energy, courage, teamwork, or skill in the uses of one's resources.

Kaplowitz has identified four different consequences of power attribution which he terms strategic, ideological, moral, and psychological consequences. Because each patient has potential power, the nurse can utilize the knowledge of these consequences to facilitate powerfulness instead of powerlessness. The consequences are dependent upon the patient's view of potential power as a stable attribute rather than something that varies from decision to decision. First, *strategic consequences* involve the notion that perceived power can lead to desired outcomes and is therefore a source of real power: the critical care patient perceives himself as a person who can control his environment and possibly his treatment outcome. Knowing this the nurse seeks ways to give control to the patient so his personal power is reinforced. The patient's opinion may be sought regarding when he desires to ambulate, be bathed, or sit in a chair. Second, *ideological consequences* result primarily from the attribution of potential power rather than exercised power. The patient who chooses to participate in his care or to comply with treatments has exercised his power. On the other hand, a patient may decide temporarily to refrain from participation in his care for various reasons, thereby still maintaining his potential for power. Third, *moral consequences* involve the attribution of responsibility and are related to external power. A patient may give power to other people or external circumstances and blame them for his behavior. In this respect the patient no longer has responsibility for his behavior. The responsibility is therefore transferred to the entity or individual who presumably caused the behavior. The nurse helps the patient assume responsibility for his own behavior. Rather than becoming angry or complacent regarding an aspect of care or treatment modality, the patient is encouraged to discuss his concerns, feelings, or needs. Fourth, *psychological consequences* involve the patient's locus of control. Patients who demonstrate external locus of control may feel they have never been in control of their own destiny. On the other hand, the internal locus of control patient may feel he has control over events in his life including the critical care unit. Knowing whether the patient is an internal or external locus of control person will help the nurse design her nursing care and teaching program.

The nurse restores her patient's control when she encourages him to express his feelings, to participate in his own care, and to make choices and decisions. For example, when a nurse permits the critically ill patient to express what he feels, then he can undergo illness as an experience that reorients feelings and strengths that are positive forces in his personality. This patient will have the power to express his feelings of frustration, anger, hostility, anxiety, or fear. He knows that his messages will be received by a listening and understanding nurse. Instead of telling the patient to rest and not to talk, his nurse encourages verbal participation. She realizes that by giving her patient the opportunity of verbalizing his concerns, needs, or desires, she restores his control and participation in his own care. She further realizes that "if a patient is approached as a person with the ultimate power of accepting or rejecting the proposed care, then the effectiveness of that care is increased and both patient and staff satisfaction is increased" (Tryon 1965, p. 121). The nurse can actively listen to her patient's concerns regarding his family, job, finances, and future. The patient will soon believe that he is a significant person within a highly technical environment. Initially, the patient may be able to participate only on a verbal level. Of course this depends upon the severity and stability of the patient's condition. Once it has been assessed that the patient is able to progress to a more active involvement, he can be encouraged to do so.

The nurse keeps in mind that the nurse-patient relationship is composed of two strangers who come together in a stressful situation. The nurse's commitment to her professional goal causes her to attach to the patient, and the patient's need for care activates his attachment to the nurse. The bonding that occurs between the two individuals is of such a nature that while the two individuals are attached, they remain two separate individuals (Carser and Doona 1978).

The nurse may unintentionally continue in her active role rather than reassess the appropriateness of her interventions. It is essential that she reassess her actions before continuing on an active level, and the case of Mr. T. shows why. Mr. T. is a patient who had open heart surgery for mitral and aortic valve replacement. At the time of his surgery, he developed cardiac tamponade. The patient's postoperative course was critical for two days. The nurse was a very active member in Mr. T.'s health care. She took total control of all nursing responsibilities. She bathed, fed, turned, and suctioned her patient. After the two-day crisis, Mr. T. began to stabilize and improve, but his nurse continued to play an active role in maintaining control. She continued to guide, direct, and plan his care. Subsequently, the staff observed that Mr. T., instead of being pleased with his new progress, was actually withdrawn and depressed. When asked how he saw himself progressing, he said, "I guess I must still be pretty sick. I can't even feed or bathe myself yet, and it has been almost five days." As the nurse began playing a less active role in Mr. T.'s care, his depression subsided. He became involved in directing and planning his own care. According to Tryon (1965), "When the patient participates in planning his own care, he assumes some responsibility for the outcome or the effect of that care. When he participates he is able to use more effectively the health resources offered him. When a particular course of action is suggested, he knows why it has been suggested, and he is able to express his feelings about it" (p. 126).

As the patient begins to participate in his own care, he obtains the power to choose or decide how he wants his nurse to participate. This implies that both participants are sensitive to each other's needs. As David (1955) points out, "If one is to have satisfactory interpersonal relationships, he must be sensitive to the feelings and attitudes of the people in his environment. The more one distorts, or misperceives the personalities of those around him, the less likely he is to make a good adjustment to his surroundings" (pp. 24–25). Hopefully, both people have gotten to know each other. The nurse must know her patient before she is able to assess his readiness to assume decision-making responsibilities. If he is ready, the nurse begins the process on a less significant level. For example, the nurse may give her patient power to decide when and how he would like certain treatments to be performed. He may choose to sleep before an IPPB treatment. If his lungs are clear and his blood gases are adequate, the nurse can approve his decision. Of course this implies that the nurse has already collected the data before giving her patient a choice. Little by little, the patient's decision-making powerfulness is increased.

The nurse can foster decision-making powerfulness when she allows her patient to choose which personal environmental props will go in his closet, remain in his luggage, go into the nightstand drawer, or be placed on top of the bedside table. His personal environmental props may be the only daily contact he has with home. Pictures of animals, children, or grandchildren become important to the patient. Furthermore, patients like their cards displayed on their table. This serves to remind them that they are significant to friends. Instead of collecting the patient's props and placing them "out of the way," the nurse can leave her patient's watch, glasses, pictures, or books within easy reach. The nurse also helps the patient achieve a type of environmental powerfulness by keeping his bedside table within reach. This may seem like an obvious intervention, but it is frequently overlooked. If the patient has received a diuretic and does not have a Foley catheter or bathroom privileges, the nurse can attempt to keep his urinal empty and within reach. The patient who is encouraged to cough can have his tissues within reach. Lastly, the patient who is told to force fluids needs his water pitcher full and close at hand.

In restoring psychological control, the critical care nurse's primary goal is to facilitate the maintenance of patient autonomy. Maintaining autonomy is done while the patient undergoes a stressful and critical life crisis. The nurse has two options in accomplishing this goal. First, the nurse can support the patient's ego as he confronts the biological threat. Second, the nurse can foster the patient's regression and allow him to submit to the crisis (Carser and Doona 1978). Needless to say the nurse invariably will seek the first alternative. Facilitating ego strength involves encouraging the patient's participation and respecting his opinion, values, and ideas.

Environmental Control. The nurse can ensure environmental powerfulness by seeing that her patient's call light is functioning. Occasionally, the light does not work, and it may not have been functioning for several days. The nurse can also have the light securely fastened in an accessible area of the patient's bed. As mentioned earlier, this may be the patient's only means of communicating with his nurse. A tracheostomy patient may also need a magic slate board near his bed. He can use the board as a way of writing notes to his nurse so that she is better able to understand his needs. This allows the patient a feeling of control within his environment.

In addition the critical care nurse can modify the hospital environment. The nurse provides environmental control through personalization of nursing care. When talking to the patient, the nurse can use his name and seek the patient's counsel when designing and implementing nursing care. The nurse also intervenes by assisting the patient to recognize and learn to use control measures. The patient is permitted to have verbal input into the scheduling of activities including family visits. Furthermore the nurse helps the patient formulate realistic goals and expectations for himself. For example, the patient may decide he would like to sit up for five to ten minutes longer or ambulate to the door or hallway instead of simply around the bed.

If the nurse strives to foster physiological, psychological, or environmental powerfulness, she may alleviate negative behavioral responses. According to Peplau (1952), "Feelings of crying or anger for the benefit of the nurse may be expressed in order to get attention. If sustained assistance or self-enhancement is not provided in other ways, patients often do use these forms of behavior to express the powerlessness that they feel" (p. 31). These feelings can be reduced if the patient can identify with a nurse who helps him to feel less threatened and more in control or more powerful. As the patient is able to identify with his nurse, he is ready to learn.

Reinforcement of Learning and Knowledge

Patient education is an effective way to increase the patient's power. Without a knowledge base, the cardiac patient feels powerlessness or a loss of control over symptoms such as angina or diaphoresis. If the coronary care patient is told what to eat or what medication to take without being informed about how a particular medication or diet relates to cardiac dysfunction, the patient is forced into lack of control over the outcome of the illness. Therefore the nurse seeks to make patient education available to the patient.

When she reinforces or promotes learning, the nurse must assess her patient's readiness to learn. He may feel anxious about acquisition of new knowledge. He may subscribe to the philosophy that "what you don't know won't hurt you." But lack of knowledge can be harmful to the future of the patient. The renal failure patient on hemodialysis who does not understand that he must restrict fluids, sodium, or potassium may die. During the initial crisis, the nurse must take extreme care in talking with the patient. Because the critically ill patient is often in a highly suggestible condition, the most insignificant remarks by the health team can make a lasting impression on the patient. Therefore, early explanations should be brief and simple.

As the patient progresses in his care, he will be exposed to certain treatments and procedures. The nurse can remember that while these procedures are routine to her, they may be new to her patient. Before the nurse decides on the type and extent of explanation required, the patient should have an opportunity to express his views of the forthcoming event. His description may be grossly inaccurate, weird, or fanciful, but if communication does not start with recognition of his perception of the situation, the most careful explanation may fail to assure him (Aasterud 1965, p. 83). Besides providing the original explanation to her patient, the critical care nurse can spend time reexplaining information that has been given to the patient by other members of the health team.

The nurse may choose to give her patient learning input on a one-to-one basis. She may spend time teaching one day and follow it with a return demonstration. This enables her to see how much the patient actually retains from the original learning session. Furthermore, it gives the patient time to assimilate his new knowledge so he can ask questions if necessary. The nurse continues to reiterate certain pertinent points in order to reinforce his learning. Once the patient seems to have a grasp of his illness, and its causes and prognosis, the nurse can bring the family into the teaching input sessions. She may even have the patient teach his own family. The nurse may simply be an observer, participating only when specific questions arise from the family. By teaching both the family and patient, the nurse provides them with equal knowledge. She knows that what one forgets, the other might remember. In any case, knowledge does give the patient a feeling of powerfulness.

Therefore a patient educational program will make the necessary information available. When critical care patients have the opportunity to increase their knowledge about their illness, treatments, and prognosis, they are in a position to make choices and ultimately to have more control over their being.

NURSING EVALUATION

Evaluation of powerlessness is based upon the patient's behavior and the nature of the nursing care he requires. The nurse assesses the various regulatory and/or cognitive behaviors signifying loss of control or powerlessness. The nurse designs her nursing care to return power and control to the patient. The nurse evaluates the effectiveness of interventions by noting whether or not the patient becomes involved in his care, makes decisions, and assumes responsibility for his decisions.

SUMMARY

Being a patient in a critical care unit is an unfamiliar experience. The patient takes his cues from those around him. When he is encouraged to ask questions, to express his feelings, and to participate in planning for his care, he will know what behavior is expected. If he is discouraged from expressing himself and from taking part in his care, he may well assume that his proper role is a passive one and he will not be able to take responsibility when he ought to. An active patient role requires more of the patient. It also requires more involvement of those working with him. But the outcome in both effectiveness of care and satisfaction of patient and practitioners makes the added investment worthwhile (Tryon 1965). The patient can only experience powerfulness as his nurse is able to restore certain controls and reinforce his new knowledge.

REFERENCES

AASTERUD, MARGARET, "Explanation to the Patient," in *Social Interaction and Patient Care*, ed. James K. Skipper and Robert Leonard, p. 83. Philadelphia: Lippincott, 1965.

BLOCH, DOROTHY, *Alienation: Behavioral Concepts and Nursing Intervention*, ed. Carolyn Carlson and Betty Blackwell, New York: J. B. Lippincott Co., 1978.

CARSER, DIANE, and MARY DOONA, "Alienation: A Nursing Concept," *JPN and Mental Health Services*, 16, no. 9 (September 1978), 33-40.

DAVID, ANTHONY, "Alienation, Social Apperception and Ego Structure," *Journal of Counsulting Psychology*, 19, no. 1 (1955), 24.

DEAN, DWIGHT, "Alienation: Its Meaning and Measurement," *American Sociological Review*, 26 (October 1961), 758.

FIELD, ELOIS, "Authority: A Select Power," *Advance Nursing Science*, 3, no. 1 (October 1980), 69-83.

FROMM, ERICH, *The Sane Society*. New York: Holt, Rinehart and Winston, 1967.

GOFFMAN, ERVING, *Asylums*. New York: Doubleday, 1961.

HACKETT, THOMAS, M.D., "The Coronary-Care Unit: An Appraisal of Its Psychologic Hazards," *New England Journal of Nursing*, 279, no. 25 (December 19, 1968), 1365-1370.

HILGARD, ERNEST, "Human Motives and the Concept of the Self," *The American Psychologist*, 4, no. 9 (September 1949), 374-382.

JOHNSON, DOROTHY, "Powerlessness: A Significant Determinant in Patient Behavior?" *Journal of Nursing Education*, 6, no. 2 (April 1967), 39-44.

KAPLOWITZ, STAN, "Towards a Systematic Theory of Power Attribution," *Social Psychology*, 41, no. 2 (1978), 131-148.

KRETCH, DAVID, RICHARD S. CRUTCHFIELD, and EGERTIN L. BALLACHEY, *Individual in Society*. New York: McGraw-Hill, 1962.

KRITEK, PHYLLIS, "Patient Power and Powerlessness," *Supervisor Nurse*, June 1981, pp. 26-34.

MCFARLAND, DALTON, and NOLA SHIFLETT, "The Role of Power in the Nursing Profession, *Nursing Dimensions*, 7 (Summer 1979), 1-13.

MASLOW, ABRAHAM, *Toward a Psychology of Being*. New York: Van Nostrand, 1968.

O'CONNOR, GARRETT, "Psychiatric Changes in the Acutely Injured," *Postgraduate Medicine*, 48 (September 1970), 210.

PEPLAU, HILDEGARD, *Interpersonal Relations in Nursing*. New York: Putnam's, 1952.

RAKOEZY, MARY, "The Thoughts and Feelings of Patients in the Waiting Period Prior to Cardiac Surgery: A Descriptive Study," *Heart and Lung*, 6, no. 2 (March-April 1977), 280-287.

ROGERS, C. R., "A Comprehensive Theory of Personality and Behavior," unpublished paper, 1948. Cited in David Krech, Richard S. Crutchfield, and Egertin L. Ballachey, *Individual in Society*, pp. 96-97. New York: McGraw-Hill, 1962.

ROY, SISTER CALLISTA, *Introduction to Nursing: An Adaptation Model*. Englewood Cliffs: Prentice-Hall, 1976.

SEEMAN, MELVIN, "On the Meaning of Alienation," *American Sociological Review*, 24 (December 1959), 783-791.

_____ , "Alienation and Learning in a Hospital Setting," *American Sociological Review*, 27, no. 6 (December 1962), 772-782.

SMITH, SYDNEY, "The Psychology of Illness," *Nursing Forum*, 3, no. 1 (1964), 36.

STEPHENSON, CAROL, "Powerless and Chronic Illness: Implications for Nursing," *Baylor Nursing Education*, 1, no. 1 (1979), 17-23.

TRYON, PHYLLIS, "Giving the Patient An Active Role," in *Social Interaction and Patient Care*, ed. James K. Skipper and Robert Leonard, p. 121. Philadelphia: Lippincott, 1965.

WILKINSON, MARCIA, "Power and the Identified Patient," *Perspective in Psychiatric Care*, 17, no. 6 (1979), 248-253.

YODER, SUSAN, "Alienation as a Way of Life," *Perspective in Psychiatric Care*, 15, no. 2 (1977), 66-71.

7
Avoidance and Denial

BEHAVIORAL OBJECTIVES

1. Define the terms *avoidance* and *denial*.
2. Identify the three components associated with direct action tendency or avoidance.
3. Discuss how defensive reappraisal or denial applies to the critically ill patient.
4. State the regulatory behaviors associated with avoidance and denial.
5. Identify four cognitive behaviors associated with avoidance and denial.
6. Design a nursing care plan that reduces avoidance and denial behaviors in the critically ill patient.

Illness is viewed by society as a weakness. The public is confronted with media showing us glowing and youthful beautiful women with peaches and cream complexions, perfect white teeth, and shiny, silky hair. Likewise men are depicted as handsome and virile with muscular tan bodies, perfect teeth, and well-groomed hair. Wellness and youth are both highly valued. Magazine and newspaper advertisements recommend various types of vitamins to protect us against illness and give us continued energy to perform our activities of daily living. Furthermore we are bombarded with advertisements regarding the advantages of health clubs, exercise programs, or jogging.

Our economy is based on the "healthy employee." Even though companies or businesses make provisions for sick leave, an individual who uses this provision may run the risk of not being recommended for promotion and/or salary increase. Individuals feel compelled to come to work regardless of how they feel. In addition, some places of employment pay their employees for a sick day only after they have been with the company six months to a year. The company may make no arrangements to replace the sick employee temporarily. As a result, fellow workers must absorb the absent person's workload in addition to their own. This situation conjures up feelings of guilt. Rather than face the reality of illness, with its feelings of guilt and lack of rewards, the individual will either avoid or deny the fact that he or she is ill.

The thrust of our culture is directed toward physical perfection and health. It is no wonder that people are taken off guard when the impact of illness manifests itself. Suddenly there exists a tremendous threat to the individual's internal being or self-system. According to Kiening (1978), "The threat to the self-system depends not only upon the actual degree of physical disequilibrium brought about by the illness itself but, more importantly, upon the alteration of the self-concept that takes place as a result of impaired physical functioning" (p. 211).

Because of the threat to his self-system, the individual has to adapt or make certain adaptive changes. The specific type of changes is dependent upon the type of illness, severity of illness, and threat to the person's self-concept. Adaptation is a lengthy and ongoing process. The individual himself changes as he adapts to illness. He is different from the way he was before and different from others who do not have his problem. The illness may force him to act entirely differently than he would in complete health. Therefore, he may resort to certain coping mechanisms such as avoidance and/or denial.

DEFINITION OF TERMS

Lazarus (1966) has identified two general categories for adapting or coping. The first consists of *direct action tendencies* aimed at eliminating or reducing the anticipated harmful confrontation that defines the threat. The second consists of purely cognitive maneuvers, termed *defense reappraisal*, through which appraisal is altered without action directed at changing the objective situation. This latter form of coping he refers to as defense mechanisms. It may seem as though there is little difference between the two categories. Nevertheless, there are differences, and these can best be seen when we apply the categories to the critical care patient.

Direct-Action Tendencies: Avoidance

Direct-action tendencies consist of actions aimed at eliminating or reducing the anticipated harmful confrontation that defines the threat. Lazarus (1966) has identified four fundamental types of direct-action tendencies, which we shall briefly examine, although we will apply only one, avoidance, to the critically ill patient. The four fundamental types are (1) actions aimed at strengthening the individual's resources against harm, (2) attack, (3) avoidance, and (4) inaction.

By taking actions to strengthen his resources against an external danger, the individual can reduce the threat by directly influencing the actual condition. He utilizes his energy against the threat, which may deplete the individual of energy needed to move him along the health continuum. He may, for example, mobilize all his energy in his trust of the doctor, but in so doing, he fails to realize that his illness or pathology may be irreversible. When he finally learns this, the patient feels failure. As a result, he may feel depression and guilt. As Lazarus (1966) points out, such failure can also affect his future behavior:

> When the individual has counted on a trusted protection to preserve him from a harm, and the protection fails in this, the reaction is likely to be extreme disappointment. The individual has learned that supports on which he has counted, and which give him a sense of security, are not to be depended upon, greatly weakening his future estimate of powers to cope with threat. (P. 259)

Other examples include preparing carefully for an exam, exercising after surgery to avoid thrombophlebitis, and restricting or eliminating fluids and sodium from the diet to prevent fluid retention. A nursing student, for example, may have studied diligently for an exam only to fail. Her method of preparation may have been the same one she used for a previous exam that she passed. This method, however, may not have suited the second exam. A postoperative open heart patient may actively do his exercises as ordered, yet for some physiological reason he may still develop thrombophlebitis. The hemodialysis patient may restrict his fluids and salt intake but nevertheless retain fluids leading to congestive heart failure and/or pulmonary edema. What do these individuals do in such circumstances? First, they examine the environment for cues in order to prepare for danger. The student may need to discuss the exam with her teacher to assure correct studying. The heart patient may need his nurse to observe or assist him in the proper methods of exercising. The hemodialysis patient may need additional treatments in order to reduce fluid retention. In each instance, these persons incorporate their environment into their world view in an attempt to lessen the potentiality of further threat.

The action tendency that is "aimed at preventing the anticipated harmful confrontation by means of an assault on the agent of harm may be termed attack" (Lazarus 1966, p. 261). Attack may be expressed overtly in both physical and verbal behavior. This is synonymous with the fight principle. A critically ill patient who is physically immobilized by tubes, cables, restraints, or pathology may resort to verbal attack. The quadriplegic patient who cannot pull out his tubes or throw something out of anger may choose to throw words in an attempt to attack those caring for him. He may use colorful language in order to elicit a negative response from the individual being attacked. No one enjoys profanity, and the quadriplegic patient realizes this. Such a verbal attack is the most aggressive act he can perform. Verbal attack is the only output mechanism of the physically immobilized patient. It may either lead to avoidance by the health team or buy him the attention he desires. The nurse can help the patient channel his energy in other ways.

A patient may use physical attack by grabbing his nurse, disconnecting his own intravenous therapy, removing his Foley, pulling off his EKG leads, or picking at his A-V shunt. Such a patient may be unable verbally to attack those guiding and directing his care, so instead he attacks the means of treatment. He believes that an attack against his equipment is an attack against those caring for him. He believes those objects to be "theirs" rather than "his," and he fails to realize that he is only attacking himself. By removing the objects of illness, he believes that he can also remove the illness himself.

Direct-action tendencies that are "aimed at interfering with the anticipated harmful confrontation by preventing contact with the agent of harm may be regarded as avoidance" (Lazarus 1966, p. 262). Physical danger may be avoided by physical action. An example of the physical action tendency is to remove oneself from the situation. If one's house were burning, one would leave. However, an individual who has certain symptoms may avoid seeing his doctor, who could identify the origin of his symptoms and perhaps discover a threatening situation.

The same individual may take emotional action to avoid the threat of a potential problem. This is flight response. Flight does not merely take place on the physical action level. One can also try to shut something out of one's mind. The patient might accomplish this goal consciously or unconsciously. He might consciously decide to avoid the threat of illness by discussing peripheral topics such as his grandchildren, rose bushes, or pet. These are relatively safe topics that pose no threat or danger.

Inaction, the fourth fundamental type of direct action tendency outlined by Lazarus (1966), is "the complete absence of any action tendency for coping with the threat. Apathy is the term used to connote the affect or attitude associated with inaction" (p. 262–263). The individual becomes convinced that there is no way of preventing a harmful outcome or situation. For example, a critically ill patient may have sustained a number of postoperative complications that serve to deplete him of his energy and his goal of returning to a previous level of wellness. Each new complication only serves to heighten the threat of impending doom. In time the patient succumbs to feelings of hopelessness and powerlessness. Both feelings foster a direct action tendency of inaction or submission. After all, he believes that no matter what he does, what his doctors do, or how hard he tries, other complications will occur. He sees no other alternative but to give up. He avoids action by submitting to inaction.

Defensive Reappraisal: Denial

Denial is a very simple psychophysiologic defense mechanism where the individual does not perceive certain stimuli. Furthermore the individual does not integrate them into a realistic idea or percept. Lazarus (1966) notes that defenses are psychological maneuvers whereby the individual may deceive himself regarding the condition of the threatening stimuli. External and internal harm is simply not anticipated. Some defense mechanisms such as denial serve to minimize the potential of threat of a stressful situation. In fact, as Janis (1983) points out, the common feature of the behavior denial is a tendency to minimize or fail to appraise correctly an undesirable personal characteristic or event. In circumstances of extreme stress, this tendency is observed in normal persons and may have adaptive value. The patient may use intellectual denial as an adaptive response. Intellectual denial of any such potential danger is referred to as minimization of the threat. Moreover, according to Janis, denial in the form of minimizing the magnitude or imminence of the threat may prove to be an adaptive type of response even when the dangers are nonambiguous, if there is little realistic basis for hope of survival.

Kiening (1978) has described denial as follows:

> Denial is a defense mechanism operating outside of and beyond conscious awareness in the endeavor to resolve emotional conflict and so allay anxiety. It achieves its purpose by disowning, rejecting, or ignoring one or more of the elements of the conflict. Obvious reality factors that the person finds painful or unpleasant are perceived as a threat to the self-structure and treated as if they did not exist. If the threat cannot be escaped or attacked, anxiety may be reduced and comfort reestablished by denying its existence. (P. 212)

Therefore, denial serves to decrease the individual's anxiety level. This is accomplished by minimizing the individual's perception of the threat. If we do not perceive an object as threatening, we do not experience internal threat.

According to Goldberger (1983) there are three types of denial: major, partial, and minimal. *Major denial* describes patients who state they experience no fear at any time throughout their hospitalization or earlier in their lives. *Partial denial* describes an individual who initially denied being frightened but eventually admits experiencing some fear. Finally, *minimal denial* applies to individuals who complain of anxiety or admit to feeling frightened. Goldberger goes on to note that denial is not an all-or-none affair. It can be massive, covering a large area of external reality as in the psychotic, or operate within a fairly specific conflictual or painful situation as in the case of an acute illness or death of a loved one. Unless supported by the environment, denial will not be successfully maintained for more than brief periods at a time.

A patient who has recently been discharged from a critical care setting may begin to manifest the same or similar symptoms that led to his hospitalization. To cope with the situation, he may deny that a potential threat has recurred. He denies fact and feelings, past or present, anything that could be too painful to acknowledge. The memory of his recent hospitalization is too vivid in his mind. He chooses to deny the threat, hoping that the symptoms will go away. If the individual is successful in his denial, there will be no threat because he has prevented any significant connection between ideas that are threatening from taking place. Action tendency may not take place because the individual no longer appraises a threat that he must face.

Another patient currently hospitalized in a critical care unit may choose to deny even while he is actually experiencing the problem or crisis. Denial can be viewed as a normal behavior. Examined from the standpoint of normality, denial may be thought of as coping behavior, that is, one of the psyche activities by which the adaptative process is brought about. As Goldberger (1983) reminds us, even though denial may take its toll, it may also serve very important adaptive functions by conserving energy and postponing action. This observation is becoming more and more frequent especially when reference is made to critically ill patients such as those suffering from myocardial infarction. Among such patients, even extreme denial is used by otherwise normal and stable people as part of coping with the illness (Goldberger 1983).

According to Kiening (1978), coping behavior can be seen as consisting of two aspects: an externally directed aspect, judged for its effectiveness in social terms, and an internally directed or defensive aspect, which serves to protect the individual from disruptive degrees of anxiety and which is judged for adequacy by the degree of comfort resulting.

Denial is a process that aims at minimizing fear and utilizes any number of other defenses, such as displacement, isolation, or rationalization. According to Hackett (1970), "Denial is interpersonal as well as intrapersonal and probably varies in extent and effectiveness depending upon who the patient addresses" (p. 42). Behaviorally an individual may exhibit denial by not paying attention to or not speaking of the threatening connotation of events. Therefore if the patient chooses to deny he is critically ill, he will also avoid the idea in thought, deed, or word. A critically ill patient who knows he or she is dying may prefer not to think or talk about it. This is not denial but avoidance (Lazarus 1983).

Coping mechanisms such as avoidance and denial are only adaptive when they allow the individual to be more comfortable and not be seriously disrupted in other outgoing activities. Before applying the concepts avoidance and denial to the critically ill patient, we must remember that avoidance and denial serve to protect the individual. Statements such as "It can't be happening to me," or "I don't believe it," are a form of denial. The individual needs time to recover from the psychological shock or threat of illness. The individual is only capable of absorbing a small portion of the threat. It is unrealistic to expect him to incorporate all of the shock at once. The function of both avoidance and denial is to reduce conflict and anxiety through alteration or distortion in perception of the threat.

THE CONCEPTS OF AVOIDANCE AND DENIAL APPLIED TO THE CRITICALLY ILL PATIENT

Patients are looked upon in a holistic way by the nurse providing patient care. The critically ill patient is viewed as a whole entity. Critical care nurses know that when an aspect of the whole is altered, other systems are also altered to compensate for various pathophysiological changes. This notion especially applies to critical care units. In these units, it is easy to lose sight of the patient as a whole. He may become a heart, lung, or kidney. In critical care units, it is easy for the nurse and doctor to minimize the danger to the patient by saying, "It's going to be all right," "Leave the worrying to us," or "You just rest." Such statements are attempts to reduce the patient's anxiety, but they may serve to perpetuate his avoidance and denial. In addition, such statements may lessen the nurses' and doctors' own fears about the threat of danger to the patient. The individual as a whole needs to be acknowledged as a living being. As a living being or system he responds to changes in a constancy of interaction with his environment. Ideally, the critical care patient adapts to the forces that shape and reshape the very essence of his being.

The individual in a holistic sense feels he has self-worth, dignity, and integrity. As Hackett (1970) notes, "It is through his sense of self-worth and identity that the individual cherishes his personal integrity. The knowledge of being a whole person is intensely private, and the patterns of behavior which individuals assume throughout their lives cannot be left behind when they become ill" (p. 260). Once the individual becomes a patient with a diagnosis of illness, he enters into adaptive activities that are based upon his perception of the sick role. This perception may include awareness of a potential threat. His reaction to the threat may be temporarily held in control by means of avoidance and denial. These two means of coping or adapting continue only as long as he does not perceive any apparent sign of danger. Illness may be a new experience to him, so his adapting mechanisms begin quickly out of fear. According to Crate (1965), "Adaptation begins when the person learns, either by diagnosis or change in function (symptoms), that he has a particular condition. This represents a threat to his self. He resorts to denial of the threatening conditions to protect himself against the impact of it" (p. 72).

Direct-Action Tendency: Avoidance

Illness, injury, or disease and hospitalization in critical care cause certain unpredictable changes to occur within the individual. It should be noted that each patient reacts differently to stressful situations. A patient can either learn from the experience and change, or else think of himself as the same as before hospitalization with no physiological change. As Travelbee (1966) notes, the nurse, too, may react to change with avoidance coping mechanisms:

> No human being can be repeatedly exposed . . . to illness, suffering and death without being changed as a result of these encounters. . . . One common outcome is to withdraw from the individual or situation producing the feeling, with indifference or detachment. Indifference or detachment become protective mechanisms in that they prevent the nurse from experiencing the full impact of the anxiety that is engendered in the situation. (P. 45)

Lazarus (1966) has identified three basic kinds of coping reaction patterns found in avoidance. These include (1) directly expressed avoidance with fear, (2) fear with avoidance expression inhibited, and (3) avoidance without fear.

Directly Expressed Avoidance with Fear. Directly expressed avoidance with fear requires appraisal of threat. The degree of threat is relevant to the strength of the avoidance action tendency and the degree of fear. For example, an individual may avoid the sick role altogether. He fails to see his physician at the onset of symptoms. Mr. J. was such a patient. He was 40 years old, married, and the father of three boys. His job combined construction and sheet metal work. It depended upon the needs of his clients. The work he did kept him outdoors and in high places. Since he lived and worked in an industrial area, smog was a continual problem. In the construction side of his business, he remained with his employees and supervised their activities. The work was hard, requiring long hours without adequate rest. He realized the dangers and pressures of his job but nevertheless continued. One day, as he was assisting two men to join together two large beams 14 stories up he became dizzy. Luckily, he was standing near the skeletal structure of a wall so he grabbed onto it. He quickly looked to see if the other men had noticed. Fortunately, their backs were turned at the time. Since no one noticed, he decided not to relate the incident. After all, he was probably just tired. During the next several weeks, Mr. J. noticed that he became dizzy at other times—when mowing the lawn and when in very high places. He also noticed that the dizziness was more frequent when the weather was hot and smoggy. Furthermore, he noticed that he coughed more frequently than in the past when he smoked or worked with his sheet metal. Again, he shrugged off the symptoms as meaningless. He was probably overworked and fatigued. Neither he nor any member of his family had ever been sick, so illness seemed to be an impossibility.

Time passed without problem until one day, when Mr. J. was working on the sixteenth floor. As usual, it was hot and smoggy during the summer months. This time he was supervising the pouring of concrete. Suddenly and without warning, he became dizzy and fell to the floor. Several men came to his aid, helped him down the elevator, and against his protest called for a doctor. His doctor insisted that he come to his office for some routine tests.

Reluctantly, Mr. J. followed his doctor's orders. After all, he had very little faith in what a few tests could determine. A chest X-ray and other diagnostic tests revealed Mr. J. had emphysema. He was told by his doctor that the dizziness was due to oxygen deficiency. This would be particularly true on smoggy days when he worked in high places. His cough was due to the irritating effect of smoking and of the metal particles he inhaled while cutting metal. He would have to eliminate these factors if he wanted to continue living a relatively normal life. Mr. J. did not believe in nor accept his doctor's diagnosis. He just decided to push the whole incident out of his mind. Construction and sheet metal work were the only things he knew, and the threat of their loss was too overwhelming even to think about. As Janis (1958) has pointed out, "The closer an anticipated threat of body danger is perceived to be, the greater will be the individual's motivation to ward off anticipatory fears by minimizing the potential danger or by intellectually denying that he will be seriously affected by it" (p. 73).

As the weeks progressed, Mr. J.'s symptoms increased in frequency. The harder he tried to avoid their presence and overcompensate, the more intense the symptoms became. It was as if Mr. J.'s manliness was being challenged. Finally the challenge became too great. Mr. J. once again passed out high above the smoggy city he loved so well; this time he did not regain consciousness until he was in a critical care unit. There he awakened to find a breathing mask on his face, EKG leads on his chest connected to a strange machine, and intravenous fluid flowing into his arm. He no longer could avoid the insignificance of his symptoms or the doctor's diagnosis and warnings. The critical care unit and technology made his illness very apparent. He realized that he had fought a vigorous yet unsuccessful battle.

Mrs. C. is another example of a patient who sought avoidance of the sick role. Like Mr. J., her avoidance was brought about by tremendous fear. Mrs. C. was 52 years old, a widow for two years, mother of two married daughters, and a grandmother of three. Mrs. C. had always been a relatively active woman, free of illness. During the past several weeks, Mrs. C. noticed her dresses were getting tight. Since she had always carefully watched her diet, she could not understand the reason for her sudden gain in weight. Nevertheless, she decided to diet for a week, hoping this would cause weight loss. After a week of strict dieting, she noticed no apparent change. Furthermore, she noticed a change in the color of her stools. She thought their clay-colored appearance was the result of her diet. Next, she began to experience high abdominal pain. Once again she avoided the threat of a potential problem by reducing the symptom to indigestion and took an antacid to alleviate the situation.

Two weeks passed, and the symptoms continued. Mrs. C.'s daughters began to notice a change in their mother. She seemed irritable and without her usual energy. In addition, they noticed the sclera of her eyes were slightly yellow. Together the daughters pleased with their mother to see a doctor. Their pleading was to no avail as Mrs. C. continued to rationalize that nothing was wrong and the symptoms would go away. Realizing their mother was a strong-willed and stubborn woman, they decided to respect her judgment and not pursue the issue. As the days turned into weeks, Mrs. C.'s symptoms became more acute. Finally Mrs. C. had to seek her doctor.

Mrs. C. was immediately admitted to a critical care unit. Her symptoms pointed in the direction of liver pathology. Because she had been symptom-free until several weeks ago, her doctors began thinking of hepatic carcinoma. Needless to say, like so many other patients, Mrs. C. had already thought of the dreaded illness cancer. A liver biopsy was ordered. For the next 24 hours, and even after the diagnosis hepatic carcinoma was confirmed, Mrs. C. avoided any discussion of her illness. She remained in the critical care unit where attempts were made to treat her ascites and control her newly developed bleeding problems.

Both Mr. J. and Mrs. C. attempted to rationalize their symptoms away. Janis (1958) describes the function of rationalization as follows:

> The rationalization defense may be conceived as a means of escape from thinking about the causes of current emotional tensions to prevent fear reaction from snow-balling. By giving himself convincing reasons as to why he is feeling somewhat upset, a person can avoid certain of the most disturbing inner cues, thoughts, or images which explicitly and vividly represent the most dreaded possibilities of suffering and loss. (P. 82)

In each case the threat was appraised. The threat was illness and possible disability due to physiological changes resulting in permanent damage. Mr. J. feared loss of manliness. To him, manliness was synonymous with being able to perform physically like younger men. It further meant directly supervising and working beside his men. He was able to lead his men successfully because they respected his ability to join them in their endeavors rather than guiding them from afar. His judgment became their own, and his decisions or desires met with their respect. All these personal factors went into the success of his business. Therefore, illness posed a tremendous threat. Mrs. C., on the other hand, feared loss of independence resulting in a forced dependence on her daughters. At age 52, she was not able to accept; consequently, she avoided thinking about the possible consequences of her symptoms. Both individuals feared loss of the physical freedom that they had always taken for granted in health. According to Kiening (1978), temporary or permanent interruption to one's health "always poses some threat to the individual's life situation. Although the fear of death or disability looms as an important factor in the patient's response to the impact of illness, there are many other needs, the fulfillment of which is jeopardized by an alteration in physical or psychological well-being" (p. 213).

Mr. J. and Mrs. C. both viewed illness and its physical restrictions or possible death as overpowering. Their only means of coping with the threat was to avoid confronting it: if a person never validates the origin of his symptoms (diagnosis), the symptoms remain nebulous. The individual has nothing concrete to fight, such as myocardial infarction, renal disease, emphysema, or a hepatic tumor. Mr. J. and Mrs. C. intellectually ran from the problem until they were forced physically to give up. Once hospitalized, they could no longer avoid their illness, but they could continue to avoid the subject by choosing not to discuss it. Mr. J. and Mrs. C. represent examples of patients who expressed avoidance with fear. The fear was manifested in the threat of illness with all its limitations and changes.

Fear with Avoidance Expression Inhibited. Fear with avoidance expression inhibited involves the same appraisal as does avoidance directly expressed with fear. Differences, according to Lazarus (1966), "lie primarily in the role of situational constraints, and secondarily, in the motivational pattern, belief systems, and age resources of the individual" (p. 320). As with directly expressed avoidance with fear, one must appraise the threat and the location of a harmful agent.

An individual may not be aware of his own avoidance. He may evaluate that the harmful agent is overpowering and can only be dealt with by avoiding a confrontation. He may also make the judgment that the means of avoiding confrontation is only limited or temporary. Mr. L. was such a patient. He was 48 years old, aggressive, dynamic, and described by friends as a "real workhorse." He was married, the father of three children, and president of a prestigious bank in the community. All his life, he had assisted other people in working out their financial problems. Twenty years of his life had been spent in service to his church, community, and family. One year before Mr. L. had experienced his own personal crisis—an acute myocardial infarction. Prior to that time, he had frequent episodes of chest pain. One year later, Mr. L. continued to experience substernal chest pain. He had noted a definite increase in the pain's frequency. Mr. L. attempted to compensate for the pain by increasing his medication and decreasing any strenuous activity. He kept both these maneuvers from his doctor and wife. He did not want his family to worry about his problems. One day Mrs. L. noticed her husband taking a nitroglycerine tablet while reading the newspaper. She thought this was rather unusual and alarming, but the pills had become an accepted routine to Mr. L.

Naturally, Mrs. L. was quite concerned. She finally convinced her husband to enter the hospital. Like Mr. J., Mr. L. became technically aware of his physical problems. An EKG was immediately taken and the staff then connected him to a cardioscope. His nurse administered intravenous therapy and oxygen via nasal prongs. Since he was free of arrhythmias, his condition was considered stable.

Mr. L.'s doctor believed he had severe coronary artery disease that warranted a coronary artery bypass. The doctors had to perform a heart catheterization in order to confirm their diagnosis. Dr. P. decided to discuss the situation with Mr. L.

DR. P.: Mr. L., how are you feeling this morning?
MR. L.: Fine, I feel silly being here.
DR. P.: Why is that?

MR. L.: I feel like nothing is wrong, and that I am occupying a bed someone else could use.

DR. P.: The angina you felt was real, and it will probably continue.

MR. L.: Say, how is your wife and family?

DR. P.: They are fine. Tom, there are some diagnostic tests I would like to do on you.

MR. L.: Oh, I don't need any tests. My problem was just fatigue. I'll be okay.

DR. P.: We need to do certain tests to make sure you'll be okay.

MR. L.: I am feeling better. How has your golf game been?

DR. P.: Not too good.

MR. L.: Let's play some golf when I leave the hospital.

DR. P.: We will talk again later. We need to talk about consent for diagnostic tests to confirm the status of your coronary arteries. It may be necessary to perform coronary artery bypass. (*He then leaves Mr. L. alone.*)

MR. L.: (*Turns on his side and begins reading a book.*)

Mr. L. appraised the threat to be a continued disabling illness. His activity was becoming more restricted and the pain more frequent. When his doctor attempted to explain various diagnostic procedures necessary in order to document the need for surgery, he avoided the issue by changing the subject to golf and the doctor's family. In all probability, he was not ready to hear about heart catheterization or the possibility of coronary artery bypass. To Mr. L., "diagnostic tests" represented more of the unknown. The reality of what Dr. P. told him did not seem to sink in because he immediately began reading his book. On the other hand, the reality could have been so threatening that he decided to put it out of his mind by reading. Some patients have difficulty seeing beyond the immediate threat of surgery. They fail to see the advantage of surgery simply because they have not been informed. For Mr. L., the advantage would be relative freedom from angina and a possible return to his previous activities.

Mr. L. may view the location of the harmful agent as the critical care unit. He remembered his first and last experience with the event. His memory has been refreshed by tubes and wires, his chest connected to cardioscope leads, his nose and mouth were covered by a mask, his arm was immobilized by intravenous therapy tubing, and his veins were bruised by repeated venipunctures. In addition to the technical environment, the idea of surgery frightened him. It is no small wonder that the patient sees the harmful agent as overpowering. The only way for him to cope is to avoid confronting it.

Other critically ill patients may react differently. Like Mr. L., they may be fearful and yet lack awareness that avoidance is occurring. Some patients believe that once out of the critical care environment, they will feel better. Such a patient seems to dissociate himself from the crisis or environment.

One patient may refuse to keep an appointment for fear of discovering the meaning of his symptoms. Another patient may refuse to take his medications or may impede routine laboratory blood work. He may view them both as unnecessary and expensive. Furthermore, he may fear side effects from the medication. Like illness itself, medications may be a new experience. A patient with chronic obstructive lung disease may refuse to take his breathing treatments. His fear and subconscious avoidance may be different from those of the postoperative open heart patient, who associates his breathing treatments with pain. Still another critically ill patient may refuse to sign a consent for an emergency procedure or diagnostic test such as lumbar puncture, biopsy, or pacemaker insertion. The threat of the procedures may be more overpowering than the results. Lastly, there are patients in critical care units who fear the various pieces of equipment either already connected or waiting in readiness to be connected. Without awareness of what he is doing, a patient may disconnect his EKG leads, intravenous therapy, Foley catheter, or A-V shunt. He may even attempt to disconnect himself from the critical care unit by trying to leave.

In all probability, these critically ill patients have strong internal values that work against avoidance. Their expression of avoidance, consequently, is only temporary. In time, according to Lazarus (1966), "If the internalized values are weaker than the original threat itself, they will not be as effective in constraining avoidance, since the danger is greater in not expressing the action tendency than in doing so" (p. 306).

Avoidance without Fear. Just as there can be fear with avoidance expression inhibited, there can also be one last type of avoidance, avoidance without fear. We have previously discussed patients who demonstrated the action tendency of avoidance out of fear. These critically ill patients were familiar with the source of their threat. One of them, for example, would know why he avoided a particular test to validate his symptoms. Avoidance without fear, on the other hand, "presupposes a situation in which the avoidance behavior is instrumental for goal gratification without the presence of any threat to the individual. The avoided object is thus not regarded as an agent of harm. Confrontation with it is avoided for other reasons" (Lazarus 1966, p. 306).

Mrs. P., a 58-year-old woman married to a disabled veteran, is an example of someone who experienced avoidance without fear. Because her husband became a paraplegic shortly after their marriage, the couple had no children. Mrs. P. has assumed responsibility for the care of her husband. In addition, she has been the sole provider for both herself and her husband, except for his small supplementary disability check. Four days previously, Mrs. P. was admitted to a critical care unit when she developed severe chest pain, diaphoresis, nausea, and shortness of breath. An EKG and serum enzyme studies revealed an anterior myocardial infarction. During the four days after her arrival, Mrs. P.'s condition remained essentially stable, in the sense that she manifested no arrhythmias, her serum enzymes were returning to normal, and she seemed to be free of pain. Mrs. P.'s only goal consisted of her need to be discharged as quickly as possible. She felt great responsibility for her disabled husband. Mrs. P. repeatedly minimized her responsibilities at home, saying, "There isn't that much to do." However, friends visiting Mrs. P. shared their observations with the nursing staff. They described her home situation as very strenuous and time-consuming. Like all good friends, they were concerned that she might return home and resume her work much too soon. Nevertheless, Mrs. P. continued to reassure her friends and nursing staff that she felt good. Mrs. P. learned that on the fifth day she was going to be transferred to a general floor rather than to a subacute unit. This piece of news naturally made her quite happy.

During the night, Mrs. P. developed chest pain. For fear of not being transferred out of the critical care unit, she did not tell her nurse. She felt quite confident that the pain was of no significance and probably represented indigestion. After all, she did not experience any other symptoms such as diaphoresis, nausea, or shortness of breath. Furthermore, the monitor pattern looked the same as before. Eventually, the pain subsided and she was able to sleep. The next morning, her nurse observed that Mrs. P. ate very little for breakfast. She felt this was unusual for her patient and decided to confront her with the observation.

NURSE: Good morning, Mrs. P. Is everything okay?
MRS. P.: Why, yes.
NURSE: Was your breakfast all right?
MRS. P.: Yes.
NURSE: I noticed that you didn't seem to eat very much this morning.
MRS. P.: Oh, that! I can't develop an appetite just lying in bed all the time.
NURSE: You do feel all right?
MRS. P.: Yes. When will I be transferred out of here?
NURSE: As soon as a bed becomes available.

Mrs. P.'s explanation was quite logical; consequently, the subject was dropped. The nurse had validated her observations. Later in the morning, Mrs. P. was transferred to a two-bed ward. Things seemed to progress nicely for Mrs. P. her first day on the floor. She had even convinced her doctors to increase her activity. The following morning, she suddenly experienced chest pain. This time, the pain seemed more severe. However, Mrs. P. still remained without fear, remembering how it went away before. Fortunately, her roommate noticed Mrs. P. clutch her chest. The roommate quickly called the nurse, who immediately notified Mrs. P.'s doctor and began carrying out his orders. These included her immediate transfer back to critical care.

Mrs. P.'s goal was a quick and speedy recovery. She wanted to return to her disabled husband. She felt that if she avoided the danger signal of pain, she could achieve her goal. The goal became the driving force behind her avoidance. Mrs. P., like many other critically ill patients, did not fear the pain when it occurred, because she did not perceive the pain as a threat. Besides, the pain came independent of other symptoms. This factor alone made it less significant to her. She successfully avoided, without fear, until the day after her transfer, when the pain and related symptoms were no longer avoidable.

Defensive Reappraisal: Denial

Each day many persons are faced with stressful events or situations. Two stressful events requiring hospitalization in critical care are myocardial infarction and open heart surgery. As Elliott (1980) has noted, individuals use denial as a coping mechanism to relieve anxiety and to help them with the painful realities of the situation. There are times when patients in coronary care either deny the nature and severity of their condition (cognitive denial) or deny having painful feelings associated with the situation (affective denial). Denial is one of the first adaptive behaviors that cardiac patients have in their coping repertoire. An individual who is suddenly confronted with the need for surgery or acute illness has had little time to prepare for the crisis. The experience is viewed as a threat. It is therefore normal for such individuals to use denial to handle the initial anxiety which the illness or injury has produced.

The first factor to take into consideration when looking at defensive reappraisal is that the "degree of primitivity of the coping process is related to the degree of threat. Since defense is a primitive reaction, it follows, then that it will occur more readily under strong threats than under weak threats" (Lazarus 1966, p. 307). Critically ill patients can enter critical care units in various stages of crisis. Therefore, the defense mechanism utilized varies in intensity. A more critically ill patient may utilize complete denial or may even dissociate from the problem, whereas a less critically ill patient may respond through partial denial. It must be remembered that "any external sign that increases a person's awareness of the proximity of a threat will tend to elicit an increase in denial tendencies" (Janis 1958, pp. 73–74).

Denial, at least partial denial, is used by most critically ill patients. Denial is used not only during the first stage of illness or following confrontation but also later on from time to time. Denial serves the purpose of functioning as a buffer after unexpected shocking news. It allows the patient time to collect himself and other less radical defenses. Once the crisis has subsided, the same patient later on in his hospitalization may be relieved to talk with someone about his prognosis and his possible death or biological loss. Greene, Moss, and Goldstein (1974) note that the individual who denies minimally does not need tremendous outside assistance to seek a physician for relief of coronary symptoms. On the other hand, when denial is major the individual will put off seeking help unless someone else pushes him into action.

Mr. F. is an example of a patient who manifested complete denial and disassociation. A 49-year-old married man, Mr. F. was a diabetic who had been frequently admitted in the past years in a diabetic coma. He had also been admitted for myocardial infarction, upper respiratory infection, and urinary tract infection. With each admission, his physical status diminished to the point where he now complained of leg discomfort (peripheral neuropathy), and he also noted visual changes. A few weeks before, while clipping his toenails, he accidentally clipped a piece of skin. He had been cautioned by his doctor about the importance of good and careful foot care. He assumed the toe would heal with no apparent difficulty. However, as the weeks progressed, the toe itself changed in color. He continued treating the toe with his own conservative means, which had little or no healing effect. Then, in addition to suffering from an infected toe, Mr. F. became ill with influenza. After a day of vomiting and diarrhea, he contacted his doctor. Knowing his patient's physiological status and diabetic history, the doctor immediately admitted him to intensive care. Fortunately, Mr. F. arrived before other complications, such as upper respiratory infection or diabetic coma, could occur.

While admitting Mr. F. to intensive care, his doctors discovered the infected toe and learned that it had been a problem for several weeks. Naturally, Mr. F. was informed of the graveness of his failure to report the infection immediately. His doctor informed him, "Debridement would be necessary. There is also the possibility you could lose your toe, or even you foot." Mr. F. assured the doctor that "Debridement would do the job." He continued to say, "It will be all right in a few days." A week passed, and his toe did not improve. It seemed apparent to all except Mr. F. that his toe would have to be amputated. Meanwhile, Mr. F. had avoided any reference to his foot. It was as if the foot belonged to someone else. He disassociated himself from its existence. He attributed the pain in his foot to peripheral neuropathy.

Mr. F.'s case illustrates a major problem of denial described by Kiening (1978):

> Denial serves only to cover or minimize the anxiety-provoking aspect of the reality that constitutes the threat. So long as the person can maintain his denial in the face of objective evidence, it serves as an effective protection against overwhelming anxiety. Its inconsistency with reality makes it a very brittle defense, however; and when it finally must come face to face with reality, it crumbles, leaving the person defenseless. (Pp. 212-213)

Mr. F. was able to face the fact that he had diabetes. He denied illness by ignoring a certain portion of the problem, his infected toe. By ignoring this aspect, he could also ignore thinking about any form of loss or possible disfigurement. Such denial is typical of the cardiac patient who attributes his chest pain to indigestion. Other critically ill patients deny their illness by focusing on such topics as constipation, hearing aids, or hemorrhoids. There are even patients who minimize their illness or at least a portion of it by saying, "It didn't hurt that much," "It wasn't so bad," or "Everything will work out for the best." Such statements may be a normal way to minimize the danger.

A second factor in regard to defense reappraisal is the absence of any visible action tendency for overcoming or reducing the anticipated harm. Rather than view denial as a specific defense mechanism, it can be regarded as a process by which other defense mechanism can be used to reduce stress. Froese et al. (1974) point out that denial is effective in reducing anxiety and suggest that a relationship may exist between the successful use of denial and morbidity/mortality in acute coronary disease as found in the coronary care unit. The ability to deny stress successfully may be a factor which enhances survival in myocardial infarction.

When pressures are great and prognosis is grave for the critically ill patient, his denial becomes a denial of the fear of death. The critically ill patient may be totally unable to accept either the sick role or the thought of potential death. According to Wu (1973), "When an individual cannot accept his illness in the presence of dysfunction or symptoms, he is exhibiting illness behavior through the use of defense mechanisms such as denial" (p. 158). Again, absence of action tendency may be the result of detachment or disassociation.

Mrs. H. represents such a patient situation. A 50-year-old woman, the mother of two, she was a hemodialysis patient. She had a history of nephrossclerosis that necessitated hemodialysis three times a week. Mrs. H. had tremendous difficulty with fluid retention and subsequent weight gain. The nursing staff had carefully instructed her about fluid restriction, dietary needs, and a sodium-potassium restriction. No matter how hard the health team worked, Mrs. H. periodically entered the hemodialysis unit in borderline pulmonary edema. At home she refused to restrict her fluid intake, to reduce her protein intake to the limits prescribed, or to restrict her salt intake. While in the hemodialysis unit, the nurses noticed that Mrs. H. referred to her A-V shunt or the hemodialysis machine as "your shunt," "your machine," or "it."

Mrs. H. seemed to dissociate herself from the problem of renal failure and hemodialysis. It was as if the machine were connected to someone else's body. She did not take action to reduce fluids, protein, or salt, because she did not perceive them to be "her" problems. Even though her headaches and fatigue were real, she still continued to deny their origin. The threat of accepting her current status as a new way of life was too overwhelming. The nurses realized the patient's dilemma and they also understood that the time was not ripe to confront Mrs. H. King (1966) addresses the problem of premature confrontation as follows:

> Confronting the patient with the focus of his denial, or with anything associated with it, can threaten this defense. When denial is threatened, internal and external perception, as well as comprehension, are blotted out to maintain the denial. Thus, large portions of reality are not at the individual's disposal, and his thinking tends to remain static or unrealistic. (P. 1010)

Instead of confrontation, the hemodialysis nurses chose to support Mrs. H. and, when possible, to remind her of reality.

In such a situation, a patient may need to deny at least part of the problem. Until she accepts her dialysis machine as a substitute for her kidneys, the nurse has nothing but her support to offer the patient. As the patient begins to identify with "her shunt" or "her dialysis machine," then the nurse can move to any additional areas of denial such as diet or medication. Nurses can follow the same pattern with other critically ill patients who use denial as their coping mechanism.

A third and last factor of defensive reappraisal concerns the location of a harmful agent. Some patients exhibit externalization of blame. They blame others for whatever illness they suffer or whatever burdensome treatment they must endure. A patient may blame his nurse, doctor, or wife, and use them as scapegoats; he displaces his inability to accept the illness onto the people he holds responsible for his care. He may also view them as responsible for his problem. Such reactions are simply an attempt by the patient to identify an agent of harm. He also feels guilty for becoming ill in the first place. He may totally defy treatments or orders by refusing to comply with instructions from his health team. Such behavioral actions, according to Kiening (1978),

> may pose more of a problem for the nurse. Because they are often acted out, these clues may not be easily recognized. Here again, the range of behavior is wide—from the quiet model patient whose underestimate of his needs may be so great that the medical staff and his family overlook his real feeling and requirement to the hostile, uncooperative patient who violates his medical orders. (P. 215)

NURSING ASSESSMENT OF AVOIDANCE AND DENIAL

The nurse assesses avoidance and denial through the critically ill patient's particular behavioral response. The responses are categorized into regulatory behavior and cognitive behaviors. Regulatory behaviors result from physiological changes, if any, associated with the problem. Cognitive behaviors are attributed to psychosocial alterations.

Regulatory Behaviors

The regulatory system involves stimuli from the external environment and from changes in the internal state of dynamic equilibrium. The regulatory behaviors are physiological responses associated with avoidance and denial. It may be that most regulatory behaviors can also be attributed to the anxiety or fear that the patient is trying to deny. The following regulatory behaviors may be manifested by the patient:

Regulatory Behaviors
Tachycardia
Tachypnea
Normal or increased blood pressure
Angina
Arrhythmias
Increased urinary catecholamines
Gastrointestinal discomfort

The patient may also experience other related physical complaints. For the cardiac patient experiencing angina and subsequent EKG changes, denial of the symptoms may only contribute to the biological crisis.

Cognitive Behaviors

The cognitive system involves inputs from internal and external stimuli which include psychological and social factors. Cognitive behaviors stem from alterations in information processing, judgment, learning, and emotion. Therefore cognitive behaviors are associated with psychosocial responses.

The range of behavior along the continuum of denial is wide. According to Kiening (1978), there are differences in behavior both in the level of awareness at which denial operates and the degree to which reality is excluded. The following are examples of avoidance and denial cognitive behaviors:

Cognitive behaviors
Rationalization
Displacement
Magical thinking
Isolation
Tunnel vision
Selective perception
Withdrawal

The patient may also experience anger. When using denial as a defense mechanism, the patient becomes angry each time someone attempts to focus on the current illness or reality. Regardless of the specific threat, denial can be manifested in many ways.

NURSING DIAGNOSIS OF AVOIDANCE AND DENIAL

The nursing diagnosis is based upon an understanding of the patient's problems and an assessment of various regulatory or cognitive behaviors. When the patient is unwilling to discuss his biological crisis, listens only selectively to what is told him, rationalizes various symptoms, engages in magical thinking, and attributes the cause of the current threat to an external source, the critical care nurse is able to make a diagnosis. The nurse attempts to identify internal and external stressors so they can be appropriately confronted, explained, or eliminated.

NURSING INTERVENTIONS IN CASES
OF AVOIDANCE AND DENIAL

The nurse intervenes in areas of both direct action tendency (avoidance) and defensive reappraisal (denial). Even though denial, as previously mentioned, can be relatively healthy, it can, as Kiening (1978) has pointed out, "at times seriously interfere with the treatment program. It may defeat the nurse's best efforts to establish a helping relationship with her patient. On the other hand, it may serve as a protection for the ego, preventing the person from becoming overwhelmed by anxiety and averting extensive emotional disorganization" (p. 213). In general, the critical care nurse's goal becomes twofold: she can protect the patient's personal integrity and she can help him to accept the illness and disfigurement.

Protection of Personal Integrity

Denial seems to establish a protective screen between the unconscious and preconscious. It is a defense that appears to work solely within the realm of the ego. For example, any illness or disease that affects the heart is likely to have an effect upon the patient's self-esteem and body-image. This is especially true for male cardiac patients who need to form some type of protection to their ego. The independent individual who is forced into a dependency role has his ego and self-esteem devastated. How the critically ill patient uses denial while in a particular critical care unit to protect himself from complete disorganization needs to be recognized by the nurse. Frequently the clues indicating avoidance-denial, whether it be therapeutic or nontherapeutic, are overlooked or ignored (Elliott 1980).

Besides being an excellent observer and assessor, the critical care nurse can be an active listener and supporter. Critically ill patients have their own personal reasons for avoidance or denial in confronting a perceived threat or harmful agent. Initially, the reason may be unknown even to the patient. Usually, his behavior is oriented toward protecting his personal integrity. The nurse must therefore listen to and support the patient. Because illness, or the discovering of a physiological dysfunction, may be a totally new experience, the patient may have no coping mechanism on which to draw. He may resort to primitive means of adapting, such as avoidance or denial. Hopefully, the adaptive mechanism chosen will only be a temporary one. The nurse can help her patient maintain his integrity while simultaneously helping him deal with the behavior action chosen. This assumes that the nurse is aware her patient is denying or avoiding. It is not unusual for patients skillfully, and perhaps unconsciously, to deny or avoid confrontation with illness. Their subtle behavior can deceive even their families. The "happy-go-lucky" patient is an example of someone who attracts health personnel into his room because of his joking or jesting. The staff may feel confident that he has accepted his illness. They described him as "an absolute joy to take care of" or a "real pleasure." The next day, the very same patient may be quiet, depressed, or even tearful. The patient needed to be jovial and project a "nothing-is-wrong-with-me" attitude. It was his way of reassuring himself that, in fact, he would be all right. His behavior served to minimize the intensity of the situation.

In working with denial of illness as a nursing problem, the nurse must first assess its existence, the extent to which denial may be harmful for the individual, and the extent to which it is therapeutic for the patient, depending upon the type, severity, and duration of the biological crisis. Denial can be acknowledged as operating but not as presenting a particular nursing care problem. During an initial biological crisis it can be an emergency brake that prevents complete disorganization in the face of a crisis with which the patient is not yet ready to handle (Kiening 1978).

The critical care nurse must identify the behavior, accept it for what it latently represents, and patiently wait for other signs that might be incongruent with the patient's original behavior. The case of Ms. S. shows how a critical care nurse intervenes to accomplish these three factors. Ms. S., a 23-year-old woman, was burned while adding lighter fluid to her cigarette lighter. While filling her lighter, she apparently spilled some of the lighter fluid on her nylon gown. After filling her lighter, she checked to see if it worked. In the process, a spark fell on her gown. The result was second-degree burns on her neck, chest, hands, and upper thighs. Since the burns were mostly second-degree, Ms. S. required pain medication over her four-day stay in the burn unit. During her four days, she remained jovial. When the critical care nurse prepared her patient for the Hubbard tank, they had the following dialogue:

NURSE: I am going to change your dressings after you return from the Hubbard tank. Before that, I'll give you some medication.

MS. S.:   Yes, give me the good stuff. I might enjoy becoming an addict.

NURSE: Do you think you are taking too much medication?

MS. S.:   No, I was just kidding. Boy, wait until Frank sees all these groovy dressings. Will he ever laugh!

NURSE: Who is Frank?

MS. S.:   He is my boyfriend. I guess he has been too scared to see me.

NURSE: Why do you think he will laugh at your dressings?

MS. S.:   Oh, because I look like a mummy.

NURSE: Is that how you see yourself?

MS. S.: No. I don't want to see myself. Maybe I can keep the bandages forever. Say, I thought you were getting me a pain medication.

NURSE: Yes, I was. We will continue talking later, Jane.

Ms. S.'s nurse gently opened the door into her serious thoughts regarding an altered physical integrity. She accomplished this goal by carefully listening to what Ms. S. was directly and latently saying. The patient was only able to cope with the threatening subject for a brief moment. Nevertheless, she brought up the subject of reality: "I don't want to see myself"; "Maybe I can keep the bandages forever." Once the door was opened, she immediately retreated to the subject of her medication. The critical care nurse, aware of Ms. S.'s behavior and needs, complied with the sudden change of topic. The nurse realized that her patient was only able to handle a small portion of the total tragedy. Ms. S. also gave her nurse clues as to her self-concept. She referred to herself as "an addict" and "a mummy." The patient may be describing herself as someone who no longer has social integrity or significance because of disfigurement. Consequently, such a person needs to be shielded from others in a mummylike fashion. These are things Ms. S.'s nurse can work on when she assesses the patient's readiness. Her nurse is also aware of a danger pointed out by King (1966), namely, that if she "attempts to force the surrender of denial through intense and untimely intervention, the patient will only strive to maintain his defense with a force equal to that exerted by the nurse" (p. 1011). The nurse can therefore pace herself with her patient. By pacing, the nurse avoids moving ahead of the patient by pursuing a threatening topic before the patient is ready. Nor does she remain behind, ignoring the topic. Once the nurse identifies what she believes to be avoidance or denial behavior, she looks for possible reasons behind such behavior. In other words, the nurse must discover what meaning avoidance or denial has for the patient.

It should be noted that what is analyzed as pathology may be the valid use of a healthy protecting mechanism. Then, too, behavior that seems like denial may not in fact be real denial. Often it happens that critically ill patients are aware of their illness and its implications, but they may choose consciously to face the crisis alone rather than add to the stress and anxiety of family members. Furthermore, confronting the patient with reality before he is emotionally ready may do more harm than good. Early confrontation of reality can cause the patient to be more adamant in his defense mechanism, thereby making the immediate situation more comfortable. The nurse knows that the patient who is already experiencing a biological crisis or disfigurement needs support and understanding rather than additional stress or confrontation (Kiening 1978).

The critical care nurse can, in many situations, accept her patient's denial or avoidance expression. However she may not be able to accept his denial or avoidance behavior toward treatment. For example, when a hemo-dialysis patient ignores his diet or refuses to take care of his A-V shunt, the nurse need not accept such activity. Instead, she can pursue the reasons behind his actions. To the patient, hemodialysis may represent an unacceptable change in life-style. He may have difficulty tolerating dependency on an inanimate object. In distinguishing forms of denial that require her intervention, the nurse can keep in mind the warning of Crate (1965): "It is not the role of the nurse to attempt to change the basic life pattern of the patient, but to support him as he moves toward a way of life that accommodates his illness" (p. 72).*

Acceptance of Illness or Disfigurement

The critical care nurse's second major goal is to help her patient accept his illness or disfigurement. The nurse must keep in mind that both avoidance and denial are stages within the adaptive process. Before the patient can accept his illness, disfigurement, limitation, or change in lifestyle, he must be aware they exist. The goals of the nurse and the critically ill patient must be compatible. The critical care nurse can assist and support her patient as he develops awareness of his problem, and she can encourage him to share in the responsibility of dealing with the problems.

Acceptance does not occur all at once. The patient may accept the fact that he is ill or has a physiological dysfunction, but he might refuse to accept a certain aspect of his illness. Moreover, as Wu (1973) points out, there may be regression in levels of acceptance:

> Having accepted the fact of his illness, the patient will engage in activities so as to rid himself of the dysfunction or symptom and regain his previous state of health. However, there is no guarantee that once the patient accepts his illness, he will maintain this position throughout the course of his illness. It is likely that with added experience and knowledge, doubts and skepticisms will arise to cause conflict and resumption of illness behavior. (P. 158)

The patient may have difficulty accepting physical dependency due to physiological limitations sustained in a burn, drug allergy, or cardiac arrest. In addition to physical dependency, the patient may have additional technical dependency on various pieces of equipment such as a hemodialysis machine or a pacemaker. The nurse can assist her patient to evaluate realistically and to find meaning in forced changes of life-style. She can support her patient as he tries to look beyond the immediate situation. The nurse can help the patient make futuristic plans that are both realistic and safe. When appropriate, she can help her patient see that his dependency is only temporary; if it is permanent, she can help him to look at alternative ways of incorporating the dependency into his new identity.

In the case of Ms. S., the nurse can continue to orient her toward reality. The patient, in pulling the pieces of her life back together, may continue to belittle herself. She may have tremendous guilt over the origin of her burns. She may feel that a stupid act created a permanent disfigurement. The nurse can then help identify and reinforce the patient's strengths, getting her to draw upon all her inner resources. In order to accomplish such a goal, the nurse must see the patient as having worth and then make a personal commitment to the recipient of her care, which means that she is willing to become involved with her patient no matter what adaptive behavior the patient may unpredictably manifest. Such a commitment is of ultimate significance in maintaining and/or restoring her patient's personal integrity.

NURSING EVALUATION

Evaluation of the patient's problem is an ongoing process. The critical care nurse assesses regulatory and cognitive behaviors supporting the diagnosis of avoidance or denial. The nurse evaluates interventions designed to protect the patient's integrity and help him to accept the illness or disfigurement. As the patient begins asking questions about the illness, treatment, or prognosis, the nurse knows that the patient is moving towards acceptance.

SUMMARY

The critical care nurse can attempt to foster her patient's personal integrity. She can get to know her patient's personal tastes, likes and dislikes, food preferences, visitor preferences, family needs or problems, and financial concerns. These assessments can become part of the nurse's personalized plan of care. As she strives to maintain or restore her patient's sense of integrity, she can facilitate his acceptance of the illness, disability, or disfigurement. In instances both of fostering integrity and of facilitating acceptance, the nurse must be prepared to accept her patient's behavior, knowing that he may suddenly see her as an agent of harm. She can realize that he has reasons, and that in time he will become aware of his own avoidance or denial. If she becomes angry at his adaptive behavior, she will spend valuable time handling her own personal guilt feelings rather than helping her patient work through his own guilt. After the patient becomes aware of his behavior, he is ready to begin accepting the illness, loss, disability, or disfigurement. What happens at this level depends upon the nurse's therapeutic plan. According to Levine (1967), "The meaning of illness and the accepted norms of behavior during an illness are culturally determined and markedly influence the outcome of a therapeutic plan. The holistic view of the individual must include the close, personal ties he has with his life beyond the predicament of illness itself" (p. 260).

The critical care nurse can continuously keep in mind that she is dealing with a whole person. The illness may have insulted her patient's physical integrity, but it has only temporarily bruised his personal and social integrity. If the nurse avoids her patient's denial, she then contributes to the damaging of his personal and social integrity. The critical care nurse who is willing to become involved with her patient through active listening and supporting can help him beyond the level of avoidance and denial into acceptance.

REFERENCES

BREZNITZ, SHLOMO, "Anticipatory Stress and Denial," *The Denial of Stress*, ed. Shlomo Breznitz, pp. 225-255. New York: International University Press, 1983.

CRATE, MARJORIE, "Nursing Functions in Adaptation to Chronic Illness," *American Journal of Nursing*, 65, no. 10 (October 1965), 72.

ELLIOTT, SUSAN, "Denial as an Effective Mechanism to Allay Anxiety Following a Stressful Event," *JPN and Mental Health Services*, October 1980, pp. 11-15.

EPSTEIN, SEYMOUR, "Avoidance-Approach: The Fifth Basic Conflict, *Journal of Consulting and Clinical Psychology*, 46, no. 5 (1978), 1016-1022.

FLASKERUD, JACQUELYN, EDWARD HOLLORAN, JANICE JONKEN, MARY LUND, and JOAN ZETTERLUND, "Avoidance and Distancing—A Descriptive View of Nursing," *Nursing Forum*, 18, no. 2 (1979), 158-174.

FOSTER, SUE, "Behavior Following Acute Myocardial Infarction," *American Journal of Nursing*, 10, no. 11 (November 1970), 2344-2348.

FROESE, ARTHUR, ERNESTO VASQUEZ, NED CASSEN, and THOMAS HACKETT, "Validation of Anxiety Depression and Denial Scales in a Coronary Care Unit," *Journal of Psychosomatic Research*, 18 (1974), 137-144.

GENTRY, DOYLE, and THOMAS HANEY, "Emotional and Behavioral Reaction to Acute Myocardial Infarction," *Heart and Lung*, 4, no. 5 (September-October 1975), 738-744.

GOLDBERGER, LEO, "The Concept and Mechanisms of Denial: A Selective Overview," in *The Denial of Stress*, ed. Shlomo Breznitz, pp. 83-95. New York: International University Press, 1983.

GREENE, WILLIAM, ARTHUR MOSS, and SIDNEY GOLDSTEIN, "Delay, Denial and Death in Coronary Heart Disease," *Stress and the Heart*, ed. Robert Eliot, pp. 143-161. New York: Futura Publishing Co., 1974.

HACKETT, THOMAS, "The Coronary Care Unit: An Appraisal of Its Psychologic Hazards," *New England Journal of Medicine*, 279, no. 25 (December 19, 1964), 1365-1367.

_____ , *Psychological Aspects of Illness*. Springfield, Ill.: Charles C Thomas, 1970.

_____ , and N. H. CASSEM, "Development of a Quantitative Rating Scale to Assess Denial," *Journal of Psychosomatic Research*, 18 (1974), 93-100.

JANIS, IRVING, *Psychological Stress*, New York: John Wiley, 1958.

_____ , "Preventing Pathogenic Denial by Means of Stress Inoculation," in *The Denial of Stress*, ed. Shlomo Breznitz, pp. 35-76. New York: International University Press, 1983.

KIENING, SISTER M. MARTHA, "Denial of Illness," in *Behavioral Concepts and Nursing Interventions*, ed. Carolyn Carlson and Betty Blackwell, pp. 211-225. Philadelphia: Lippincott, 1978.

KING, JEAN, "Denial," *American Journal of Nursing*, 66, no. 5 (May 1966), 1010-1013.

LAZARUS, RICHARD, *Psychological Stress and the Coping Process*. New York: McGraw-Hill, 1966.

___ , The Cost and Benefits of Denial," *The Denial of Stress*, ed. Shlomo Breznitz, pp. 1-30. New York: International University Press, 1983.

LEE, DOUGLAS, "The Role of Attitude in Response to Environmental Stress," *Journal of Social Issues*, 22, no. 4 (1966), 83-91.

LEVINE, MYRA, "The Four Conservation Principles of Nursing," *Nursing Forum*, 6, no. 1 (1967), 46.

___ , *Introduction to Clinical Nursing*. Philadelphia: F. A. Davis, 1969.

SCHULTZ, DUANE, *Sensory Restriction: Effects on Behavior*. New York: Academic Press, 1965.

THOMAS, SUE ANN, ELLEN SAPPINGTON, HERBERT GROSS, MARGARET NOCTOR, ERIKA FRIEDMANN, and JAMES LYNCH, "Denial in Coronary Care Patients—An Objective Reassessment, *Heart and Lung*, 12, no. 1 (January 1983), 74-80.

TRAVELBEE, JOYCE, *Interpersonal Aspects of Nursing*, Philadelphia: F. A. Davis, 1966.

WAGSTAFF, GRAHAM, "Behavioral Correlates of Repression-Sensitization: A Reconciliation of Some Conflicting Findings, *Indian Journal of Psychology*, 52 (1977), 195-201.

WAINSTEIN, E. A., *Denial of Illness*. Springfield, Ill.: Charles C. Thomas, 1955.

WU, RUTH, *Behavior and Illness*. Englewood Cliffs, N.J.: Prentice-Hall, 1973.

8
Loneliness

BEHAVIORAL OBJECTIVES

1. Define the terms *lonesomeness, aloneness,* and *loneliness.*
2. List the functions of loneliness.
3. Describe how existential loneliness or real experience applies to the critically ill patient.
4. Describe how loneliness anxiety or fear of aloneness applies to the critically ill patient.
5. Identify three regulatory behaviors associated with loneliness.
6. Identify four cognitive behaviors associated with loneliness.
7. Describe ways in which the nurse can minimize existential loneliness.
8. Describe how the nurse can minimize loneliness anxiety.

The experience of loneliness is an old experience. Throughout the ages people have had to cope with the agonizing problem of loneliness. Nevertheless, loneliness is an increasingly pervasive factor in modern society (Potthoff 1976). Because of this, loneliness has gained increasing recognition within the past several years. Professional groups have studied loneliness and its application to infants, prisoners, isolated adults, and aged individuals. We live in a mobile society where people tend to move toward and away from each other with great rapidity. As a result, relationships have a tendency to be only temporary. Consequently, people feel the void of friendship loss. To guard against the feeling of voidness and the loneliness that results, people shy away from involvement beyond the superficial level. In the process of avoiding the thing they fear, these people become even more lonely. Possibly this is why there are so many singles organizations and lonely hearts clubs.

Nursing literature traditionally has examined loneliness as it pertains to psychiatric patients, to death and dying, and to care of the aged patient. Today nurses need to examine loneliness as it applies to another part of our patient population, those needing hospitalization in critical care units. Even though tremendous stimuli surround the critically ill patient, he can still experience the overwhelming feeling of loneliness. The nurse realizes that "the patient is the most important person in the hospital. He is, therefore, the center of much attention from all kinds of people. In spite of this he is probably the loneliest person in the hospital. People come and go, but few really encounter him as a person" (Hurlburt 1965, p. 229).

The experience of loneliness varies greatly but there is a core experience or feeling state which is always similar. Furthermore loneliness is experienced not only when we are alone, but whenever there is an absence of emotional relatedness (Applebaum 1978). Many times individuals are not aware of their own loneliness. There are circumstances in which loneliness occurs that we cannot control. The loss of a loved one and separation due to hospitalization are such experiences. In each instance, we lose contact with significant others in our daily lives. It may only be at this time that we realize how important the contact has been with the significant other in our environment. According to Hoskisson (1965), "It is only when we are aware that we require contact with another human being or an environment, that we are aware of loneliness. Sometimes loneliness is apparent and sometimes not, so that we can well be alone without this need and in the limited sense we are not lonely, although all of us from the cradle to the grave need human contact" (p. 26). Once the individual becomes aware of the absence of contact, he may choose to deny his loneliness. The individual may choose not to be aware of being lonely out of the necessity to avoid it.

Virtually everyone in our society daily spends time alone. Over a lifetime this adds up to many years of solitude. We are predisposed to think of aloneness as undesirable and as necessarily leading to loneliness. However, solitude can also be a time for reflection, rest and self-renewal (Larson, Csikszentmihalyi, and Graef 1982, p. 40). Even though loneliness permanently or temporarily severs the individual from contact or human relationships, it can also, as Moustakes (1961) points out, provide an opportunity for the individual to learn new things about himself that can help in coping with future experiences of loneliness:

> [The] solitary state gives the individual the opportunity to draw upon untouched capacities and resources to realize himself in an entirely unique manner. It can be a new experience. It may be an experience of exquisite pain, deep fear and terror, an utterly terrible experience, yet it brings into awareness new dimension of self, new beauty, new power for human compassion, and a reverence for the precious nature of each breathing moment. (P. 7)

DEFINITION OF TERMS

Before focusing solely on loneliness, it is important to distinguish among lonesomeness, aloneness, and loneliness. The critical care patient will experience all three at different times during the hospitalization. The nurse needs to be aware of their existence.

Lonesomeness

The feeling of lonesomeness is not an unusual experience. It happens to each of us at various times in our lives. Lonesomeness, according to Peplau (1955), "implies being without the company of others but recognizing a wish to be with others" (p. 1476). A patient can experience lonesomeness when he is out of contact with others. For example, isolation may require separation from family and friends. The patient in isolation with staphylococcal infection, hepatitis, or leukopenia is physically separated from others. On the other hand, a patient surrounded by staff and other patients can also feel lonesome. The individual acknowledges his need to feel close to other people and can frequently express this feeling. He may assume responsibility for reversing the feeling by requesting more patient-family or nurse-patient contacts. If ambulation is possible, the patient may extend himself on a social level. His social encounters with other patients may extend himself on a social level. His social encounters with other patients may even have a therapeutic effect on both people. They may share their concerns and possibly even their feelings of lonesomeness.

Aloneness

Aloneness is often considered to be a negative state whose only positive aspect is that people who are able to overcome its terrible effects may experience a strengthening and greater integration of their personality; the implication is that adversity is positive for the individual and the solitude is necessarily a form of adversity (Suedfel 1982). There are individuals, however, who choose to be alone. The creative individual who paints, writes, invents, or discovers retreats from the presence of others. Being alone gives these individuals time to contemplate. It is possible to be alone without being lonesome. The individual can choose to be alone in order to accomplish his goal.

On the other hand, a patient may experience aloneness against his will. The patient feels aloneness when making decisions that have a future effect upon himself and his family. A patient who must sign a consent for cardiac catheterization after being told of the possible complications will feel alone. The patient who signs his preoperative consent for bilateral nephrectomy and/or A-V shunt implantation knows that he alone must make the final decision. The patient's family, nurse, and physician all have a role in the decision, but it is the patient who stands alone. The hospital usually gives him the consent form to sign the day or evening before the event. This gives the patient time, in his aloneness, to think through his decision. He may not want to be alone, but his body has given him no other choice.

Loneliness

Potthoff (1976) points out that loneliness is the feeling of not being meaningfully related. It involves the deep hurt of isolation and separation. When the individual experiences intense feelings of loneliness, the first wish is that it would go away. Some of the causes of loneliness can be changed, controlled, or eliminated. However a devastating event such as injury, illness, or disease cannot be quickly changed. The latter causes of loneliness must be endured by the patient and family.

According to Sodler and Johnson (1980), loneliness is an experience that is subjective and internal. One of the most salient features of loneliness is a special kind of feeling that seems to encompass the entire self. Unlike sensation or localized feelings, the feeling of loneliness is total. In addition the feeling of loneliness has a cognitive element. There is also the realization that loneliness constitutes a distinctive form of self-perception. Loneliness is a form of acute self-awareness.

The critical care nurse knows that anxiety usually accompanies loneliness. It is often experienced as separation anxiety and need not be confused with loneliness. Loneliness represents a feeling that a loss has already occurred. The ability of the unconsciousness to contain contradictory feelings permits the two behaviors to occur simultaneously (Applebaum 1978).

Loneliness can be precipitated by a change in the individual's achieved social relations or by a change in the individual's desired social relations (Peplau and Caldwell 1978). Loneliness signifies severed ties and absence whereas our ordinary spatial expectations are oriented toward coherence and connection. Severe loneliness can signal confusion and emptiness, and it can make an individual feel out of place (Sodler and Johnson 1980). The loneliness and fear of the critically ill patient becomes our fear and concern. When we begin to encounter the patient's fear and loneliness, we also begin to encounter our own. Not every individual, whether the patient or nurse, desires this kind of encounter; most persons avoid it as much as possible.

Ellison (1978a) notes that the experience of loneliness appears to have several components, namely, emotional, perceptual, motivational, and behavioral components. Loneliness is characterized by intense emotional pain. It is frequently expressed in physical symptoms such as the empty feeling in one's stomach.

Dynamics of Loneliness. Loneliness involves a central experience of isolation. Isolation, whether it be emotional or social, refers to the lack of a satisfying relationship. The two dynamics of loneliness consist of belonging and understanding. A lack of the sense of belonging is the first dynamic quality of loneliness. It is characterized by a lack of assurance that one really belongs and is wanted (Ellison 1978a).

The second dynamic of loneliness involves a lack of understanding. The person may feel as if no one understands. The lonely person has either been deprived of a meaningful relationship or is unable to form one. There is an inability to share intimate concerns with another person who responds with interest, empathy, and appropriate affection. Loneliness that originates from a perceived lack of relationship with someone who not only accepts but also understands may be experienced by individuals with or without significant others (Ellison 1978a). Therefore loneliness involves a lack of positively experienced intimacy with another person who is perceived as significant and who desires the relationship.

Functions of Loneliness. Moustakes (1961) proposes that loneliness involves a unique substance "of self, a dimension of human life which taps the full resources of the individual. It calls for strength, endurance, and sustenance, enabling a person to reach previously unknown depths and to realize a certain nakedness of inner life" (p. 8). He goes on to indicate the positive functions of loneliness:

> The individual in being lonely, if let be, will realize himself in loneliness and create a bond or sense of fundamental relatedness with others. Loneliness rather than separating the individual or causing a break or division of self, expands the individual's wholeness, perceptiveness, sensitivity, and humanity. It enables the person to realize human ties and awareness hitherto unknown. In loneliness one is definitely alone, cut off from human companionship. (P. 47)

Moustakes believes these positive functions are possible because there is

> . . . a power in loneliness, a purity, self-immersion, and depth which is unlike any other experience. Being lonely is such a total, direct, vivid existence, so deeply felt, so startingly different, that there is no room for any other perception, feeling, or awareness. Loneliness is an organic experience which points to nothing else, is for no other purpose and results in nothing but the realization of itself. (P. 8)

Loneliness serves the function of helping the individual look within himself. As he looks toward himself, he communes with himself. "He discovers life, who he is, what he really wants, the meaning of his existence, the true nature of his relations with others" (Moustakes 1961, p. 102). As the individual reaches completion of his loneliness experience, he realizes its purpose. Awareness of being lonely tells a person that he has grown, matured, and reached out for others in a deeper and more vital sense.

Just as loneliness can have long-term positive functions, it can also have negative side effects. Loneliness can become unbearably immobilizing. It is this potential immobilizing side effect of loneliness that concerns the critical care nurse. Loneliness as it applies to critical patients has not been examined in previous nursing literature. We will examine two types of loneliness, as Moustakes defines them. First, there is the loneliness of self-alienation and self-rejection, which is not true loneliness but a vague and disturbing anxiety. We call this aspect of loneliness by the term *loneliness anxiety*. Second, there is *existential loneliness*, which inevitably is a part of human experience.

THE CONCEPT OF LONELINESS APPLIED
TO THE CRITICALLY ILL PATIENT

Existential loneliness is an intrinsic and organic reality of human life, in which there is both pain and triumphant creation emerging from a long period of desolation. The existential person is fully aware of himself or herself as an isolated and solitary individual, while a person suffering loneliness anxiety is separated from his or her feeling and knowing self (Moustakes 1961). Existential loneliness is the real experience of the individual. Loneliness anxiety is more diffuse, and many times the critically ill patient experiences it after the initial crisis or real experience. Needless to say, the patient can simultaneously experience both types of loneliness. The difference lies in the intensity of the experience. Existential loneliness is the real experience of the here and now. The question, "Will I live or die?" is an expression of existential loneliness. Loneliness anxiety, on the other hand, involves more focus on fear of aloneness and fear of future implications.

Existential Loneliness: Real Experience

Existentialists take as their starting point the fact that humans are ultimately alone. None else can experience our thoughts and feelings; separateness is an essential condition of our existence (Perlman and Peplau 1982). The experience of existential loneliness has been treated extensively. It is the realization of one's essential aloneness in the world. It can be a brief or extensive encounter that leads to a state of exhiliration and ultimately to a greater acceptance of reality. Existential loneliness begins in infancy and recurs with each step in the individuation process. It arises as a reaction to a growth process and disappears when the new growth has become an integral part of the character structure (Applebaum 1978). As Wolfe (1961) notes, existential loneliness is an essential condition of creativity, that out of the depths of grief, despair, and the shattering feeling of total impotency springs the urge to create new forms and images and to discover unique ways of being aware and expressing experience.

The existential position separates secondary loneliness following loss from the primary loneliness of being human and having knowledge of one's potential death (Satran 1978). Therefore existential loneliness refers to one's sense of separateness from a mutuality with meaning in life and God (Ellison 1978a). As mentioned earlier, existential loneliness represents the real experience of a critically ill patient. The real experience, or existential loneliness, has two major components: the threat of illness and the loneliness of both psychological and physiological pain.

Mr. D. was a 45-year-old patient who experienced existential loneliness. He entered the hospital's emergency room late one evening in severe respiratory distress. A history revealed that Mr. D. had experienced shortness of breath upon the slightest exertion, fatigue, and peripheral edema for the past several months. A physical examination revealed mitral stenosis. Mr. D. was quickly admitted into the hospital's coronary care unit and separated from his tearful wife. Diagnostic tests confirmed the presence of severe mitral stenosis and the surgical team informed Mr. D. and his wife that surgery would be mandatory. Because Mr. D. seemed to be apprehensive about the possibility of surgery, his doctors decided to wait two days to give the health team the opportunity to prepare Mr. D. physically and psychologically for the event. The nurses instructed both Mr. and Mrs. D. regarding his post-operative admittance into ICU, the possible length of stay in ICU, the various routine procedures and treatments to be done, and the health team's general expectations of Mr. D. during his hospitalization. The nurses attempted to prepare Mr. D. for the eventual soreness in his chest and throat, his forced immobility, and the strange pieces of equipment that would be stationed around his bed. In addition, nurses told Mr. D. that his wife or son would be the only people admitted to visit him, and that their visits would be limited. Mr. D. and his wife were given the opportunity to express their expectations of the health team.

Most of the preparation and teaching done by the health team was based upon theory and related practice involving the team's experience with other open heart surgical patients. Their experience was not based on "real experience," since they themselves had not experienced the surgery.

Two days later, doctors replaced Mr. D.'s mitral valve. Immediately after surgery, he was admitted into ICU. There the wires and tubes connected to his body during surgery were now neatly attached to the appropriate pieces of equipment around his bed. His endotracheal tube was connected to a volume respirator; EKG leads were connected to the cardioscope; an artterial line and a central venous pressure manometer were connected to a manifold; a chest tube was connected to water seal drainage or gomco suction; a Foley catheter was connected to a urometer; a pacemaker was attached to Mr. D.'s chest as a precautionary measure; and the IV tubing was threaded through an IVAC machine. His nurses frequently checked those pieces of equipment, which provided data regarding his biological status.

Mr. D. sleepily awakened to find himself in a noisy and strange environment. He heard people talking around him, but did not know if they were talking to or about him. He wanted to respond verbally, but there was something in his mouth that made it impossible. He tried to move his body, but the pain, wires, and tubes curtailed such mobility. His only recourse was to try to withdraw into sleep. Even sleep was difficult because of all the noises within his immediate environment. Just as he seemed to drift off into sleep, he was suddenly awakened by a tube being threaded down his throat. As he began coughing, he moved his hands towards his chest in an attempt to support his sutures. His face expressed the pain he felt. Mr. D. wanted his wife to be present, but he remembered his nurse saying she could only be with him for short periods of time. Mr. D. repeatedly gestured towards his throat indicating his desire to have his endotracheal tube removed. The nurses realized that his growing alertness made him more intently aware of his sore throat and sutured chest. When his blood gases became normal, the nurses expedited the removal of his endotracheal tube. During the next two days, Mr. D. requested more frequent visits by his wife and son. Once again, the nurse attempted to explain why such visits would not be possible. The nurse began noticing that Mr. D. seemed quieter than usual. He seemed to lie in bed with his eyes closed. During the morning of the fourth day in ICU, Mr. D. and his nurse had the following conversation:

NURSE: Is there anything wrong, Mr. D.? You seem so quiet.

MR. D.: (*With tears in his eyes*) It isn't important.

NURSE: What isn't Mr. D.?

MR. D.: No one really knows what it is really like until you experience it yourself.

NURSE: What do you mean?

MR. D.: Open heart surgery.

NURSE: Go on.

MR. D.: No one really knows how bad the days after surgery will be until the person experiences it himself. I was told I would have pain in my chest but I wasn't told how bad it would be. It really hurts! It really hurts!

NURSE: Yes, Mr. D. We can prepare you to expect the pain but not the degree of intensity. What else is bothering you?

MR. D.: Everyone pays more attention to my wires and tubes than to me. I don't feel like my body is my own. People talk around me, and I don't know if I should respond. I keep hoping I'll wake up to find out it was all a bad dream.

NURSE: The worst part is all behind you, Mr. D. The main thing is what can we do to help you now?

MR. D.: Get me out of here so I can see more of my family and friends. I miss them.

NURSE: Maybe we can let your wife sit with you for longer periods of time. You no longer have all the equipment around your bed. You are doing so much better that maybe we can have you transferred out of ICU.

Mr. D. experienced both aspects of existential loneliness. His real experience involved the threat of illness and both psychological and physiological pain.

As Potthoff (1976) has pointed out, "the ultimate loneliness is the pain of feeling that there is no depth which speaks to our depth, there is no integrity which upholds us on our integrity, there is no responsiveness in relation to our deepest needs and highest aspirations. In our aloneness there is only a void" (p. 11).

The Threat of Illness. Our bodies are deeply involved in our functioning as persons. As Potthoff (1976) indicates, we are externalized through our bodies; we communicate through our bodies; we learn through our bodies.

Whenever illness comes, it represents an interruption in one's life and more importantly life's goals. Events cannot go on as usual because immediate and future goals must be postponed. Illness has its own specific goals which may or may not be altered or controlled. Individuals experience illness under different circumstances. Individuals may be hospitalized in critical care for a short or prolonged period of time. In the midst of hospitalization in critical care there are strange persons, noises, and procedures. All of these separate the individual from his usual surroundings and create feelings of loneliness (Potthoff 1976).

Illness with its threat to biological integrity is a real experience. It is real in the sense that the threat involves potential loss of all or part of a function or organ, or of life itself. The real experience of illness causes existential loneliness. Illness may be either an old or new experience to the patient. In either instance, the illness with its threat creates loneliness. It involves separation and isolation from the secure and the familiar. Such was the case with Mr. D. He entered the hospital complaining of shortness of breath and hours later was told he had severe mitral stenosis. Next he was informed that surgery would be necessary. Mr. D.'s apprehension was noted by the health team, and because of this his surgery was postponed for two days. During the two-day period, the health team assessed his physical and psychological status. Even though the nurses told him what to expect after his surgery, he realized the experience would be real only to him. He was prepared to the extent that he had a limited experience with illness over the past several months, but he had not experienced surgery.

Mr. B. on the other hand, represents a patient whose encounter with illness was a totally new and potentially lonely experience. He was a 27-year-old man who had experienced second- and third-degree burns over a large portion of his body. He was in his backyard busily preparing his barbecue pit for a quiet afternoon of eating and visiting with members of his family. He cautiously lighted the charcoals he had earlier soaked in lighter fluid. As the charcoals were turning a gray color, Mr. B. decided to add a last splash of liquid lighter fluid. While he did this, an explosion occurred. People yelled, children cried, and Mr. B. screamed for help as his clothes burned. An alert man came to the aid of Mr. B. and quickly suffocated the flames. As the crisis subsided, Mr. B. was admitted to a burn unit where emergency care and treatment could begin. To Mr. B., the experience was real. The event thrust him into the threat of illness involving loss of bodily part, or even of his life. Unlike Mr. D., who had experienced some illness over the past several months, Mr. B. had been free from illness. Suddenly and unexpectedly, a quiet afternoon with his family had turned into a holocaust involving the loneliness of hospitalization and long, involved treatment.

The list of patients like Mr. D. and Mr. B. who share the real experience of illness could continue. Take for example the individual who, on a Sunday morning while driving to church, becomes involved in a serious automobile accident. He is admitted into ICU with multiple fractures, lacterations, and possible subdural hematoma. Another example is the individual who went into a grocery store to buy a loaf of bread and was shot by a thief. If he survives the gunshot and surgery, he also will awaken to find himself in a critical unit. Yet another example is the relatively healthy individual who took an antibiotic when he had a cold, developed a drug reaction, and found himself hospitalized for acute tubular necrosis. The above patients, including Mr. D. and Mr. B., experienced existential loneliness as it relates to the real experience of illness with its many threats, including threat to life itself. The potential threat to life can be a lonely one to the patient. Illness is not only a physical event; it also becomes a psychological event. The illness and threat of loss or disfigurement create both a psychological and physiological pain. Both types of pain are real experiences to the individual and therefore create feelings of loneliness. As Mr. D. said to his nurse, "No one really knows." The critical care nurse can instruct her patient with theories and related experiences, but she cannot share the direct experience of the event itself. This is the event that becomes the real experience of the critical care patient himself. He alone must endure the illness or surgery.

In summary, disease and illness seems to facilitate experiences of isolation and loneliness. Removal of individuals from familiar belongings, family, and community networks foster loneliness. The critically ill patient becomes more dependent and desires meaningful relationships. These patients because of the nature of their illness, injury, or disease can experience intense loneliness (Ellison 1978a; Satron 1978).

The Psychological Pain. Loneliness is a prolonged state of psychological pain or anguish caused by a sense of separation. It is a feeling of being a nonentity, of nonbeing, of nothingness, experienced in the depths of one's being (Polcino 1979). Psychological pain occurs when the individual must maintain a separateness from others. The separateness of existential loneliness involves three components: separateness from contact with significant members of one's life, separateness from one's body, and separateness from one's values and ideas. According to Peplau and Caldwell, (1978), "A cognitive analysis emphasizes people's desires and preferences concerning social relations, rather than assumed human needs for contact. Loneliness exists to the extent that a person's network of social relationship is smaller or less satisfying than the person desires" (p. 208).

Mr. D. experienced all three components of psychological pain, especially separateness from contact with significant others and separateness from his body. First, he experienced the separateness from contact with significant members of his life. When he was transferred to coronary care, he temporarily left behind his tearful wife. Upon entering CCU, he assumed the new role of patient. Mr. D. represents those patients who are first admitted into the hospital and then admitted into a subculture of the hospital, namely critical care. The individual who discovers he has a disease, illness, or surgical needs finds himself isolated or separated from fellowship. He is now different, and the difference may only be in his temporary label, "patient."

Once the individual receives the label of "patient," he has a distinction all his own. This distinction represents failure, not success. The patient joins a protective community of the people who have the same label. As his diagnosis is confirmed, he receives a more specific distinction. He is now a burn patient, a renal patient, a cardiac patient, a respiratory patient, a liver patient, or a patient with an infection. This last distinction removes the patient from the larger community to a more specific community: ICU, CCU, hemodialysis, isolation, or a burn unit.

Mr. D. was first admitted to CCU and then, after surgery, into ICU. He became separated from significant members of his life. Ideally, as Moustakes (1961) points out, "The experience of separation or isolation is not unhealthy any more than any condition of human existence is unhealthy. Ultimately each man is alone but when the individual maintains a truthful self-identity, such isolation is strengthening and induces deeper sensitivities and awareness. In contrast, self-alienation and estrangement drive one to avoid separation" (p. 34). The critical care nurse can help her patient maintain his self-identity by personalizing his care. She can offer something more than his label or diagnosis by providing him with the identity he had in the nonhospital community: his name. This can lessen the loneliness he feels.

Burnside (1971) has described the particular loneliness of the hospitalized patient:

> When a person is hospitalized, he becomes more acutely aware of his human separateness. The disease, the trauma is happening to him, and no one else can experience this for him. There is no escape from his body capsule. In the hospital, the opportunity for relating is minimal. He is surrounded by strangers who relate to him in the most intimate way, yet with an aura of detachment. Loneliness becomes overwhelming. Physical stress leaves him helpless, as bodily functions are out of control. (P. 395).

The hospital environment creates feelings of separateness and isolation. Patients see it as sterile and frightening. The patient, like Mr. D., is thrown into a world of unfamiliar sights, sounds, and faces. His stretcher passes through the sterile baize or green corridors. He sees faces rushing past him, unaware of his presence. He becomes aware of the bleak whiteness of laboratory coats and uniforms. He hears strange voices talking in an unfamiliar technical language, charts clicking as nurses place them in a rack, and phones ringing. As he continues his trip toward his new home, he becomes increasingly aware of his loneliness. As his feeling mounts, his stretcher bangs through the double doors and into the critical care unit. Strangers neatly lift and tuck him into his bed. It is here that the patient receives various procedures and treatments. He looks around to see beds lined up in an orderly fashion. His food arrives in the same neatly organized manner. This neat categorical arrangement of beds and food does not represent his personal preferences.

Patients like Mr. D. become aware of the hospital's impersonal rules and regulations. His family is limited in the length and frequency of their visits. Friends may be temporarily discouraged from visiting. He does not understand the frequent medications, IVs, and the taking of his vital signs. He feels a sense of disrespect for the integrity of his wishes. He senses a lack of genuine human warmth and understanding. He feels surrounded by superficial smiles, words, and encounters. Needless to say, all these factors contribute to the critically ill patient's feeling of loneliness. Within this setting, the patient tries to maintain his identity, but this is difficult, because just as he feels separated from significant members within his environment, he also feels a separation from his own body.

Mr. D. experienced separateness from his own body. He felt that everyone was more interested in his tubes and wires than in him as a person. He heard people talking in his environment, but he did not know if they were talking about or to him. He may have felt like an object. His feeling of separateness from his own body was demonstrated by his statement, "I don't feel like my body is my own." Mr. D.'s feelings are not unique. Other critical care patients experience similar loneliness. The patient feels that he is the subject of various tests, procedures, and treatments. His body may become the place for research or application of new treatments. The patient with burns on both legs, for example, may receive two different ointments on his burns. One leg may receive the traditional treatment and the other the experimental ointment. A new drug that increases cardiac output may be used in the treatment of congestive heart failure. The infection control team may offer a new approach to the handling of a particular infection. The patient feels that his body is a test tube or a commodity. Doctors or technicians may refer to him as "an interesting renal (or cardiac, or hepatic, or respiratory) patient." He may feel like one big kidney lying in bed. He becomes totally separated from his diseased system, which now takes precedence over all other symptoms.

Separateness from significant others and from one's body are the two most significant components of psychological pain in existential loneliness. The individual is unable to derive security from his family, and he experiences a sense of unrelatedness with his own body. He entered the hospital with a feeling of relatedness to family and self, but when he became a critical care patient, he relinquished control over both.

The critical care patient may also be separated from others by his values or ideas. His beliefs regarding health care and its delivery may be totally different from those of his nurse or physician. He may feel compelled to surrender his ideas in the face of his serious plight. Mr. D. wanted more frequent visits with his family, but his nurse reminded him of the unit's rules and regulations. The newly diagnosed myocardial infarction patient may find it difficult to remain immobilized if he has always maintained an active life. The patient with acute tubular necrosis cannot understand why he must restrict fluid intake. The patient with a staphylococcal infection in his incision cannot understand why he must have three consecutive negative cultures before he can leave isolation. Each patient realizes that in order to reach the goal of wellness, he must submit to the decisions made by others.

The psychological pain of loneliness can also be attributed to blaming one's self or the situation. Self-blame can be associated with withdrawal and the blaming of others. The latter can create further separateness from significant others. Blaming others for one's current situation can be associated with greater hostility and resentment. Another cause of psychological pain is the feeling of hopelessness. The psychological pain of loneliness is compounded when the individual is unable to see future change. Hope of alleviating loneliness is closely linked to both perceived control and stability. The patient's feeling of hope can be the greatest when the causes of loneliness are altered and controlled (Peplau and Caldwell 1978).

The Physiological Pain. There are three ways in which the critically ill patient responds to physical pain. He may choose to ignore the pain, to react to the pain realistically, or to overreact to the pain. In the first instance, the individual may avoid or ignore pain because he feels that it will limit or immobilize him, reducing his ability to interact with his environment. He feels that if he submits to the pain, he will not be able to participate in activities with his family or friends. Essentially he avoids the loneliness he assumes his pain will create.

Mr. D. followed the second way in which a patient reacts to the lonely experience of pain by reacting realistically. His nurse attempted to help him anticipate the pain in his chest and throat, but she could not describe the real experience. Mr. D. alone had to experience the loneliness of pain. He wanted to sleep in order to awaken and discover he had only dreamed the surgical event. The pain he experienced was real and tangible. He could only inform others when it occurred and hope that the medication would relieve it.

Lastly there are those patients who overreact to their pain. The same type of pain that one patient can ignore or react realistically to may seem so intolerable to another patient that he can only respond by overreacting. A patient overreacts in an attempt to gain his nurse's attention and to decrease his loneliness. Smith (1964) describes how extreme pain can lead to avoidance behavior:

> The more pain the patient experiences, the more he becomes preoccupied with the avoidance of further pain. His defenses become phobically organized in that all of his fears may become focused on the needle or the pill or some treatment procedure. One or another of these factors is perceived as the source of all discomfort; it is therefore regarded as something that must be avoided, regardless of the consequences insofar as the illness itself is concerned. (P. 41)

Many of the patients with whom critical care nurses work have experienced major surgery. To them coughing, turning, deep breathing, or dangling is painful. After attempting supportive measures or medications, the nurse may be forced to suction the patient, and the suctioning episode may create more physical pain than if the patient had coughed on his own. In this case, the patient had become immobilized by the fear of physiological pain to the point that he wanted to avoid it. Another patient may have his call light on the exact moment he knows he can have another injection or pill. If the nurse is late in bringing the medication, the patient reacts with anger or hostility. In doing so, the patient not only alienates the provider of his care, but he also pushes himself further into psychological loneliness.

Regardless of its origin, physiological or psychological pain can be unbearable. According to Burnside (1971), "If the alleviation of pain is one goal, then one may need to mitigate the aloneness or loneliness that may be concurrent with the pain" (p. 395).

Loneliness Anxiety: Fear of Aloneness

Loneliness anxiety can be a feeling that comes to a person when there seems to be no one who cares about what happens to him. The feeling is expressed as self-pity, thus making the individual think only of himself and the things expected from other people (Williams 1978). Loneliness anxiety results from a fundamental breach between what one is and what one pretends to be, a basic alienation between person and person and between person and surroundings. Loneliness anxiety has also been described as a system of defense mechanisms that distracts people from dealing with crucial life questions and that motivates them constantly to seek activity with others (Perlman and Peplau 1982). It can involve a transient situational disturbance. Loneliness anxiety can occur as reaction to any recent loss, endured during enforced physical isolation, separation from loved ones, loss of body part, loss of self-esteem, or loss of attachment figure (Applebaum 1978).

In its application to the critically ill patient, loneliness anxiety implies fear of aloneness. The patient realizes that he alone must experience the unknown. This involves fear of aloneness in his new critical care environment and in the vagueness of his new or altered future. He alone must go through the admission rituals, and he alone must integrate the necessary changes of his future into his being. Loneliness anxiety, like existential loneliness, involves two major component parts: fear of aloneness in one's environment and fear of aloneness in one's future. The patient may not communicate these fears, thus pushing himself further into the loneliness and aloneness he fears. In his mind, he is in the process of becoming a cardiac or respiratory cripple, disfigured, or machine-dependent.

Fear of Aloneness in the Environment. The fear of aloneness in the environment begins the minute a patient arrives in critical care. The critical care environment consists not only of various supportive devices but also of the health team. Even though there are people in his environment with whom he interacts, the interaction may have little significance, because, as in existential loneliness, the patient experiences a separation from the significant people in his life. Those who remain are strangers. The strangers make him realize his aloneness in a foreign, technical world. Because his internal feelings are diffuse, he may not overtly communicate the process of loneliness anxiety. The patient may not even realize that the gnawing feeling in the pit of his stomach is not an impending ulcer, but rather impending loneliness. The patient will also feel aloneness coupled with loneliness. He alone is the one experiencing the pain that brought him to the hospital. Others can ask him questions about his pain or prescribe an analgesic, but he alone endures the frustration of pain. He alone is subjected to the numerous admission questions. He alone must experience the continual poking and probing of the admitting physician. His liver and abdomen are palpated; his chest is percussed; his eyes, ears, and nose are examined; and his cardiac status is assessed. He alone must experience the initial diagnostic procedures necessary to confirm the data obtained from the doctor's poking and probing. He alone is subjected to the intrusion of various needles and tubes. He alone must lie under the X-ray machine, or breath rhythmically into a volume respirator, or remain motionless as an EKG machine records his cardiac rhythm. He alone must be told what all the poking, probing, and intrusive tests showed. He alone hears the frightening diagnosis acute tubular necrosis, serum hepatitis, disseminated intravascular coagulation (DIC), acute myocardial infarction, acute pancreatitis, pulmonary emphysema, or second- and third-degree burns over 40 percent of his body. He alone experiences the potential threat to his life. All of these experiences occur in a strange environment. The critically ill patient experiences the fear of aloneness.

Fear of aloneness and separateness can occur simultaneously. According to Ellison (1978a), the motivational and behavioral effects involve attempts to overcome the separateness and to effect a mutual relationship. The lonely person is thought to become perceptually sensitive to potential relationship and potential rejection. His fear may cause him psychologically to constrict or curl up. The patient realizes that it is his own, not someone else's body being discussed. All of us at one time or another have experienced the "curling up" phenomenon. A child who becomes frightened at night, for example, may physically curl up into a protective ball rather than call her parents. There are times when adults react in a similar manner. In the event of a physical threat, such as flying objects or a possible auto accident, we instinctively protect ourselves by curling or bending our bodies away from the threat. This is a defense we utilize to protect ourselves against unwanted harm. The defense response is a normal one.

The critical care patient also experiences the same phenomenon. Because of the various tubes, needles, or equipment restricting his physical mobility, he may be unable physically to curl up or constrict into a protective ball; instead, he constricts psychologically. Like physical constriction, psychological constriction is also a defense mechanism. The patient's anxieties and fears cause him to turn within himself. Such behavior does not reduce his loneliness, for within himself he discovers that his own being is threatened by illness and potential loss of life. The frailties of his own body do not provide him with the antidote to his loneliness, security. His fear of aloneness makes him less responsive to his environment. He may be totally unaware of what is happening. The process of being constricted greatly reduces the patient's intake system. He does not hear, see, or feel his environment. He may not realize that a family member has been at his bedside for two consecutive days. He may not realize that his attentive nurse has been actively observing his care. He may not realize that his physician has been conscientiously monitoring his progress. Above all, he may not realize that he is surrounded by people who care about his well-being.

The critically ill patient may feel continually isolated. The emotional isolation can only be overcome by the reestablishment of the lost relationship or the establishment of a new one of a similar nature. This kind of loneliness is generally experienced as a sense of utter aloneness whether or not significant others are available (Ellison 1978a).

It is only as the patient begins to uncurl or become less constricted that his intake system increases. He becomes increasingly more aware of his immediate environment, activities within it, and his placement within it. As he looks around his environment, he discovers only unfamiliar faces and he suddenly feels a tremendous void in his life. This void is loneliness anxiety. Even though he is physically close to the staff and other patients, his loneliness makes him feel "a world apart from others—a frightening world. The person is lost and, in fact, feels much like the child who lost his parents in a crowd" (DeThomaso 1971, p. 113). Again the loneliness creates anxiety within the patient. Some of his reactions toward family members reflect this anxiety. Nurses quite frequently hear their patient say, upon seeing a family member, "Well, where have you been?" "Have you been here all this time?" "It's about time you showed up," or "I have missed seeing you." Family members may be shocked by the patient's remarks because during the initial crisis, he seemed to respond to their presence. The family may not have realized that the patient was heavily sedated. The nurse can frequently instruct the family that they should make their presence known to the patient. Many times, a family member will quietly sit at the patient's bedside, afraid to announce himself for fear of causing the patient harm. He or she, thinking that the patient is sleeping, may not approach the patient's bed. This can do more harm than good: the patient may feel abandonment by those he loves or needs the most. As a patient becomes less constricted, he senses a loss in relatedness to others, and this feeling leads to estrangement.

The time spent being psychologically constricted decreases involvement with those around him. His nurse may know him better than he knows her. Her face is still unfamiliar to him. Consequently, he feels lonely. As DeThomaso (1971) points out, loneliness may result from unsatisfying relationships with others, or "may also ensue when satisfying relationships have been established but severed because of separation, death or illness" (p. 113). The patient again experiences the painful feeling of aloneness. The "painful experience of loneliness denotes the sensation of feeling alone and at the same time having the awareness that one needs a connection with his fellowman. Loneliness is not only a factual acknowledgment of being by oneself, but it indicates an urgent desire to re-enter human contact" (p. 114). One way in which the patient can fill the voidness or loneliness he feels for human contact is by becoming acquainted with the nurse.

It must be remembered that the critically ill patient may not be able to communicate his fears of aloneness. It is difficult for him to explain the vague psychological process of "curling up" or the emptiness he feels. These are diffuse feelings based upon anxiety. He may not realize that both feelings represent loneliness. The patient may feel that his manliness or her independence is based upon an ability to cope and tough it out. Because the patient does not feel a part of his environment, he fears aloneness in it. It was mentioned earlier that the people in his environment are strangers. Therefore, it is only when communication takes place between the patient and his nurse that he ceases to be surrounded only by strangers. When the patient knows his nurse, his fear of aloneness in his environment may diminish.

Fear of Aloneness in the Future. Loneliness signifies a failure to achieve one's own standards for social relations and a failure to conform to social norms. More important than the patient's fear of aloneness in his environment is his fear of aloneness in his future and in the future of his family. He fears the transitional aloneness of moving from the sick role to the well role. The patient may actually fear the aloneness of these changes. Initially, he may not realize that he does not make the changes totally alone, that he does have the support of his family and health care. This realization often comes later in his hospitalization. In the beginning, however, he alone must be the one to accept these changes and incorporate them into a new lifestyle. The transition toward change is a lonely one. The changes may mean he cannot be as active as before, he cannot travel as extensively as before, or he cannot return to his previous job. Only the patient can know the meaning change has for him. His family can assist him in the transition, but he alone must make the decision to accept or reject change. Within the lonely process of either accepting or rejecting change, the patient goes through the psychological pain of mourning. As stated earlier, the patient, in his anxiety, goes through the process of becoming a cardiac cripple, a respiratory cripple, or machine-dependent. He may not realize that the changes do not render him a cripple. Mr. T. is an example of a patient who experienced the fear of aloneness in his future.

Mr. T. was a young, dynamic executive. His wife described him as a devoted father and husband, an active participant in his community, and a hard-working man. At the relatively young age of 45, he commanded a large organization. Mr. T. has always worked long hours under tremendous pressure. Recently he had experienced brief episodes of chest pain. He attributed the pain to anxiety and exhaustion. As the weeks progressed, the pain became more frequent and more intense. Again he chose to ignore the symptoms and to continue his aggressive pace. He thought the pain was due to indigestion, so he began taking antacids, but his pain continued. One day, he experienced other symptoms besides chest pain. While leading a conference, he suddenly became short of breath, diaphoretic, and slightly cyanotic. He was immediately rushed to a local hospital. It was in CCU that doctors diagnosed his problem as acute myocardial infarction.

Even though Mr. T. was told he had sustained a myocardial infarction, he did not seem to respond. Instead, he requested his briefcase, a telephone, and permission to be visited by his business associates. His nurses and doctors tried to explain the significance of rest. The more his doctor attempted to convince him of their position, the more agitated he became. To Mr. T., the competitive world and the pressures of business were his life. He had never before experienced illness or restrictions, and he did not seem to want to learn how to deal with them. The health team had no alternative but to sedate him. Even in his sleep, he could not achieve complete rest. His mind was preoccupied with business meetings and impending transactions. Each time he awakened, he asked when he would be allowed to go home. When told he would remain in CCU at least two more days and would then spend two weeks in either intermediate care or on the general floor, he again became agitated.

MR. T.: Can't anyone understand that I have got to get out of here? I don't have time to be sick.

NURSE: Mr. T., you are a sick man.

MR. T.: Sick! I can't be! I have too many business dealings to handle.

NURSE: I thought you said you had business associates.

MR. T.: Yes, I do.

NURSE: Why can't they handle the business while you are recovering?

MR. T.: I am the only one who can handle everything.

NURSE: You know, Mr. T., you can't continue with your current pace. You'll need to start sharing some business responsibilities.

MR. T.: No one seems to understand, and I don't want to spend more time explaining it. Enough has been said.

NURSE: All right, Mr. T., if you should want to talk again I'll try to be a better listener next time.

MR. T.: (Looks at the nurse who had turned and walked away from his bed.)

Throughout the next two days, Mr. T.'s physical condition stabilized, but psychologically he seemed withdrawn. This was a complete reversal of the behavior he exhibited after his admission into CCU. Because it was such an abrupt change, his nurse decided to confront Mr. T. about his behavior:

NURSE: Mr. T., what is wrong? You seem so quiet.

MR. T.: Oh, nothing.

NURSE: I'll try to be a good listener.

MR. T.: (Looks at his nurse and smiles.) I don't know if anyone can help me. (Silence.)

NURSE: Continue.

MR. T.: It's just that so much has happened over the past several days. One day I am in control of my business, and the next day I am in CCU with a coronary. I am told I'll have to change my pace of living. (*Silence.*)

NURSE: Is it the change itself or the uncertainty of a new future that bothers you?

MR. T.: It is both. I worry about my family and what my illness means to them. I worry about my business. I worry about having to sit in a chair the rest of my life.

NURSE: Who said you would need to sit in a chair the rest of your life?

MR. T.: That is the feeling I get.

NURSE: No, that is the last alternative. The changes involve slowing down, not stopping altogether. You do need to relax. You need the help of your business associates and family. You'll be able to continue in your business.

MR. T.: Maybe I'll talk to Tom, my partner, and see about sharing some of the responsibilities.

NURSE: That sounds much better. Once you leave CCU, perhaps you can have Tom visit you.

MR. T.: Thanks for your help and care.

Initially Mr. T.'s fear of aloneness manifested itself as denial. The thought of any restrictions was foreign to him. Mr. T. was not unique in his behavioral response. Patients may react to the loneliness of change in several ways. Their reaction demonatrates a type of mourning process. The patient may quietly accept the changes, deny the need for change, become angry about future changes, or withdraw further into loneliness. Mr. T. seemed to experience three of these behaviors. First, he seemed to deny illness and the need for change by attempting to continue with his hectic pace. When he could not convince his doctors or nurses that he was well enough to return to work, he became angry. He felt he was the only one who could solve all the problems. He did not think anyone would understand his concerns, and therefore he alone quietly worried about the future of his family and business. This was best demonstrated by his statement, "Enough has been said." Such a statement coupled with his angry behavior pushed him further into the thing he feared the most—aloneness.

Ironically, the patient may reject help from others—the same others with whom he wanted to have a sense of relatedness—because illness and the unfamiliarity of the illness experience, including forced dependency and passivity, are such a threatening experience. Mr. T. finally communicated his fear of aloneness in his future to the critical care nurse. Once he communicated his fears, he no longer experienced aloneness. Someone else in his immediate environment had become aware of his internal thinking. More specifically, the nurse was able to discover his misconception about the future. To Mr. T., changes in his future involved sitting in a chair and becoming a cardiac cripple. His nurse immediately clarified this misconception and helped him to seek alternatives. This process can only occur when the patient decides he no longer can tolerate his loneliness and seeks to communicate his fears.

The critically ill patient, regardless of his reasons for being in critical care, seeks to eliminate feelings of either existential loneliness or loneliness anxiety. The critical care nurse can realize that the patient's own desire for relatedness becomes the vehicle through which she may guide him out of his loneliness.

NURSING ASSESSMENT OF LONELINESS

The nurse assesses loneliness through the patient's behavioral response. The behavioral responses are categorized into regulatory behaviors and cognitive behaviors. Regulatory behaviors lead to physiological responses. Cognitive behaviors are psychosocial in nature.

Regulatory Behaviors

The regulator involves input, processes, effectors, and feedback loops. It involves stimuli from the external environment such as the critical care unit and from changes in the internal state of dynamic equilibrium. The following regulatory behaviors are physiological responses which can be associated with loneliness:

Regulatory Behaviors
Loss of appetite
Weight loss
Fatigue
Sleeplessness
Tachycardia

Cognitive Behaviors

The cognator system involves inputs from internal and external stimuli which include psychological and social factors. The specific aspects of the cognator mechanism consist of perceptual/information processing, learning, judgment, and emotion. The cognitive behaviors associated with loneliness are psychological responses and consist of the following:

Cognitive Behaviors
Anxiety
Depression
Apathy
Lack of interest
Withdrawal

According to Potthoff (1976) pain, fatigue, anxiety, and worries about family, work, and finances often coincide with illness and hospitalization. When the patient realizes he is ill, there is a feeling of separateness from familiar people and things which are part of his usual life. The result is a strangeness in illness which leads to loneliness.

NURSING DIAGNOSIS OF LONELINESS

The nursing diagnosis is a statement of the current problem. Regulatory and cognitive behaviors coupled with stressors causing the problem combine to help the nurse make the diagnosis of loneliness. Internal stressors involve fear of loss due to illness, injury, or disease; separation from significant others; age; or medications. External stressors can be attributed to the immediate critical care unit with its unfamiliar noises and strangers. All the above stressors combine to cause loneliness.

NURSING INTERVENTIONS ASSOCIATED WITH LONELINESS

In nursing situations, the critical care nurse does not deal directly with the patient's loneliness but rather with his defenses against experiencing the pain of loneliness—the plausible structure he has erected to cover up the problem and hide it from himself and from others (Peplau 1955). The patient who feels alone and isolated from others may feel threatened by the potential loss of his boundaries. In other words, he fears the loss of his ability to discriminate between the subjective self and the objective world around him. The nurse helps her patient maintain a sense of boundary.

Existential Loneliness: Real Experience

The critical care nurse can help her patient overcome existential loneliness by minimizing the threat of illness and minimizing both psychological and physiological pain. Each part of existential loneliness or real experience should be understood in terms of its boundaries.

Minimizing the Threat of Illness. Boundaries of illness become manifest as the patient shares in detail those events that led to his hospitalization. He goes into lengthy detail telling the minute-by-minute activities prior to the crisis. The nurse can realize that the patient needs to discuss these events because the experience is real to him. The details may seem rather tedious and boring to the nurse, but their expression minimizes the patient's loneliness. He has shared his concerns and thoughts with someone else. Relating the details has two functions. First, it gives the patient an opportunity to work through the guilt he feels for having become ill. Guilt and the threat of one's illness can be a very lonely experience. The patient may make statements such as, "I hate to have the men work overtime at the office for me," "My wife really depends on me," or "My husband has never had to manage both the house and children alone." All these statements imply feelings of guilt. The nurse intervenes to minimize the individual's guilt feelings by allowing him to share what makes him feel guilty. Second, the nurse helps her patient identify strengths of the family members who remain at home and of the business associates who can take over his workload. The critical care nurse can encourage the patient to share his feelings of guilt with the family. The patient may need direct reassurances from those for whom he feels the guilt.

When the patient shares the details of the prehospitalization crisis, he is actually seeking support and clarification. When he shares details, the patient is indirectly asking if he could have precipitated the problem. In listening to her patient, the critical care nurse may learn that prior to his MI he was running up three flights of stairs while simultaneously carrying groceries. Another individual may have been working long hours under extreme pressure prior to his MI. Other factors, such as diet, age, or activities, must also be considered. The hemodialysis patient who does not limit his fluid, sodium, or potassium intake may find the boundaries of his illness extending into crisis. Therefore, one must teach him the significance of proper diet. The hemodialysis or cardiac patient's spouse may join him in certain diet restrictions. This patient's experience remains real but need not be a lonely one. In sharing activities that led to his biological crisis, the patient also asks, "Will it happen again?" He wants to know the boundaries of his current illness. All patients, regardless of their reason for being in critical care, hope that the boundaries will not extend to permanent loss of function, of organ, or of life itself. The mere thought of such a possibility makes the patient lonely.

The nurse's goal is to move the critical care patient toward developing expanded rather than constricted boundaries of illness. She can teach her patient the positive stages of healing and therapy. A cardiac patient can learn his physiological boundaries in terms of scar tissue. The critical care nurse can teach her patient the stages of healing, the amount of time spent within each stage, and the levels of possible activity in each stage. The burn patient can learn in a similar manner. After the initial crisis has subsided, the nurse can teach him the stages of wound healing, methods of treatment, including grafting, and the length of time in rehabilitation. The hemodialysis patient realizes that dialysis is now a vital part of his life. His nurse can support his new life-style and help him remain productive. Each critical care patient can learn the possible time boundaries in which his illness will reach some level of stability. This includes the healing process and its various stages. The critical care nurse can minimize the threat of illness by providing her patient with realistic but positive boundaries. The patient will realize that as he progresses through the stages of healing, he will soon be returning to his family and work. Consequently, the real experience of crisis diminishes, and the new experience of restoration begins. Besides minimizing loneliness by helping her patient to look realistically at boundaries of his illness, the nurse can also minimize both psychological and physiological pain.

Minimizing Psychological Pain. The three components of psychological pain, as mentioned above, are separateness from contact with significant others, separateness from the body, and separateness from one's values and ideas. The critical care nurse can attempt to minimize psychological pain by fostering her patient's relatedness to significant others, to his body, and to his values and ideas.

The nurse realizes that critically ill patients feel more secure knowing that their significant others are nearby. Sullivan (1953) refers to "the human need for contact and tenderness in order for one to be equipped to negotiate the stages of development satisfactorily. With a deprivation of human relatedness, a person must defend himself against total annihilation of self through a substitutive production of fantasies which can not be shared by others" (cited in Gupta 1971, p. 23). Relatedness occurs on two levels. First, there is physical relatedness. Second, there is relatedness to the critically ill patient's illness, injury, or disfigurement. The nurse can attempt to foster physical relatedness. She can use her judgment in permitting more frequent visits by the significant members of the patient's family. Some patients and their families benefit from being physically close to one another. Physical closeness helps to diminish the patient's feeling of loneliness. The need for such physical closeness may be paramount in the initial stage of illness. When the critically ill patient is admitted into critical care, a family member can be permitted to remain visually close. As each treatment or diagnostic procedure is completed, the family member can be encouraged to move from visual to physical closeness. If at all possible, the nurse can place a chair beside the patient's bed, so that the family member and the patient can experience both visual and physical closeness to each other.

It should be noted that everyone experiences loneliness at some time or stage in life. Each person needs to maintain a meaningful relationship with others. When the patient is hospitalized in critical care he can experience an unfulfilled need for relationship with others. The result is isolation and stagnation. These feelings of loneliness can be relieved by relating with others. There are degrees of loneliness and each individual has his own method of coping. The specific methods utilized, whether they be functional or dysfunction, will have an influence upon nursing interventions (Williams 1978).

Usually only the patient's immediate family—parents, spouse, and older children—can visit. If the patient has small children at home, he has difficulty maintaining a sense of relatedness to them. The spouse can keep the patient informed as to events at home. Children can record their voices into a tape recorder, for example, and the patient can record his voice and make personal statements to each child. If the children's mother is hospitalized, the father can bring one of the children's favorite books to their mother. The mother can read a portion of the story into the tape recorder; then, during the family's nighttime routine, the children and father can listen to their mother read to them. Encouraging such family contacts is yet another way in which the critical care nurse can minimize the psychological pain of separateness. Another way in which she fosters physical relatedness is to send something home from the hospital, a picture of the hospital, a sugar container, or a letter. Besides recording their voices, children can be encouraged to write letters and draw pictures. The nurse can then place the children's drawings around the patient's environment.

Relatedness to significant others also involves becoming related to their illness, injury, or disfigurement. In order to facilitate such relatedness, the nurse can include the patient's family in her briefings. The nurse and other members of the health team can explain what the illness, injury, or disfigurement implies, the treatment plan, and the nursing care. The nurse may first give one-to-one instruction to the patient. Once she assesses his comprehension and readiness, she can encourage him to teach his spouse, but she will of course be present to explain, interpret, or clarify any misconceptions. The patient may be unable to teach his own spouse, and the nurse must be ready to assume the responsibility. The teaching plan must be initiated early in the patient's hospitalization. If not accomplished early, the patient and his spouse may not attain a sense of relatedness to the illness. The nurse's goal is to facilitate relatedness through knowledge. The patient and his spouse can together share the experience, thus minimizing both individuals' feelings of loneliness.

The second way in which the critical care nurse minimizes psychological pain is by facilitating the patient's sense of relatedness to the boundaries of his own body. The nurse can help her patient to be a part of the diagnostic and therapeutic regime that is happening to his body. When she attaches various wires and tubes to his body, she can explain their meaning to him. If the wires and tubes are attached without meaningful explanation, the patient will not achieve a sense of relatedness to them. While attaching the EKG leads to her patient's chest, for example, the nurse may learn what the patient already knows about EKGs and cardioscopes. Once she assesses his experiential knowledge, she can refer to the cardioscope as "his." In addition, she can refer to the purpose it has to him personally—to record his cardiac rhythm continually. The nurse can personalize each procedure or treatment performed by relating the experience to his body. The health team can examine the critically ill patient as a whole, rather than as a specific organ. The nurse may encourage her patient to listen to his chest and heart sounds. She may also explain to him his EKG pattern and give him a strip of his own rhythm. The critical care nurse's goal is to foster in her patient a sense of relatedness to his body; therefore, all discussions around the patient's bed must include the patient. This comprehensive attitude will enable the patient to feel that he is not simply an object in a strange environment.

The last way in which the nurse can minimize psychological pain is by giving a sense of relatedness to the patient's values and ideas. She can help to make the patient become aware of boundaries, in terms of limits or restrictions. Although he desires to be active, he will have to comply with the counsel of the health team. Boundaries or limits define those activities that the patient can do and those activities that he must temporarily postpone. The nurse can emphasize the word *can* rather than *cannot*. The word *cannot* signifies a loss to the patient, a loss that perpetuates his feeling of loneliness. In most instances, the patient will return to a relatively stable level of wellness and need not make major changes, and ideally he can then resume some of those activities temporarily postponed. The nurse and patient can discuss limits that the current crisis has dictated. In looking at the limits, the nurse can help her patient find meaning in them. She can find meaning that is personal and relevant to her patient, in contrast to the impersonal rules and regulations that earlier created existential loneliness. For example, the nurse can explain to the patient in isolation why he must be separated from other patients. To the patient with acute pulmonary edema, she can explain why diuretics are given and why fluids are limited. To the burn patient, she can explain the painful necessity of daily trips to the Hubbard tank. Besides finding meaning in the boundaries or limits, the nurse can encourage her patient to participate in his care. This participation may only be on a decision-making level. Nevertheless, the nurse can realize that no decision is ever too insignificant if the patient has played an active role in that decision. The decision may involve devising a flexible schedule or a routine of care. This would be of paramount significance to the burn patient or the isolated patient, because each faces a period of hospitalization longer than that of other critically ill patients. The patient and nurse will gradually look at postponed activities. Again, the patient is free to discuss his feelings with his nurse. He need not experience the loneliness of his thoughts; now he can share them..

Minimizing Physiological Pain. The critical care nurse assesses when the patient is experiencing pain and intervenes to alleviate it. She realizes that a patient may complain of pain in his foot, chest, finger, hand, leg, or as Peplau (1955) expresses it, "any other organ that could be called into service to indicate the pain of loneliness" (p. 1479).* As mentioned previously, a patient may react in one of three ways to pain. He may ignore the pain altogether, react to it realistically, or overreact. Regardless of his reaction, pain is a real experience to the critically ill patient and cannot be ignored. The nurse must assess the meaning of pain to her patients who choose to ignore it and who choose to overreact to it. The degree of intensity is not the important factor; what matters is how the individual reacts.

The nurse may discover that the patient who overreacts to pain is seeking her attention. She can intervene to provide the patient with attention by making purposeful communication contacts with him. She can talk with him about things that are on his mind, following in any direction the patient should choose. Through communication, the nurse can attempt to move the patient out of his isolation and existential loneliness. In so doing, she can be guided by Gupta's (1971) observation that "Persons who are in a state of deep isolation and loneliness can communicate and be communicated with only in the most concrete terms; one cannot break through their isolation with abstraction" (p. 23). Keeping this in mind, the nurse starts where her patient is and moves accordingly. The mere fact that she is present and not doing something to him demonstrates her caring. She can simply listen to her patient talk. He can usually perceive the boundaries of his thoughts. His mind can focus on any physiological pain he feels.

It is imperative that the nurse spend just 10 or 15 minutes giving him her full attention. A consistent amount of time each day will provide the key that unlocks the door of his loneliness and minimizes his physiological pain. While sitting at his bedside, the nurse can touch him. Sitting demonstrates a genuine interest in the patient. Touch can be most effective in helping a lonely patient; there are times when touch accomplishes more than words. Touch can be a sincere gesture of warmth and understanding. The attention derived through touch and verbal communication can help the patient who has a tendency to overreact to pain.

The critical care nurse's goal in intervening to alleviate existential loneliness is twofold. First, she minimizes the threat of illness. Second, she minimizes both psychological and physiological pain. The critical care nurse can next intervene to alleviate the loneliness anxiety of her patient that causes fear of aloneness.

Loneliness Anxiety: Fear of Aloneness

In helping her patient cope with his loneliness anxiety, the critical care nurse has two goals. First, she can intervene to foster the patient's relatedness to his environment. Second, she can develop the patient's relatedness to his future. Both goals involve the establishment of boundaries.

Fostering Relatedness to the Environment. The critical care nurse fosters environmental relatedness by helping the patient to establish boundaries of location. The patient needs to know the proximity of his critical care unit to other departments. If the patient is scheduled for a lung scan, he may want to know how far away he must venture from his more familiar territory. A patient who is scheduled for a valve replacement or coronary artery bypass can be permitted and encouraged to tour ICU where he will stay after surgery. If he makes such a visit, the patient may see another patient who has just experienced similar surgery. He can become familiar with the equipment around his bed and be reassured that it is all normal. He has the opportunity to react to what he sees and to ask questions; in his mind, reality can replace fantasy. Furthermore, it is a tremendous asset if the wife or husband can visit with the patient. Together they can discuss what they saw. The patient need not feel loneliness in his thoughts, because he can share them with his family. Allowing the patient to look at the environment gives him a reference point and a sense of relatedness.

The patient in isolation may want to know the relationship of his room to the nurses' station. This knowledge will give him a sense of security. Even though he cannot see the station, he knows exactly where it is. A more ideal situation would be to have, as do many coronary care units, closed-circuit television transmission from the nurses' station to the patient's room. Some agencies have the patient under television surveillance. The critical care nurse can also experience a similar surveillance, permitting the patient to see his nurse, talk to her, and know that she is really "out there."

The patient also needs to know his boundary of location in relationship to the other patients. He may need to have his territorial boundaries defined. This would include the relationship of his bed, nightstand, bedside table, and chair to others. He learns how close other patients are, should he want to talk. Once he knows his physical relationship or boundaries to objects within his environment, he feels a sense of territorial relatedness and ownership. The patient's desire for physical boundaries may even reach outside the hospital. Patients frequently want to know the major streets surrounding the hospital. They may especially want to know what streets run parallel to their bed. This type of information gives the patient a proper perspective of his relationship with the "outside world," and it also gives him an idea of where he is in relationship to his most favorite location—home. Knowing where he is in relationship to home helps reduce some of the feelings of loneliness.

The nurse must realize that the patient's bed becomes his only reference point. He views everything from this central position. Therefore, the critical care nurse can define the patient's boundaries of location in relationship to his bed. The patient then becomes oriented to the dimension of his physical boundaries, whether they be curtains, objects, walls, streets, or other departments. The nurse must also realize that a patient may be so afraid that he forgets to ask what street runs parallel to him, where the family room is located, where his nightstand is located, or where the bathroom is located. The nurse can assume the responsibility for establishing his boundary of location.

Fostering Relatedness to the Future.   After the patient and/or nurse have established appropriate boundaries of location, she can then help to establish his boundaries of future. In order to have a sense of relatedness to his future, the patient must believe that a future exists. The nurse can emotionally reassure her patient that a future does exist. She and other members of the health team then help the critically ill patient derive meaning from the future. If the patient feels his life will not have meaning, he will succumb to the role of cripple. The health team can work with the patient and his family to look realistically at any changes that can be made in their life-style. Each supports the other, reducing feelings of loneliness anxiety. The nurse can intervene to help her patient focus on the positive aspects of his future. He soon realizes that the boundaries of his future are not limited. With realistic guidance from the health team, the patient can realize that the loss is not as overwhelming as anticipated. He no longer fears aloneness in his own future. Instead, he has a sense of relatedness to it and a sense of significance in it.

NURSING EVALUATION

Evaluation of the patient's problem and nursing care is an ongoing process. The nurse assesses regulatory and cognitive behaviors supporting the diagnosis of loneliness. Interventions designed to minimize loneliness are evaluated for their effectiveness. Effectiveness is measured by the alteration of regulatory and cognitive behaviors. It should be noted that the cognitive behaviors may not totally disappear until the patient is transferred from critical care and/or reunited with significant others.

SUMMARY

The critical care nurse can assist her patient in formulating boundaries of illness, location, and future. She can help him maintain a sense of relatedness to others through meaningful communication by utilizing a variety of therapeutic techniques. All of these actions can lead the patient out of his world of isolation and loneliness. As Hurlburt (1965) reminds us, "No one whether it be doctor or nurse can go away with the satisfaction that he or she has given comprehensive care, if only the physical needs of the patient have been met. To do only this is to deny the humanization of a fellow human being. To encounter another person at his or her point of deepest need is one of the greatest privileges of any human encounter" (p. 299).

REFERENCES

APPLEBAUM, FLORENCE, "Loneliness: A Taxonomy and Psychodynamic View," *Clinical Social Work Journal*, 6, no. 1 (Spring 1978), 13-20.

DETHOMASO, MARITA, "Touch Power," *Perspectives in Psychiatric Care*, 9, no. 3 (1971), 112-118.

ELLISON, CRAIG, "Loneliness: A Social-Developmental Analysis," *Journal of Psychology and Theology*, 6, no. 1 (1978a), 3-17.

——, "Understanding Loneliness," *Life and Health*, 93, no. 4 (October 1978b), 13-16.

FLANDERS, JAMES, "A General Systems Approach to Loneliness," in *Loneliness: A Sourcebook of Current Theory, Research, and Therapy*, ed. Letitia Peplau and Daniel Perlman, pp. 379-405. New York: John Wiley, 1982.

FRANCIS, GLORIA, "Loneliness: Measuring the Abstract," *International Journal of Nursing Studies*, 13 (1976), 153-160.

——, "Loneliness: Measuring the Abstract II," *International Journal of Nursing Studies*, 17 (1980), 127-130.

——, "Loneliness: The Syndrome," *Issues in Mental Health Nursing*, 3 (January-June 1981), 1-5.

FROMM-REICHMANN, FRIEDA, "Loneliness," *Psychiatry*, 22 (1959), 1-15.

GUPTA, MADELEINE, "An Interruption in Loneliness: The Use of Concrete Objects in the Promotion of Human Relatedness," *Journal of Psychiatric Care*, 9, no. 4, (July-August 1971), 23.

HOSKISSON, J. B., *Loneliness*. New York: Citadel Press, 1965.

HURLBURT, KATHRYN, "The Loneliness of Suffering," *Canadian Nurse*, 61, no. 4 (April 1965), 299.

JONG-GIERVELD, JERRY DE, and JOSEPH RAADSCHEILDERS, "Types of Loneliness," in *Loneliness: A Sourcebook of Current Theory, Research and Therapy*, ed. Letitia Peplau and Daniel Perlman, pp. 105-119. New York: John Wiley, 1982.

LARSEN, REED, MIHALY CSIKSZENTMIHALYI, and RONALD GRAEF, "Time Alone in Daily Experience: Loneliness or Renewal?" in *Loneliness: A Sourcebook of Current Theory, Research and Therapy*, ed. Letitia Peplau and Daniel Perlman, pp. 40-53. New York: John Wiley, 1982.

LOUCKS, SANDRA, "Loneliness, Affect, and Self-Concept: Construct Validity of the Bradley Loneliness Scale," *Journal of Personality Assessment*, 44, no. 2 (1980), 142-147.

MIJUSKOVIC, BENJAMIN, "Loneliness and a Theory of Consciousness," *Review of Existential Psychology and Psychiatry*, 15, no. 1 (1977), 19-31.

MOUSTAKES, CLARK, *Loneliness*. Englewood Cliffs, N.J.: Prentice-Hall, 1961.

PEPLAU, HILDEGARD, "Loneliness," *American Journal of Nursing*, 55, no. 12 (December 1955), 1476-1481.

PEPLAU, HILDEGARD, and MARYLA CALDWELL, "Loneliness: A Cognitive Analysis," *Essence Issues in the Study of Aging, Dying and Death*, 2, no. 4 (1978), 207-220.

PEPLAU, LETITIA, MARIA MICELI, and BRUCE MORASCH, "Loneliness and Self-Evaluation," in *Loneliness: A Sourcebook of Current Theory, Research and Therapy*, ed. Letitia Peplau and Daniel Perlman, pp. 135-151. New York: John Wiley, 1982.

PERLMAN, DANIEL, and LETITIA PEPLAU, "Theoretical Approaches to Loneliness," in *Loneliness: A Sourcebook of Current Theory, Research and Therapy*, ed. Letitia Peplau and Daniel Perlman, pp. 123-134. New York: John Wiley, 1982.

POTTHOFF, HARVEY, *Understanding Loneliness*. New York: Harper and Row, 1976.

POLCINO, ANNA SISTER, "Loneliness—The Genesis of Solitude, Friendship, and Contemplation," *Hospital Progress*, August 1979, pp. 61-65.

REISMAN, DAVID, *The Lonely Crowd*. New Haven, Conn.: Yale University Press, 1969.

RUSSELL, DANIEL, "The Measurement of Loneliness," in *Loneliness: A Sourcebook of Current Theory, Research and Therapy*, ed. Letitia Peplau and Daniel Perlman, pp. 81-104. New York: John Wiley, 1982.

SATRON, GEORGE, "Notes on Loneliness," *Journal of the American Academy of Psychoanalysis*, 6, no. 3 (July 1978), 281-300.

SKIPPER, JAMES, *Social Interaction and Patient Care*. Philadelphia: Lippincott, 1965.

SLATER, PHILIP, *The Pursuit of Loneliness*. Boston: Beacon Press, 1970.

SMITH, SYDNEY, "The Psychology of Illness," *Nursing Forum*, 3, no. 1 (1964), 41.

SODLER, WILLIAM, and THOMAS JOHNSON, "From Loneliness to Anomia," in *The Anatomy of Loneliness*, ed. Joseph Hartog, Ralph Audy, and Yehudi Cohen, pp. 34-64. New York: International Universities Press, 1980.

SUEDFELD, PETER, "Aloneness as a Healing Experience," in *Loneliness: A Sourcebook of Current Theory, Research and Therapy*, ed. Letitia Peplau and Daniel Perlman, pp. 54-67. New York: John Wiley, 1982.

SULLIVAN, HARRY S., *Interpersonal Theory of Psychiatry*. New York: Norton, 1953.

TANENBAUM, DAVID, "Loneliness in the Aged," *Mental Hygiene*, 51, no. 1 (January 1967), 91-99.

WILLIAMS, LULA, "A Concept of Loneliness in the Elderly," *Journal of the American Geriatrics Society*, 26, no. 4 (April 1978), 183-187.

WOLFE, *The Hills Beyond*, cited by Moustakes, *Loneliness*, p. 33.

YOUNG, JEFFREY, "Loneliness, Depression and Cognitive Therapy: Theory and Application," in *Loneliness: A Sourcebook of Current Theory, Research and Therapy*, ed. Letitia Peplau and Daniel Perlman, pp. 379-405. New York: John Wiley, 1982.

ZILBOORG, GREGORY, "Loneliness," *The Atlantic Monthly*, 161, no. 1 (January 1938), 45-54.

9
Psychological Immobility

BEHAVIORAL OBJECTIVES

1. Define *psychological immobility*.
2. Describe how the three environmental factors affect the critically ill patient.
3. Discuss how organ image influences the critically ill patient.
4. Describe two role disturbances as they affect the critically ill patient.
5. Identify three regulatory behaviors associated with psychological immobility.
6. Identify four cognitive behaviors associated with psychological immobility.
7. Design a nursing care plan that will facilitate psychological immobility.

An individual in a critical care unit attempts to maintain a holistic self-image in which the many facets of physical, social, or psychological being are of equal significance. Individuals take for granted their physical, social or psychological being until they are in disequilibrium. The biological systems involved then become the focal point of the individual's attention. His preoccupation with what he has previously taken for granted is normal human behavior. Such behavior, according to Olson (1967), "is an integrated developmental process of action and interaction of the physiology, personality, society, and culture of the individual. All human behavior grows through a series of interrelated and independent age-related life-stages" (p. 794).* When one body system loses equilibrium, all other systems also become in-

---

*Copyright, American Journal of Nursing Company. Reprinted, with permission, from *American Journal of Nursing.*

volved. Normally the individual mobilizes patterns of defense to reestablish or maintain equilibrium. An individual who trips over a throw rug, for example, mobilizes his entire body toward maintaining or restoring equilibrium to keep him from falling. If he succeeds, he will simply stumble, but if he fails, he will try to get himself in a state of readiness to be protected from injury as he falls.

Individuals, including critical care patients, mobilize patterns of behavior either to protect themselves or to reestablish normalcy. Behavioral responses indicate to the critical care health team the way in which the individual is maintaining psychological equilibrium or mobility. According to Auger (1976), "The process of isolating behavior as a quality separate from all other qualities of the individual is intended to develop an abstract formulation of behavior in order to identify the areas of commonality and uniqueness. Behavior can be viewed as a complex system with a surrounding environment that operates according to certain rules that can be specified" (p. 32). Furthermore the defense a patient uses may depend upon how the patient perceives illness. If he perceives illness as a threat to his being, he will respond as he does to any threat. According to Wu (1973), "Like health behavior a moderate degree of perceived severity and serious consequences increase the likelihood that actions will be taken. However, if the individual experiences severe threat associated with the symptoms, he is likely to become immobilized with fear" (p. 145).

The individual's behavioral response to various situations, including illness, indicates that person's ability to assess the significance of those situations to his or her own self. A person's own altered physical or psychological being is more significant to him than the alterations of the person dying in the bed in a room nearby. One has more ego involvement with one's own body and the many biological threats it encounters than with those confronting other patients in the environment. Illness and the necessity for hospitalization in critical care represent a severe threat and can reduce an individual's ability to psychologically cope in a positive direction. What may result is psychological immobility and behavioral responses to that immobility. Psychological immobility can be either temporary or permanent. Temporary psychological immobility can be a normal behavioral response found in the avoidance-denial aspect of illness. Once critical care patients acknowledge their illness and accept its implications, they can move from psychological immobility to mobility. Permanent psychological immobility, which may result from an inability to behaviorally cope with illness or from a position deliberately chosen in relation to the illness, makes the individual a psychological cripple.

DEFINITION OF PSYCHOLOGICAL IMMOBILITY

According to Bellak (1952), "Psychological immobility exists when a patient who principally is physically well enough to function occupationally and socially has fears or symptoms or attitudes which make him an invalid"

(p. 4). Carnevali (1970) believes that "immobilization is a concept which can be applied in a wide variety of patient situations. At first thought, the word may evoke ideas of bedrest, casts, paralysis, or lack of motion in joints and muscles. The concept has greater utility, however, if it is not viewed in such a limited sense" (p. 1502).* Primary physical immobility caused by acute illness often leads to secondary psychological immobility. As Olson (1967) points out, physical immobility may be caused by both the illness itself and the restrictions imposed by supportive devices that limit activity:

> Immobility reduces the quality and quantity of sensory information available to the organism and reduces the ability of the individual to interact with his environment. We maintain contact with the environment through the senses and seek to control behavior in various aspects of the environment by responding to the perceived sensory stimuli. The process of perception requires the interpretation of complex stimulus. Immobilization reduces the efficiency of the sensory processes and the individual suffers sensory deprivation. (P. 795)*

The individual may experience psychological mobility if he feels a loss of personal worth or dignity. If his illness has altered a biological system internally or externally through loss, injury, or disfigurement, he may feel less than whole. Depending upon the degree of loss, injury, or disfigurement, the individual may give up or may reach a steady state of immobility. Coupled with his feelings of loss in personal worth or dignity is his feeling of fear, which can serve to immobilize the critically ill patient. Such fear, or fright, can cause freezing, a type of psychological immobility. As Bowlby (1960) explains, fright "is the subjective experience accompanying at least two related instinctual response systems—those leading on the one hand to escape behavior, and on the other hand to alert immobility, or freezing" (p. 96).

Psychological immobility can arise as a result of physical immobility due to supportive devices, loss of a bodily part, estrangement from familiar and supportive surroundings, and estrangement from meaningful people such as family members. The critically ill individual is forced to submit to the domination of one or more biological systems in disequilibrium. Many patients in critical care can cope with the threats created in illness by adapting and incorporating necessary changes in their biopsychosocial beings. Some patients, however, cannot cope with illness. As previously mentioned, this inability can be temporary or permanent. Such an inability can be the result of a psychological response to the illness itself or to new changes in roles imposed by the illness. In either case, the individual copes, especially if the situation or future outcome is threatening, by freezing or becoming psychologically immobile.

THE CONCEPT OF PSYCHOLOGICAL IMMOBILITY APPLIED TO THE CRITICALLY ILL PATIENT

A physically injured individual is distressed both physically and psychologically. What is involved is the individual's perception of his environment and illness. The relationship of the individual to the environment is described as a problem of perception. Perception has been defined as the way a person relates to the environment (Baj and Walker 1980).

Antecedent events become cues that indicate to the individual which behaviors are appropriate to a given situation. Antecedent events predict the consequences of various adaptive and ineffective responses in which an individual might engage. Behavioral designing to facilitate psychological mobility involves arranging an environment to produce and maintain specified behaviors in particular situations. This may not always be possible or realistic in critical care. The environment may not always be arranged to accommodate the patient. Biological crisis necessitates immediate action directed toward restoring biological mobility.

Illness severe enough to warrant hospitalization in a critical care unit can create feelings of fear, which may be intense enough to overshadow positive coping means. Positive coping signifies that the patient is able to adapt to his illness. He may experience temporary psychological immobility by refusing to participate in his care or by resisting rehabilitation. Once the initial crisis subsides, he no longer experiences his previous immobility. On the other hand, there are times when psychological immobility occurs in overwhelming situations, where the stress exceeds the coping ability. Frequently, critical care nurses see psychological paralysis when a stressful experience advances upon a patient and his family (Carnevali 1970). The patient may become immobilized because acute illness threatens life itself. Coupled with fear of death, the individual fears powerlessness and abandonment.

Psychological immobility has three precipitating causes. First of all, the environment may be so intense that it totally intimidates the patient, who becomes immobilized by what he sees going on around him and by what he fantasizes could happen to him. Secondly, illness itself, which threatens his biological being, can cause psychological immobility or paralysis. The patient may not want to participate in his care because he fears his biological integrity will not withstand the therapy. In this instance the individual becomes organ-oriented. We will discuss organ orientation, or image, later. Lastly, the individual may become immobilized if he is confronted with role disturbance, forcing him to adapt to a new role.

Environmental Factors

The critical care patient as a behavioral system is dependent upon the external critical care environment. The system may achieve instability by excess or deficits within the external environment. Stressors within the environment consist of the critical care unit itself, the use of supportive devices, and the critical care health team.

The environment of the critical care unit has a significant impact on the health care team as well as on the patient. The knowledge explosion and advances in the diagnosis and treatment of disease have created an overwhelming technological and bureaucratic system of health care (Baj and Walker 1980). Therefore the critical care environment may facilitate psychological mobility or immobility. Anyone who has ever walked through a critical care unit immediately senses its environmental stresses or tensions, and a patient who arrives in such a unit makes a similar assessment. The manner in which he is admitted can dispel or enhance his feelings of environmental fear. If the environment is a relaxing one, the patient may feel it is conducive to his psychological mobility, but if the environment is hectic, noisy, and stressful, it can communicate anxieties to an already anxious patient that can immobilize him. He sees things that only enhance his fears. For example, an emergency may occur in the unit. People run, alarms sound, and voices call out for medications, defibrillation, and other threatening techniques. All other patients alert to the problem may react by becoming fearful that the same or a similar experience might happen to them. Happily, the critical care unit can also serve to reassure the patient. He realizes that if an emergency should occur, he is in expert hands. He should make the patient feel secure and motivated toward achieving wellness, although such security and motivation is not always possible. Nevertheless the patient is uncertain as to the purpose or direction of the surrounding numerous activities upon arrival in the critical care unit.

In order to become psychologically mobile, the patient must feel motivated. According to Vernon (1969), "Motivated behavior involves awareness of and prompt reaction to particular features of the environment. In withdrawal and flight, for instance, some aspect of the environment is perceived as threatening danger, injury or pain" (p. 12). The individual can become motivated by external stimulation. Motivation may not always be in a positive direction; it may take the form of avoidance or flight. Because of his illness, the patient cannot flee the stressful environment. He may, however, withdraw or avoid thinking about its seriousness or implications. In this respect, temporary psychological immobility can have a positive effect, since, as Vernon (1969) points out, it "enables the individual to protect or defend himself from the danger and injury. Avoidance and flight are characteristically associated with the emotions of fear and anger respectively, and the relationship is so close that frequently it is impossible to distinguish motivated behavior from emotions" (p. 49).

Shortly after the patient's arrival in a critical care unit, he must part with familiar possessions and family members. He has to exchange his clothes for a hospital gown, and he finds himself in a strange bed surrounded by strangers—other patients and nurses. As his personal possessions are removed and his family leaves, the unfamiliar and the unknown close in upon the individual. Everyone in his immediate environment is a stranger, and at a time when he most needs support and familiarity, little seems to be available. His nurse's contact with him centers on admitting the patient and connecting him to various pieces of supportive equipment.

Supportive devices within the environment also contribute to psychological immobility. The degree of physical immobilization caused by various supportive devices depends upon the type and severity of disease, illness, or injury. Obviously, some critical care units may require fewer supportive devices than others. Hemodialysis, for example, utilizes one cumbersome piece of equipment, the hemodialysis machine. Coronary care, intensive care, burn care, and respiratory care involve more monitoring devices. In these units, wires and tubes connect the patient to machines. The more wires and tubes there are, the less mobile the patient is. He may finally gather together enough courage to turn in bed, but his machines may beep or buzz at him in defiance. He becomes frustrated at having to inconvenience his nurse, who must come to his bedside to terminate the beeping and buzzing. The patient may choose to remain physically immobile. Other patients may take out their frustrations on their nurses. As Carnevali (1970) points out, "major or persistent minor frustrations can cause a patient to give up further effort at any independence of thought or action—this is passive immobilization. Others subvert their frustrations into hostility against the helping figures; this in turn seems to place restraint on the effective and therapeutic intervention that is possible between them" (p. 1505).* Instead of getting angry at himself, the patient expresses anger toward his nurse. He may rationalize that she was responsible for connecting him to all the restricting pieces of equipment.

Physical mobility tends to enhance one's psychological mobility. As we move through our environment, we make emotional contact with people or objects within that environment. The contact seems to stimulate or motivate us toward making additional contacts. Normally while we lie in bed, our senses make psychological contact with the environment. We turn from side to side, side to back, back to side, and back to stomach. Our physical mobility allows us to attain a combination of alternative positions. With each turn, we become aware of new sounds or visual images. If we turn toward a window, we become aware of cars on a nearby freeway, dogs barking, or a neighbor leaving for work. A sudden unfamiliar noise creates both physical and psychological mobility or energies. We turn toward the noises, realizing that there are no physical boundaries to or consequences of such mobility. But the critical care patient does not have such physical mobility. If he physically turns in an attempt to make visual and auditory contact with his environments, the machine buzzes. For fear of disturbing the wires and tubes, he decides to remain physically immobilized. Therefore, visual contact with his immediate environment is limited to the movement of his eyes while lying on his back. He can no longer verify strange sounds with his eyes. One fre-

*Copyright, American Journal of Nursing Company. Reprinted, with permission, from *American Journal of Nursing*.

quently sees this type of patient lying on his back, eyes staring at the ceiling or the foot of his bed, his hands clenched at his side. All the supportive devices serve as constant reminders of his illness and its severity. The intensity of the environment and the supportive devices create feelings of fear within the individual. The fear tends to reduce the patient's ability both to hear what is happening around him and to make appropriate interpretation of the sounds.

The nurse is the third environmental cause of psychological immobility. Her contribution is not, of course, intentional, but she can cause the patient psychologically to give up. The nurse, as we have noted earlier, becomes the most significant person in the patient's environment. She has the power to control the patient's environment and to reduce or eliminate those factors contributing to his psychological immobility. The process begins the moment a patient arrives in critical care. At first she has to keep him alive, which she does by attaching the necessary machines or supportive devices, administering emergency treatments, and coordinating the hospital's admitting process, including no small amount of paperwork.

The nurse may become involved in conversations at the patient's bedside that may or may not pertain to him. Nevertheless conversations that the patient hears may upset him. The reactions of others are often anxiety-arousing. Having to trust one's life to the hands of complete strangers, becoming hospitalized in critical care and helplessly dependent upon others are psychologically distressful (Mattsson 1975).

The tremendous amount of activities or responsibilities placed upon the nurse can push her into a goal-directed, rather than a patient-directed, attitude. The patient may get the feeling that everyone seems to be more concerned with supportive devices and admission procedures than with him. He may also get the impression that his condition is more critical than he thought, because he cannot realize that much of what appears to be chaos is really normal. A hurried nurse may unintentionally convey to the patient her own feeling of anxiety or sense of urgency, since she knows the consequences of his illness and the potentially life-threatening problems that it might cause. Once the chaos of admission procedures and crisis has subsided, the patient may be left alone with his thoughts. But what thoughts! His senses have been assaulted, his body is not "right" and he is hooked up to strange machines; it is no wonder that the patient becomes psychologically immobile.

Illness: Organ Image

Organ image is the mental picture the patient assigns to his or her specific biological problem. For example, critical care patients may view themselves as a heart, a kidney, or a lung. The patient's organ image is reinforced when members of the health team focus on his altered biological systems rather than on the individual by name. Therefore, patients see themselves from an organ image point of view rather than as a whole.

Behavior that is not stressed because of illness is organized and patterned. The result is that patients utilize their energy in a stable and consistent manner. Behavioral responses are flexible and appropriate to the problem-force environment. This reflects a dynamic process of equilibrium or adaptation among the various subsystems. Physical stress such as illness, injury or disease can produce psychological immobility.

Mattsson (1975) notes that the psychological component of traumatic injury may be like any other internal injury in that the specific site is not always immediately evident and it may take some type of skilled observation and continuous monitoring to determine precisely where and how badly one is hurt. Psychological healing becomes inadequate if the necessary aggressive or antiaggressive responses remain too weak or become too strong.

Psychological immobility may begin when the patient arrives in a critical care unit or it may begin when doctors diagnose his illness. Critically ill patients react to their diagnosis in several ways: one may not hear it; another will not understand; another may become immobilized. The last response can be temporary or permanent. Temporary immobility allows the patient to get himself psychologically organized. It must be remembered that "emotional stress responses may peak and wane, allowing patients to return to their usual pattern of emotional mobility, but here, too, there are instances where emotional immobilization is not only prolonged, but increasing" (Carnevali 1970, p. 1506). A critical illness can bring about two psychological responses. A patient may simply freeze, out of fright, or he may become preoccupied with the diagnosis, disease, or surgically altered organ. In this second response, the patient becomes organ image–conscious. There are times during the initial crisis of illness when the patient is unable to incorporate environment events. Organ image, whether it is related to myocardial infarction, renal failure, ketoacidosis, chronic obstructive pulmonary disease, or a serious burn, reduces the individual's receptiveness to environmental stimuli. Organ image is a stressor that reduces environmental intake and contributes to psychological immobility. Some patients become terrified by their illness and events surrounding hospitalization.

The terror created by the traumatic events leaves the patient initially frightened and helpless. This state of distress is generally followed by emotional numbness which can lead to depression. Even when a patient has made a fast and satisfactory biological recovery, the threatening experience can continue to haunt him. The patient finds himself uncertain about his beliefs and attitude toward himself (Mattsson 1975).

According to Bowlby (1965), "Fright is the subjective experience accompanying at least two related instinctual response systems—those leading on the one hand to escape behavior, and on the other hand to alert immobility or freezing" (p. 96). The critically ill patient is unable to escape his new situation physically. Instead he may choose to escape psychologically. On the other hand, the individual can psychologically freeze. Both choices, according to Bowlby, are "conceived as systems built into the organism and perpetuated by heredity because of their survival value. The systems governing freezing seem almost to require some external conditions for their activation. Amongst those to which they appear to be naturally sensitive are loud noises, sudden visual changes, physical pain, and mere strangeness" (p. 97).

Anything unusual or unfamiliar in the patient's external environment can frighten him. He may request transfer before he is physically ready for such a move. The patient's request to flee his strange environment may be his only way of coping with a new situation. As Bowlby points out, his reaction to illness and environmental strangeness is on an elemental level:

> At this elemental level of instinctual behavior, the individual does not structure his universe into objects interacting causally to produce situations, some of which are expected to prove dangerous and others harmless. On the contrary, so long as he is operating on this level, his responses are rapid and automatic. They may or may not be well adapted to the real situation. The individual flees or remains immobile not because he has any clear awareness of danger but because his flight or freezing responses have been activated. (P. 97)

The critical care patient can physically flee in one of two ways. He can sign himself out of the hospital or attempt to leave quietly when no one is watching.

Mr. D., a 45-year-old merchant marine, was admitted to intensive care. He had been on vacation visiting some friends when he suddenly became ill. He complained of a severe headache, dizziness, blurred vision, nausea, and chest pain. It was originally thought that Mr. D. had experienced a myocardial infarction, but an EKG did not reveal any significant changes. His blood pressure was 220/160, and an X-ray revealed a descending thoracic aortic aneurysm. The patient was immediately started on Nitroprusside IV drip to regulate his blood pressure. Because of the nature of his physiological problem, nurses had to take Mr. D.'s blood pressure frequently. Mr. D. did not like this treatment, and his behavior revealed his dissatisfaction with his stay in critical care. The doctors decided to inform Mr. D. about his diagnosis and its implications for future surgery.

DOCTOR: Mr. D., does your head still hurt?

MR. D.: Yes, but not as much. Does that mean I'll be leaving soon?

DOCTOR: No, Mr. D. There are a few things I want to discuss with you.

MR. D.: Like what?

DOCTOR: Well, your hypertension and its cause. Do you remember that we took an X-ray shortly after your admission?

MR. D.: Yes.

DOCTOR: That X-ray revealed a descending thoracic aortic aneurysm.

MR. D.: So what does that mean?

DOCTOR: It means a weakening or ballooning of the major artery. The situation is most critical. This is one of the reasons why you have hypertension.

MR. D.: So what do you do with the weakened area?

DOCTOR: We will need to remove it surgically.

MR. D.: Why can't I continue with my medications and not have surgery?

DOCTOR: Without surgery, your life will be in danger. The aneurysm can rupture. If that happens, then it's all over.

MR. D.: I see. How long would I have without surgery?

DOCTOR: That depends on keeping your blood pressure down, strain at work, and your activities.

MR. D.: I would rather go home.

DOCTOR: We'll talk about it again later.

Mr. D. was then left alone to contemplate the possibility of surgery. He wanted a more conservative intervention such as medication rather than surgery. After he was told the implications of his illness and his immediate need of surgery, he changed the subject. Instead of wanting surgery to rectify the situation, he "would rather go home." The idea of surgery was frightening, and he wanted to flee.

This is a normal reaction to a diagnosis that requires changes in life-style, limitation of activity, or surgical intervention. Many critical care patients only talk about going home, and eventually they submit to the prescribed surgical intervention. Submission to changes in life-style or limitation of activity may not take place as quickly. Mr. D., however, continued to talk about going home. His verbal desire to flee increased to the point that it turned into demands. On the following afternoon, Mr. D. put on his clothes and demanded that his doctors release him. Fortunately, his blood pressure had gone down since his admission. Much discussion between the doctors, nurses, and Mr. D. could not convince the patient of the seriousness of leaving before surgery could be performed. Mr. D. signed a consent and left the hospital. Other patients may not be as obvious in their demands, as the next example illustrates.

Ms. T., a 23-year-old woman, was admitted to critical care with a drug overdose. She had apparently become disturbed over a conflict with her boyfriend. As a result, she took an overdose of Doriden. For two days, Ms. T. was totally dependent on various pieces of equipment and her nurse. On the third day, the nurse removed her endotracheal tube, respirator, and cardioscope. Ms. T. became more alert and active. She had made a previous attempt on her life only one year before, and she knew from previous experience that when she was completely alert, she would have to move to the psychiatric unit. She did not want to go there. While the nurses worked with other patients, Ms. T. pretended to be asleep. In the evening, Ms. T. made her attempt to flee the unit. She quietly removed the IV tubing from its bottle, placed the tubing in her pocket, and quickly walked toward one of the two doors leading out of the unit. Luckily, an alert intern reading charts at the nurses' station noticed Ms. T. As the two saw one another, Ms. T. bolted toward the door, but the intern caught her. Fortunately for Ms. T., her escape was terminated. Unfortunately for Mr. D., his escape could not be terminated. Both patients demonstrated escape by physically fleeing the crisis situation. Other patients unable to physically flee their illness freeze psychologically.

Illness is a hazardous event. According to Rapaport (1965), "The hazardous event creates for the individual a problem in his current life situation. The problem can be conceived of as a threat, a loss, or a challenge. The threat may be to fundamental, instinctual needs or to the person's sense of integrity. . . . A threat to need and integrity is met with anxiety" (p. 25). Illness involves loss of function or of all or part of an organ. The individual becomes preoccupied with the organ or system involved, which previously he had taken for granted. As Olson (1967) points out, one's body image has considerable psychological importance:

> One of the fascinating paradoxes of human condition is that the human body, which units and identifies man as a biologic specie, gives rise, in each of us, on a psychological level, to a body-image that is one of the subtly unique features of the individual's personality. A person's conception of his own body as a whole and of different parts of the body contributes greatly to his conception of his own personality and of his relations with other people. (P. 794)

Patients in critical care do become preoccupied with their disease or surgically altered organ. Some patients become preoccupied to the point of physically immobilizing themselves. They are fearful of carrying out necessary rehabilitative maneuvers for fear of overtaxing the sick organ. In other cases, patients have improved biologically to the point of attaining greater mobility, but their psychological condition has reached a steady state of immobility. The psychological block prevents greater physical mobility.

The degree of psychological immobility depends not only upon the individual's previous coping ability but also upon the severity of his illness. Loss of function may represent a temporary situation in which there is minimal biological alteration. Such is the case in illness like acute tubular necrosis, cerebral artery spasm resulting in temporary unilateral weakness, myocardial infarction with minimal EKG and serum enzyme changes, and pneumonia. In such cases there is temporary loss of function, but good treatment and care may restore the function. When function does not return to the sick organ, the patient experiences loss of a part, such as loss of one kidney due to pathology or injury, loss of myocardial tissue due to several infarctions leading to congestive heart failure, or loss of lung tissue due to chronic obstructive lung disease or lobectomy. Similarly, loss of function can result from conditions such as hepatic failure due to cirrhosis, or right-sided hemiplegia due to a CVA. In some instances loss of a part can result in loss of a whole organ, as in lobectomy, pneumonectomy, bilateral nephrectomy, bilateral amputation above the knee, quadriplegia or paraplegia, or skin loss due to burns.

An organ that is partly or entirely lost usually has tremendous ego value to the patient. Its loss psychologically immobilizes him, preventing him from progressing beyond his condition at the time of the initial loss. Even if a sick organ regains part of its functions or strength, or if a pacemaker, respirator, or hemodialysis machine can substitute for the organ, many patients cannot bring themselves to recognize biological improvements or biological substitutes. All they see is a future of limitations or controls.

Mr. J. is an example of a patient who experienced loss of a part. He entered coronary care complaining of severe substernal chest pain, nausea, vomiting, diaphoresis, and shortness of breath. This was his third admission in two years. An EKG revealed acute myocardial infarction. Mr. J. did notice that his tolerance for fatigue had greatly diminished. He no longer was able to work the long hours in his business that he previously worked. Lately he noticed that he experienced shortness of breath for no apparent reason. Mr. J. was familiar not only with his coronary care environment but also with the consequence of his sick organ. For three days after his arrival in CCU, his condition remained critical. He experienced hypotension and shortness of breath. His doctors feared cardiogenic shock and impending congestive heart failure.

Upon his arrival in CCU, staff members attached a cardioscope to Mr. J., and he also received oxygen by mask and IV. Only the cardioscope directly monitored his sick organ. Mr. J. realized this from his previous admission, and he frequently watched his own rhythm. He remembered that on his previous admission, he had developed arrhythmias. As he developed cardiogenic shock and cardiac failure, he required additional supportive devices, including IPPB to facilitate breathing, CVP, a Foley catheter to monitor hourly output, Swan-Ganz to monitor pulmonary artery pressure (PAP) and pulmonary capillary wedge pressure (PCWP), and additional IVs with vasopressor medications. This equipment was new to the patient. The nurses began noticing that Mr. J. lay rigidly immobilized in bed. He seemed to be afraid to move. In addition, he was preoccupied with both his cardioscope and IVs. Every time the nurses approached Mr. J.'s bed, he wanted to know how his monitor pattern looked to them, what his enzyme studies showed, how his blood pressure was responding to medications, and if his EKG showed any improvement. During the next three days, Mr. J.'s biological status stabilized to the point that vasopressors and hourly monitoring of his urinary output were not necessary. Even with less intense focusing on Mr. J.'s sick organ, he nevertheless continued to preoccupy himself with anything related to it. Mr. J. and his nurse had the following conversation:

NURSE: Mr. J., since you are doing so well, I'm going to increase your activity.
MR. J.: How?
NURSE: I'll have you do part of your bath and maybe shave yourself.
MR. J.: Do you think that is wise? You know how sick it has been.
NURSE: What is "it"?

MR. J.:   My heart. Why don't you continue to bathe me, and I'll do it another time.
NURSE: I'll bathe you today, and you can shave yourself.
MR. J.:   I think you had better do that as well. You know, my condition is more severe this time.
NURSE: Are you afraid something will happen?
MR. J.:   It could. I might not survive the next one. You just bathe me. All this talk is tiring.
NURSE: All right, but we'll talk about your need to increase activity tomorrow.

Mr. J.'s biological condition had improved enough that he could participate in his own care and become more actively involved. Instead he wanted to withdraw from any physical involvement. His attention focused on his sick organ, to which he referred as "it" or his "condition." As Bellak (1952) notes, the critically ill patient's "attitude toward the sick organ may so change that it, itself, becomes anthropomorphized: he thinks of it as something independent, something that needs special care. The patient's attitude towards his organ (and thus, towards himself), may become that of an overanxious mother towards a child—always worrying, always overprotecting" (p. 3).

Some critical care patients become organ image–conscious. The burn patient sees his skin in a completely different way. The hemodialysis patient attributes a new image to the sick or surgically removed organ. Patients who need rehabilitation to breathe, to walk, or to move without overtaxing a severely damaged heart may physically or psychologically refuse to participate. The patients may fear that rehabilitation will impair their biological process, and they fear the sick organ is not ready for such activity. Instead they are content in not testing the organ. These people reach a steady state of psychological immobility; such patients are often referred to as cardiac or respiratory cripples.

These critical care patients are often physiologically capable of achieving much more than they are psychologically willing to attempt: here is where the role of the nurse is vital. Realizing that her patient may become preoccupied with the organ involved, she can provide subtle support for the sick organ rather than intently focusing upon it. Much of what the health team does during a crisis focuses intently on the diseased system, to the exclusion of all else. It is understandable that the patient himself focuses on a sick organ. He may organize his future around his current feelings toward the organ. A cardiac or respiratory patient, for example, may decide that the risks are too great, and he will choose to give up, when in fact he is physically capable of achieving more than his mind allows.

The loss of an entire organ, or of its function, can result from severe pathology or surgical intervention. The burn patient's skin is replaced with grafts. The cardiac patient has various alternatives. If his conductive tissue is lost, he uses a pacemaker. Diseased valves and coronary arteries are replaced. He could, in the last resort, have a heart transplant. The renal patient might acquire kidney transplants. If this is not possible, he could have hemodialysis. The pulmonary patient may be maintained on a volume respirator, or he may have a lung transplant.

Surgical intervention may involve the transfer of specific parts—one's own body arteries,—or it may involve a total removal, but no matter what the surgical intervention may be, the idea itself can psychologically immobilize the patient. The nature of the threat posed by surgery is described by Bellak (1952) as follows:

> Surgical operation stands as a major threat to anyone who must undergo it. It carries certain similar danger for all. These realistic dangers may be listed as: the threat of life itself, the loss of important body parts or functions, the danger of chronic invalidism, postoperative pain or suffering, the delay of important plans, questions concerning the surgeion's skills and competence, economic dislocation due to the period of unemployment and the expense of the operation, hospital care and postoperative treatment. (P. 53)

The critical care nurse can prepare her patient thoroughly for surgical intervention, and this preparation should include not only explanation of the physical and/or technical aspects of surgery, but also a realistic evaluation of the patient's future.

The cardiac patient can anticipate being free of much or all of his pain. The renal patient can look forward to a relatively new life-style made possible by renal transplant. It is imperative that the nurse be realistic in mobilizing the patient toward a positive outcome. As Bellak (1952) notes, the patient's psychological acceptance of his sick organ or surgical procedure is "directly related to his concept of illness. When the patient is given a diagnosis he has to absorb the information in terms of the knowledge he has of it, and in terms of the knowledge the doctor gives him" (p. 2).

The critical care nurse keeps in mind that illness has a different connotation for each patient, but each patient may experience a period of psychological immobility. In some cases, the immobility is only temporary; in other situations, it becomes a permanent way of life. The individual may reach a steady state of psychological death. The critical care patient may eventually give up and accept roles others have given him, or may manufacture his own, for example, the role of invalid or cripple.

Role Disturbance

At the psychological level there is an increase in the patient's efforts toward maintenance and repair of his self-image, self-identity, and self-integrity. The patient attempts to maintain his psychological balance. He wants to get back on his feet, resume his normal activities, and be in his own familiar territory (Mattsson 1975).

A critical illness may force role alterations upon on individual. The forced role disturbances necessitate that one's behavior be altered to fit the new situation. Two types of role disturbance may occur in critical care: sick-role disturbance and social-role disturbance. Each role change may lead to self-conflict whereby the individual feels insecure with his or her own body and its real or artificial boundaries.

Self-conflict resulting from sick-role disturbance may affect a critical care patient who has been healthy until forced by a major illness or injury to assume a new role. Unlike the chronically ill patient who may have had time to adjust to the sick role, a critical care patient may be assuming a totally new role. The events that occur after his arrival in a critical care unit, and his uncertain future, are vague and unknown. The patient may not know what is expected of him as a sick person. His only orientation to illness may be through magazine articles, relatives, or television programs. He may not understand the more simple things around him, such as the call light, the bed control, and the bedpan. The more complex supportive devices, such as the cardioscope and the respirator, may be totally beyond his comprehension. Since the patient is connected to various supportive devices, thereby confirming the presence of a biological crisis, he loses the connection with the supportive assistance of family. All that is familiar to him has been replaced with unfamiliarity. His personal family has been replaced with a new hospital "family" of nurses, doctors, technicians, and other patients. His home has been replaced by a new "home": the coronary care, hemodialysis, intensive care, burn, neurological, or respiratory care unit. His familiar bedroom has been replaced by a strange bed with various control devices. Needless to say, the patient experiences feelings of psychological immobility.

Critically ill patients experiencing their first illness become preoccupied with certain aspects of it. Consider, for example, the situation of one first-time coronary patient as described by Bellak (1952):

> The first coronary attack with its overwhelming pain and the accompanying feeling of possible death, is a severe trauma for the patient. Once the acute danger situation is passed, the patient starts to realize the nature of his affliction within the framework of his established reaction pattern, to danger situations. He may feel that he is doomed and his attitude towards life will change. (P. 36)

Although the hemodialysis patient may not be new to the sick role, he becomes preoccupied with his dependency on an external object. The laryngestomy patient may become anxious when he realizes that his tracheostomy is permanent. Unfortunately, the sick role creates anxiety. According to Hellmuth (1966) "Anxiety strengthens latent dependency which is likely to well up when a patient recuperates from a critical illness. The anxiety may blow out of proportion to the degree of impairment really present and therefore lead to disturbed perception of nursing or medical recommendations. The staff may view the patient's condition more or less disabling than he does himself" (p. 772).

Even if an illness stabilizes to the point of allowing greater physical mobility, the patient may remain psychologically tied to his sick role. He feels insecure about the future and may be unable to plan for it constructively. The nurse and family must intervene before this point to facilitate movement away from sick-role disturbance and toward a well role.

There may be an additional problem, however: social-role disturbance. Although the patient may be able to move physically out of the critical care unit, he may be psychologically tied to the security it offers. Some of the dependency stems from social-role disturbance, which usually manifests itself after the crisis of illness has subsided. By this time the patient begins thinking about his future and the future of his family, especially if the illness has imposed future limitations, dependency on others or on an inanimate object, or a possible reversal of roles. The hard-working man who enters a critical care unit with myocardial infarction, right-sided weakness due to cerebral artery spasm, or hypertension will have to curtail some of his activities. He may spend 16 hours a day constantly exposed to the stresses and strains of making decisions. Work has become the essence of his existence. Curtailment of his activity may be beyond his comprehension. After a certain degree of pressure from his family and doctor, the patient will agree to limit his workload for a period of time. In all probability, he will find himself able to establish limitations, but, as he feels better, he will attempt to resume his full work schedule. According to Bellak (1956), "With some persons, the work habit is a firmly established pattern and a relatively conflict-free area of the ego. It is important, therefore, to know the degree of work stability, the extent to which work has been a predominantly satisfying experience, and the emotional factors that have operated both in the patient's concept of work and in his self-concept as a worker" (p. 486).

All individuals want to feel that they are productive and contributing toward some goal for either themselves or their family. Work becomes a vehicle for achieving such a goal. Society forces us to evaluate the work effectiveness of those around us by assessing the number of their material possessions. A major illness imposes limitations on the individual that render his feeling of productiveness temporarily or permanently ineffective. The individual may sense a loss of self-esteem and dignity. It must be remembered that "the increased self-esteem that accrues through the dignity of being productive, the rewards and satisfactions inherent in achievement, and the opportunity for gratifying social relationships make work itself a primary technique in the restoration of the patient" (Bellak 1956, p. 488). The individual who must curtail or reduce his work schedule may become depressed. As a result, he might withdraw from all work, becoming a psychological cripple. In all probability such an individual is either afraid to or unable to differentiate pertinent duties from irrevelant ones that could be handled by someone else. Both the nurse and the patient's family can help out in this situation. It is necessary that the nurse learn what the patient's prehospitalization values and life-style were.

Concern for loss of social activities presents another terrain for fruitful nurse and family intervention. For example, the cardiac patient who experienced a myocardial infarction or arrhythmias during sexual intercourse may fear the same problem will recur, and he may feel too inhibited to discuss sexual matters with his doctors or nurses. Fortunately, critical care nurses and physicians now recognize that this area is vital to the patient's total rehabilitation. If the subject remains locked away in the supply closet, unspoken frustrations develop between husband and wife. Sexual awareness should be a vital part of the nurse's and doctor's rehabilitation plan. Hopefully, psychological immobility toward sexual intercourse can be openly discussed and worked through prior to the patient's discharge.

If the patient fails independently to verbalize his or her concern regarding future sexual activity, the health team can initiate this conversation. Prior to discharge, patients normally receive instruction about activity, diet, or medications; this briefing can include discussion of sexual activity. The cardiac patient who fears angina during sexual intercourse can be instructed to take a nitroglycerine tablet prior to intercourse. The hemodialysis patient may feel energetic and sexually inclined shortly after his dialysis treatment. Regardless of the critically ill patient's biological problems, the health team must include sexual awareness in its care plan.

Dependency on an external object, like work or sexual limitations, can also create role disturbances. Each individual likes to think of his own body as being autonomous. The healthy individual makes social contact through the process of sensory and motor interaction with his environment, and he has the freedom and physical capability for this interaction. Suddenly, major illness strikes, and he finds himself not only limited by physical immobility but possibly dependent on an inanimate object. The cardiac patient may be dependent on a pacemaker. The respiratory care patient may be dependent upon a permanent tracheostomy and/or respirator at home. The hemodialysis patient is dependent upon a hemodialysis machine, which he must use regularly at a hospital. Such dependency on supportive devices may psychologically immobilize the individual until he realizes their significance.

A final cause of social-role disturbance is role reversal. As Cummings (1970) points out, the critical care patient most affected is probably the male hemodialysis patient:

> Three main aspects of the male role in our culture—breadwinner, disciplinarian, and decision maker—seem to be particularly vulnerable to encroachments of kidney disease and dialysis. When the wife must leave the home, when she assumes the role of dispenser of rewards and punishments, when she must make the major decisions connected with management of the home—these are circumstances which cannot help but demote the patient in his own eyes. (P. 72)

Such a patient has to cope with both the financial chaos of major illness and major social role changes. He feels guilty about his physical inability to assume responsibility for his family, his wife's sudden need to work, and his creating a tremendous financial burden for the entire family. It is not unusual to have such a patient give up and become psychologically crippled, failing to use what physical potentials he has. There are similar problems when the wife is the one disabled. If the family is young, the wife feels guilty about her inability to meet the family's needs. Her husband must now assume some of the household responsibilities. If the children are at an age where they can help, the responsibility rests on their shoulders.

Social-role disturbance is not unique to the hemodialysis patient. All critically ill patients who experience a major illness necessitating future limitations or restrictions may have social-role changes. No matter what the patient's physical problem is, he must be supported so that he will not reach a steady state of psychological immobility. Nurses and family members must encourage him to move beyond his current limitations and to develop his remaining potentialities. The critical care nurse and the family become the primary motivating factors.

In summary, the specific insult may consist of a blow to the individual's psychological integrity, self-autonomy, faith in self and others, orientation to pleasure, need to control others, hopes for the future, or whatever is of psychological significance to the patient at a specific time (Mattsson 1975).

NURSING ASSESSMENT OF PSYCHOLOGICAL IMMOBILITY

The critical care nurse assesses psychological immobility. The responses can be categorized into regulatory and cognitive behaviors. The primary behaviors manifested will be cognitive responses rather than regulatory.

Regulatory Behaviors

The regulator system involves stimuli from the external environment and from changes in the internal state of dynamic equilibrium. The regulatory behavior or physiological responses in psychological immobility consist of the following:

Regulatory Behaviors
Fatigue
Anorexia
Loss of weight
Numbness of body part

Cognitive Behaviors

The cognator system involves inputs from internal and external stimuli which include psychological and social factors. The specific aspects of the cognator mechanism consists of perceptual/information processing, learning, judgment, and emotion. The cognitive behaviors are psychological responses which in cases of psychological immobility consist of the following:

Cognitive Behaviors
Withdrawal
Depression
Anger
Lassitude
Apathy
Memory disturbance

NURSING DIAGNOSIS OF PSYCHOLOGICAL IMMOBILITY

The nursing diagnosis is a statement of the current problem. Regulatory and cognitive behaviors coupled with stressors causing the problem combine to help the nurse make her diagnosis. The problem is psychological immobility. For the patient experiencing psychological immobility, internal stressors consist of organ image and role disturbance. External stressors include environmental factors such as supportive devices, noises, and staff. Internal and external stressors can combine to cause psychological immobility.

NURSING INTERVENTIONS TO FACILITATE PSYCHOLOGICAL MOBILITY

The critical care nurse realizes that disease, illness, and injury create instability and psychological immobility. The nurse, together with other members of the health team, witnesses situations in which some loss of function, part, or whole has created imperfection in the patient. The imperfection affects the patient's ability to gain, transmit, or utilize environmental information. The goal of the critical care health team is to reduce psychological immobility.

The critical care nurse can be a major force in moving the patient toward psychological mobility. She can help him cope with the strange noise and machines of the critical care environment, the crisis of major illness, and the possibility of social-role changes. The patient may make progress in one area only to regress or become immobilized in another area. The nurse can attempt to move him beyond his current illness level toward wellness. This involves a stabilizing process, which has been described by Sutterley (1973) as follows:

> The stabilizing process is a self-regulating process that is characteristic of living open systems. All living systems tend to maintain steady states among many variables, seeking a balance between adjusted interlocking processes or subsystems which process matter, energy or information. The steady state is not static in most respects, for the parts or subsystems are often in constant flux. (P. 72)

The principle stabilizing force in a patient's environment is his critical care nurse. She can make his transition from the familiarity of home into the uncertainty of critical care and technology a smooth one. The admitting process need not be traumatic for the individual, if his nurse keeps in mind that the impact of illness has already traumatized or immobilized him. She can assess those factors in his environment that can create psychological immobility, including the atmosphere of critical care, the supportive devices, and the nurse herself. The nurse can create a critical care environment unclouded by continual impending crisis. She does this by creating a facilitating environment in which the patient feels secure and confident that his biological crisis will be resolved. She needs to motivate her patient by assessing those areas that hamper his mobility. Carnevali (1979) suggests that "the nurse who is knowledgeable about factors in the patient's situation which tend to foster immobilization will be alert to cues indicating that he is having difficulty in coping with problems in this area. She will also seek out and modify the potentially immobilizing factors within the patient and his environment which lend themselves to her control" (p. 1053).*

Environmental Factors

A critical care nurse can influence the patient's environment by minimizing unfamiliar noises, creating a familiar environment, explaining and removing supportive devices as soon as possible, and providing family contact. Unfamiliar noises and supportive devices are part of critical care units. Instead of keeping equipment around the patient's bed, the nurse can remove it. Volume respirators, for example, are usually kept near patient beds even when no longer needed. Removal of unused pieces of equipment makes the patient feel he is moving towards wellness and increases psychological mobility.

The nurse provides familiarity when possible. Familiarity with one's environment leads to behavioral stability and psychological mobility. Familiarity may be accomplished by placing some of the patient's personal possessions in the nightstand beside the bed. Cards, pictures of family members, and personal items can be placed within physical and visual contact.

It is even more important to provide greater family access to the critically ill patient. The family can provide tremendous input regarding the patient's previous coping patterns. The critical care nurse must keep in mind that, as Bellak (1956) notes, "the patient exists in the context of a family environment. . . . Even superficial . . . examination of family relationships frequently discloses clues to unsound familial attitudes toward the patient and his illness, which exacerbate the patient's own invalidizing attitudes" (pp. 488–489). In other words, the patient will not achieve psychological mobility if his family forces him into a cripple role.

The nurse must assess the reaction of family members to the individual's illness and their readiness for him to assume more than the cripple role. Through her assessment the nurse may discover that the family erroneously feels responsible for the patient's hospitalization. The critical care nurse can help the family look realistically at their feelings. Next she can help the family accept the patient's illness and its limitations. Together the nurse and family can motivate the patient, but motivation toward psychological mobility can only occur when he senses meaning in his own existence. People who are significant to the patient are the only ones able to provide this force.

Illness: Organ Image

The critical care nurse fosters psychological mobility by assessing the significance of the illness on the patient. There are times when some critically ill patients enjoy the sick role and the attention focused on the sick organ. The patient may find security in the dependency role wherein others attend to the patient's various needs. The notion of being placed in the center of the health care stage makes some patients feel significant. For some patients, illness coupled with the immediate need to be hospitalized implies the threat of death. Therefore these patients actively seek to achieve a level of biological and psychological stability so that they may return to the familiar territory called home. The critical care patient is motivated to avoid further disease or illness which can limit present and future activities. Bellak (1956) indicates how the patient's attitudes may change with time:

> Gradually the meaning to the patient of his illness undergoes certain changes. His initial diffuse anxiety is replaced by a more personalized concept. The nature of the pathology and how the illness looks and feels to him take on special meaning to the patient on conscious, preconscious, and unconscious levels. . . . He learns to live with his illness and achieve some degree of acceptance of it. (P. 488–489)

The critical care nurse must be open to the anxieties, frustrations, and threats of existence experienced by the critically ill patient. The burn patient is anxious when confronted with a whirlpool treatment including debridement and dressing change. The pulmonary patient is anxious when weaned from a volume respirator. Likewise, the hemodialysis patient may become fearful about dependency on a machine and its future financial cost. The nurse also attempts to make the patient feel less intimated by the illness.

A critically ill patient who continues to feel intimidated by illness cannot find meaning in it. Instead, the patient may retreat to invalidism or become a psychological cripple. To avoid immobility and to facilitate psychological mobility, the nurse actively helps the patient identify accomplishments and assets. Organ image may cause patients to focus their entire attention upon the sick organ to the exclusion of other variables. Furthermore, some patients are forced to expand in areas which they fear might place the sick organ in jeopardy. For example, the pulmonary patient may be afraid to increase his physical mobility and therefore his distance from the main support system, namely, the volume respirator. Furthermore, the patient fears transfer out of the respiratory care unit and into an intermediate or general care unit. Rather than viewing the transfer as a positive statement regarding the state of the sick organ, the patient looks upon it with a degree of fear. To patients, transfer implies learning what is expected of them in a different setting and meeting strangers who are unfamiliar with their personal care. The cardiac patient may be afraid to ambulate for fear of experiencing angina or extending the current infarction. The burn patient may experience psychological immobility if there are complications, if grafts are rejected, if overwhelming pain is experienced, if family or friends fail to be supportive, or if body image is so altered that people relate to the patient as if he or she were a different person. In each instance, critical care patients must sense their own biological and psychological readiness for mobility.

Nursing interventions need to take into account the fact that the psychological task is simultaneously simplified and complicated by the spontaneous healing mechanisms and potentials provided by nature. While the interactional nature of the treatment situation may be complex, its complexity is simplified by the fact that all participants are expected to be working in the same direction toward a common, mutually rewarding goal. That goal is the patient's maximum recovery (Mattsson 1975).

Role Disturbance

Crisis can strip away conventional roles. If the individual has not developed an internal sense of identity or self, any loss of conventional roles may contribute to a feeling of loss of self. Such a loss further contributes to the patient's feeling of nonexistence or nothingness. On the other hand, the biological crisis may facilitate the individual in developing a more enduring sense of identity. Role disturbance may be the most difficult area in which the critical care nurse works. Her role is mainly supportive and facilitative. She can attempt to move her patient out of the dependency role into a role in which he can be as self-sufficient as his condition permits. What happens at home between the patient and his family is out of her jurisdiction. The exception may be in hemodialysis, where the nurse sees her patient frequently on an outpatient basis and can assess home problems and discuss possible solutions. In the near future, critical care nurse specialists will make home visits and assess potential problems at first hand.

According to Mattsson (1975), the therapeutic intervention involves such fundamental questions as how the patient and others can best change their own behaviors, and how they can alter and influence each other's behavior in order to help the injured individual toward optimal psychological survival and mobility.

NURSING EVALUATION

Evaluation of the patient's problem and nursing care is an ongoing process. The nurse assesses various regulatory and cognitive behaviors supporting the diagnosis of psychological immobility. Interventions designed to minimize psychological immobility are evaluated for their effectiveness. The critical care nurse facilitates psychological mobility by minimizing unfamiliar noises, creating an environment that is familiar, explaining and removing supportive devices, providing family contact, assessing the significance of the illness to the patient, and fostering role acceptance.

SUMMARY

The critically ill patient draws upon the stabilizing force of his nurse to provide psychological mobility. The nurse attempts to draw upon her patient's ego strength, which, according to Bellak (1956), "is reflected in the nature of the self-image, the quality of reality testing and adaptation, the capacity to cope with life stresses, the patterns of control and frustration tolerance, and the nature of interpersonal relations" (p. 486). The critical care nurse seeks ways of eliminating or reducing the environmental factors, organ image, or role disturbance that lead to psychological immobility. Her goal is to facilitate the patient's attainment of psychological mobility.

REFERENCES

AUGER, JEANINE, *Behavioral Systems and Nursing*. Englewood Cliffs: Prentice-Hall, 1976.

BELLAK, LEOPOLD, *The Psychology of Physical Illness*. New York: Grune and Stratton, 1952.

BELLAK, LEOPOLD, and FLORENCE HASELKORN, "Psychological Aspects of Cardiac Illness and Rehabilitation," *Social Casework*, 37 (1956), 486.

BOWLBY, JOHN, "Separation Anxiety," *The International Journal of Psychoanalysis*, 61, (1960), 96.

CARNEVALI, DORIS, "Immobilization—Reassessment of a Concept," *American Journal of Nursing*, 70, no. 7 (July 1970), 1502.

CUMMINGS, JONATHAN, "Hemodialysis—Feelings, Facts and Fantasies," *American Journal of Nursing*, 70, no. 1 (January 1970), 72.

HELLMUTH, GEORGE, "Psychological Factors in Cardiac Patients," *Archives of Environmental Health*, 12 (June 1966), 772.

MATTSSON, EIRA, "Psychological Aspects of Severe Physical Injury and Its Treatment," *The Journal of Trauma*, 15, no. 3 (1975), 217-233.

OLSON, EDITH, "Immobility: Effects on Psychosocial Equilibrium," *American Journal of Nursing*, 67, no. 4, (April 1967), 794.

RAPAPORT, LYORA, "The State of Crisis: Some Theoretical Considerations," in *Crisis Intervention*, pp. 22-31. New York: Family Services Association of America, 1965.

ROBERTS, SHARON, "Psychological Equilibrium," in *AACN's Clinical Reference for Critical Care Nursing*, ed. M. Kinney, C. Dean, D. Packa, and D. Voorman, pp. 331–341. New York: McGraw-Hill, 1981.

SUTTERLEY, DORIS, *Perspectives in Human Development*. Philadelphia: Lippincott, 1973.

VERNON, M. D., *Human Motivation*. Cambridge: Cambridge University Press, 1969.

WU, RUTH, *Behavior and Illness*. Englewood Cliffs, N.J.: Prentice-Hall, 1973.

10

Depersonalization

BEHAVIORAL OBJECTIVES

1. Define the terms *dehumanization* and *depersonalization*.
2. Identify the origin of depersonalization and dehumanization.
3. State five regulatory behaviors associated with depersonalization.
4. State six cognitive behaviors associated with depersonalization.
5. Design a nursing care plan that fosters personalization.

Human beings live in a changing world that requires changes in the organization of the self if self is to be maintained. Depersonalization may be the most significant stress factor in critical care. Although the patient spends a great deal of time having physical needs treated, he may not be recognized as a person (Kleck 1984). The individual accepts the condition of his care sometimes without thought.

According to Levy and Wachtel (1978), we take action with relatively little thought about what we are doing. We live without observing ourselves. However there are times when we are aware of ourselves as actors and seem to be observing ourselves as we are acting. The degree and type of heightened self-observation varies within and between individuals. The experience can be mild or intense, pleasant or unpleasant, and transient or long lasting.

Human beings have the capacity to make choices and the desire to exercise this capacity. The human nervous system, including the brain, has the capacity to police its inputs, to determine what is and what is not significant for it, and to pay attention to and reinforce or otherwise modify its behavior in the process of living. In this sense, the human being is a participant in and producer of his or her own value-satisfaction. As Cantril (1964) points out, people perceive only what is relevant to their purposes and make their choices accordingly. He notes further that "Man wants security both in its physical and its psychological meaning to protect gains already made and to assure a beachhead from which further advances may be staged. Man wants some surety that one action can lead to another, some definite pretension which provides an orientation and integration through time" (p. 130).

The critically ill patient, however, often finds himself in a situation of shifting values and orientation. According to Spiegel (1964), "In our society . . . the person who is acutely injured tends to produce a shift from individual to collateral values, and from orientation of Doing to Being" (p. 296). This can hold true when the patient and nurse in a crisis situation become consciously aware of physical trauma due to disease or injury. If the nurse is aware only of her patient's illness or injury, she excludes him as a total being. The nurse can focus upon more than the critically ill patient's illness. She can assess her patient's behavior in an attempt to see how he transcends the immediate situation. His illness may have forced him to reach a steady state of permanent damage or limitation. Depersonalization may occur as a symptom in many psychiatric syndromes especially in patients with depression (Blue 1979). The critical care nurse can attempt to facilitate the patient's movement beyond his current crisis, because the nurse realizes that the patient is dynamic, always in the process of becoming. The nurse avoids viewing the patient only as an illness and thereby causing him to feel dehumanized or depersonalized.

DEFINITIONS OF TERMS

The two terms that need to be defined are *dehumanization* and *depersonalization.*

Dehumanization

Dehumanization, which is often coupled with depersonalization, can be defined as the result of divesting the person of human capacities and functions until he becomes less than a human being. It frequently occurs in a situation where one person or group is responsible for making the day-by-day decisions regarding the comfort and welfare of others. Anyone who is responsible for the care, maintenance, support, or supervision of dependent people should be alert to the possibility of dehumanization (Vail 1964). It is quite possible that the process of dehumanization begins subtly once a patient enters a critical care unit. According to Travelbee (1964), "it well may be that once the individual assumes the role of nurse or the role of patient a wall goes up between these two human beings until, unless this process is interfered with, both perceive the other as an abstraction or a set of abstractions" (p. 71).*

Depersonalization

Depersonalization is a complex syndrome found in emotional disorders. It is a trying and exceedingly difficult syndrome to bring into remission, much less cure. Patients may complain of a changed way of experiencing internal reality and the concreteness of the external world (Torch 1978).

One experience shared by critically ill patients is the impact phase, the initial encounter with the critical situation. This phase renders the patient in a state of shock. The initial emotional encounter may occur at the time of the physiological crisis or whenever the person becomes consciously aware of his illness. Lee (1970) describes the effects of this encounter as follows:

> In the wake of a strong stimulus there is a threat of impending disaster and the task is to regain homeostasis. Anxiety permeates the atmosphere and finds its outlet in automatic and poorly controlled behavior. Sensation and emotion are not distinguishable. Feelings tend to be relegated to another level of experience, peripheral or unconscious, and subjective experiences of all involved seem to evince a profound numbness, strangeness, unreality. The state is called depersonalization. (P. 578)

In depersonalization there is an absence of the self-image. The persistent need to apprehend a self results in ceaseless and useless self-scrutiny. There is a feeling of change throughout, of estrangement from the self, and usually, though not always, a feeling of total change in subjective perception of the external world (Torch 1978).

Even though depersonalization involves a disturbance of object relations, it is an experience pertaining to the way one sees the physical and mental self. In the first case, the person will complain that his body, or rather certain parts of the body, do not feel like his own. Whenever the depersonalization extends to the mental self, there is a feeling of unreality, of being "outside the self." The personalized patient will think, react, and act, but his experience is that of a detached spectator who is observing another person's performance (Jacobsen 1971).

Depersonalization is thought to be a defense against internal impulses and thoughts that emerge in the ego, while derealization is a defense against threats from the external world that resonate with the ego's store of repressed memories and painful experiences. Therefore in depersonalization and derealization there is a loss of the ability to imaginatively place or represent oneself in objects that are perceived, including one's own body as a percept (Levy and Wachtel 1978).

According to Torch (1978), depersonalization involves distinct feelings

*Copyright, American Journal of Nursing Company. Reprinted, with permission, from *American Journal of Nursing.*

of unreality which shade most of the patient's clinical picture. The feelings of unreality exist with the feeling being perceived in a nondelusional and ego-dystonic manner that have an "as if" quality to them. In addition there is a perplexing and curious subjective report of a change in affect. The patient will remain quite able to experience discomfort in his depersonalization.

Lastly, some believe that in depersonalization there is a blocking of sensory pathways due to the inhibition of the reticular activating system (RAS). In depersonalization, the RAS brings about changes or images by altering the rate of elaboration of fresh aspects of the images (Levy and Wachtel 1978).

THE CONCEPT OF DEPERSONALIZATION APPLIED TO THE CRITICALLY ILL PATIENT

According to Levy and Wachtel (1978) depersonalization has two main features. First, it involves a sense of unreality involving one's person or the external object world (derealization). Second, there is a feeling of being split off or detached from oneself or one's body, which is experienced as observing oneself behave. The split has been described as split between body self-representation and mental self-representation, or between the participating self and the observing self. Regardless of its specific features, depersonalization can be a frightening experience, and one to which the patient in critical care can suddenly become a victim. It often happens, for example, that during the patient's initial stay in critical care, the first priority is care of his physical problem. Then, as his condition stabilizes and the patient becomes more alert, he suddenly realizes that the staff does not know him as a person (Kleck 1984).

The Origin of Depersonalization and Dehumanization

Fleeting experiences of depersonalization may develop when persons suddenly find themselves in a strange and unfamiliar environment. The environment may be strange because of its sounds, unusual looking equipment, and unfamiliar faces. The patient may suddenly realize that he does not belong to this environment. Depersonalization is a subjective mental phenomenon having as its central feature an altered awareness of the self. It can occur in a variety of psychological states accompanied by extreme anxiety. Admission into critical care unit with all its stressors is such a psychological state. The illness, disease, or injury that leads to hospitalization in a critical care unit can be a life-threatening experience. Depersonalization is, like fear, an almost universal response to life-threatening danger. It develops instantly upon the recognition of danger and vanishes just as quickly when the threat to life is past (Noyes and Kletti 1977).

Shortly after the patient arrives in a critical care unit, people may perceive him as an exciting new disease or illness. Unintentionally, the nurse may, as Travelbee (1966) points out,

> . . . perceive an illness instead of the human being who is ill, or she may stereotype all patients and endow them with a cluster of characteristics they do not possess such as assuming that all patients are dependent and acting on this assumption without further reflection. The human being is not perceived, only his endowed characteristics. Such a process is termed the process of human reduction. (P. 36)

The process of human reduction, or dehumanization, takes place when persons see an individual as an illness instead of a human being with an illness. The patient may be referred to as "Dr. Jones's acute pulmonary edema," "the old fossil in bed 3," "the GI bleeder," or "the infected burn case."

Depersonalization appears to be an adaptive mechanism that combines opposing reaction tendencies, the one serving to intensify alertness and the other to dampen potentially disorganizing emotions. The use of defense mechanisms against the threat of extreme danger or anxiety is understandable. When confronted with life-threatening danger such as severe trauma, multisystem disease, or complications, the patient may soon become an observer of what is taking place and remove himself from danger. Detachment appears to be a major adaptive mechanism which, in the depersonalized state, is seen in bold relief (Noyes and Kletti 1977).

An individual patient does not equate himself with his illness. If this were so, then treating or caring for "the illness" would satisfy the human being. In fact, we generally perceive illness as something one *has*, not something one *is*. To perceive an individual as an illness is to ignore his humanity, and individuals so perceived are well aware that they have been dehumanized. Such individuals may be grateful of the attention given their illness, but they will also feel resentment toward those who have dehumanized them (Travelbee 1966).

As mentioned previously, dehumanization or depersonalization can begin when a critically ill patient arrives in the hospital. Usually the patient enters the hospital in a state of crisis. Nurses generally know the type of patient requiring their care. For example, the admitting care and treatment of the coronary patient entering CCU is clearly defined, as is that for the burn patient, who enters a Hubbard tank and then the burn unit, or the renal patient entering hemodialysis. The admitting care and treatment may be somewhat more diverse in ICU. Nevertheless, the nurse knows there are certain procedures she will perform for those patients arriving in units where the patient's problems are well defined. Because the patient is usually in a crisis situation, the nurse can direct her goal toward crisis intervention. She can assess her patient's physiological condition through observation and technological feedback. For example, the nurse may begin gathering her data by connecting her patient to a cardioscope, starting an IV, monitoring venous pressure, taking vital signs, inserting a Foley catheter, administering O_2 by mask, and requesting a chest X-ray, an EKG, or laboratory studies. As all this takes place, the environmentally shocked patient begins to feel like a task or an object. So much attention placed on equipment and techniques makes him wonder if he is the same person he was before the illness or crisis. He finds it difficult to believe that "these things" are happening to him, and soon he is in a depersonalized state. This is especially true if the patient becomes a chore or a task. Should the nurse withdraw and direct her energy toward her bureaucratic duties, she will fail to perceive the uniqueness of her patient. If the nurse treats her patient as an object or thing, according to Travelbee (1966), he may refuse her assistance, not because he regards the assistance as valueless, but because he feels that he is viewed as valueless, and he resents being dehumanized.

Attention to electronic equipment and continual surveillance of EKG patterns, blood gases, arterial pressure, or dialysis exchange are necessary for the care of these patients, and the ability to operate the machines, interpret laboratory values, and recognize life-threatening arrhythmias should be part of the critical care nurse's armamentarium. Even though these aspects of care may help reduce mortality, they do not necessarily ensure excellence of technique. Instead they may serve to depersonalize the patient. Dehumanization and depersonalization of the patient increase in relation to the number of people perceiving him as an illness rather than as a human being. Various people may enter his territory to listen to his transient friction rub or increasing rales, check his peripheral vascular circulation, examine his burns, or irrigate his A-V shunt. The patient, now an object, feels that he is a collection of disassociated parts rather than an integrated whole.

Some view depersonalization according to how an individual handles either external or psychic trauma. Depersonalization has been referred to as a defense in its own right and may be the result of a breakdown of defenses. If the patient feels that he is a collection of dissociated parts, he may use fantasy. The patient may say, "This is not real," or "This is not happening to me." The denial of the reality of the body and the self banishes dangerous needs and impulses. Likewise the denial of the reality of the outside world enables the individual to detach himself from its dangers (Levy and Wachtel 1978).

The critically ill patient who becomes depersonalized may create a substitute world in which he puts his faith. He may withdraw into sleep to avoid being looked upon as an object; this becomes his escape mechanism. The most common emotional response an individual feels when subjected to the frustration of dehumanization is anger. He may express anger openly and directly, to whoever provokes him, or subtly and indirectly, especially if he fears retaliation. The patient may also substitute anger objects; he might express hostility toward his wife, even if she is not the cause of his anger, or he may become angry at the cleaning lady instead of his nurse. Fear of becoming further depersonalized might keep him from demonstrating anger toward his nurse: he may fear total alienation from all nursing personnel, and he realizes that his nurse is one of the primary people in his critical care environment who can help him reach some level of stability and wellness.

The following case studies and situations illustrate depersonalization and dehumanization. In each example, one can see the patient's desire to be treated as a unique human being. Each, however, felt that he was treated as a unique specimen, or object. Although staff members may have thought they answered the patient's questions or met his needs, it appears that they may have met only their own needs.

Case 1. Mr. J. was a 44-year-old man who entered the hospital with severe substernal chest pain radiating down both arms, diaphoresis, shortness of breath, nausea, and color changes. This was Mr. J's first hospitalization. After he came to the emergency room, he was admitted to CCU. Because of the seriousness of his condition, the nurse immediately connected him to a cardioscope, inserted an IV, and administered O_2 by mask. Next, a doctor arrived to make his overall diagnostic evaluation. Subsequently, he ordered a chest X-ray, an EKG, and blood work. One by one, the various technicians arrived to carry out their assigned tasks. Meanwhile Mr. J. lay quietly in bed with his eyes closed. He had received 10 mg of morphine sulfate for his chest pain and had been instructed not to talk; he was told to try to sleep. This proved difficult, however, while so many people did things to him. Each person had failed to tell him what they were looking for or what they expected to find.

After two hours, Mr. J.'s pain continued. His cardioscope pattern showed marked S-T elevation and frequent multifocal ectopic beats. The nurse called this to the attention of Mr. J.'s doctor, who immediately ordered a xylocaine drip. When Mr. J. noted an additional bottle threaded through an IVAC machine, he asked his nurse, "What's that one for?" The nurse responded, "Oh, it's just some medication for your heart. You have occasional ectopic beats." The patient responded with a quiet "oh." He then closed his eyes and turned his head away.

Later a team of cardiologists entered CCU to see Mr. J. After discovering that he was asleep, they stood at the foot of his bed and discussed his case. The doctor told his interns, "This man has had a massive anterior infarction. It is one of the worst MIs that I have seen. If he sat up, he would probably lose part of his heart." The doctors all laughed. "We might anticipate that he could go into congestive heart failure. Anyway his condition is extremely critical," continued the doctor. They then left the patient. Moments later Mr. J.'s nurse approached his bed to check his xylocaine drip and vital signs. Mr. J. opened his tear-filled eyes and said, "I guess they thought I was asleep. I didn't want to disturb them. What's a massive anterior infarction and congestive heart failure? Is it true a part of my heart will be lost or fail if I sit up? It sounds terrible. I had better have you call my wife."

Case 2. Mrs. E. was a 55-year-old woman in acute respiratory distress. She was admitted to ICU for observation and possible tracheostomy. Mrs. E. was extremely fatigued, and the slightest exertion caused severe shortness of breath. She was extremely anxious. After Mrs. E. was partially settled in her new home, her doctors entered the room and mumbled a quick hello. Next, without even a brief introduction, they let down the side rail and pulled up her patient gown in order to listen to her unique lung sounds. After listening to her characteristic emphysemic wheezing, they left her alone, failing to raise her side rail and to return her gown to its previous place. She lay there exposed and without the energy to pull down her own gown.

Later Mrs. E.'s nurse and doctor approached her bed carrying a piece of paper that they showed to Mrs. E., saying that it was a consent to perform a tracheostomy.

MRS. E.: A consent for what?

DOCTOR: A tracheostomy

MRS. E.: What is that?

DOCTOR: It is a little hole the doctor puts in your throat to help you breathe. Just sign here next to the "X."

MRS. E.: I can't see without my glasses.

DOCTOR: Here is the "X."

MRS. E.: Where?

DOCTOR: Really! Here, I'll just put your hand over the spot. Then you sign your name.

MRS. E.: (*Following her nurse's orders, the patient quickly signs her name.*) Is that all?

DOCTOR: Yes. (*Together the doctor and nurse leave.*)

Mrs. E. was left alone to contemplate the idea of a hole in her throat. She had many questions, but everyone seemed too busy to answer them. She told herself that after the procedure she could ask all her many questions. Unfortunately, Mrs. E. did not know that unless her trach cuff is deflated, she would still be unable to ask questions.

Situation 1. Two nurses in ICU are sitting outside a patient's room, where he can hear them. They are in the process of giving and taking report. The two nurses think the patient is asleep.

NURSE 1: I'll give you the report on bed 3.

NURSE 2: Okay. He is that old guy with renal failure.

NURSE 1: Yes. He drove me up the wall today.

NURSE 2: I know what you mean. The old fossil did the same thing to me last night. Why are they keeping him here anyway?

NURSE 1: I don't know. Anyway, his care is essentially the same. You know those renal patients are all alike.

NURSE 2: Okay. How is Mrs. Lovely? I really like her.

The report continues on with Mrs. Lovely. Note that "bed 3" was not even accorded the dignity of a name. Instead he became "that old guy with renal failure," and "the old fossil."

Situation 2. The setting is CCU, and the nurse is sitting in front of the master EKG machine. She hears an alarm and goes to check the patient.

NURSE: (*Enters the patient's room. Says nothing to the patient, who is awake.*)
PATIENT: (*Looking at the nurse*) Did I do something wrong?
NURSE: (*Continuing to look at the cardioscope and not at the patient*) No, it's the crazy machine.
PATIENT: Can I help in any way?
NURSE: (*Continuing to look at the machine*) No, just lie still and don't move. (*She then leaves the patient alone.*)

If the nurse were to return to her patient's bedside, she would probably find him lying in the same rigid immobilized position. He is afraid to move for fear the box in the corner will buzz, causing his nurse to enter his room unnecessarily. He does not want to take any more of her valuable time than absolutely necessary.

In each case study and situation, the critical care patient experienced some element of depersonalization and dehumanization. Mr. J. and Mrs. E. were treated as specimens under a microscope. Neither patient felt included in his or her own care. The doctors talked about them as if they were a heart and a set of chronic lungs. Mrs. E. was stripped of her personal and private dignity when she was left alone with her chest exposed. The patient in ICU with renal failure relinquished his dignity when the nurses failed to refer to him by name. According to Travelbee (1966), "Sterotyping all patients and endowing them with a cluster of characteristics they do not possess is another way of dehumanizing individuals. All of these perceptions have one common characteristic—they all ignore truth" (p. 36). The truth may be that the renal patient in bed 3 acts like an "old fossil" because his BUN is 180 and his creatinine is 6.3. "An understanding of the likeness and differences amongst all human beings can guide one's perception of human beings and their behavior. Another determinant of perception of others is the value of worth accorded each human being" (Travelbee 1966, p. 31).

The fact that the patient is in a critical care unit means that he is forced to make an adjustment. In a time of physiological crisis, this process becomes an intensely personal one fraught with threats of abandonment, of a loss of goodness, and of his ability to accomplish it. The renal failure and the pulmonary or cardiac problem may be "old hat" to the critical care nurse, but to the critically ill patient they represent a new experience. Because he has not had these problems before, and he has no frame of reference from which to judge his physiological state, he therefore depends upon his nurse's judgment. If she perceives him an object, however, then he cannot find in her the human quality he desperately needs. Instead he perceives depersonalization and finds little comfort or satisfaction from her care.

The patient experiencing depersonalization detaches himself from a threatening internal or external reality by living out an unconscious fantasy of being dead, asleep, or an inanimate object. Some have suggested that depersonalization occurs when higher-level defenses such as repression fail. Depersonalization seems to reduce the individual's anxiety level. The possible reason why anxiety is experienced with depersonalization is that depersonalization may be an inherently inadequate defense mechanism. This implies that the defense fails and the precipitating anxiety is consciously experienced (Levy and Wachtel 1978).

Depersonalization can occur subtly and unintentionally. It is easy, for example, to forget a patient's name and inadvertently substitute his room number or diagnosis for it. This is a simple error, but an unintentional slip can become a set pattern of behavior. More obvious depersonalization and dehumanization techniques are to refer deliberately to a patient as "an old fossil," "an old grump," or "the fat lady in room 4." Regardless of whether the depersonalization technique is conscious or intentional, the consequence is the same: the patient is demoted to the level of object or thing. It is worth repeating that people in the health profession may not realize that depersonalization is taking place. The staff becomes concerned with carrying out the necessary and often life-saving technical procedures. Their concern may become so intense that they ignore the behavioral "me" aspect of the individual. Critical care nurses must be sensitive to the human element of their patient.

The Human Design: Humanization

The relationship between nurse, patient, and family is more beneficial and satisfying when it is based upon personalization and humanization of caring. Before discussing how personalization can occur in a highly technical environment, we need first to discuss humanization and how it takes place. As Travelbee (1966) points out, "it requires little thought, effort, or emotional involvement on the part of the nurse to view human beings as "patients." The "patient" is an abstraction, a set of expectations personified by tasks to be performed, treatments to carry out, an illness, or a room number. People relate to other human beings, not to abstractions" (p. 35). Cantril (1964) notes that "Human beings want to experience their own identity and integrity, more popularly referred to as the need for personal dignity. Every human being craves a sense of his own self-constancy, an assurance of the repeatability of experience in which he is a determining participant. He obtains this from the transaction he has with other individuals" (p. 1). It is the nurse who can provide positive transactions for the critically ill patient.

It must be pointed out that the nurse herself is human and often needs protection. Like the patient, she is capable of making mistakes. She may not always say the correct words or express her feelings. Nevertheless, the critical care nurse can look beyond her immediate technical interventions to nurse the "me" quality of her patient. The "me" refers to those unique attributes the critically ill patient brings with him when he enters the hospital. In realizing that her patient strives to transcend the self, the nurse can attempt to help him rise above the limitations of his immediate illness. To do this, the nurse has to focus on the patient as person rather than the patient as illness, avoiding the tendency to examine the disease or illness as the central focal point.

The concept of humanization can help the nurse to understand how her patient copes with his illness or diagnosis. It is such knowledge and its application in her care that humanizes her approach to a particular patient. From the patient's point of view, his problems are unique. For example, the patient who has chronic glomerulonephritis resulting in renal failure and ultimate bilateral nephrectomy has never experienced being dependent upon a hemodialysis machine. He has no previous experience from which he can draw strength or hope for the future. His nurse and her human caring can provide strength and encouragement to transcend the crisis. He may temporarily choose to transcend the crisis by escaping the situation through denial, anger, or rejection, and the nurse must realize that this is a human quality.

Touch can be a humanizing experience. In a sample of 225 coronary care patients conducted by Lynch et al. (1977), it was observed that a significant reduction in ventricular arrhythmias occurred following pulse palpation. The data suggest that significant changes in ventricular arrhythmias can occur as a result of even minimally arousing psychosocial interactions.

According to Travelbee (1966), "The commonalities of human experiences are based on the assumption that every human being undergoes certain experiences during the process of living and reacts to these experiences in a way that can be comprehended or understood by another" (p. 30). A nurse aware of this assumption realizes that her humane guidance can help her patient move beyond any form of negative behavior. She knows that he is always in the process of becoming, evolving, or changing. In addition, he has a distinguishing characteristic of being able to remember the past and to anticipate the future while living in the present. The nurse may attempt to draw upon her patient's positive past experiences, which could be incorporated into her patient's future. A patient with an acute myocardial infarction, for example, may be an avid fisherman and golf enthusiast. The nurse can help him understand that he can still participate in these activities in the future. She can describe these activities as an asset, for they may facilitate the patient's physical and psychological well-being.

The more immediate and important goal is to help the patient transcend the present crisis situation. He must feel secure enough to accept that he still has a future. This type of security comes through a trusting relationship with his critical care nurse, one that she can encourage through her ability to humanize the patient. Humanization makes the patient feel significant. The nurse can make him feel as if he is the most important patient in the critical care unit. Even though she may spend only 10 minutes with him, if she gives him her undivided attention it may seem to the patient like 30 minutes. According to Gotshalk (1966), the human being is a high-grade psychological system that interacts with other beings in psychological terms. A person is a biophysical system exhibiting in his open relations with others a pattern of stimulus response. He is a responding agent or a reagent. The human design signifies that the critical care patient, besides being a high-grade physiological-psychological system, is also a social being.

NURSING ASSESSMENT OF DEPERSONALIZATION

The critical care nurse assesses depersonalization through the patient's behavioral response. The responses can be categorized into regulatory and cognitive behaviors.

Regulatory Behaviors

The regulatory system involves inputs, processes, effectors, and feedback loops. It involves stimuli from the external environment and from alteration in the internal state of dynamic equilibrium. The regulatory behaviors are physiological responses. In assessing depersonalization, the regulatory behaviors are difficult to determine. Possible regulatory behaviors consist of the following:

Regulatory Behaviors
Numbness of body part
Inability to move (catatonic state)
Increased heart rate
Increased respiratory rate
Fatigue
Loss of appetite
Dizziness
Flatness of visual and auditory stimuli

Cognitive Behaviors

The cognator system involves inputs from internal and external stimuli, which include psychological and social factors. The specific aspects of the cognator mechanism consists of perceptual/information processing, learning, judgment, and emotion. The cognitive behaviors are psychosocial responses.

The depersonalized patient scans his nearly blank internal environment. It is at this stage, however, that the depersonalization syndrome separates into two distinct entities with most patients remaining immobilized by the feelings of unreality (Torch 1978). The cognitive behaviors associated with depersonalization consist of the following (Levy and Wachtel 1978; Torch 1978):

Cognitive Behaviors
Obsessional thinking
Low self-esteem
Doubt
Insecurity
Depression
Anxiety
Giddiness
Uselessness
Loss of affective responsiveness
Remoteness
Feeling of being dead

According to Torch (1978), the veil that separates the depersonalized patient from his world contains so many components that it becomes nearly impossible to repair damage that could cause depersonalization, because of the strewn wreckage of various metaphysical remnants that the patient has in his repertoire. Refocusing of the insecurity on the self and the self in the world may be a secondary response to trauma and anxiety.

NURSING DIAGNOSIS OF DEPERSONALIZATION

The nursing diagnosis is a statement of a particular problem. In this instance the specific problem is depersonalization. The diagnosis is made by assessing various regulatory and cognitive behaviors. The behaviors originate from internal or external stressors. When the patient feels extremely threatened by his illness, injury, or disease, he may discover that previously used defense mechanisms are now ineffective. The anxiety or stress this produces causes the patient to detach or dissociate from the situation. The result is a feeling of being depersonalized.

NURSING INTERVENTIONS TO FOSTER PERSONALIZATION

Coupled with humanization is the tremendous need to help personalize the critically ill patient. It is difficult to help another human being help himself, because all of us live in two worlds, "the" world and "my" world. According to Zderad (1969), "the world is the outer common world of everyday experience, the shared world where men live and work and play together, where nurses nurse patients. My world is an inner private world, my own unique view of the world" (p. 655). The critical care nurse cannot be concerned with the outer objective world; she must treat her patient as a unique individual. To accomplish her goal she can attempt to see the world as he does. In order to provide personalization, she can reach out to her patient and be sensitive to his inner world, putting herself into her patient's place without losing her sense of objectivity. The nurse who can provide personalization is able to sense her patient's confusion, his anger, his fear, or his feeling of isolation.

Furthermore, the critical care nurse must realize that the patient wants to experience a sense of his worth and to protect his personal identity and integrity. The patient wants to know he is valued by others, and that others will somehow communicate that his own behavior and its consequences make some sort of difference to them. This transaction confirms a patient's sense of identity and provides him with a sense of personal worth and self-respect (Cantril 1964).

The abundance of technical equipment in critical care units can give the appearance of depersonalization. Sometimes the nurse must give a significant portion of her time to the respirator, chest tube, pacemaker, and other devices and tests. She may finish making her hourly assessments only to discover that they are due again. The time spent in these assessments is vitally necessary for the recovery of the patient, but it is also vitally necessary that the nurse maintain a balanced stance vis-à-vis her patient. She must temper the aggressiveness required by her technical assessments with awareness of her patient's personal integrity. Even though the nurse is hourly collecting her data, she can and should provide personalized care.

Patient dependency, a constant factor in care of the critically ill, further accentuates the need for personalization. In critical care units, where time is of utmost significance, the nurse must move quickly to establish a therapeutic relationship with her patient. She can realize that the first criteria for a successful relationship is trust, and if her initial approach fosters personalization, the patient may allow her to move from his "the" world into his "my" world.

This is what the French philosopher Gabriel Marcel calls the I-thou quality of a relationship. Patients in this type of relationship feel that critical care nurses do not see them as objects in a highly technical environment. Instead they sense a commitment for their entire well-being. The "my" world of the patient represents his inner feelings and thoughts, including fears, frustrations, or anxieties. Because of their I-thou relationships, both nurses and patient are placed in a unique position. They form a close and intense association during the crisis period that is founded not only on trust but also on openness.

According to Sobel (1969), a nurse with an open attitude regards the patient as another human being, not as an object of psychological treatment. Openness addresses itself to the highest level of maturity that exists potentially in each human being. It acknowledges that the patient himself must resolve the many aspects of the human struggle involved in going through a life-threatening event. When the nurse makes this acknowledgment, she may finally be able to be herself with the patient.

The following case study and situation illustrate how nurses personalize their approach by being open to the critically ill patient. Each nurse focuses her attention directly on the patient, explaining what she will be doing to him and including him in his own care.

Case 3. Mr. B. was a 50-year-old man admitted to ICU with acute GI bleeding. Mr. B. had had bloody emesis and tarry stools for the previous two days. He had no previous history of GI bleeding or ulcers, and he was not taking any medication that could induce bleeding. After Mr. B.'s arrival by stretcher, he was lifted into his bed. As soon as he was comfortably situated in bed, his nurse approached him.

NURSE: Hello, Mr. B. My name is Sally, and I will be your nurse this evening. (*She places her hand in his and gently squeezes it. With her hand in his, she subtly checks the color of his nail beds and the palm of his hand.*)

MR. B.: Sally! Okay! You can call me George. (*He squeezes Sally's hand in return.*)

NURSE: Are you fairly comfortable now, George?

MR. B.: Well, not exactly. I have some pain here. (*Points to his stomach.*)

NURSE: How long have you had the pain there? (*Points to the same spot.*)

MR. B.: It just started a couple of days ago.

NURSE: Did you notice whether the pain occurred at any particular time during the day?

MR. B.: No. It just came on suddenly. Then I started throwing up blood, and my bowel movements were black and had a terrible odor.

NURSE: All right, George, Dr. J. will be in to see you shortly. He will probably ask you similar questions. Do you feel nauseated now?

MR. B.: No.

NURSE: All right. Just in case, I'll place an emesis basin by your head and attach the call light on your side rail. I am going to leave you to get a few things that we'll need after the doctor sees you. All of these things are routine. I'll explain what they are when we are ready. Is there anything I can get you before I leave, George?

MR. B.: No, but thanks.

NURSE: You're welcome.

The nurse leaves the room and discusses Mr. B.'s symptoms with Dr. J. Dr. J. then orders a nasal gastric tube, IV, a cardioscope, and O_2 by mask. The doctor leaves the nurse to obtain a history and physical from Mr. B. Fifteen minutes later, Dr. J. completes his interview and instructs the nurse to carry out the above orders. The nurse reapproaches Mr. B.'s bed, organizes the equipment, and explains the order of each procedure, from simple to complex. She instructs Mr. B. regarding the routine purpose of the cardioscope, O_2 by mask, and IV therapy. She realizes that insertion of the nasal-gastric tube can be a traumatic and complex procedure to some patients. Therefore, she has chosen to save this procedure for last. She further realizes that Mr. B., who already is fatigued, may need to rest after its insertion. She takes time to explain the purpose of the nasal-gastric tube, its location, and care of the tube. In addition, she has prepared Mr. B. for what he is expected to do during insertion of the tube. He is told to sit in a high Fowler position and swallow water as the tube is advanced.

NURSE: George, sometimes when the dentist is working in your mouth, do you feel like gagging?

MR. B.: Yes.

NURSE: You may feel the same way when I begin passing the NG tube. This is why you may want to swallow water.

MR. B.: Okay, I'll try.

NURSE: All right, George. You relax now, and when you are ready to begin, we'll start. The main thing, George, is to try to relax.

MR. B.: I think I am ready. I just keep drinking the water.

NURSE: Yes, I'll tell you when to swallow as I advance the tube.

MR. B.: Okay. Let's do it.

NURSE: All right. (*She inserts the NG tube and begins to advance it.*) Now, George, begin swallowing. Swallow. Good, George. Keep swallowing. Swallow. We are just about finished. Swallow. There—it's in, George.

MR. B.: Wow, I never swallowed so fast or hard in my life.

NURSE: You did a beautiful job. You can try to relax now. I'll be irrigating your tube with iced saline. This will decrease the bleeding by causing vasoconstriction. Do you understand what this means?

MR. B.: Yes.

NURSE: It may make you feel cold. Just let me know, and I'll get some extra blankets.

MR. B.: Thanks. I'll try to rest. Thanks for taking your time with me.

The nurse immediately established a personal relationship with Mr. B. by introducing herself as Sally, identifying herself as his nurse, and explaining that she would be with him the rest of the evening. The two started on a personal level by using first names, and the nurse made him feel secure, because he knew someone would be watching out for him. Sally included Mr. B.

into his care, explained the procedure to him, related it to something from his past (the dentist), and paced herself according to his readiness for the tube. In this way, she took a technical procedure and personalized it to his individual need. She involved him in his own care and made him feel significantly by "taking her time." Through proper pacing of her interventions, she carried out the least threatening procedure first, and saved the most difficult one for last. As a result, she demonstrated her ability to be sensitive to his needs rather than her own.

Situation 3. The nurses in ICU are making their morning rounds for report. The routine of the unit is to take and give report at the patient's bedside. It is 7:00 A.M., and the night shift is reporting off. They are standing beside Mrs. H., a 24-year-old woman who delivered a baby girl three days ago. Since that time, Mrs. H. has developed a pulmonary embolism. She has been having considerable pain breathing. She is also quite anxious about her other two children, her husband, and her new baby.

NIGHT NURSE: Good morning, Mrs. H.
MRS. H.: Good morning.
NIGHT NURSE: Did the medication I gave you help the pain?
MRS. H.: Yes, but after a couple of hours the pain returned.
DAY NURSE: I'll check with Dr. X. today about your medication and pain. Maybe he can give you something else.
NIGHT NURSE: You are scheduled for a lung scan today. Do you know what that is?
MRS. H.: Yes. I had one after I was transferred here.
DAY NURSE: Do you have any questions about the test?
MRS. H.: No, other than the time I'll be going.
DAY NURSE: I'll call and check. It depends on how many such tests have been scheduled today. In the meantime, would you like your morning care before or after the lung scan?
MRS. H.: I think before; then I can rest when I return.
DAY NURSE: Okay. That's fine. How has your diet been working out?
MRS. H.: It's okay. The pain is what bothers me.
DAY NURSE: Some of the pain is normal. I'll check with the doctors as soon as they make rounds.
NIGHT NURSE: I called the nursery and your baby is doing fine. The nurses say she is a doll.
MRS. H.: Thank you for calling. That relieves my mind.

The nurses then continue to make their morning rounds and maintain the same personal interaction with each patient. In this situation the nurses demonstrated personalization by including Mrs. H. in their morning report. They treated her with personal warmth and dignity. By planning her own care with her, they made her feel significant. Both nurses focused their attention on the areas that seemed to be concerning Mrs. H., her pain and her baby. The night nurse independently called the nursery to see how Mrs. H.'s baby was doing. She anticipated that her patient would want this information early in the morning, and the information seemed to relax Mrs. H. The nurses listened to what Mrs. H. said and supported her with feedback that her messages regarding pain were received and would be looked into sometime during the morning. The day nurse offered information regarding Mrs. H.'s daily activities. She gave Mrs. H. a choice in making decisions regarding sequential order of her care and then accepted her decision.

As Mrs. H.'s condition improves, she may be allowed to make other decisions. With the doctor's approval. Mrs. H. may be taken by wheelchair to see her baby, in coordination with her husband's visit. This is another way of personalizing the patient's care. The openness between both the nurses and Mrs. H. showed respect on the part of the nurses for Mrs. H.'s individualness. Mrs. H. and the nurses are open systems exchanging energy with each other. As Gotshalk (1966) has described it, this sort of energy exchange, "a kind of give and take on the physical level, is the elementary framework of all the concrete interaction of the human being with her surroundings" (p. 36). Through openness the nurses focused directly upon the patient, her problems, and her needs. They could provide personalized care, because they had information that was specific to her. They had entered her "my" world.

It is safe to state that nurses are the individuals most responsible for the critically ill patient's emotional well-being. The nurse acts as stabilizer in an ever-changing and uncertain environment. Because she remains continuously with the patient, she sees the many dimensions of her patient's personality as well as changes in his physiological status. She is the one who works with the patient's negative and positive behavioral manifestations. One dimension of a personalized nurse-patient relationship involves human compassion for the critical care patient. Human compassion does not imply a loss of the nurse's identity but rather a deeper understanding of her patient's identity.

The most important role a nurse can play in fostering personalization is to be open. According to Sobel (1969), openness means that the nurse will talk to the patient while she takes care of his medical needs. It means that the nurse will meet and respond to the patient's face and eyes. It means the nurse will feel free to exchange thoughts, ideas, and feelings on a human level with her patient. It means that she will think about and feel what the patient is going through without turning away from it and/or without rushing in to do something about painful circumstances that she may not be able to alter.

Efforts toward personalization should begin the moment the critically ill patient arrives in a critical care unit. The attitude with which he is received can determine how he will respond toward those in his new world. The staff's attitude can point the patient toward a feeling of personal uniqueness or toward a feeling of anonymity. The patient's illness is unique to him. Therefore, it is quite easy for him to magnify his anxiety out of proportion to the reality of the situation, and the nurse's attitude can create either a facilitating or disabling environment. At the time of admission, the nurse's first intervention can be to introduce herself. Nurses often forget such a simple thing in the busy minutes that follow a patient's arrival. The exchange of names becomes one way in which the nurse may initiate personalization. In meeting people on a social level, we normally introduce ourselves as Sally Jones, or Ms. Jones. The informal or formal approach depends on the comfort of the individual. The patient may then respond by saying, "I am Geoge Smith," or "Mr. Smith." In most critical care units, nurses use first names because the intense nature of the environment quickly brings people into a close relationship. In the process of being introduced socially, we usually extend our hand as a gesture of wanting to affirm the introduction. The critically ill patient can expect no less than the same social-personal respect. The entire introductory process may take a matter of seconds, but the effects can be long-lasting. The admitting critical care nurse is usually the nurse longest remembered. In many respects, she is the individual who initiates most of the patient's care, and she is the person in whom the patient invests his trust.

Besides the initial exchange of names, the nurse can further acknowledge her patient's individuality by explaining the various procedures and diagnostic tests he will experience within the next few hours. She can attempt to personalize the sometimes impersonal tests to her particular patient, keeping in mind that the procedures might be totally unique to him. For example, the nurse in Case 3 explained each procedure to her patient, Mr. B. She personalized the explanation by correlating the information with something meaningful from his past.

After she has completed the initial diagnostic work and assessed the seriousness of the critically ill patient's condition, the nurse can begin to learn the personal indiosyncrasies of her patient by listening to him, observing his actions, and talking with him about his work, leisure, hopes, and dreams. These approaches become a vehicle for getting to know his "my" world. A structured means of obtaining information about the patient's "my" world is through a nursing history form, which asks for specific information and provides a useful goal-directed tool for gaining pertinent personal data. There are times, however, when the patient does not reveal his views of the "my" world, even in a nursing history. For example, pain may separate him from others or absorb his full attention; worries and fears may immobilize him. When his defenses do not permit him to share concerns with others, or when he is simply withdrawn, the critical care nurse must seek alternative ways of knowing her patient. From these other ways she can learn his view of reality.

One thing that the nurse can do to know her patient is to incorporate empathy into her care. The nurse's ability to empathize becomes a human movement toward oneness with the other and helps her to achieve personalization in her care. As Zderad (1969) notes, "both the patient and she will become more whole in their humanness by increasing their understanding; by developing their capacities to imagine, to perceive, to feel, to respond; and by making real their individuality and their interrelatedness" (p. 662). The nurse can further achieve openness by allowing the patient to participate in the decision-making process of his care. For example, in Situation 3 where the ICU nurses were making their morning rounds, the nurses included Mrs. H. in the planning of her own care. The nurses asked Mrs. H. whether she wanted her morning care before or after her lung scan. The decision was a simple one, but to the patient it was a significant one. During the initial crisis, of course, the nurse makes all pertinent decisions, but as the patient stabilizes, he can be included in decision making on a simple level. The decisions or choices to be made by the patient have already been screened by the patient's nurses; a nurse would not allow her patient to make a choice or decision that cannot be accommodated because it is inappropriate or unrealistic. This would only serve to make the patient lose faith in the honesty and integrity of his nurse. Once the patient makes a choice or decision, it must be carried out. This will cause the patient to feel that his opinion is wanted, respected, and—most important of all—accepted.

In most critical care units, the area around the patient's bed is usually very small. In an open unit, the only object in the critically ill patient's territory besides his bed may be a nightstand, which normally serves to hold gloves, suction catheters, irrigation solutions, or other impersonal objects. The nurse can utilize some of the nightstand for her patient's personal belongings: pictures, clocks, toilet articles, books, or cards. Pictures are most important for patients who have young families or grandchildren. The nurse can get into her patient's "my" world by talking about his pictures. The patient may enjoy discussing peripheral topics such as his family or grandchildren rather than himself, because he may feel threatened by his illness. Asking about a patient's picture makes the patient feel that the nurse is interested in him. Furthermore, pictures add a personal, imaginative touch to the patient's "the" world. Patients, especially the critically ill aged, also enjoy having a clock by their bed. In some critical care units there are no windows, and if the lights remain on 24 hours a day, the patient may never know when it is day or night. A clock, or even a calendar, can help the patient maintain a sense of time.

Another means of fostering the personalization of the critically ill patient is by involving his family. Acute crisis often serves to bring together family members. Their reactions may range from quiet dread to generalized excitement. In the confusion of the crisis, they are probably unable to evaluate the situation reasonably. The patient usually appreciates personal interest shown by his family members. He likes to know that his family is near. An acutely ill patient may need a family member simply to sit by his side and hold his hand, and a perceptive nurse can assess this need and act accordingly. Critical care nurses often have to spend what seems to be hours with a patient's family answering the same or similar questions. By simply taking the family to the patient's bedside and explaining what is happening they can save much time. Once the foundation has been established between the nurse and family, the nurse can keep the family informed of changes in care or status. Sometimes a particular aspect of the patient's care changes, and uninformed family members might perceive that the patient is worse. If the family members communicate their anxiety to the patient, he will believe himself to be worse. This situation can usually be avoided if the nurse personalizes her relations with the family as well as her care of the patient.

NURSING EVALUATION

Evaluation of the patient's problem and nursing care is an ongoing process. The critical care nurse assesses regulatory and cognitive behaviors supporting the diagnosis of depersonalization. Interventions are designed to foster personalization and prevent depersonalization or dehumanization. Depending upon the severity and duration of the biological threat, the cognitive behaviors may not totally disappear until the patient is transferred out of critical care.

SUMMARY

Nurses can and should personalize their care of critically ill patient. Personalization should begin the moment a patient arrives in a critical care unit and continue until he is transferred out of the unit. The first step is a simple name introduction. Personalization continues as the nurse becomes aware of her patient's "my" world. The key to a personalized approach lies in the nurse's evaluation of her attitudes and beliefs toward her patient. She must see him as a unified and orderly whole, a social unit, trying to master his internal biological crisis and to cope with his unfamiliar environment. Once the nurse has achieved this perspective, she can deal with her patient as a person, not as an illness.

REFERENCES

BLUE, RICHARD, "Use of Directive Therapy in the Treatment of Depersonalization Neurosis," *Psychological Reports*, 45 (1979), 904-906.

CANTRIL, HADLEY, "The Human Design," *Journal of Individual Psychology*, 20, no. 2 (November 1964), 133.

CLEMENCE, SISTER MADELEINE, "Existentialism: A Philosophy of Commitment," *American Journal of Nursing*, 66, no. 3 (March 1966), 500-505.

COMBS, ARTHUR W., and DONALD SNYGG, *Individual Behavior*, rev. ed. New York: Harper & Row, 1959.

DAVIS, MARCELLA, "Socioemotional Component of Coronary Care," *American Journal of Nursing*, 72, no. 4 (April 1972), 705-709.

GOTSHALK, DILMAN W., *Human Aims in Modern Perspective*. Antioch Press, 1966.

HASPEDIS, BETTY, "The Nursing Service Administration Creates and Activates a Caring Climate," *Nursing Clinics of North America*, 4, no. 4 (December 1969), 690.

JACOBSEN, EDITH, "Depersonalization," in *Depression*, ed. Edith Jacobsen, pp. 137-38. New York: International Universities Press, 1971.

KLECK, HENRY, "ICU Syndrome: Onset, Manifestations, Treatment, Stressors, and Prevention," *Critical Care Quarterly*, 6, no. 4 (March 1984), 21-28.

LEE, JANE M., "Emotional Reaction to Trauma," *Nursing Clinics of North America*, 5 no. 4 (December 1970), 578.

LEVY, JUDITH, and PAUL WACHTEL, "Depersonalization: An Effort at Clarification," *The American Journal of Psychoanalysis*, 38 (1978), 291-300.

LOEN, MARILYN, and MARIAH SYNDER, "Psycho-Social Aspects of Care of the Long-Term Comatose Patient," *The American Association of Neurological Nurses*, 2, no. 4 (December 1979), 235-237.

LYNCH, JAMES, SUE THOMAS, DAVID PASKEWITZ, AARON KATCHEN, and LOUNDES WEIR, "Human Contact and Cardiac Arrhythmia in a Coronary Care Unit," *Psychosomatic Medicine*, 39, no 3 (May-June 1977), 188-192.

NOYES, RUSSELL, and RAY KLETTI, "Depersonalization in Response to Life-Threatening Danger," *Comprehensive Psychiatry*, 18, no. 4 (July-August 1977), 375-384.

SOBEL, DAVID, "Personalization in the Coronary Care Unit," *American Journal of Nursing*, 69, no. 7 (July 1969), 1442.

SPIEGEL, J. P., "Attitudes Toward Death and Disease," in *The Threat of Impending Disaster*, eds. Grosser, Wechsler, and Greenblatt, p. 296. Cambridge, Mass.: M.I.T. Press, 1964.

TILLICH, PAUL, "What is Basic in Human Nature," *American Journal of Psychoanalysis*, 21-23 (1962), pp. 115-121.

TORCH, E. M., "Review of the Relationship between Obsession and Depersonalization," *Acta Psychiatric Scand*, 58, (1978), 191-198.

TRAVELBEE, JOYCE, "What's Wrong with Sympathy," *American Journal of Nursing*, 64, no. 1 (January 1964), 71.

——, *Interpersonal Aspects of Nursing*. Philadelphia: F. A. Davis, 1966.

VAIL, DAVIS, "The Danger of Dehumanization," *Mental Hospitals*, 15 (November 1964), 599.

ZDERAD, LORETTA T., "Empathetic Nursing: Realization of a Human Capacity," *Nursing Clinics of North America*, 4, no. 4 (December 1969), 655.

11

Transfer Anxiety

BEHAVIORAL OBJECTIVES

1. Define the terms *anxiety* and *transfer anxiety*.
2. Discuss how transfer within critical care units affects the critically ill patient.
3. Identify the three components associated with transfer within critical care units.
4. Discuss how transfer out of critical care units affects the critically ill patient.
5. Identify the three components associated with transfer out of critical care units.
6. State six regulatory behaviors associated with transfer anxiety.
7. State five cognitive behaviors associated with transfer anxiety.
8. Design a nursing care plan that will reduce transfer anxiety.

Anxiety is a part of our daily lives. It is usually experienced when we are confronted with stressful situations. New situations or encounters can arouse fears of the unknown whereas familiar situations can cause feelings of avoidance. In such instances, people frequently describe their anxieties as "butterflies in my stomach," "a case of the jitters," or "nervousness." Such normal feelings are usually transitory. Once the stress situation has passed, the individual expresses feelings of relief or elation. It has been said that our culture creates a pressure cooker environment. Portnoy (1959) points out that as society progresses, so do our pressures:

> Anxiety-producing factors in our culture grow progressively more numerous and intense, while anxiety-relieving agencies have become sharply and increasingly less

effective. Perhaps more fundamental are the increasing strains and pressures experienced by individuals living in a period characterized by great complexity, cultural disunity, and instability, rapid change and the mingling of varied and differing cultures (p. 307).

Much has been written about the concepts of anxiety. According to psychoanalysts, anxiety begins at the time of birth and continues until death. Because it is an internal feeling, anxiety may be difficult to identify and pinpoint. It is diffuse and may know no boundaries. Sometimes anxiety may serve to protect us—alarming us about a situation yet unexperienced. People sometimes refer to this type of situation as a feeling of "impending doom." A nurse often feels this way about her critically ill patient. Her feelings may be labeled *intuitive anxiety*, and it makes her alert to the situation and the possible dangers therein. On the other hand, there are some situations in which a person feels anxiety but is unable to identify what it is about the situation that makes him anxious. Moreover, he may be unable to function within the situation.

Not only do individuals differ in their reaction to anxiety, but psychoanalysts themselves differ in their approach to anxiety. Many mental health professionals regard anxiety as a painful, debilitating, even catastrophic condition that cries for alleviation. Anxiety as a malignancy, however, is a limited concept. It considers the emotion only in the extreme intensity in which it disrupts behavior. Moderate anxiety may in fact energize the organism and improve performance (Levitt 1980).

Anxiety can be caused by external environmental threats, particularly when, as noted by Schwarzer, van der Ploeg, and Spielberger (1982), the individual may have no control over the outcome:

> Anxiety refers to an unpleasant emotional reaction that results from the perception or appraisal of a particular situation as threatening. If an individual in any given situation perceives environmental demands as potentially dangerous, or as exceeding his competence and resources, the person-environment transaction will be judged stressful. Environmental demands are more likely to be perceived as threatening by an individual if future damage or loss is anticipated and no adequate coping strategy is available. (P. 3)

Let us consider a nurse who has worked in obstetrics for the past ten years and is asked one evening to rotate or float temporarily to intensive care. She may be comfortable, confident, and independent in her old role as obstetrical nurse and scared to death in her new role as intensive care nurse. The larger environment remains a constant; it is only the smaller, immediate environment of intensive care that has changed. The nurse's internal security or integrity may be threatened, and she will feel uncomfortable, insecure, and dependent.

The critically ill patient faces continual anxiety, which begins the minute he enters a critical care unit. The individual's anxiety focuses on fear of the unknown environment and the threat to his physical integrity. Once the threat to his physical integrity subsides, the individual becomes less anxious and more comfortable within his own familiar surroundings. In addition to familiarity within his surroundings, he also becomes more familiar with the staff providing his care. His increasing comfort, like that of the obstetric nurse, becomes threatened again if he is forced into another anxiety state, transfer anxiety. Although critical care personnel usually give much attention to alleviating the patient's internal anxiety and fear, they tend to give little attention to anxiety aroused when the patient leaves hs increasingly familiar and secure surroundings. This is transfer anxiety, a very special form of separation anxiety.

It must be remembered that both the nurse and patient become intensely involved with one another. Critical care units offer patients continuous exposure to health personnel. A goal in such units, as Adreoli et al. (1971) note, is consistency of patient care and staff involvement: "Consistent patient assignments minimize and provide the reassurance fostered by seeing familiar faces. Not only does this facilitate orientation, but it also augments the development of effective therapeutic relationships" (p. 147). Normally the critical care nurse spends her time in the here and now. This means that she focuses her attention on recognition of complications associated with the patient' illness. Furthermore, she attempts to recognize and understand the patient's behavior and its psychological meaning as it effects how he copes with illness. Little is done in preparing the patient for his eventual graduation from the critical care environment. However, the nurse can focus her attention beyond the here and now into the future of prepared transfer.

The critical care nurse often believes that once the patient is ready for transfer her responsibility towards him diminishes. While the patient is in critical care, the nurse's goal is to protect him from threats to his physical integrity and to facilitate his biological movement out of the critical phase of illness. Once this goal is accomplished, the nurse turns her attention toward the more acute illness of other patients. She tends to see preparation for eventual transfer out of a critical care unit as an acute situation. Just as entrance into a critical care unit can be traumatic for the individual, his exit can also be a traumatic experience—traumatic in the sense that his psychological integrity can become threatened. He has placed tremendous confidence in the critical care nurse and fears that other nurses will not meet his needs or expectations. Transfer anxiety, whether conscious or unconscious, has the potential of becoming a problem in critical care units. We will first discuss its definition and meanings, and then we will apply the concept to critical care patients.

DEFINITION OF TERMS

Levitt (1980) notes that anxiety is timeless and has an enormous impact on human life. Almost every corner of human endeavor is thought to be affected somehow by anxiety. Anxiety is not only our official emotion; it is the primary focus of a concerted effort aimed at the improvement of human life. A definition of *transfer anxiety* and its components cannot be made without first examining general meanings attributed to the larger concept *anxiety*.

Anxiety

Anxiety as an emotional state is often referred to as *A-state*. Transitory or state anxiety (A-state) may be conceived of as a complex, relatively unique emotional condition or reaction that may vary in intensity and fluctuate over time. A-state may be conceptualized as consisting of unpleasant, consciously perceived feelings of tension and apprehension, with associated arousal of the autonomic nervous system. Therefore the term *anxiety* or *state anxiety* is used to refer to the emotional reactions evoked in individuals who interpret specific situations as personally threatening (Spielberger 1972; Solomon-Hast, 1981).

Anxiety is a conceptualized as a reaction to a perceived threat. The threat results from an anticipation of a personally important loss or failure. Among other factors, the strength of the anxiety reaction should be determined by the perceived degree of threat which itself depends on particular personality characteristics and environmental conditions. (Becker 1982).

Threats to the critically ill patient's biological integrity occur the moment he experiences illness. The threat and anxiety aroused continue until he learns that his biological system has reached stability. Even after that time, he has fleeting moments of anxiety. The patient who experiences his first myocardial infarction becomes anxious when he thinks about the possibility of another insult to his heart. The patient who is admitted for his second coronary artery bypass in three years becomes anxious when he reflects on the surgery, the postoperative pain, and future needs of additional surgery. The alcoholic patient admitted for bleeding esophageal varicosities realizes that without adequate rehabilitation he will return to a critical care unit in an even greater state of crisis and debilitation.

The anxiety phenomenon is viewed as apprehension initiated by a threat to some value which the individual holds essential to existence. It has been noted that the capacity to experience anxiety is innate, while reactions to particular events or stimulus conditions evoking it are largely learned. Anxiety becomes abnormal if reactions are disproportionate to the objective danger, but not the subjective danger, and repression is involved. Anxiety at a low level is useful and is associated with mastery over oneself with the environment. Anxiety serves the purpose of making an individual aware of an existing or potential threat (Johnson 1979).

Threat to the individual's self-system occurs as he views himself in relationship to past, present, and future changes. Such threats focus upon his psychological integrity. For example, the burn patient becomes anxious when he realizes the possibility of physical disfigurement. The diabetic patient who loses a leg due to infection experiences anxiety when, like the burn patient, he views his altered body image. Anxiety becomes an energy, one that hopefully serves to motivate the individual. Anxiety that the patient experiences when his biological integrity or self-system integrity is threatened can be perceived indirectly, by its effect.

We expect individuals who experience threats to their biological integrity and self-system to be anxious. As Portnoy (1959) points out, this is normal anxiety: "It is man's nature to have anxiety in the face of certain kinds and degrees of threat. In brief, it is the ultimate expression of our being human. We experience normal anxiety in the face of death, old age, and illness as we recognize our factual helplessness" (p. 310). Because anxiety is multi-dimensional, it takes many forms. One such form is transfer anxiety.

Transfer Anxiety

Transfer anxiety is very similar to separation anxiety. It is anxiety experienced by the individual when he moves from a familiar, somewhat secure environment to an environment that is unfamiliar. For patients moving out of critical care units, it involves separation from the close surveillance of monitors and machines. It also involves interpersonal separation from those nurses and doctors who maintained personal surveillance.

Bowlby (1960) discusses three conditions of anxiety that are components of transfer anxiety: primary anxiety, fright, and expectant anxiety. Primary anxiety "is thought of as an elemental experience and one which, if it reaches a certain degree of intensity, is linked directly with the onset of defense mechanisms" (p. 92). In discussing primary anxiety, Bowlby refers to the instinctual system, composed itself both of behavior and of the hypothetical internal structure that, when activated, causes the behavior. The behavioral response includes both the motor behavioral pattern and its physiological and psychological concomitants. Wherever an instinctual system activates and is unable for any reason to reach termination, a form of anxiety results. In some cases the environment may fail to provide the terminating condition. A critical care patient may not be adequately prepared for transfer from a familiar into a unfamiliar environment. He does not have the opportunity to begin the normal termination process. For healthy individuals, termination is a relatively simple and nonthreatening experience. Most persons can independently choose the time when they wish to initiate the termination process. Because of their independence, they have more control over the situation; their termination experience is not blocked, and anxiety need not exist. In illness, however, the individual moves into a dependency relationship with his environment and nurses. He has minimal control over events within his environment, including commencement of the termination process. If not properly prepared, the termination process can become blocked, and transfer anxiety develops.

Primary anxiety may be built-in or inherited. It can be detected on the basis of hospital interpersonal experiences in which termination was a part of the eventual outcome. The particular responses to primary anxiety, however, are learnable and vary from individual to individual. According to Levitt

(1980), these reactions may be task-irrelevant—that is, having a tendency to disrupt performance, such as feelings of inadequacy, fear of failure, or desire to quit the situation—or task-relevant—that is, facilitative of performance, since they move the individual to reduce anxiety by completing the task successfully.

The critically ill patient may unconsciously block the termination process. He feels relatively secure in his current environment. Without realizing it, he may be bound to his nurse by a number of instinctual response systems, each of which is primary, that together have high survival value. The patient depends on his nurse's knowledge and skill in providing his care. He hopes that she will prevent further threats or loss to his biological integrity. Besides intervening as protector, the nurse represents the human element in her patient's technical environment. It is her human quality of caring that emotionally attaches the patient to her. Just at a time when the individual's emotional dependence reaches a high, he may suddenly be forced to terminate the relationship by leaving the unit. The abrupt termination causes rupture of the attachment he holds for the unit and his nurse, and this rupture leads to transfer anxiety.

The second condition of anxiety identified by Bowlby (1960) is fright, the subjective experience accompanying at least two related instinctual response systems—one leading to escape behavior, and the other to immobility or freezing. Like all instinctual response systems, those governing escape and freezing are built into the organism and perpetuated by heredity because of their survival value. The patient admitted to a critical care unit may experience fright. He enters a strange and foreign world filled with strange pieces of equipment that make unique sounds. Instead of feeling secure in such a protective environment, he may instinctively be motivated to escape.

The individual may escape by withdrawing, but more often he escapes by initiating his own transfer process on a verbal and/or nonverbal level. The patient may verbally express his readiness or desire to be moved. It is not unusual to hear a patient say, shortly after his arrival into a critical care unit, "When do I get out of here?" or "Well I guess this will be my home for a couple of days." Still other patients may tell their nurse how good they feel, how much they feel they have improved, or how ready they are to leave the hospital. The patient may be seeking reassurance that he is in fact improving and will be leaving the unit shortly. But whether he realizes it or not, the critical care patient is verbally initiating his own transfer process.

The patient may also initiate transfer on an action level. He may feel he has improved to the point that he no longer needs to remain in bed, to use his oxygen mask, or to use his cardioscope. Consequently, he removes the EKG leads or climbs out of bed. These clues are move obvious than the verbal kind and can be handled directly. It is quite possible that the patient no longer needs his cardioscope and bedrest restriction. Therefore, the nurse may intervene to have them discontinued as soon as biologically possible.

Nurses usually react in disbelief to verbal or nonverbal clues. A nurse may be surprised by her patient's behavior until she realizes that in all probability he is frightened, and his fright feeds upon the coming and going into his personal environment of numerous people and machines. Such activities serve as a constant reminder of how sick or critical he is. Therefore, he escapes by initiating his own transfer from the critical care environment, because a real transfer would mean his condition was improving.

Fright can also cause the critically ill patient to freeze emotionally. Feeling secure in his highly technical and protective environment, he may regard the critical care unit as a haven of safety that terminates escape responses and brings a sense of security.

Bowlby (1960) also discusses what he terms *expectant anxiety.* As soon as the individual, whether infant or adult, has reached a stage of development in which some degree of foresight is possible, he is able to predict situations as dangerous and to take measures to avoid them. The individual facing an inadequately planned transfer experiences expectant anxiety. He fears that he is likely to lose his haven of security. To transfer means leaving a familiar and somewhat predictable environment. In return he moves into a new environment where the expectations are not clearly defined in his mind, and where fear of the unknown creates internal anxiety. Let us now apply these concepts of transfer anxiety to care of the critically ill patient.

THE CONCEPT OF TRANSFER ANXIETY
APPLIED TO THE CRITICALLY ILL PATIENT

According to Kristie (1979), hospitalization is often an anxiety-provoking experience. Because illness is an unknown entity and interferes with the individual's normal life pattern, it is a threat. The hospital itself is a threat because it produces a feeling of helplessness and isolation from the patient's usual method of meeting needs.

As Klein (1968) points out, critical care units are

> notable for the continuous EKG monitoring, the frequent treatment procedures, and the immediate application of life-saving techniques when catastrophies threaten. Another characteristic of these units is the intensive care nurse and physician interaction with the patient. Nurse's observations are regarded as important. An overall result is that the patient is being looked after to an extraordinary degree. (P. 104)

Such looking after by both equipment and health personnel leads to dependency. The individual may feel anxious about his illness but secure in a closely monitored and protected environment. As the transfer potentially threatens his security, the individual experiences additional anxiety.

Hospitalization in critical care places the patient in an unknown or unfamiliar setting. It is an event which increases anxiety in nearly all individuals. Increased anxiety is often precipitated by stresses such as separation from family and familiar surroundings, fear of the unknown, and inability to completely comprehend the complex nature and consequences of illness (Johnson 1979).

The critical care patient moves away from his familiar territory into an unknown and unfamiliar setting. The patient who is prepared for transfer is able to respond with courage and can call upon his internal strengths to meet or endure the threat of change. All too often, the critical care nursing places emphasis upon the acute phase of illness. We focus on the shock of diagnosis, anxiety over illness and survival, total dependency, fear of equipment failure, and fear of rejection by significant others. We place little if any attention upon helping the individual to transfer successfully out of a critical care unit. Transfer anxiety is generated by two different types of transfer: it occurs when the individual is transferred from one critical care unit to another, and when the patient is moved from a critical care unit to an intermediate or general floor.

Transfer within Critical Care Units

Normally we think of transfer anxiety as occurring when a patient moves out of a critical care unit. However transfer anxiety can occur within the units themselves. For example, a patient experiences anxiety when he is moved from one bed to another within the same unit, or when he is moved from one critical care unit to another. Transfer within the unit can lead to primary anxiety, fright, or expectant anxiety.

Mr. J. is an example of a patient who experienced all three conditions of transfer anxiety. He was admitted to an eight-bed intensive care unit in severe pulmonary distress. The schematic drawing in Figure 11.1 shows Mr. J.'s relationship to the nurses' station before and after transfer. At the time of Mr. J.'s arrival, the only available bed was in position 3. Because of Mr. J.'s hypoxic condition, he was extremely disoriented, agitated, and

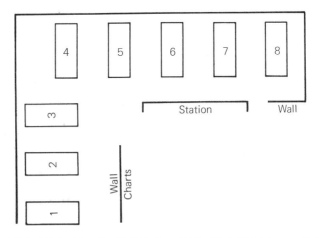

Figure 11.1 Schematic drawing of Mr. J.'s critical care unit.

combative. Hand restraints only served to enhance his agitation and his desire to remove all the wires and tubes. The nurses decided his bed position was excellent because it could be seen from the nurses' station. Furthermore, there was enough room around the bed to absorb various pieces of equipment without infringing upon the territorial rights of Mr. J.'s neighbors. Mr. J. was the epitome of a well-monitored patient. Wires led to cardioscope, a Foley catheter connected to a urometer, intravenous tubing led to an IVAC machine, lines monitoring arteries and veins connected to a manifold, a nasal-gastric tube connected to an intermittent suction apparatus, and a volume respirator connected to an endotracheal tube.

At the end of 72 hours, the health team decided a tracheostomy would be necessary. Mr. J.'s blood gases were still unstable, and tenacious secretions made a tracheostomy necessary. Mr. J. remained under close surveillance for several days. During this time his behavioral picture changed, and he became less agitated, confused, and combative. He had become accustomed to the various pieces of equipment and their unique noises. More important, he had become familiar with the faces of his nurses. His biological and psychological needs were being fulfilled, and he no longer felt a threat to his integrity. As Mr. J.'s biological picture improved, the staff disconnected and removed some of his equipment. The nurses made him feel he was in a people-oriented environment. They spent time weaning him off the volume respirator and comforted him when he became fearful about not being able to breathe. Because the nurses were in close proximity to his bed, he rarely used his call light. Mr. J. knew his condition was improving because various procedures and treatments were occurring less frequently. As his blood gases and clinical picture stabilized, he noticed the nurses spending less time at his bedside.

Early one morning, without warning or preparation Mr. J. and his bed were moved to position 8 (see Figure 11.1). To the left of Mr. J. was a green wall; at his feet, another green wall; and to his right was another patient's bed. Mr. J. was not sure why he was moved so abruptly and without an explanation. The patient to Mr. J.'s right had had a coronary artery bypass on the previous day. Mr. J. heard the nurses discussing his new neighbor's critical condition. The environment around the neighbor was full of equipment. Because the nurses did not want Mr. J. watching or worrying about his neighbor, they pulled the curtain along side his bed. Although the object of this intervention was to protect him, it only served to make Mr. J. feel isolated and rejected. He no longer felt the close observational proximity with his nurse. He could no longer call his nurse with a wave of his hand, nor could he raise his voice above a whisper. His tracheostomy was still in place, and he simply did not have the energy to place his finger over its opening and speak in an inaudible whisper. The only recourse was to use his call light. Within a four-hour period, the nurses noted that Mr. J. had used his light ten times. This was most unusual for Mr. J. Furthermore, they noted that he was becoming more agitated and irritable. For the eleventh time, Mr. J. put on his call light. The critical care nurse decided to go to his bed.

NURSE: Mr. J., What can I do for you?

MR. J.:   (*With his finger placed over the tracheostomy*) What can you do for me? That's a laugh.

NURSE: What do you mean, Mr. J.?

MR. J.:   No one seems to care about what they can do for me.

NURSE: Yes, we care about you.

MR. J: No, you don't, otherwise you wouldn't have moved me to this hole. (*Points to his surroundings.*)

NURSE: What do you mean, hole?

MR. J.:   This place! I feel isolated like you are trying to hide me.

NURSE: No one is trying to hide you.

MR. J.:   What if I need to be suctioned? Who will see me when the curtains are pulled? I am still a sick man.

NURSE: Mr. J., you are doing much better. We needed your bed for a more critically ill patient.

MR. J.:   Aren't I critically ill when I still have a tube in my throat?

NURSE: You are improving to the point where the tracheostomy tube will be removed.

MR. J.:   When will that be?

NURSE: Soon, but I can't tell you when. In the meantime would you feel better if I pulled back the curtains?

MR. J.:   Yes. I would feel better if I had my original bed.

NURSE: We will try to make you comfortable here.

Mr. J. experienced all three components of transfer anxiety: primary anxiety, fright, and expectant anxiety.

Primary Anxiety.   The primary focus of critical care is to provide a high level of technical surveillance and immediate treatment for clinical problems. When admitted to critical care, the patient is given a special place. Even though he may be bombarded by stimuli from monitoring alarms, continuous lighting and constant flow of staff, he becomes accustomed to the sight and sounds revolving around him. If the patient is separated from his original space where he has gained knowledge about the unit and security, he can experience primary anxiety. Mr. J. was prematurely separated from his haven of safety and security and moved to a place in the corner. In bed 3 he had the security of close surveillance by his nurse. He knew that when a need such as suctioning presented itself, his nurse would be in a state of readiness to intervene. The patient still thought of himself as critically ill. This feeling was reinforced by his equating illness with a "tube in my throat." The transfer came earlier than the patient anticipated and created a blockage. Bowlby (1960) explains how such a blockage can lead to anxiety:

No matter what the nature of the blockage, it is postulated, if an instinctual response system is activated and unable to reach termination, changes occur both in behavior (namely in psychological and physiological functioning) and also in the subjective experience of the individual himself. When it rises above a moderate level it gives rise to the subjective experience of anxiety. (P. 96)

Mr. J., like other patients transferred to a less-strategic area in a critical care unit, may not be able to adjust to termination of certain aspects of his care. In other words, Mr. J. considered himself still critically ill. The nurse, on the other hand, felt his condition had improved to the point of allowing transfer to an area where continuous surveillance might not be possible. The nurses were functioning on one level and the patient on another.

When the patient first arrives in a critical care unit, he relinquishes control over his body. According to Davis (1972), "The very nature of the illness requires that all, or nearly all, bodily functions and care be assigned to others. It requires little imagination to appreciate that when a patient is suddenly and completely divested of control of his body, he may experience this as a fundamental threat to his ego, even when he knows that it is being done to help him" (p. 707).* Mr. J. had relinquished control over his biological system to machines and nurses. For several days, they had given him close attention; suddenly he was moved, without an explanation, to a corner bed surrounded with walls and curtains. Not only was he relocated, but the number of personal nurse-patient contacts was greatly reduced. No explanation was given for the reduction in nursing and technical surveillance. He could only fantasize that the nurses were "trying to hide" him. He did not interpret the move as a graduation or recognition of improvement in his biological adaptation to the respiratory problem that led to his hospitalization. The experience, instead of being a positive, supportive one, became clouded with negativism. Mr. J. became agitated and restless. His nurse intervened when she feared that his behavior might precipitate another pulmonary crisis.

Fright. According to Solomon-Hast (1981), the patient may be preoccupied with the multitude of external and internal stimuli confronting him to the point that he fails to see his own progress. External stimuli can originate from supportive devices, other critically ill patients, and critical care staff. Internal stimuli can evolve from internal concerns or fears such as fear of dying, fear of helplessness, or fear of a damaged self-concept. Consequently the multitude of external and internal stimuli cause the patient to perceive the environment as threatening.

As Spielberger points out, when the individual perceives a situation as threatening, irrespective of the presence of real danger, it is assumed that he will respond to it with an elevation of A-state. In other words, the individual will experience an immediate increase in the intensity of an emotional state characterized by feelings of tension and apprehension and by increased autonomic nervous system activity.

During an acute illness, the patient cannot fight because of severe debilitating episode and cannot flee because of being confined to the critical care unit. The result is that expected coping mechanisms become ineffective in handling the current illness. Initially the patient is unable to cope with the critical care environment. He becomes anxious until he feels secure with the nursing staff. Once a beginning level of security is established in critical care, the patient experiences fright when he is moved to another bed within the unit.

Mr. J. also demonstrated fright behavior. He wanted to escape the primary anxiety of premature separation by returning to his original bed. He also wanted to escape the fright of not being suctioned as needed. He labeled his new location within the unit as a "hole." He showed his fright by increasing the frequency of using his call light. The nurses were comfortable with his stable biological status; consequently, they spent less time in his care. The patient, on the other hand, did not understand or interpret their actions as positive. Instead, he thought they were avoiding him.

The nurses should have established a time structure with the patient: for example, a nurse could have returned to his bedside every half-hour to assess his respiratory status, comfort, or needs. Gradually, the nurse could extend the time structure. With each assessment made, the nurse can verbally assure the patient that his condition is stable, reassuring the patient that the nurse is still assessing him and that her assessment finds him stable.

Expectant Anxiety. Mr. J. also experienced expectant anxiety regarding his new role. At the time of his transfer, he considered himself critically ill. He expected the nurse's surveillance to be the same or at least similar to that received in bed 3. He depended upon the nurses. Within a matter of seconds, the patient was thrust into the role of independence. Everyone but the patient thought he had improved to the point of providing a controlled amount of his own care. The nurses had the advantage of knowing the expectations of his transfer and new role. The patient did not know the expectations; therefore, the transfer only created anxiety.

Mr. J.'s anxiety is not unlike that of other patients who are transferred to another area within the same unit. These patients are forced to adapt psychologically to a new territory and a new level of wellness. The adaptation may not be a prepared one. In adapting to his new territory, the individual must learn the meaning of strange noises emanating from his new neighbors as well as those coming from his own immediate environment. The patient must also adapt biologically to a higher level of wellness. This new level involves less dependency on others and more on himself. As Shannon (1973) points out, adaptation is an ongoing process:

> Adaptation to disease does not end when the acute phase of the illness is over, but rather this adaptation process is continuous and complicated. In the convalescent phase, the individual is mentally and physically more free to carry the burden of making a change by himself, but in the acute phase of his illness he must rely on the nurse to help him make the necessary adjustment. (P. 364)

The patient may not be ready to terminate his secure territory or his dependency relationship with the staff. Rather than experience the primary anxiety of separation from his haven of security, he may refuse to be transferred. In this instance, according to Shannon, the critical care nurse "should not push, force, or try to change the patient, but she should develop a relationship in which he can use her as a guide as he makes the necessary changes within himself through the normal process of adaptation" (p. 365).

Patients may vary in their response to transfer. One patient, like Mr. J., may interpret transfer as avoidance behavior. Another patient may interpret the change as a sign of deterioration in his progress. As an example, consider the patient whose wound, drain, or tracheostomy cultures are positive for staphylococcus. At one moment, he is lying by other critical care patients, and then he is whisked into a separate room. Biologically his condition is improving, but his new infection makes isolation necessary. The isolation experience may only serve to make him feel more alone or even frightened; he loses the open space, where he can maintain visual contact with the nursing staff. The transfer, as with Mr. J., leads to primary anxiety, fright, and/or expectant anxiety. Transfer into isolation may come at a time when the individual is just getting comfortable in a critical care unit. Suddenly, without warning, he is moved to a private room. Nurses who previously approached his bed with smiles now either talk to him from the doorway or enter his room in gowns and masks. He does not feel the same degree of interpersonal ties that he felt before. His contact with significant others, including his family, is reduced. Like Mr. J., such an individual may become frightened that a need or aspect of care will not be fulfilled. He may see the environment as threatening. Such a relationship between the individual and his immediate environment can cause anxiety, since the two are closely interrelated.

Like critical care patients who experience transfer anxiety when they are moved to a new location within the same unit, a patient may experience the same anxiety when he is moved from one critical care unit to another. Mrs. P. experienced transfer anxiety when she moved from intensive care to coronary care. She was a 45-year-old mother of two admitted into the hospital with a history of coronary artery disease. Her angina attacks had increased in intensity, frequency, and duration. It was virtually impossible for her to do housework without experiencing some degree of pain. She had been told by her doctor that diagnostic studies such as cardiac catheterization would be necessary to determine whether she needed a coronary artery bypass. Mrs. P. avoided the diagnostic studies because she feared that she might require surgery. An independent and active person, she did not want to leave her family or work. The thought of surgery and of postoperative convalescence made her postpone hospitalization all the more.

As her angina attacks increased, the need for hospitalization became more apparent. After coaxing from her family and physician, she entered the hospital for cardiac catheterization. The test confirmed her physician's suspicions and Mrs. P.'s fantasies that open heart surgery would be necessary to relieve the stenosed coronary arteries. The doctors explained to both

Mrs. P. and her husband that surgery should be performed immediately. They were reassured that the possibility of complications had greatly been reduced, and they were further reassured by the information that the team of cardiac surgeons who would be operating on Mrs. P. performed several successful coronary artery bypasses a week. Mrs. P. finally agreed to have the surgery. Doctors told her that the usual postoperative stay in the intensive surgical care unit was two to four days, and that she would be expected to become independent and self-sufficient as soon as possible.

On the following morning, Mrs. P. successfully endured open heart surgery. She entered intensive care after four hours of surgery. Her postoperative biological status was stable, and she grew in her ability to be independent. The nurses encouraged her to do as much of her care as possible. Everyone commented on how well she was progressing and noted that in all probability, she would be transferred to a general floor within three days. She no longer needed an arterial line, Foley catheter, or central venous pressure measurements. These signs alone encouraged her that transfer from the noisy busy environment of intensive care would soon be a reality. Everything progressed normally until the third day, when she developed an arrhythmia. Her cardioscope showed multifocal PVCs. A lidocaine drip was ordered to control the ectopic beats. The lidocaine seemed to control her ectopic beats, but she developed atrial fibrillation.

It was decided that transfer to coronary care would be necessary. Here the coronary care nurses could better monitor her arrhythmias. Mrs. P. could not understand why she was moved to coronary care nor why there was a sudden change in what she was permitted to do. No longer was she encouraged to be independent and self-sufficient. Instead, she was encouraged to depend on the nurses for everything. This signified to Mrs. P. a regression in her biological status. Furthermore, the nurses were all new to her. When she questioned her nurse about the change in location and activity, she was told not to worry, that her heart had an irregularity that could best be treated in coronary care. Later that same day, nurses noticed that Mrs. P. was watching her monitor. After watching for several minutes, she began to cry. It was at this point the nurse decided to talk with Mrs. P.

NURSE: What's wrong, Mrs. P.

MRS. P.:   Oh, nothing.

NURSE: Something must be bothering you to make you cry.

MRS. P.:   (*Wiping her tears*) Does being in here mean that my surgery was a failure?

NURSE: No, Mrs. P., not at all. Quite the contrary: your surgery was a success.

MRS. P.:   Then why is everyone suddenly so concerned with my heart? Isn't that why people are put in coronary care, because of their hearts?

NURSE: Yes. You were transferred here because your heart was beating irregularly.

MRS. P.: So what does that mean?

NURSE: It involves observation and treatment with medication. The arrhythmia sometimes occurs after coronary artery bypass surgery.

MRS. P.: How long will I be here, and how long will I be in bed?

NURSE: Until the medication converts the arrhythmia into a normal rhythm.

MRS. P.: What happens if it never does?

NURSE: Let's wait and give the medication a chance.

MRS. P.: Okay. Do the nurses in ICU ever work in CCU?

NURSE: Yes. Would you like some of them to visit you?

MRS. P.: That would be nice if they have time.

Mrs. P. experienced primary anxiety of separation from one critical care environment and movement into another. The patient had expected to transfer to a general floor, not to another unit, and transfer to coronary care served to frighten her. Instead of feeling fortunate to be in another haven of security, she wanted to know how long her stay would be. The transfer seemed to signify a surgical failure and also the end of a newly gained control over her environment and care. After moving toward independence, she was suddenly forced into a dependency role. Furthermore, she knew what was expected of her in intensive care but she did not know what to expect in coronary care. Her level of independence was determined by the arrhythmias. Once this stabilized, the patient could leave coronary care.

Patients like Mrs. P. often cannot see beyond their immediate crisis. Mrs. P. was frightened about what would happen if the arrhythmias never convert. Her transfer led to premature separation from interpersonal relationships with the nurses. She and her ICU nurse had established a rapport; each knew what to expect from the other. The interpersonal closeness was indicated by her comment, "Do the nurses in ICU ever work in CCU?" The transfer also created fright because it brought a perceived threat to her newly revascularized heart. Like so many other critical care patients, Mrs. P.'s heart became the essence of her being. Any danger to it was a threat to her life. In this respect, coronary care has always been perceived as a threatening environment. Mrs. P. knew what to expect postoperatively, but she had no knowledge of what to expect from the complication. Although she discussed this possibility with her health team, she believed that its occurrence was not very likely. Everyone around her seemed confident that the arrhythmia would disappear as suddenly as it appeared, but such reassurances did not necessarily remove her sense of anxiety regarding the transfer.

Another patient for example is Mr. A., a 57-year-old man who was helping his wife move the furniture when he suddenly developed severe substernal chest pain, shortness of breath, and diaphoresis. His wife quickly called an ambulance, and he was rushed to the emergency room of a nearby hospital. In the emergency room, he developed several episodes of ventricular fibrillation necessitating repeated defibrillation. Finally the ventricular fibrillation converted to sinus tachycardia with frequent ectopic beats. Doctors felt that immediate transfer to coronary care could be achieved without a crisis, and they moved Mr. A. there rapidly. It was in coronary care that an EKG revealed a severe anterior myocardial infarction with frequent ectopic beats.

Mr. A. was kept under strict observation. The emergency cart remained out of sight but near his bed. The nurses monitored him frequently in an attempt to anticipate any potential problems. During the next several days, Mr. A. experienced cardiogenic shock. His blood pressure never rose above 70–80/50. Because of his lowered arterial pressure, the nurse and doctors became concerned about his deteriorating renal status. Since his original arrival in the unit, his urine output had been minimal. The staff hoped that as his cardiac output improved, so would his renal perfusion and status. The environment around Mr. A. was extremely controlled. The staff limited his activity and visits by his immediate family. His wife was able to visit her husband only for brief moments.

Mr. A. remained in coronary care for two weeks. During this time, he totally depended upon the nurses to maintain his physical and psychological integrity. Several times within the two weeks, Mr. A. expressed concern over his diagnosis of myocardial infarction. He seemed to feel more threatened by his cardiac problem than by his growing renal problem. This may be common for a cardiac patient because, as Reiser (1951) notes, a cardiac problem is perceived as especially threatening:

> The diagnosis of a cardiac lesion may constitute an overwhelming psychological threat, and many of the symptoms, such as dyspnea, orthopnea, and anginal pain may be alarmingly sudden in onset and productive of severe anxiety. The cardiac patient is confronted with a closely interrelated system of physiologic and psychologic stresses that are in large part inseparable. The anxiety engendered by the disorder may tax both cardiac and psychologic reserve and exert an unfavorable influence upon the medical course and response to therapy, as well as upon the total personality function. (P. 781)

Within a week after his initial infarction and cardiogenic shock, Mr. A.'s blood pressure returned to normal. His renal status, however, did not improve as hoped. A total of two weeks had passed since the initial crisis of myocardial infarction, arrhythmias, and cardiogenic shock. Mr. A.'s problem now focused on the growing concern for his lack of renal function, diagnosed as acute tubular necrosis. His cardiac status had improved but he still needed critical care, so it was decided that he should be transferred to intensive care. His doctors believed the renal problem could best be assessed and treated in intensive care.

Mr. A. had experienced two weeks of closeness within a relatively small and quiet unit. Then he was moved with a minimal degree of hurry to a busy and noisy environment of intensive care. As his stretcher was pulled next to his new bed, Mr. A. said, "This place is much larger and noiser than coronary care. What are all those pieces of equipment at the head of my bed? My bed in coronary care didn't have all that stuff. I don't think I am going to like it here." The nurses tried to relieve his transfer anxiety by reassuring him that he would continue to receive the same excellent care. Once in bed, he began asking questions about his cardioscope. Again the nurse tried to alleviate his anxiety by identifying the parts of his cardioscope and answering his numerous questions. The critical care nurse realized that, as Andreoli et al. (1971) point out, leaving the relative security of a CCU unit is likely to create a special kind of transfer anxiety:

> Most patients find the atmosphere of the coronary care unit and its specialized equipment comforting and reassuring as compared with other intensive care units. Within this unit there is usually a high nurse-patient ratio. The patient receives the constant attention that his acute illness demands and becomes accustomed to this. He establishes close interpersonal relationships with the staff. Termination of the established therapeutic relationships may produce notable psychologic reactions that could influence his physical condition. (P. 150)

Even though Mr. A. was told he would receive excellent care, he no longer experienced close observation by the nurses. He still had his cardioscope, but it was only checked when an alarm sounded. At all other times, Mr. A. felt that it was only a piece of equipment decorating his environment. His new environment was confusing. He noticed several more nurses, but they all seemed to be preoccupied with other patients. Each time a nurse did approach his bed, she did not check his monitor, but instead she checked something under his bed. One morning, while his nurse was assisting him with his bath, Mr. A. initiated the following conversation:

MR. A.:   Things are sure different here than in CCU.
NURSE: What do you mean?
MR. A.:   I was told I would be observed closely.
NURSE: You don't think you are being observed in here?
MR. A: No. The only time I feel I am being observed is when my alarm buzzes. Then a nurse comes to my bedside.
NURSE: Why do you want a nurse to check your monitor?
MR. A.:   That's why I came to the hospital—because of my heart. Instead the nurses keep looking under my bed.
NURSE: Your heart has improved to the point where it does not require as close observation as it did in CCU. The nurse is checking your urine output.
MR. A.:   You mean my heart has improved?
NURSE: Yes. Now we are more concerned with your kidneys.
MR. A.:   Are they improving?
NURSE: Yes. Your urine output is improving.
MR. A.:   Good.

Although Mr. A. had been transferred from coronary care to intensive care, he remained emotionally in coronary care, where he had developed interpersonal relationships and knew what was expected of him. His emotional dependency on coronary care was demonstrated by his initial obsession with the cardioscope and by his need for close surveillance. To him, his primary problem remained his heart. He expressed fright when his nurse failed to check his monitor as frequently as had been done in coronary care. In all probability, he never really heard the explanation for his transfer. Mr. A., like so many other patients who transfer from one unit to another, had just begun to accept his illness when a complication occurred. The complication forced him to accept still another dimension of illness.

It may be quite normal for a patient who is transferred from CCU to ICU to continue to think that his cardiac status needs surveillance and to wonder why his nurse is preoccupied with his urinary output, blood gases, or electrolytes. Nevertheless, his feelings of primary anxiety, fright, and expectant anxiety are less acute than those of a patient who is transferred from a critical care unit to a general floor. A patient who transfers within the same unit, or from one unit to another, still finds a haven of security. He still experiences the close surveillance of both nurses and monitoring equipment. Both these factors greatly reduce his transfer anxiety.

Transfer out of Critical Care Units

Minckley et al. (1979) point out that even when the patient's physiological status has stabilized so that he can be transferred out of critical care, the patient's psychological adaptation may be behind or unstable. In addition, the critical care staff may unintentionally create a dependent patient who is not prepared to leave the safe environment. The focus of nursing care in critical care is on the here and now rather than on a future time when the patient will be transferred to a less intensive care setting. The patient experiencing anxiety may feel as though his sense of being and identity are threatened. Therefore the patient may leave the unit fearful that another biological crisis will occur. Transfer from a critical care unit to a general ward can create acute feelings of primary anxiety, fright, and expectant anxiety. Primary anxiety arises when there is a blockage in the termination or separation process. Such a blockage has to do with the type of transfer, the timing of transfer, and the interpersonal relationships severed.

Primary Anxiety. When the patient's biological problem stabilizes, various stress-related physiological, behavioral, and attitudinal changes also diminish. The behavioral changes occur because the patient feels a sense of security and protection within the critical care environment. However, when the patient is transferred without adequate preparation from the protective environment, he once again experiences anxiety and stress (Minckley et al. 1979). Most of the patients in critical care are connected to a cardioscope and/or other monitoring devices that are detached when the patient is ready for transfer. Removal from these devices often provokes anxiety. Detachment of the cardioscope may cause the myocardial infarction patient to fear that an arrhythmia will go unnoticed. Other patients have similar fears about removal of supportive devices or treatments such as chest tubes, arterial line, Swan-Ganz line, or IV therapy; or about a decrease in the number of laboratory tests or medications. Therefore transfer from a critical care unit such as coronary care, respiratory care, or intensive care to an intermediate care unit moves the patient from a dependent to an independent existence. In critical care the patient receives close nursing surveillance. Once transferred out of critical care, the patient moves into the environment where technological and nursing support are less intense. Abrupt or ill-prepared transfer leads to primary anxiety.

Primary anxiety occurs when the patient does not have the opportunity to transfer gradually. The transfer process may be abrupt: a patient may be told only minutes before that he is to be transferred to a two- or four-bed ward. He may not have sufficient time to go through the normal termination process, to say good-bye to his nurses and fellow patients, to receive reassurances from the nurses that his condition is stable, or to have his family notified of the transfer. Notification of the family is most important. All too often families go to the bed of their loved one only to find it empty or occupied by a stranger. They quickly seek out a nurse to discover the location of their loved one. It is not infrequent to have a family member become so anxious that he or she bursts into tears upon learning the patient has been safely transferred. If the transfer is done quickly, the patient may be informed that his bed is needed for an emergency or for someone who is critically ill. The patient may not appreciate such as explanation, because he still considers himself as being critically ill.

According to Klein and Rabkin (1981), primary anxiety associated with premature separation can cause the patient to respond in three ways: protest, despair, and detachment. *Protest* is similar to an anxiety attack and is characterized by pleading, clinging, and demanding. If the patient realizes that transfer is eminent, he may request additional nursing care when his condition does not require it. Another patient may refuse to leave critical care or seek reentry into critical care after he has been transferred to an intermediate care setting. The stage of *despair* is comparable to the feeling of depression. The patient who is abruptly transferred because the room is needed for a more critically ill patient can experience despair because he has little, of any, time to adjust to the idea of a new less intense environment. Such patients can experience feelings of abandonment. They manifest these feelings by constant use of their call light, requests for pain medication, or requests for additional nursing care. The *detachment* stage can manifest itself as withdrawal behavior. The patient withdraws from meaningful interaction with the staff for fear that, like the critical care team, they also will abandon him.

Abrupt transfer does not give the patient time to assimilate the positive characteristics of his transfer. He may view the entire process as rejection, as indicated in a study of Klein (1968) that examined the transfer process of coronary care patients:

> Although the transfer was intended to be a sign of getting well, the patient's feeling of rejection by those who had been caring for him was far more frequent. This feeling appeared to be related to several factors. The patients were often transferred abruptly without choice or warning because other emergency admissions needed the space. Secondly, when the patients were moved from a private room to a four-

bed unit, it was seen by the patient as a form of demotion. In the ward area they were often surrounded by critically ill patients and this was interpreted as a contradiction to the statement "you're getting well." (P. 107)*

Abrupt transfer creates primary anxiety, in which the sequence of events in normal termination process are blocked. To avoid feelings of rejection, the nurses who have taken an active role in the patient's care should visit him, helping him to continue to feel significant in their eyes. They can inquire about his progress and answer questions he may have about his new environment or treatments. He may feel more comfortable sharing his concerns with familiar faces, and the nurse can then share his concerns of fears with his new health team. As he is able to increase his physical activity, his new nurses can encourage him to return to the critical care unit and visit with his original nurses. The patient need no longer feel rejection.

Normally the transfer from coronary care, for example, occurs three to five days after myocardial infarction or as the need for constant monitoring is diminished. While the patient views the transfer as evidence of biological improvement, he nevertheless experiences feelings of anxiety. A study by Toth (1980) measured the anxiety level of MI patients on the day of transfer from CCU. The experimental group received structured pretransfer teaching while the control group received unstructured pretransfer teaching. The anxiety level of the experimental group was lower than that of the control group on all physiological parameters tested. It seems that when the patient is adequately prepared for transfer, anxiety levels are reduced.

Primary anxiety can also be created by the timing of a transfer. Most patients do not have the opportunity to decide when they want to move and it would not be realistic to leave such matters entirely in patients' hands, since some may elect to remain in a critical care unit until discharge. Transfers that occur late in the evening or at night are generally more anxiety-provoking than those that occur in the daytime. The transferred patient does not have the opportunity to become territorially acquainted with his new environment. "Adapting to a hospital environment and trying to locate familiar landmarks is difficult under the best of circumstances. Middle-of-the-night transfers, which may be for administrative conveniences, increase the stress for patients" (Davis 1972, p. 708). A daytime transfer allows the patient to locate his closet, bathroom, and call light as well as to meet his new roommate and nurses. He has daylight to adjust to his unfamiliar environment and make it familiar, and he has the opportunity to lay territorial claim. Such a process helps to reduce feelings of transfer anxiety. Middle-of-the-night transfer can lead to confusion. The aged patient's vision is greatly diminished in the daytime let alone at night, and he may hallucinate in unfamiliar surroundings. An object such as an intravenous pole may take on human form. Such anxieties and fear can create a biological crisis. It is not unusual to readmit a patient into critical care who has only been transferred one or two days.

*Copyright 1968, American Medical Association.

The final contributing factor to primary anxiety is disruption of the patient's interpersonal relationships. The transfer may create a rupture in the social bond between nurse and patient. Suddenly the patient finds himself in an environment where there is less nursing surveillance. In some instances he may only see a nurse when she distributes his medications, whereas previously he was continually surrounded by nurses. It is not unusual for the patient to experience feelings of abandonment, loss, or insecurity. He had placed his entire trust in the judgment and knowledge of his nurses and doctors. Together the nurse-doctor-patient team "weathered the storm." This factor alone creates an intimate bond between the three people. The patient may experience anxiety because he feels that he is still in need of or dependent upon a similar close relationship with his nurse. Many critical care patients who are transferred, particularly cardiac patients, feel "deeply threatened and in need of a strong dependable relationship, within the framework of which reassurance can be offered to alleviate the anxiety stirred up by the symptoms and the fears of their heart disease" (Reiser 1951, p. 781). In all probability, his health team did not prepare the patient for the decreased need in nursing surveillance. He needs to be informed that his care will not be as intense. It must be emphasized that he has reached a point of improvement, and that he no longer requires intensive care or observation.

Fright. The second condition associated with transfer anxiety is fright. In a critical care unit, the patient may have been dependent upon not only the nurses but also upon wires, tubes, or pieces of equipment. As we have seen above, critical care patients may be connected to nearly a score of mechanical or electrical wires. Each piece of equipment produces its own noisy yet reassuring sound to the patient, who knows that his support system is working and will sound an alarm if it fails. Each patient feels secure in the knowledge that if all is going well externally, everything must be fine internally.

The nurse's goal is to reduce fright as much as possible. The coronary artery bypass graft (CABG) patient with high anxiety levels can run a greater surgical risk than patients with low anxiety. According to Johnston (1980) anxiety can be a significant predictor or determinant of various forms of physical and psychological duties which influence the success of the surgical procedure. Anxiety levels do not decrease after a surgical intervention because the patient experiences continuing threats of hospitalization, separation from significant others, and invasive procedures. For the surgical intensive care patient who is already experiencing anxiety, the threat of transfer out of a protected environment creates additional anxiety and more specifically fright. There are two external forces, his nurse and his equipment, that can serve to reassure the patient.

As the patient steadily improves, the staff can reduce treatments and remove pieces of equipment. This can serve to reassure the patient that he is getting well. If the termination process has taken place gradually, the patient may accept the fact that he is improving. This is usually the case with the respiratory patient who is gradually weaned off the volume respirator.

Another patient may not have his wires or tubes removed until seconds before a transfer, and he may wonder why, when just seconds before he needed his cardioscope and other devices, they have suddenly been discontinued. In all probability, they could have been discontinued earlier. The cardiac patient in particular may fear that any irregularity in his heart will not be detected. As Reiser (1951) points out, "The monitoring device becomes a significant object to the acutely ill cardiac patient and he is very dependent on it for a sense of security. The exact purpose of the monitor can be clarified to the patient so that his fear of his heart not functioning without it will be dispelled" (p. 781). The respiratory patient, if transferred with his tracheostomy tube, may become anxious about the frequency of being suctioned. He may feel he needs the same amount of suctioning as he did in intensive care. This type of patient has to be taught how to expectorate his own secretions, and he should be told that he may have very little if any secretions. In other words, he needs reassurance that he is progressing normally and safely.

Mrs. K., a 73-year-old woman, experienced fright after her transfer from intensive care. She was initially admitted in severe respiratory failure. She had a long history of illness, including chronic obstructive pulmonary disease. Shortly after Mrs. K.'s arrival in the unit, doctors decided to perform a tracheostomy and connect her to a volume respirator. The decision was difficult to make because the staff realized she would become dependent upon the respirator, thus creating a difficult weaning process. Mrs. K. also depended upon her nurses. She made frequent requests of the nurses, demanding much of their time. Mrs. K. remained in intensive care for five weeks. During that time her condition gradually improved to the point that she could tolerate being out of bed for one hour and off the respirator while on a T-tube for as long as three hours. She could not, however, tolerate having her nurse out of her presence for more than 15 or 20 minutes. The nurses tried to establish limits on her behavior, but each time they tried Mrs. K. cried, making her nurse feel guilty.

After two weeks, Mrs. K. transferred to a general floor. She still had her tracheostomy, although she had been successfully weaned off the respirator. Two days later, one of the intensive care nurses decided to visit Mrs. K. The nurse had just walked into her room when Mrs. K. began crying.

NURSE: What's wrong, Mrs. K.?
MRS. K.:   Everything!
NURSE: What do you mean?
MRS. K.:   They could care less if you lived or died around here.
NURSE: Who, Mrs. K.?
MRS. K.:   The nurses. They all seem to avoid me.
NURSE: What makes you feel they are avoiding you?
MRS. K.:   Well, they never want to answer my light. Instead an aide or someone else answers my light.
NURSE: What is it you want when you ask for a nurse?
MRS. K.:   Oh, I don't know. Sometimes I forget. Maybe I have

NURSE: them get water, juice, or a blanket. Maybe I want them to see if I need suctioning.

NURSE: As I recall, Mrs. K., you know pretty much when you need to be suctioned.

MRS. K.:   Yes.

NURSE: Why don't you make a list of things you want your nurse to do. Then you will be calling her less often, and I suspect she will respond. You are doing so much better, Mrs. K., you really don't need someone watching you all the time.

MRS. K.:   You think so.

NURSE: Yes. I'll check with you tomorrow to see how things are going. (*She leaves the room and talks with Mrs. K.'s nurse about setting limits.*)

Mrs. K. expressed fright over the decrease in nursing surveillance. She was still dependent upon her nurse for observational care. The nurse's presence seemed to reassure her, although seeing the nurse too often would· only reinforce Mrs. K.'s beliefs that she is still critically ill.

Nurses can anticipate potential areas of fright prior to a patient's transfer from intensive care. Feelings of fright arise when a person does not know what to expect in a given situation. If nurses would prepare patients for transfers by explaining what they can expect and what new staff members will expect from them, transfer anxiety can be greatly reduced.

Expectant Anxiety.   The last condition that might lead to anxiety is the patient's expectation of his transfer. First, a patient will expect his care to continue in the same vein. Second, he will continue to think of himself as critically ill. The patient may have difficulty accepting abrupt changes in his care or treatments. According to Klein (1968), the basic change in his treatment "usually results in less medication and increased physical activity. A gradual progression is viewed positively by the patient, but all too often he goes from complete bed rest in critical care to up at liberty on a step down or intermediate care unit. Abrupt changes in diet are also frequent in the new environment" (p. 107). The patient may not have been prepared to be more independent. As is the case with sudden removal of pieces of equipment, the patient may have difficulty accepting or understanding abrupt changes in his physical mobility. Only minutes before, he was immobilized by wires, tubes, and an order to remain inactive. Now he is suddenly expected to go to the bathroom on his own, ambulate, or completely bathe himself. The patient may wonder whether his biological system can function with abrupt changes in medication, diet, or activity.

The individual who is admitted to a critical care unit brings not only an illness, injury, or disease but a mental set about each. The mental set will influence the manner in which the patient assumes the patient role (Johnson

1979). The mental set includes certain expectations regarding the unit, treatments, and staff. Once the expectations are learned, the patient may have difficulty transferring those expectations into an intermediate care setting.

The patient may have difficulty integrating himself into his new environment. He knows only what was expected of him in critical care. According to Levitt (1980), therefore, he becomes tense and anxious. Tension may have two meanings with reference to anxiety and stress. Tension means a vague feeling of disquiet, a restlessness, a diffuse, unidentified wanting to do something that is a consequence of anxiety occurring at a level below conscious awareness. In this sense, tension is an intervening variable, a state that links unconscious anxiety to manifest behavior. Anxiety and tension may arise because the individual still looks upon himself as critically ill. His presence in critical care continually reinforced this concept of himself. The fact that he is about to be transferred means that the health team no longer considers his condition as critical, but because he is still physically housed in a critical care unit, with wires and tubes coming from many parts of his body, he considers himself critical.

Illness threatens the patient's sense of biological and psychological integrity. He must sidetrack his past expectations and formulate new and possibly more meaningful ones. The nurse must remember that this internal struggle may force the patient to consider himself ill longer than is actually the case. Davis (1972) notes "that by the time a patient is transferred to the general floor the staff's perception of him has usually shifted from seeing him as a critically ill patient to one who is recovering and getting better. The patient, on the other hand, may still perceive his situation to be highly precarious and, in effect, still think of himself as on the brink of death" (p. 706).* Again the patient may not realize that his biological problem is healing, and that he is simply convalescing until discharge. The patient can be prepared for alteration in aspects of his care and the expectations of his new equipment. Such knowledge will help him fit into his new setting.

NURSING ASSESSMENT OF TRANSFER ANXIETY

Behavioral manifestations of transfer anxiety can be assessed on an ongoing basis before and after transfer from critical care. The critical care nurse has the opportunity to observe the patient in a variety of situations over a specific period of time (Solomon-Hast 1981).

The critical care nurse assesses transfer anxiety through the patient's behavioral response. The responses are categorized into regulatory behaviors (physiological responses) and cognitive behavior (psychological behaviors).

Regulatory Behaviors

The regulator system involves stimuli from the external environment and from changes in the internal state of dynamic equilibrium. The regulatory behaviors are physiological responses. Research on the effect of psychological stress in the body and the course of illness has shown that emotional stress can activate the autonomic nervous system response of fight or flight. An abrupt or unprepared for transfer out of critical care can create unnecessary stress. The release of epinephrine and norepinephrine produces the following regulatory behaviors:

Regulatory Behaviors
Increased heart rate
Increased systolic blood pressure
Increased pulse pressure
Increased demands for O_2 by myocardium
Angina
Arrhythmias
Decreased gastrointestinal motility
Increased respiratory rate
Dilation of bronchioles
Dilation of pupils
Diaphoresis
Tremors

These regulatory behaviors can have a negative effect upon the patient's physiological status. Therefore the critical care nurse seeks ways to lessen their occurrence.

Cognitive Behaviors

The cognator system involves inputs from internal and external stimuli which include both psychological and social factors. The cognitive behaviors are psychosocial responses. The cognitive behaviors associated with transfer anxiety consist of the following (Solomon-Hast 1981; Spielberger 1972);

Cognitive Behaviors
Worry
Anxiousness
Tension
Overexcitement
Restlessness
Reduced perceptual field
Distorted time sense with focus on the present
Fatigue

The cognitive response to anxiety is a reaction to some form of stress.

NURSING DIAGNOSIS OF TRANSFER ANXIETY

The nursing diagnosis is a statement of the current problem. Regulatory and cognitive behaviors coupled with internal-external stressors combine to help the nurse make her diagnosis. The specific problem is transfer anxiety. Internal stressors consist of the fear of dying, fear of separation from significant others, and fear of biological or social loss. External stressors consist of a threatening yet protective environment with unfamiliar technology, strange noises, frequent intrusive procedures, and unfamiliar faces. Each stressor has different significance for the critically ill patient. Nevertheless all stressors can combine to contribute to transfer anxiety.

NURSING INTERVENTIONS AND TRANSFER ANXIETY

Like the patient, critical care nurses also experience anxiety as a result of stress experienced in the work situation. The nurse's personal experience of anxiety may be influential in deterring meaningful interaction with patients (Johnson 1979).

In order to minimize transfer anxiety, the nurse can begin her work the moment a patient arrives in a critical care unit. We usually become so involved in the immediate admitting crisis that we sometimes fail to prepare the patient for his eventual transfer. Such a reaction on the nurse's part is understandable; however, sometimes the critical care nurse continues to perceive the patient on a biological level. She, like the patient, fails to move beyond the threat to his biological integrity. She may see him as a biological entity, rather than as a human being with a biological problem. The nurse can begin to reduce the conditions that lead to the three components of transfer anxiety: primary anxiety, fright, and expectant anxiety.

Primary Anxiety

Nurses can decrease the patient's anxiety by planning the transfer well ahead of time and discussing it with him. This will minimize the distruption that occurs as a result of the transfer. Transferring the patient during the day allows the patient to orient himself to the new environment. The patient needs to know where his personal belongings, beside drawer, bathroom, call light, and nurses' station are located. When the patient has been prepared for transfer, the pretransfer feeling of security can be sustained throughout the process of adjusting to a new environment (Minckley et al. 1979).

Primary anxiety will diminish if the patient's transfer is planned. What this implies is that the nurse can control as much as possible the type, timing, and degree of disruption in interpersonal relationships caused by the transfer. The first consideration is the type of transfer. As Nehren (1965) points out, the termination process begins upon arrival: "Theoretically, termination for the patient begins for him at the time of his first contact with the nurse, doctor, hospital, or community agency. At this time the staff can focus their health teaching upon the day when the patient no longer will be dependent on them" (p. 110).* The patient can be prepared regarding his medical progress. Knowledge of what to look for in his own condition would let him know that a higher level of wellness and transfer are imminent. Critically ill patients look at objects within their environment to give them clues regarding their biological status: their cardioscope, intravenous bottle, arterial line, Swan-Ganz line, chest tubes, Foley catheter, endotracheal tube, tracheostomy tube, or volume respirator. Other signs may become apparent to the patient: decrease in pain, reduction in the number of venipunctures for laboratory studies, decrease in number of blood gases drawn, absence of arrhythmias, reduction in medication, or increase in urinary output. Of course the significance of each one of these signs must be interpreted and identified for the patient. The cardiac patient, for example, needs to be informed about the rhythm he sees dancing across his cardioscope. If a patient receives medication such as lidocaine for ectopic beats, this must be explained. When the intravenous bottle containing lidocaine is removed, the nurse can reassure her patient that the arrhythmia has subsided and that his rhythm has stabilized.

The patient can be taught recognition of changes in his own rhythm. This does not imply that he should continually take his pulse. It simply implies that the patient can be able to identify what he calls "palpitation" or "skipped beat." He would no longer feel the need to depend upon an external device to monitor an arrhythmia. The nurse can stress, of course, that such arrhythmias probably will not occur. A cardiac patient who was initially admitted with shortness of breath necessitating oxygen and with substernal chest pain necessitating medication will perceive that, as his cardiac integrity stabilizes, he no longer experiences shortness of breath or pain. These factors alone may suggest to the patient that transfer is close.

The burn patient will have physical signs of involvement or failure. Unlike the cardiac patient, whose internal injury manifests itself through EKG studies, monitor patterns, or serum enzyme levels, the burn patient's signs are external. He has only to look at the outward appearance of his body to note changes. However, because of all the dressings, creams, or grafts, he may not be able to identify positive signs of progress or healing. A nurse working in a burn unit has a unique responsibility to prepare her patient for transfer. He may go home rather than to an intermediate care unit. The type of transfer he receives will in all probability be well planned. The approximate date may not be predicted as easily as for the cardiac patient. Besides noting changes in his burns, the patient may also see gradual removal of various pieces of equipment. This becomes an encouraging force that can motivate the burn patient.

The patient in respiratory crisis will be encouraged when his weaning time off a volume respirator increases from minutes to hours. He will acknowledge it as a real sign of imminent transfer when the machine is finally wheeled away. Prior to this time, he should be kept informed of changes in his blood gases—particularly of those results that indicate a sign of progress. Such knowledge makes his care and treatment more meaningful. He may even be able to predict what his blood gases will be according to the way he feels. An awareness such as this may reassure the patient when he is transferred out of critical care. He knows the signs of potential threats to his biological integrity as well as the signs of progress that indicate transfer, and he can feel more self-sufficient and in control.

Besides needing awareness of physical or environmental signs of readiness to transfer, the patient also needs verbal reassurances that his transfer is appropriate. In other words, rather than telling the patient, "We need your bed," or "A patient who is more critical than yourself needs the bed," the nurse can say, "You have improved to the point where you no longer need close observation." She can present the transfer in a positive manner, reinforcing the transfer as being something he and his family have been waiting for. Critical care nurses can refer to the transfer as Cassem (1970) characterizes it, "as graduation from critical care, stressing that the patient is leaving because he no longer needs intensive care or constant surveillance and that the worst has been passed successfully. Transfer can become an opportunity for anxiety reduction rather than a new threat to recovery" (p. 324).

In summary, transfer can become a source of stress. The patient may experience less intense nursing care and the removal of monitoring devices. Nursing staff and family feel relieved that the patient is no longer critically ill. As Schwartz and Brenner (1979) point out, because the family has been actively involved with the patients during the initial crisis, they may spend less intensive time with the patient. The patient feels as if he has been left alone to experience another new situation. Therefore the family also needs to be included in the transfer process.

A second area in which the critical care nurse can reduce primary anxiety is the planning of the timing of transfer. When at all possible the patient can be transferred in the daytime. As mentioned previously, this allows the patient to get oriented environmentally and lay territorial claims to the space around him. This is most imperative for patients who experienced some environmental confusion in critical care. Moreover, the patient who is transferred with a tracheostomy or an A-V shunt needs time to become secure within his new environment. If the patient feels threatened or insecure, the stress can lead to biological problems. According to Klein (1968), "Investigation has suggested that adrenergic activity may be an etiologic factor in ischemic heart disease and in arrhythmias following myocardial infarction. The present findings suggest that psychological stress in the immediate postinfarction period may increase adrenergic nervous activity and contribute to a variety of cardiovascular complications" (p. 108). Nighttime transfer, which does not permit adequate patient orientation to his environment, should be avoided.

Occasionally a patient may be transferred from one hospital to another late in the evening. Mr. F. is an example of such a patient. He was 33 years old, spoke only German with very few English words, and had only been in the United States for a few weeks. Mr. F. suddenly became dizzy and fainted. A friend with whom he was visiting accompanied him to the emergency room of a small hospital. He was then admitted to a general floor. There an EKG revealed complete atrial-ventricular disassociation. Doctors immediately inserted an external pacemaker. A history revealed that his brother had severe coronary artery disease and had received a permanent pacemaker at the age of 31. The patient's doctor decided to transfer Mr. F. to a larger hospital where cardiac catheterization could be immediately performed. It was 8:30 P.M. when the decision was made. The nurses in coronary care realized that by the time he actually arrived in their unit it would be 10:30.

At exactly 10:30 P.M., Mr. F. arrived in coronary care. By the time he was admitted, processed, and connected to all the necessary wires and tubes, it was time for the night shift to go on duty. The patient barely had a chance to recognize his nurse's face when he had to integrate into a new group. The language barrier created additional problems. The nurses had difficulty explaining the normalcy of admitting procedures. Furthermore, they noted Mr. F. seemed to be experiencing anxiety but they felt helpless to try to alleviate it. In the meantime his friend had gone home, 40 miles away, and promised to return after his cardiac catheterization. Again the nurses tried to explain the procedure, but their efforts only seemed to increase Mr. F.'s anxieties and frustrations. Tests revealed severe coronary artery disease. All seemed to go well until three hours later, when the patient had difficulty raising his right arm and foot. What words the nurses were able to understand now became slurred. Mr. F. had experienced right-sided CVA with subsequent aphasia. The patient was now in a strange environment and in a partially numb body.

The timing of this patient's transfer and diagnostic tests was questionable. Had he been transferred earlier, to permit increased familiarity with his environment and staff, his anxieties may not have been so intense. Unfortunately the patient had more than a language problem; he also had aphasia. It is difficult to assess whether his problem could have been totally avoided but, in the light of what is known about the effects of stress and anxiety upon biological integrity, we can speculate that it might have been.

The last area in which the nurse can reduce primary anxiety concerns the severing of interpersonal relationships. The patient has placed his total trust in the skills of the critical care nurses. Therefore, according to Nehren (1965), "In planning for the termination process, the nurse's primary objective is to help the patient to sustain his integrity as a human being when he is experiencing the loss of the nurse as a significant person in his hospital life. This will result in a prepared rather than perplexed termination" (p. 112).

Although a close relationship usually develops between the nurse and patient, this is particularly true for the burn patient, who may remain hospitalized in the burn unit for two months. The severity and location of his burns usually create a longer period of forced dependency than is the case with most critical care patients. He depends on someone to bathe him, change his dressings, relieve his pain, feed him, and listen to his complaints and fears. His nurses probably get to hear his life story; and the patient will come to regard his nurse as his companion in the fight for survival. After enduring the crisis stage, they weathered the complications associated with burns. Next, they surmounted the patient's reactions to threats against his psychological integrity. Lastly, they succeeded in supporting successful grafting. Now the burn patient faces a threat to his social integrity: he must part with his valued helper and companion. His nurse can make thorough preparation for his transfer home. It will be necessary to wean the patient psychologically from his relationship with his nurse and to prepare him for acceptance into his new social setting. If the nurse has maintained an accepting attitude throughout the patient's stay, he can make the transfer with minimal anxiety. This implies that the family has had a vital role in the patient's biological-psychological survival.

Most patients, unlike the burn patient, do not have the additional threat of physical disfigurement to increase their fear of transfer. No one may be able to recognize their physical problem. A positive nurse-patient relationship can make the transfer easy. Good preparation by the nurse may alleviate blockage and primary anxiety during the transfer. Her preparation can influence his attitude toward the relocation. He must be made to feel that his nurses are not abandoning him and that other nurses will be assisting him in the rehabilitation phase of his illness. It is impossible to remove feelings of loss totally when leaving the unit, but loss can be minimized if patients have the opportunity to say good-bye to the nurses, and if nurses visit the patient in his new home. Whenever possible, a nurse from the floor to which he is being transferred can come to the critical care unit to meet the patient. Then at least one face will be familiar to the patient.

Fright

The second condition associated with transfer anxiety is fright, which occurs when the patient goes from a very dependent and restricted environment to one of total freedom. Such a transition may occur with no intermediate steps between dependent and independent, with no resting point at interdependence. The transfer patient may also experience fright when staff members discontinue his mechanical devices seconds before his transfer. The patient may feel his "lifeline" or "umbilical cord" is being abruptly severed. In order to avoid fright associated with reduced mechanical surveillance, a patient's nurse can gradually remove such objects of illness a day before his transfer. A transfer order often comes one to two days before the actual transfer. It may take this long to obtain a bed. If the patient is well enough to be transferred to a floor that has no cardioscope or other devices the patient has needed, the health team can disconnect the equipment when the order to transfer arrives. The patient can have at least a few hours to a day to see that his biological systems are not dependent upon such supportive devices.

Schwartz and Brenner (1979) note that previous research has shown that for the MI patient transfer from CCU may actually increase stress and cardiovascular complications. Changes in the environment and interpersonal relationships contribute to the patient's stress. Movement to an intermediate care unit seems to alleviate some of the stress. Larger hospitals are incorporating ways of alleviating fright in the transfer process. They are creating weaning areas to provide intermediate care of previously critical patients. These weaning units, called "constant care" or "continuous care" units, provide the patient with continued, but lesser, surveillance. The patient nevertheless feels secure in knowing that someone close at hand is informed about his particular needs. The intermediate care unit gives the patient time to adjust to more activity, changes in diet, reduction in medication, and possible removal of supportive equipment. The nurse in such a unit can offer her patient support as he resolves losses incurred during his illness. Such adaptation is not always possible in critical care units, where the environment itself may threaten the patient and cause him to remain temporarily in the denial and avoidance phase of adaptation.

Expectant Anxiety

The last condition leading to transfer anxiety has to do with expectations. In preparing the patient for transfer, the nurse must determine that he knows what is to be expected of him. He needs to know that his activity will be increased. He will be assuming more direct responsibility for his own care. Furthermore, she can know that the treatment plan may change drastically. No longer will his nurse monitor vital signs every two or four hours. He may no longer need IPPB treatments every three or four hours. These are all signs that he is improving. The patient can be kept informed of his daily progress, so that when transfer comes he will already realize that his improved state will enable him to do more on the general floor.

Solomon-Hast (1981) has identified four nursing interventions to reduce transfer anxiety: orientation, listening, acknowledgment, and information. One way to reduce the patient's expectant anxiety is to have a nurse from the floor or intermediate care unit explain new routines prior to his leaving critical care. Orientation therefore includes nursing actions aimed at familiarizing the patient with the surroundings of, first, the critical care unit and then, when transfer occurs, the intermediate care unit. When the patient is oriented to the people around him, he begins to establish trust with individual nurses. Davis (1972) believes that "to minimize the socioemotional disruption in the transfer of the patient from critical care, whenever possible, the ward nurse should be introduced to the patient and his family while he is still in critical care. This would provide an opportunity for the nurse from the general floor to explain to the patient and his family what the atmosphere and routines on her ward are like" (p. 709). Having a three-way conference with the critical care nurse, the patient, and the intermediate care nurse would provide for continuity of care. The second intervention noted by Solomon-Hast (1981) is listening. Listening includes encouraging verbalization of the feelings associated with the illness experience, prehospital events, and pretransfer needs. When the patient verbalizes his feelings, the nurse listens for themes that can be incorporated into a future teaching program. Acknowledgment, the third intervention, includes clarifying and identifying the patient's reaction to anxiety. Sharing feelings or perceptions helps to reduce expectant anxiety. Information, the fourth intervention, directs the nurse's action toward providing specific facts to the patient. Information facilitates an understanding of the illness process, expectations while in critical care, and expectations of the noncritical care environment when transfer takes place.

Therefore transfer anxiety is reduced through an organized plan to control primary anxiety, fright, and expectant anxiety. It involves educating the patient about his own health. The individual receiving information about himself can formulate an idea about his progress rather than being left to his fantasies. When possible, the nurse-physician-patient team can establish a target date for transfer. This may be possible in coronary care, where the average stay may be five days, although there will be patients like Mrs. K. who remain in a critical care unit for five weeks. For these patients, setting a transfer target date would be unrealistic. As each predicted transfer date passed, the patient would feel a sense of failure. Therefore, these patients need day-to-day goals of improvement and motivation. Accomplishment of such goals, for example, staying off the respirator 45 minutes instead of 30, would give the patient signs of improvement and would indicate forthcoming transfer. The family can be notified of the patient's transfer. If it is possible to connect a phone at the patient's bedside, he can make the call himself. However, this may be an impossibility in most critical care units, where the unit secretary, clerk, or nurse can quickly make the phone call. It is a nice gesture that informs both the family and patient that their nurse is interested and cares about them both. Such a gesture reinforces the patient's positive concept of people-to-people nursing.

NURSING EVALUATION

Nursing evaluation of transfer anxiety is an ongoing process. The critical care nurse assesses regulatory and cognitive behaviors supporting the diagnosis of transfer anxiety. Interventions designed to alleviate transfer anxiety are evaluated for their effectiveness. The nurse minimizes transfer anxiety through an organized plan including orientation, listening, acknowledgment, and information. The goal is to reduce primary anxiety, fright, and expectant anxiety.

SUMMARY

Patients in crisis are willing to accept restrictions that accompany critical care. According to Klein (1968), "The threatening aspects of critically ill patients evoke a readiness in most patients to accept such intensive care, at least for a brief period, even though it requires extraordinary passivity and a dependence upon other people beyond that usually acceptable to an adult" (p. 104). The patient becomes comfortable and secure in his carefully monitored environment. Once forced to leave, he becomes anxious about transferring into the world of the unknown. Proper preparation, including teaching the patient about himself, will enable the patient to transfer with a minimum of anxiety.

REFERENCES

ANDREOLI, KATHLEEN G., VIRGINIA K. HUNN, DOUGLAS P. ZIPES, and ANDREW G. WALLACE, *Comprehensive Cardiac Care*, 2nd ed. St. Louis: C. V. Mosby, 1971.

BACKER, KATHERINE, and PATRICIA McCOY, "Group Sessions as a Method of Reducing Anxiety in Patients with Coronary Artery Disease," *Heart and Lung*, 8, no. 3, (May-June 1979), 525-529.

BECKER, PETER, "Towards a Process Analysis of Test Anxiety: Some Theoretical and Methodological Observations," in *Test Anxiety: An Overview of Theory and Research*, ed. Ralf Schwarzer, Henk van der Ploeg, and Charles Spielberger, pp. 3-9. Hillsdale, N.J.: Lawrence Erlbaum Associates, 1982.

BOWLBY, JOHN, "Separation Anxiety," *The International Journal of Psychoanalysis*, 41, pts. 2-3 (March-June 1960), 89-112.

——, *Separation: Anxiety and Anger*. New York: Basic Books, 1973.

CHRISTOPHERSON, BERNICE, and COLLEEN PFEIFFER, "Varying the Timing of Information to Alter Preoperative Anxiety and Postoperative Recovery in Cardiac Surgery Patients," *Heart and Lung*, 9, no 5 (September-October 1980), 854-861.

DAVIS, MARCELLA, "Socioemotional Component of Coronary Care," *American Journal of Nursing*, 72, no. 4 (April 1972), 707.

DEPREEVW, ERIC, "From Test Anxiety Research to Treatment: Some Critical Considerations and Propositions," *Test Anxiety: An Overview of Theory and Research*, ed. Ralf Schwarzer, Henk van der Ploeg, and Charles Spielberger, pp. 155-163. Hillsdale, N.J.: Lawrence Erlbaum Associates, 1982.

FREUD, SIGMUND, *The Problem of Anxiety*. New York: Norton, 1963.

GOTT, KOON, "Patient's Anxiety in Coronary Care Unit," *The Nursing Journal of Singapore*, 17, no. 2 (November 1977), 58-61, 64.

JOHNSON, M. "Anxiety/Stress and the Effects on Disclosure between Nurses and Patients," *Advanced Nursing Science*, 1 (July 1979), 1-20.

JOHNSTON, MARIE, "Anxiety in Surgical Patients," *Psychological Medicine*, 10 (1980), 145-152.

KERR, NORINE, "Anxiety: Theoretical Considerations, *Perspectives in Psychiatric Care*, 16, no. 1 (1978), 36-46.

KLEIN, ROBERT, "Transfer from a Coronary Care Unit," *Archives of Internal Medicine*, 3 (August 1968), 104-107.

KLEIN, DONAL and JUDITH RABKIN, *Anxiety: New Research and Changing Concepts*. New York: Raven Press, 1981.

KRISTIE, JANET, "Anxiety Levels of Hospitalized Psychiatric Patients throughout Total Hospitalization," *JPN and Mental Health Services,* 17, no. 7 (July 1979), 33-42.

LEVITT, EUGENE, *The Psychology of Anxiety*. Hillsdale, N.J.: Lawrence Erlbaum Associates, 1980.

LITIN, EDWARD. "Emotional Aspects of Chronic Physical Disability," *Archives of Physical Medicine and Rehabilitation*, March 1957, pp. 129-142.

MINCKLEY, BARBARA, DIANE BURROWS, KAREN EHRAT, LILAH HARPER, SHIRLEY JENKIN, WILTON MINCKLEY, BRENT PAGE, DONNA SCHRAMM, and DONNA WOOD, "Myocardial Infarct Stress of Transfer Inventory: Development of a Research Tool," *Nursing Research*, 28, no. 1 (January-February 1979), 4-10.

NEHREN, JEANETTA, "Separation Anxiety," *American Journal of Nursing*, 65, no. 1 (January 1965), 110.

PEPLAU, HILDEGARD, "A Working Definition of Anxiety," *Some Clinical Approaches to Psychiatric Nursing*, ed. Shirley Burd and Margaret Marshall, pp. 323-327. New York: Macmillan, 1963.

PORTNOY, ISADORA, "The Anxiety States," in *American Handbook of Psychiatry*, Vol. 1, ed. Silvano Arieti, p. 307. New York: Basic Books, 1959.

POWERS, MARYANN. "The Apprehensive Patient," *American Journal of Nursing*, 67, no. 1 (January 1967), 58-63.

REISER, MORTON, M.D., "Emotional Aspects of Cardiac Disease," *American Journal of Psychiatry*, 107, no. 10 (April 1951), 781.

SARNOFF, IRVING, "Anxiety, Fear and Social Affiliation," *Journal of Abnormal and Social Psychology*, 62, (1961), 356-363.

SCHWARTZ, LINDA, and ZARA BRENNER, "Clinical Care Unit Transfer: Reducing Patient Stress through Nursing Interventions," *Heart and Lung*, 8, no. 3 (May-June 1979), 540-546.

SCHWARZER, RALF, HENK VAN DER PLOEG, and CHARLES SPIELBERGER. *Test Anxiety: An Overview of Theory and Research*. Hillsdale, N.J.: Lawrence Erlbaum Associates, 1982.

SOLOMON-HAST, ANNE, "Anxiety in the Coronary Care Unit: Assessment and Intervention," *Critical Care Quarterly*, 4, no. 3 (December 1981), 75-82.

SPIELBERGER, CHARLES, *Anxiety Current Trends in Theory and Research*. New York: Academic Press, 1972.

TOTH, JEAN, "Effect of Structured Preparation for Transfer on Patient Anxiety in Leaving Coronary Care Unit," *Nursing Research*, 29, no. 1 (January-February 1980), 28-34.

WILLIAMS, JAMES, JOHN JONES, NICHOLAS WORKHOVEN, and BARBARA WILLIAMS, "The Psychological Control of Preoperative Anxiety," *Psychophysiology*, 12, no. 1 (January 1975), 50-54.

12
Sensory Overload

BEHAVIORAL OBJECTIVES

1. Define the terms *sensory process, sensoristasis,* and *sensory overload.*
2. Describe the four properties associated with the phenomenal field.
3. Apply the four properties to the critically ill patient.
4. Describe five regulatory behaviors associated with sensory overload.
5. Identify four cognitive behaviors associated with sensory overload.
6. Create a nursing care plan that reduces sensory overload taking into consideration the four properties.

Considering the implications of sensory overload research for the common experience of overstimulation in today's technologically advanced society, it is surprising that there has been only a handful of experimental studies on the effects of overload. Despite the limited data base, however, people agree regarding the maladaptive effects of sensory overload (Goldberger 1982).

Our daily activities expose us to a variety of stimuli in the external world. Some have meaning, whereas other stimuli are meaningless. At my desk, I am aware of cars on a nearby freeway, the roar of an airplane engine, a helicopter flying overhead, a neighbor yelling at her small child, dogs barking, the siren of a police car or an ambulance, television sounds from an adjacent room, birds singing outside the window, and my pencil as it moves across the paper. We learn to allow selective admission of those stimuli that have meaning. This is accomplished through an elaborate sensory screening process. I can often screen out the distant background noises, but if they become too distracting, I can move—change my environment—to a more suitable location. When an individual becomes ill, he loses his ability to change his environment. He may relinquish his ability to deal with his physical environment. The nature of his illness may render him immobile. If his environment becomes too intense, he is unable to choose another location. His environment may foster or perpetuate injury and destruction. There is no doubt that the environment evokes emotional and psychological responses and has important therapeutic potential.

The environment of a critical care unit may not always meet the basic needs of the patient. According to Taylor (1971), the basic needs of an ill and often anxious individual are the same, whatever the degree of illness or the type of treatment required; but as a general rule, the more ill the patient, the more he will be dependent upon the hospital staff to satisfy these needs. Therefore, staff in critical care units can be the most concerned for the basic needs of a patient over and above the specific therapy necessitated by the patient's illness or injury. Some physiological problems seem to be related to the unique environment of the critical care units. As we move ever more quickly into the era of technology, we can quickly lose sight of the emotional impact various pieces of equipment have on the patient. His environment becomes machine-oriented. What we find is an unintentional byproduct of technology: environmental overdose.

Modern technology has given the critical care team sophisticated monitoring and life-support devices. Furthermore technology has prompted changes in nursing and medical interventions. Because of the increasing use of technology, the nurse needs to be aware of and accommodate the patient's privacy, spatial, and territorial needs. It should be noted that the sensory overload or environmental overdose experienced by the critically ill patient may not seem as immense as that experienced by the city dweller, but we must remember that the physically healthy city dweller is able to change his environment, whereas the patient is a captive member of his environment. It must also be remembered that illness alters an individual's perceptions. He may no longer be able to differentiate meaningful from meaningless stimuli, because the sounds are all new or foreign to him. In our desire to assist our patient, we often create an environment that is too much, too soon, and too fast. The patient is then subjected to the world of environmental overdose or sensory overload.

DEFINITION OF TERMS

Sensory Process

In order to understand environmental overdose, it is helpful to define first what is meant by *sensory process*—how human beings use their senses. Naturally built into the sensory process are reception and perception.

Our behavior is based on responses initiated by the direct contact of objects with our skin and taste receptors, and by energy traveling to our eyes, ears, and nose. All this information about objects and events around us has to be correlated with information from several different types of internal receptors. These receptors are responsive to changes in the position of limbs, movements of our whole body and head, and important aspects of our internal physiology. Thus, due to the correlation between internal and external environments, we can make judgments about the movements of objects even though we are also moving. It may seem that there is little information about an environment, either internal or external, of which we are unaware. Although our sensory processing probably includes a greater number of differentiations than that of any other single species, there is still much information to which we are not responsive (Alpern 1967). The sensory process includes reception and perception. Reception pertains to the biological aspect of sensory process: hearing, vision, smell, taste, touch, and sense of position in space.

As Mueller (1965) explains, all senses are selectively receptive to environmental changes:

> One modality may respond to radiant energy whose wavelengths are restricted to one region of the electromagnetic spectrum while another system will respond to another restricted region (for example, the visual system may respond to wavelengths between 400 mu and 700 mu, while the temperature will respond to wavelengths in the infrared region). One system may respond to relatively slow pressure changes (e.g., tactile sense) while another will respond to very rapid pressure changes (the ear). One sense may be specially sensitive to chemical stimuli in gaseous form, another to chemicals in liquid form. Sometimes the sensitivities may overlap (for example, both the tactile sense and the auditory sense will respond to pressure oscillation in the range from 20 cps to 1,000 cps); sometimes the sensitivities do not overlap (e.g., the sensitivities of the eye and the joint receptors). (P. 115)

Under all circumstances, there are factors within the environment that activate each sense system. Some systems may be activated more than others. Nevertheless, all senses can be altered by one's physical environment. The alteration occurs as a result of incoming stimuli. The brain has an elaborate system that monitors all incoming and outgoing stimuli.

Lindsley (1965) points out that, because of its strategic location at the crossroads for incoming and outgoing messages and its apparent ability to sample all such activity and to develop from it a more lasting influence in a form of alerting and attention, the reticular system appears to provide a common mechanism for the foregoing sensory conditions and their effects. The reticular activating system, together with the diffuse thalamocortical projection system, provides a mechanism capable of general arousal and alerting and also a specific attentional mechanism. According to Lindsley, the centrifugal control of afferent sources permits the level of activity aroused in the cortex and the reticular formation to regulate the sensory input. It may be that as the number of stimuli increases in frequency and intensity, the centrifugal cortical system is unable to regulate the amount of incoming stimuli. Too many stimuli enter the patient's internal environment too rapidly, creating behavioral responses and changes.

Lindsley also proposes that the reticular system offers a mechanism that may account for the types of behavioral changes seen in sensory overload. He suggests that the strategic location of the ARAS (ascending reticular activating system) at the crossroads of input and output systems permits it to sample and monitor all such activity. He further proposes that in doing so, it becomes adjusted or attuned to certain levels of activity, and its own response level is projected upon the cortex, where it influences perception and learning and no doubt plays a role in the control and is adjusted to the familiar. If one overloads the reticular system with sensory input, the system meets an unfamiliar situation, and only within limits can it adjust to this change. Manipulation of the external environment leads to sensory overload or environmental overdose. Manipulation or change in environmental stimuli alters human perception.

Perception reflects the psychological aspect of the sensory process. It involves selection and organization of incoming stimuli. Attention becomes the selective part of perception. If the patient is distracted by too many stimuli, his attention jumps from one stimulus to the next. The stimuli are not organized. Until they become organized, they have no meaning. We act according to what we perceive. Our actions lead to new perceptions, and these lead to new acts. The cycle continues throughout life. We must understand the process by which we as human beings become aware of ourselves and our world. Our awareness stems from perception and the behavioral responses it elicits. Too many incoming stimuli and distorted perception may cause the patient to become confused.

Sensoristasis

Schultz (1965) defines *sensoristasis* as follows:

> Sensoristasis can be defined as a drive state of cortical arousal which impels the organism (in a waking state) to strive to maintain an optimal level of sensory variation. There is, in other words, a drive to maintain a constant range of varied sensory input in order to maintain cortical arousal at an optimal level. Conceptually, this sensory variation-based formulation is akin to homeostasis in that the organism strives to maintain an internal balance, but it is a balance in stimulus variation to the cortex as mediated by the RAS (Reticular Activating System). (P. 30)

Some activities require a greater degree of cortical arousal than others. For example, driving a car requires more cortical arousal than riding a bus. While driving a car, the individual can vary sensory input by changing lanes, turning on the air conditioner, singing, honking the horn, or listening to the radio. If sensory stimulation falls below an optimal level, the individual seeks alternative stimuli or alternative ways of varying the stimuli. In this way the individual restores sensory equilibrium. Prolonged exposure to a sensory restricted environment may have long-term effects. As Mitchell (1973) points out, "A decrease in optimal sensory level appears to affect the development or normal perception and response in the growing organism. For example, children reared in extremely restricted environments demonstrate abnormal social and perceptual behavior when placed in a normal situation" (p. 198).

There are times when patients are unable to seek alternative stimuli. Their illness or limitations may limit contact on an action level with the environment. On the other hand, there are times when the patient's sensory environment contains excess stimuli. In these instances the patient seeks to reduce additional cortical arousal or input.

Sensory Overload

Environmental overdose and *sensory overload* are synonymous terms. Sensory overload implies that two or more modalities are in action simultaneously at levels of intensity greater than normal, and that the combination of stimuli is usually introduced suddenly. Sensory overload involves multisensory experiences. Too many incoming stimuli confuse the patient. According to Lindsley (1965), an excess of stimulation from two or more sense modalities, especially a sudden, intense barrage from afferent and corticofugal sources, as in surprise or fear, may block the reticular formation, causing behavioral immobilization and general confusion. As Baker (1984) notes, when sensory overload disrupts processing of information, a decrease of the meaningfulness of the environment results.

THE CONCEPT OF SENSORY OVERLOAD APPLIED TO THE CRITICALLY ILL PATIENT

Critical care is an intimidating environment to most individuals. The critical care nurse needs to develop an awareness of the perceptual incongruencies within this setting. The pathologic effect that perceptual changes may have on the helping relationship, and the measures the nurse takes to reduce the overwhelming impact of the environment need to be assessed in order for patient recovery to be successful. The overall atmosphere created by the various sensory stimuli might be severe enough to classify critical care as what Gowan (1979) terms a *high-load environment*.

All behavior is completely determined by, and pertinent to, the perceptual field of the behaving organism. The perceptual field has also been called the personal field, the private world, the behavioral field, the psychological field, the individual's life space, and the phenomenal field. The field of perception is responsible for the individual's behavior. According to Lindsley (1965), the phenomenal or perceptual field always has at least four properties—fluidity, intensity, direction, and stability—each of which will be discussed below. Naturally there are areas of overlapping within each property.

Patients in ICU, CCU, respiratory care, and burn units may experience more sensory overload than hemodialysis and isolation patients.

Fluidity

In critical care the patient generally receives physical overstimulation and emotional deprivation. Sensory overload or physical overstimulation are caused by sensory stimuli from painful procedures and technology. All these factors contribute to what Gowan (1979) terms a *paranoiagenic environment.*

The phenomenal field is continually changing. To the individual this field represents reality. The individual becomes involved in fluidity the moment he becomes ill: he is pushed into a fluid environment that leads him into environmental overdose. Without a degree of fluidity, the individual would be unable to adjust to the changing circumstances in which he must live and find need satisfaction. This capacity for change in the perceptual field also makes learning, reasoning, remembering, forgetting, and creating possible. What happens to the individual who becomes ill and is thrust into an actively fluid environment?

Prior to his illness, Mr. P. was a citizen, husband, provider, and father. He was a unique individual, and it was his identity, his personal belongings, his personal possessions, and his personal accomplishments that made him unique. He had responsibility and prestige within the community. He was capable of integrating into his being the events in his environment and adapting as indicated. Suddenly Mr. P. became ill. His senses became bombarded with all types of stimuli, both meaningful and meaningless. His anxiety and the flooding of stimuli caused him to have tunnel vision and distorted perception. Because Mr. P. was critically ill, he was taken to a local hospital in an ambulance. In the ambulance he was even more aware of his serious condition. The attendants busily worked on him; his wife sat crying in the front seat; and his pain grew in intensity. The noise of the wailing siren alone created a feeling of sensory overload. After what seemed like an eternity, Mr. P. arrived at the emergency entrance. There a team of blurred images in white received him. He was quietly pushed into an emergency treatment room and placed on a padded table in the center of the room. More blurred images of people continued to move in and out of his environment. We have all experienced standing in front of mirrors that project a distorted image of ourselves as short, tall, thin, fat, and blurred persons. Mr. P., in his newly created and rapidly changing environment, felt as if he were seeing those around him in this way. We might perceive people and objects in the environment to be normal; however, the patient perceives the same people and objects in a distorted manner.

While lying on a hard table in a strange sterile environment, he was admitted into the hospital environment. He had to organize himself and be organized into the social role of being a patient. He was presented with a system of social control designed to teach him how to conform and submit to the so-called sick role. He became a "patient" with a diagnosis and a room, bed, and admission number. To prove his social acceptance, the hospital assigned him a wristband, neatly typed and securely fastened around his wrist. This was his new identity.

Quite often the admission process neglects the patient's psychological needs. We become administratively concerned with giving the patient access to the use of a bed and facilities of the hospital. He, on the other hand, may be more concerned about whether he is going to die, what his wife must feel, and his financial obligations. These concerns create additional feelings of sensory overload. His doctors ask questions, poke, probe, and order various laboratory tests. After making their initial assessment, they then decide to which critical care unit he will be admitted.

In Mr. P.'s case, once the decision had been made to transfer him to a critical care unit, he faced another bombardment of stimuli. Transferred from his padded table to a cold stretcher, his senses were again flooded with impending anxieties about where he was going. When he heard the doctors say "intensive care," the fluidity of his perceptual field allowed him to remember that intensive care is where only the critically ill patients are placed. Before he had time to dwell on the subject, he was quickly maneuvered out of the treatment room and down a series of corridors. The twisting ride through the hospital reminded Mr. P. of his recent ambulance ride. At least this time there was no siren, only the rapid footsteps of his escort. He entered an elevator and arrived at yet another floor, where he was skillfully threaded down the hall to his final destination. He became aware that he no longer knew where he was. He was frightened to realize that he had lost his wife. Naturally, he felt the need for her presence, if only to know that she was down the hall, not at the other end of the hospital.

Inside the critical care unit, Mr. P. became aware of new sounds and blurred images. He was wheeled beside his bed. There, numerous hospital employees began moving in and out of his room. They robbed him of his sense of privacy and exhausted him. Again he experienced sensory overload. He wanted and needed this care, but there was too much going on. As a result of feeling intrusion, he became confused about the nurses. He saw them as blurred images. Quite frequently nurses are shocked that their patient does not remember them. Although the admitting nurse may have spent time admitting her patient, to the patient she is a stranger because he was unable to perceive her as anything beyond a blur.

A patient who has undergone coronary artery bypass awakens in pain with tubes in every orifice. In addition, he is surrounded by mechanical noises coupled with the hushed noise of the health team bustling around his bed urgently collecting hemodynamic data. Needless to say the patient experiences increasing overstimulation. Ballard (1981) investigated the number of items signifying physical sensation and meaningless input. Noise, especially unfamiliar noise, created sensory overstimulation and also caused sleep deprivation. Patients complained about noises from the oxygen unit or mask and from other patients. One aspect of sensory overstimulation or overload that ranked high among the subjects was the physical discomfort resulting from their surgical intervention. Being in pain ranked second and being thirsty was ranked third.

As he lies in bed, the patient may perceive fluidity in his environment, but he perceives himself to be a static person in that environment. Events are rapidly happening around him. He knows that the people and machines are collecting data, but they do not alter his internal environment. He may still experience the same intensity of pain, concerns, fears, frustrations, and anxieties that he did upon his arrival. Therefore, his internal environment does not have the same fluidity as his external environment. He may feel static due to immobility. He is literally tied to his bed by various cables and tubes. His immobility interferes with his ability to alter the environment in an attempt to reduce incoming stimuli. He is unable to disconnect his cable, tubes, or wires and find another location in the critical care unit. He would certainly be considered confused.

Another reason that he cannot perceive fluidity is that he is unable to derive meaning from all the scientific data collected and analyzed around him. He does not understand the professional jargon. He may recognize that his external environment is changing at a much faster pace than his internal environment; he is unable to interpret his cardioscope pattern to know whether his cardiac status demonstrates fluidity in a positive or negative direction. The patient is unable to keep up with the number and frequency of incoming sensory stimuli. His senses and their ability to perceive become distorted. He may blow things out of proportion: one nurse may become two. His doctor may assume unusually large features.

The patient's response or behavior is an indication of what he perceives at the time he is taking in stimuli. Nurses can remember this when they teach a patient. A lengthy discussion about the patient's environment, including such things as his bed control, light, nightstand, IV pole, cardioscope, and call light may be too much all at once. Minutes later the patient may ask, "Where is my light?" "What is that box with the light moving across the screen?" or "What's in that bottle?" The patient has experienced sensory overload or environmental overdose. He was given too much of what he needed. His ears heard bits and pieces of the total, his eyes saw only what they were able to at the time, and he selectively perceived only what he wanted.

Nurses have frequently experienced the problem of having just instructed a patient about remaining in bed only to find him in the bathroom minutes later. Obviously his perceptual field did not permit him to learn or remember. If the situation is too fluid, the patient is unable to assimilate and internalize the changes before moving to another level of change. Information that comes too quickly causes the patient not to remember what he selectively heard.

Initially the patient may not feel as if he is a member of his critical care environment. This is due to lack of involvement. Immobilized by pain, dressings, or machines, he has been told to rest. Other people do things to and for him. He feels like a static entity within a fluid environment. Not until he is asked to become a member of his environment does he feel it is his environment. The membership dues are his participation in the environment. It is through involvement and participation that he begins to feel internal fluidity. His involvement can only occur with reduction of incoming stimuli. As the incoming stimuli are reduced, he can see a relationship between internal and external environmental fluidity. Prior to this time, environmental overdose created disinterest in his external environment.

Intensity

The intensity with which one experiences events in the perceptual field is a function of differentiation and levels of awareness. Our environment becomes more intense as our anxiety and unfamiliarity with events in it increase. The properties of the perceptual field are closely interrelated. As the fluidity increases, so does the intensity. The rapid changes in the patient's internal and external environment create an intense atmosphere. Unfortunately, critical care environments may move the patient toward physiological and psychological degeneration at a time when he needs to draw together all his resources in order to stay alive. The degeneration takes the form of sensory overload unintentionally created by machines and staff. The patient in a critical care unit has a fantastic amount of sensory input in the form of pain, noise from machines, nurses and doctors talking, multiple intrusive procedures, and frequent examinations. Together they create an intense environment.

The physical layout of critical care together with the use of life-support devices and diagnostic equipment can have a detrimental effect on the perceptual experiences of the patient. In addition they may have a negative effect upon the patient's recovery phase. Besides the stress associated with environmental congestion, there are problems related to the frequent disturbance of patients for various procedures and treatments. As Gowan (1979) points out, these disturbances result in symptoms related to sensory overload and signify or harmful violation of the patient's spatial needs.

Soon after the patient's arrival in his new environment, nurses connect him to various pieces of machinery. The amount and type will depend upon his problems and unit. It is conceivable that the ICU, respiratory care, isolation, or burn patient could have several pieces of equipment. The hemodialysis and CCU patient may have machines or supportive devices peculiar to their needs. Any or all or the following machines could be connected to the patient: a cardioscope, a respirator, an arterial line, a CVP, an N/G tube, a Foley catheter, a hypothermia blanket, a Swan-Ganz, and IVAC and chest tubes. As Abram (1965) notes, "These devices, in spite of their necessary life-saving functions and their reassuring qualities to some patients, are perceived by others, especially those patients with poor reality ties, as threatening and ideal objects upon which to project their fears" (p. 665).

Moreover, as Baker (1984) has pointed out, a barrage of equipment tends to create stress in interpersonal relationships: "Mechanical devices and overuse of space contribute to the crowding of the unit. When crowding reaches a certain level, interactions among people intensify, contributing to greater stress. Physical closeness tends to magnify an already constant and high load of tension experienced by staff" (p. 68).

In critical care, patients are encumbered by multiple tubes, intrusive lines, arterial lines, Swan-Ganz lines, oxygen masks or ventilatory machines, and cardioscope leads or wires. Furthermore each patient is isolated, insecure, immobilized, depersonalized, and in pain. Lights are constantly on, and strange machinery surrounds the patient. Constant interruptions for nursing interventions and high noise levels contribute to sensory overload (Ballard 1981).

The machines can be most distressing to the critically ill patient. This is especially true for the patient who has several pieces of equipment around his bed. The more pieces of machines around him, the more intense he feels the situation to be; and the more incoming stimuli he experiences. A cardiac patient may become preoccupied with visual display of his rhythm. He may become disturbed if the auditory beeper is used. This is a device that beeps with each heart beat. The nurse can be at another patient's bed and follow her patient's cardiac status by means of this device. In time the patient learns his own auditory rhythm and becomes frightened if the rhythm changes. It is no small wonder that patients have developed arrhythmias watching their own monitor. As Taylor (1971) points out, "Any patient is likely to attempt to assess his own clinical state from the information available, and this may be both incorrect and frightening" (p. 51).

Machines create environmental overdose by the noises they make. The cardioscope beeps and buzzes with any changes both significant (rhythm change) and insignificant (interference). The buzzing sound varies with each cardioscope. The cardioscope alarm may buzz if the patient simply turns himself. It is as if the machine angrily buzzes in defiance of the patient's independence. At night the patient sees a glow of his rhythm moving across the oscilloscope. The volume respirator and patient together make rhythmic noises. The machine cycles as it is instructed to by dial settings. It hums along until it meets resistance or changes in pressure. Then it sends out its alarming message. The IVAC machine monitors a set number of IV drops. With each drop, it makes a click and the patient can look forward to hearing 20 clicks per minute. Besides a clicking sound, there is also a glow of light as the machine detects the number of drops per minute. If the soluset chamber or bottle becomes empty, the machine sings a high soprano sound. The high-pitched sound is quite piercing, even to the nurse. The oxygen makes a hissing noise like a snake as it moves along the tubing. The nasal-gastric tube connected to an intermittent suction device also makes a click-click noise. The clicking can be rapid or slow. A hypothermia blanket makes a humming and vibrating noise. The hemodialysis machine also has a humming sound as well as various alarms that indicate trouble. Together these sounds resemble a modern symphony. Unlike the nurse, who finds significance with each click, beep, buzz, or hum, the patient can make no sense of these sounds. They are instead a source of sensory overload and irritation.

Furthermore, as Baker (1984) notes, the noisiness of a sound increases with its duration. For example an alarm lasting a minute is obviously perceived to be noisier than one lasting ten seconds. Sounds that reach a high peak very abruptly (alarms going off on ventilators and IVACs) are judged to be noisy. Whether a sound is intermittent or continuous also affects perceived noisiness. The patient's hearing will adapt to continuous noise from the humming of certain machines. Likewise the same patient may be disturbed by intermittent noises from ringing telephones, dropped items, or loud voices.

The frightening sounds of the machines and the patient's distorted perception of them become the objects of fantasies and hallucinations. A nurse found one patient standing in front of his cardioscope looking at the screen. He was frantically trying to turn the dials. When asked what he was doing, he replied quite seriously that he was getting a funny line of interference on his television screen. He simply wanted to find another station with a better picture. Another patient awakened during the night and thought there was a large animal standing over his bed. He became extremely restless and apprehensive. It was not until the nurse discovered the source of his concern that she could alleviate his fears. It seemed that with certain lighting effects, his volume respirator resembled an animal. Still another patient mistook his IVAC machine for his nurse and became quite angry when the machine did not answer his questions. The list of fantasies and hallucinations could continue. Machinery, while having a significant role in patient care, can also have detrimental side effects.

Coupled with sounds of equipment in his immediate environment, the patient must face other noises: telephones ringing, charts clicking, food tray carts, nurses talking loudly, other patients moaning in pain, or people laughing. Woods and Falk (1974) note that the noise stimuli elicited from personnel have been found to be greater than those from the machines and various treatments. Some noises can be quite injurious to the critically ill patient. These are sounds or movements that create what Haslam (1970) calls *startle reflex*. How many of us have stood at a patient's bedside and accidentally dropped an IV bottle or bedpan? It has been found that a sudden unexpected sound such as a pistol shot produces widespread changes in bodily activity. There is a rise in blood pressure, a rise in intracranial pressure, and an increase in perspiration. The heart and respiratory rates increase simultaneously with a decrease in peristalsis and the flow of saliva and gastric juices (Landis and Hunt 1931). These responses could be detrimental to the neurological, respiratory, or cardiac patients. A nurse might create the same startle response by simply touching the patient. If she quietly approaches the patient's bed and attempts to take his blood pressure without fully awakening him, the patient may awaken with a startle.

Other patients also can be a source of environmental overdose. As a patient looks at his neighbor, he tries to tell himself that the neighbor looks more critical than himself. He tries to reassure himself that things will be better. It is quite possible that the neighbor is indeed more critical. The neighbor may make noise by talking in his sleep, snoring, screaming in pain, or yelling in anger at the staff. All the neighbor's noises, coupled with the patient's own and those already in the larger environment, create sensory overload. If the patient's neighbor does become more critical, the atmosphere will grow more intense with doctors and nurses running to the neighbor's bed, additional pieces of equipment being wheeled into place, groaning and moaning by his neighbors, and orders flying at a machine-gun pace. Needless to say, nearby patients sense a growing intensity in the environment. The intensity may continue until suddenly the area around the involved patient becomes silent. The doctors and nurses no longer run; they slowly walk away from the scene. Then someone pushes a stretcher alongside his neighbor's bed, and finally the silent body is removed. It is no wonder that patients not directly involved in the crisis curl up in a protective cocoon and withdraw. Other patients erroneously identify with the dying patient. Quite frequently nurses will note an increase in heart rate of patients in close proximity to the crisis who have received an overload of environmental stimuli.

The perpetual daylight of critical care units also contributes to environmental overdose. If nurses are asked why the lights are always on, they usually reply, "I don't know; it has always been that way." Of course, this does not make it correct. In the privacy of our bedroom, we sleep with the lights off. We know the time of day by changes in lighting. In a perpetually bright unit, the patient never knows whether it is day or night. He might see a clock or read his watch and learn it is 2:00, but he will not know whether it is A.M. or P.M. The perpetual daylight fosters a sense of time dissociation and confusion. Naturally there are patients who must be observed continually in well-lighted areas. Not all critical care patients need such observation. The lights and the various sounds convey to the patient a feeling of urgency, which simply reinforces his feeling of intensity within the environment. No matter what the cause of increased sensory input, it does cause physiological and behavioral changes in the patient.

According to Haslam (1970), "The most conclusive physiologic effect of noise on the individuals is that it causes a marked interference with sleep, rest, and relaxation. This effect is of significance in that it could retard convalescence and, consequently, prolong a patient's hospitalization or delay the advancement from an acute situation into a less stressful state" (p. 717).

Combs and Snygg (1959) point out that behavior is always determined by the nature of the perceptual field at the instant of behaving. It follows that, at whatever level of awareness perception exists in the field, it will affect the individual's behavior. When we perceive clearly and sharply, behavior is correspondingly direct and efficient. When we perceive only vaguely, the behavior is also likely to be fuzzy and inaccurate. If the patient must perceive an intense world around him, he will only receive half-pictures. The critical care patient who has distorted perception due to sensory overload will have behavioral manifestations of confusion and disorientation. He will become confused about his location, the reasons for his being there, the time of day, and the date. Since his perceptions of people and objects are vague, it is understandable that distortions occur, such as the volume respirator taking on the image of an animal. It is conceivable that patients can be confused, restless, agitated, or paranoid for reasons other than anoxia.

Direction

The perceptual world of the critical care unit can contribute to a stressful, frightening, and generally unpleasant experience for patients. Furthermore it may adversly affect the helping relationship so vitally significant during the patient's recovery phase (Gowan 1979). Although the content and form of organization vary from individual to individual and from time to time, the perceptual field always has direction (Combs and Snygg 1959). Although it is usually organized and meaningful, this is not necessarily true for a critical care patient. Initially, data from his environment are meaningless to him. Clicks, buzzes, hums, and occasional crashes fill his external environment. None of this relates to his internal environment. The cardiac patient in CCU does not understand his cardioscope, the wires connecting him to the box, or the strange pattern he sees running across the screen in rhythmic fashion. The emphysema patient in ICU does not understand the details of his volume respirator or arterial line. He only knows that the noisy machine that clicks and buzzes helps him breathe. The patient in hemodialysis initially does not understand the function of his machine. He understands that it takes the place of his kidneys, but beyond this the workings of the machine are meaningless. The patient may only hear half an explanation or see half the picture. People do not behave according to the facts as others see them. They behave according to the facts as they themselves see them. What governs behavior from the point of view of the individual himself are his unique perceptions of himself, of the world in which he lives, and of the meanings things have for him (Combs and Snygg 1959).

The stage of resistance that follows the fluidity and intensity phase constitutes the individual's return to normal or adaptation. However, after repeated exposure to the stressor, the acquired adaptation is again lost. The individual can enter the stage of exhaustion, which occurs as long as the stressor is severe enough and applied for a sufficient length of time (Ballard 1981).

The patient tries to find meaning in the meaningless. A patient in a confused state may stand at his bedside against orders. Another patient may pull out his CVP infusor, IV, Foley catheter, cardioscope leads, or his nasalgastric tube. Both patients perceive themselves to be correct in their actions. Their behavior is purposeful; it always has a reason. The first patient simply wanted to stand and void. The latter patient became irritated by all the wires and tubes. He simply decided he did not need them any longer. Sometimes the patient's reasons are vague and confused, in which case his behavior is equally vague and uncertain; sometimes the meanings are clear and definite.

The first patient realized he could not void in a prone position and chose to alter his environment independently in order to accomplish his goal. His reason may be perfectly logical to him, but his nurse views it as inappropriate. His nurse fears that her patient will unintentionally injure himself. To the patient everything he does seems reasonable and meaningful at the time he does it. Combs and Snygg (1959) point out that "when we look at other people from an external, objective point of view, their behavior may seem irrational because we do not experience things as they do. At the instant of behaving, each person's actions seem to him to be the best and most effective acts he can perform under the circumstances" (p. 17).

Events in the patient's external environment have meaning. The volume respirator, hemodialysis machine, cardioscope, arterial line, and chest tube all have meaning to the staff. To the patient they are expensive pieces of machinery. The function of each is an unknown. The patient needs to feel that his body is achieving organization, that things are adjusting in a positive direction. The direction he seeks is a higher level of wellness, a level directed away from the overwhelming sensory stimulation. He wants to return to the security of his home, his family, or his friends.

Basically all people are goal-directed, no matter what the goal. If the patient does not see meaning in events around him or if he does not sense internal fluidity, he succumbs to sensory overload and withdraws. By withdrawing, he passively accepts what is happening. The other alternative he has is to take control of the situation by pulling out the various tubes and wires connected to his body. After all, to the patient they do not seem to be doing the job. Furthermore, he does not view them as being part of his body, and he may no longer choose to be immobilized by a shroud of tubing and wires. His reasons are logical to himself. However irrevelant or irrational his behavior may appear to an outsider, his behavior from his point of view is purposeful, relevant, and pertinent to the situation as he understands it. He perceives that his behavior has direction and meaning.

Stability

Although the perceptual field is highly fluid, it is by no means unorganized; the organization of the field necessarily gives it a degree of stability. To live successfully, each of us needs an organized, stable, predictable field (Combs and Snygg 1959). Unfortunately, critical care environments do not always have predictable or stable perceptual fields. There are times when the environment has greater fluidity. The care of the patient has some predictability; the nurse can assess and predict potential problems for each patient, and this enables her to have a sense of readiness when a crisis occurs. While anticipating the unexpected, she knows there are basic routines that remain relatively stable with each patient. She knows the routine treatment of the MI, open heart, neurological, respiratory, or burn patient. But she must realize that while care can be predictable, her patient may not remain stable.

Initially the patient's condition can change from moment to moment.

He can be stable one hour and be critical the next hour. A patient with mitral valve replacement can be essentially stable and within an hour show signs of cardiac tamponade. The new myocardial infarction patient may seem to be stable and then suddenly develop cardiogenic shock, heart failure, or ventricular fibrillation. The burn patient may be oriented and alert one day and the next day be combative and confused. All patients have internal fluidity, which leads to behavioral and physiological instability.

NURSING ASSESSMENT OF SENSORY OVERLOAD

The critical care nurse assesses sensory overload through the patient's behavioral response. Sensory overload can produce a variety of psychedelic effects. Individuals appear to have an optimal level of stimulation. According to Ludwig (1972), laboratory findings help to account for alterations in consciousness found in a number of intriguing clinical conditions, all of which are associated with the common denominator of increased exteroceptive stimulation. Behavioral responses of the critically ill patient can be categorized into regulatory and cognitive behaviors.

Regulatory Behaviors

The regulatory system involves input, processes, effectors, and feedback loops. It involves stimuli from the external environment and from changes in the internal state of dynamic equilibrium. The regulatory behaviors are physiological responses and consist of the following (Baker 1984):

Regulatory Behaviors
Sweating hands
Constriction of peripheral blood vessels
Flutter in chest
Fidgetiness
Tachycardia
Increased cerebral blood flow
Numbness
Anorexia
Hyperventilation
Galvanic skin response
Increased blood cortisol and cholesterol

Cognitive Behaviors

The cognator system involves inputs from internal and external stimuli which include psychological and social factors. The specific aspects of the congator mechanism consist of perceptual/information processing, learning, judgment, and emotion. Sensory overload can be comparable to ICU psychosis since both cause a global clouding of consciousness. Sensory overload results from a potentially reversible impairment of the ability to maintain attention and cognitive processes. The patient's ability to think, perceive, and remember decreases (Ballard 1981). The cognitive behaviors associated with sensory overload consist of the following (Ludwig 1972):

Cognitive Behaviors
Perceptual disorders:
Hallucination
Sound distortion
Disturbed sense of time:
Time expansion
Otherwordly feelings:
Unpleasantness
Floating in space
Feelings of loss of control
Somatic effects
Diminished reality testing:
Paranoia

NURSING DIAGNOSIS OF SENSORY OVERLOAD

The nursing diagnosis is a statement of the current problem. Regulatory and cognitive behaviors coupled with stressors causing the problem combine to help the nurse to make her diagnosis. The overall problem is sensory overload. The external stressors contributing to sensory overload are environmental. Specific environmental stressors consist of noise from supportive devices, patients, or staff; painful procedures; and lights. Internal stimuli can be the patient's perception of his immediate environment and his ability to censor incoming stimuli.

NURSING INTERVENTIONS
TO REDUCE SENSORY OVERLOAD

It is evident that the nurse is responsible for the optimal functioning of her unit. Part of her responsibility is to control the environment for the well-being of her patient, including the reduction of unnecessary sensory stimuli. The nurse must remember that she cannot create an environment to meet all needs. As Gelwicks (1966) points out, one "can never create a physical environment which will be all things to all people. The meaning of a particular environment, its emotional impact, and the consequences for an individual's behavior are significantly influenced by the physical and socioeconomic environment to which he has been accustomed prior to being admitted to the hospital" (p. 93). Patients who live in a sensorially oriented environment may not experience overwhelming sensory overload; although overload will be present, they are better able to cope with the situation. Other patients coming from less hectic environments will experience greater degrees of environmental overdose. Because the patient experiences sensory overdose in his perceptual field, the nurse uses the field's properties to reduce excess stimulation.

Fluidity

Every organism is in a complex interaction with its physical environment. In order to keep the detached human being physically and mentally well, it is important to establish an environment that will help keep him human as well as functionally efficient (Gelwicks 1966). From the moment an illness strikes, the patient must interact with his physical environment in a way that is different from his usual daily encounters. The change starts the moment he is placed in the ambulance and continues until his discharge from the hospital. In between these points, he is exposed to interactions of different degree of complexity. Each interaction creates changes, because those things involved in the interaction all have fluidity. Some of the interactions are meaningful to the patient, whereas others are meaningless. Because the patient's perceptual field will not allow him to differentiate events while in crisis, the nurse has the responsibility to differentiate the two.

The nurse can begin sensory reduction the moment her patient arrives in the emergency room. This implies that her actions must be purposeful. She does not enter and leave his environment just to see what exciting things are happening or to stare at him. Usually the atmosphere around a critically ill patient is busy with people moving briskly into and out of his perceptual field. At this time, the nurse can become a constantly organized stimulus in her patient's fluid world. She can remain with him and administer to his physiological and psychological needs. The nurse can begin her purposeful interaction with a simple introduction. She can say, for example, "Hello, my name is Nancy." In the process she extends her hand and shakes his. This simple and brief interaction accomplishes two goals: she has created warmth in a seemingly sterile and cold environment, and she is able to assess the color of his nail beds, and warmth of his skin, and evidence of perspiration in the palm of his hand, which may be due to anxiety. Next, without touching the patient, she makes a visual assessment, which tells her how quickly she needs to obtain other physical data such as vital signs or an EKG pattern, or how rapidly she should seek a respirator or other emergency equipment. If her visual assessment indicates that the patient is stable, she can calmly and purposefully obtain additional data.

Sometimes it seems as though nurses try to obtain all their data within the first five minutes after the patient's arrival. Naturally there are some situations that require such speed. Nursing actions often create a sense of drama and mystery in which overdramatic flurry in obtaining data can lead to sensory overload. Our drama reflects the opening scene of a play. If the actors run around in chaos, the play will be disorganized. Actors who are confident and purposeful make for a smooth-running play. The emergency room is analogous to the first scene of a play. It sets the pace for either a smooth or chaotic hospitalization. It is here that the patient feels he is entering either an organized caring environment that will lead to wellness or a disorganized one that will lead to destruction. Like the actors, nurses must be groomed to move in a purposeful and organized manner.

Within the fluidity stage of sensory overload, meaningful touch is known to be significant, although studies on the precise physiologic responses to touch are inconclusive. In a study by Knable (1981) of four curarized patients in a shock trauma unit, nurses touched the patients in handholding or pulse taking. All four patients showed changes in heart rate regardless of their level of consciousness. Three patients exhibited rate decreases while the fourth had an increase. Several nurses claimed touch in the form of hand-holding really made them want to help the patient and seemed to break down barriers. McCorkle (1974) found in her study of critically ill patients that touch facilitated quick rapport and revealed a greater number of positive facial expressions in the experimental group but no change in the monitored heart rate.

The nurse can extend her interaction to include the family. The family needs to know how their loved one is progressing and vice versa. Such awareness will serve to reduce the anxieties, fears, and concerns that constitute additional incoming sensory stimuli. Furthermore, if the admitting crisis has subsided and if the patient is simply waiting to be transferred to a critical care unit, it is possible to let the immediate family see him. The family has real meaning to the patient. The family is the only familiar thing in his new physical environment. The nurse may reduce stimuli by having a family member talk with the admission office, removing one additional person from entering the patient's perceptual field.

The nurse can further reduce stimuli from strangers by transporting the patient from the emergency room to a critical care unit herself. Normally when the patient is not in crisis, attendants do the transporting, but they may not know the patient and may become insecure in his presence. Their goal is to get rid of him and the responsibility. The nurse, on the other hand, knows the patient and his needs. She has confidence in her knowledge. She knows how quickly the patient must be transported to ensure his safety. The ride between the emergency room and the critical care unit is like the transition between the scenes or acts of a play. The patient is getting ready for the next act.

Intensity

Inside the critical care unit, the patient will meet yet another nurse. Because he is again in an unfamiliar environment, his perceptual field becomes distorted. His image of the new nameless nurse is blurred. Like the emergency room nurse, the critical care nurse gives herself a name identity, let us say,

Karen. Hopefully Karen has been informed of the patient's impending arrival. She can assemble ahead of time all the various pieces of machinery, wires, and tubes necessary to initiate him into his physical environment. Such organization minimizes her need to move in and out of his environment, thus causing sensory overload.

The critical care nurse knows that intense relationships often develop between the nurse, patient, and their families in critical care. Feelings of shock, grief, helplessness, fear, and frustration often accompany these relationships and may tend to categorize some of the reactions that occur in response to the highly stressful environment (Gowan 1979).

A patient who is not in severe crisis can have only one nurse admitting him into the unit. The nurse must take the time to reduce stimuli and make his first encounter in the unit a positive warm one. Obviously one nurse will create enough stimuli. A one-to-one ratio gives the two people an opportunity to interact. The nurse can, as DeMeyer (1967) advises, make every effort to "create an environment that will contribute to, rather than distract from, the physical and emotional function of the patient" (p. 268). She can create a relaxed environment, free of extraneous sensory input, and she can do this through stimulis reduction. Stimulis reduction involves controlling unnecessary auditory stimuli from machinery, staff, and other patients. It also involves visual reduction of meaningless stimuli.

Environmental noise can be a possible hazard to the patient. Noise can elicit a stress response. Such a response is associated with autonomic and endocrine changes. Consequently, unnecessary noise could clearly augment the stress and trauma suffered by the patient who has had recent illness, injury, or surgery. Noise, as we have already seen, comes in a variety of packages. Some packages take the shape of inanimate objects in the patient's physical environment. These objects are stationary and remain continually in the patient's physical environment. Other packages are carried by what resembles lead feet. They make their own unique sounds that can be heard all over the unit.

First, there is the machinery found at the patient's bed. The machines click, clank, buzz, and hum along. If at all possible the nurse can use judgment in deciding the capability of her patient to deal with his equipment. The cardiac patient, for example, may spend all day watching his rhythm, afraid that the nurse will miss an important arrhythmia. His observations make him anxious. His nurse can turn the monitor around or cover it with a towel. She can reassure him that another nurse is watching his rhythm at the nurses' station. As Baker (1984) notes, the use of centralized monitoring system can help to control noise from supportive devices. For example, one person can monitor the cardioscope and obtain rhythm strips at the central console. Furthermore ventilators or IVAC (IV-regulating) machines can be kept away from the patient's head. The outflow valve from a ventilator can be turned away from the patient's ear, reducing sound by 10 dB(A). If a nurse anticipates potential ventricular fibrillation and places a defibrillator near her patient's bed, he will ask what the machine does and wonder why it is near his bed. Its presence will create anxiety. She can reduce this anxiety, however, if she is careful to keep the machine out of the patient's sight. Another patient may be in the process of weaning from his volume respirator. If he seems to be tolerating his pulmonary independence, the nurse can move the machine away from his immediate environment, close enough to maintain his security but far enough not to be a visual stimulus. Equipment can be used only as needed.

The extraneous noises of monitors and other sophisticated machinery in the environment serve to heighten the anxiety of the patient. The nurse needs to employ essential verbal and nonverbal communication if she is to allay the patient's apprehensions and facilitate his recovery (Knable 1981). Redding, Hargest, and Minsky (1977) note that high noise levels have been shown not only to have adverse physiological and psychological effects on patients but also to increase the error-proneness of critical care personnel. Additional studies can lead to measures that will reduce the noise levels in critical care.

The nurse must make every effort to allow for periods of uninterrupted sleep. At night, alarms can be channeled to buzz only at the nurses' station. Some critical care units do not have alarms on their EKG machines. Instead the nurse listens for the EKG paper running as a rhythmic strip is recorded. Other units still have the traditional buzzer at the patient's bedside and nurses' station. The alarm creates a startle response in both the nurse and patient. The more critical patient will have his own nurse closely monitoring him, and she can turn off the alarm sound and depend upon her eyes to note changes.

There are pieces of machinery that have flashing lights. The cardioscope, for example, has a light that flashes with each QRS complex; the IVAC machine light flashes with each drop of IV solution. The nurse cannot stop the click-click-click of the IVAC machine but she can block its flashing light, as well as the light on the cardioscope. Taping over the lights will in no way alter the function of either machine or endanger the patient's well-being. If all the noises from the machines continue to annoy her patient and interrupt his sleep, she can give him a set of disposable earplugs. These earplugs will eventually be a standard part of the critical care unit's admission set for use whenever the environment is noisy. Patients who have various pieces of equipment can be put in a group so that less critically ill patients can get adequate rest, and the nurse can place patients with hearing problems next to each other or next to a patient with various machines.

The nurse can further reduce visual stimulation by turning off overhead lights. Lights, as we discussed earlier, create sensory confusion, cause patients to lose track of time, and interrupt their sleep. Besides turning off the lights, the nurse can give her patient eye patches or a blindfold to wear. Like the earplugs, these will reduce overstimulation. They also may become standard equipment at the patient's bedside. It is not necessary to leave the lights on continuously. There may be only two patients out of six or ten whom one must observe for color changes. The nurse can have the flexibility within her unit to place such patients side by side. Critical care unit personnel must have autonomy to make independent changes as the intensity of the environment changes. Unfortunately, hospitals discourage nurses from making such changes on a frequent basis because they create administrative or admitting changes. The patient's wristband, addressograph stamp, and chart must all be changed. The administrators give more thought to administrative policies, procedures, rules, and regulations than to the internal and external needs of the patient.

The nurse can minimize environmental intensity and overdose by assessing which pieces of machinery should enter the patient's immediate physical environment and which should remain in the periphery. She can block visual stimulation and reduce auditory stimuli from machines, other patients, staff members, and lights.

In summary, Gowan (1979) has identified five nursing interventions that can reduce sensory overload by offering meaningful sensory input:

1. Dimming the lights at night
2. Organizing interventions to provide for uninterrupted sleep
3. Providing clocks and calendars to foster orientation
4. Using bright colors for curtains, walls, and linen
5. Placing monitoring equipment outside the patient's immediate environment.

A far-sighted way of controlling environmental overdose and intensity is to admit the critical care nurse to planning committees that decide design of critical care units. Nurses are familiar with design problems. They should be consulted as to design and location of the unit. Nurses in ICU, hemodialysis, respiratory, neurological, or burn units realize that, like CCU, these units also need carpets, drapes, and pictures. The carpets reduce the loud noises created by heavy feet, carts, and machines. Drapes or movable soundproof partitions reduce effects of visual and auditory overload. Baker (1984) points out that keeping patients separated in enclosed rooms markedly reduces distracting noise from surrounding patients. Hearing noise from other critically ill patients may contribute to misinterpretation, anxiety, fear, and confusion.

Direction

The nurse can instill in her patient a sense of goal-directedness. The patient needs to know that his physical environment is organizationally directed toward a level of wellness. If he continuously experiences environmental overdose he will not derive meaning from the environment. Combs and Snygg (1959) note that each of us is constantly searching his field for details and meanings that will better enable us to satisfy needs. This process, which is called differentiation, involves a continual change in the perceptual field caused by the constant rise of new characters into figures and the consequent lapse of other characters into the ground. It is through differentiation that change in the perceptual field, and hence change in behavior, occurs. According to Combs and Snygg, "It is the differentiation an individual is able to make in his perceptual field that determines the nature of his perceptions—both the direct perceptions of concrete events apprehended through our sense organs and the perceptions of complex events understood only through the medium of abstract thought" (p. 30).

The nurse attempts to explain the function and purpose of the equipment and avoids the use of technical jargon (Gowan 1979). Initially, the nurse must differentiate details in the patient's perceptual field. The environment is new and foreign to him. In time he becomes more aware of his environment, and his nurse helps him derive meaning from the previously meaningless stimuli. He grows in his ability to differentiate independently the direction of his internal and external environment. The nurse fosters this direction by teaching the patient those things pertinent to him but does not overload him with extraneous and meaningless information. Meaningful data include explanation of his physical environment, physiological change, and behavioral responses to change in both. By selective teaching, the nurse can reduce the possibility of teaching overload.

Stability

The nurse can help the patient achieve stability through effective communication. Effective communication between patients and staff in critical care is often altered due to increased stimuli from mechanical devices, a variety of noises, increased degrees of tension and stress, chaos from excessive traffic, poor staffing patterns, and architectural design (Knable 1981). Nevertheless the nurse can overcome these obstacles so that communication is maintained among the staff, family, and patient.

The nurse's goal regarding stability of perceptual field is simply to reinforce it. As the patient approaches physiological and behavioral stability, the nurse can evaluate the appropriateness of her nursing interventions. Since his condition is no longer critical, she can reduce the number of technical stimuli. The patient will interpret this reduction as a sign of progress towards affirmative direction and stability.

NURSING EVALUATION

Evaluation of the patient's problem and nursing care is an ongoing process. The nurse assesses regulatory and cognitive behaviors supporting the diagnosis of sensory overload. The interventions designed to reduce sensory overload are evaluated for their effectiveness. Depending upon the severity of sensory overload and behavioral response, the nurse may not see improvement until the patient is transferred to a less intense environment.

SUMMARY

The nurse has at her disposal the means of reducing environmental overdose. She realizes that she, herself, is a primary source of overload. The critical care nurse knows that her patient's perceptual field becomes affected in illness. Furthermore, she understands that the environment of critical care units can create psychological hazards. It is possible, however, for the units to provide optimal surveillance while simultaneously not providing environmental overdose. The hectic atmosphere of crisis is not conducive for relaxation, but with more astute observations and a concerted effect by nurses, it is possible to reduce environmental overdose.

REFERENCES

ABRAM, HARRY, "Adaptation to Open Heart: A Psychiatric Study of Response to the Threat of Death," *American Journal of Psychiatry*, 122, no. 6 (December 1965), p. 665.
——, "Psychological Aspects of the Intensive Care Unit," *Hospital Medicine*, 109, (December 1969), 94-95.

AIKEN, R. J., "Quantitative Noise Analysis in a Modern Hospital," *Archives of Environmental Health*, 37 (1982), 361-364.

ALPERN, MATHEW, *Sensory Process*. Belmont, Calif.: Brooks-Cole, 1967.

BAKER, CAROL, "Sensory Overload and Noise in the ICU: Sources of Environmental Stress," *Critical Care Quarterly*, 6, no. 4 (March 1984), 66-80.

BALLARD, K. S., "Identification of Environmental Stressors for Patients in a Surgical Intensive Care Unit," *Issues in Mental Health Nursing*, 3 (1981), 89-108.

BARRY, M. J., "Sensory Alterations, Overload and Underload: Making a Nursing Diagnosis," in *Current Practice in Nursing Care of the Adult*, Vol 1, ed. M. Kennedy and C. Pfeifen, pp. 33-45. St. Louis: C. V. Mosby, 1979.

BENTLEY, S., F. MURPHY, and H. DUDLEY, "Perceived Noise in Surgical Wards and in Intensive Care Area: An Objective Analysis," *British Medical Journal*, 2 (1977), 1503-1506.

CARLSON, DUANE, "Noise Control Program Is Quiet Success," *Modern Hospital*, 105 (December 1965), 82-85.

COMBS, ARTHUR W., and DONALD SNYGG, *Individual Behavior,* rev. ed. New York: Harper & Row, 1959.

DEMEYER, JOANNA, "The Environment of the Intensive Care Unit," *Nursing Forum*, 6, no. 3 (1967), 268.

DUFFY, ELIZABETH, "The Concept of Energy Mobilization," *Psychological Review*, 58 (1951), 30-39.

GELWICKS, LOYIS, "Best Function Needs Right Environment," *Modern Hospital*, 106, no. 3 (March 1966), 93.

GOLDBERGER, LEO, "Sensory Deprivation and Overload," in *Handbook of Stress: Theoretical and Clinical Aspects*, ed. Leo Goldberger and Shlomo Breznitz, pp. 410-418. New York: Free Press, 1982.

GOWAN, NANCY, "The Perceptual World of the Intensive Care Unit: An Overview of Some Environmental Considerations in the Helping Relationship," *Heart and Lung*, 8, no. 2 (March-April 1979), 340-344.

HASLAM, PAMELA, "Noise in Hospitals: Its Effect on the Patient," *Nursing Clinics of North America*, 5, no. 4 (December 1970), 717.

HAYEK, FRIEDRICH, *The Sensory Disorder*. Chicago: University of Chicago Press, 1963.

ITTELSON, W. H., "Experiments in Perception," *Scientific American*, August 1951, 2-7.

KNABLE, JACKIE, "Handholding: One Means of Transcending Barrier of Communication," *Heart and Lung*, 10, no. 6 (November-December 1981), 1106-1110.

KORNFIELD, DONALD, "Psychological Hazards of the Intensive Care Unit," *Nursing Clinics of North America*, 3, no. 1 (March 1968), 41-51.

LANDIS, C., and W. A. HUNT, *The Startle Pattern*. New York: Farrar, Straus & Giroux, 1931.

LEVITT, LYNN, and GLORIA LEVENTHAL, "Effect of Density and Environmental Noise on Perception of Time, the Situation, and Others," *Perceptual and Motor Skills*, 47 (1978), 999-1009.

LINDSLEY, DONALD, "Common Factors in Sensory Deprivation, Sensory Distortion and Sensory Overload," in *Sensory Deprivation*, ed. P. Solomon, p. 176. Cambridge, Mass.: Harvard University Press, 1965.

LUDWIG, ARNOLD, "Psychedelic Effects Produced by Sensory Overload," *American Journal of Psychiatry*, 128, no. 10 (April 1972), 114-117.

MCCORKLE, R., "Effects of Touch on Seriously Ill Patients," *Nursing Research*, 3, (1974), 125.

MITCHELL, PAMELA HOLSCLAW, *Concepts Basic to Nursing*. New York: McGraw-Hill, 1973.

MUELLER, CONRAD, *Sensory Psychology*. Englewood Cliffs, N.J.: Prentice-Hall 1965.

NOBLE, M. A., "Communication in the ICU: Therapeutic or Disturbing?" *Nursing Outlook*, 27 (1979), 195-198.

PUTT, A., "Effects of Noise on Fatigue in Healthy Middle-Aged Adults," *Communicating Nursing Research*, 8 (1971), 24-34.

REDDING, JOSEPH, THOMAS HARGEST, and STEPHEN MINSKY, "How Noisy Is Intensive Care?" *Critical Care Medicine*, 5, no. 6 (1977), 275-276.

SCHULTZ, DUANE, *Sensory Restriction: Effects on Behavior*. New York: Academic Press, 1965.

SEIDLITZ, P., "Excessive Noise Levels Detrimental to Patients, Staff," *Hospital Progress*, 62 (1981), 54-64.

SUEDELD, PETER, *Restricted Environmental Stimulation*. New York: John Wiley, 1980.

TAYLOR, D. E., "Problems of Patients in an ICU: The Etiology and Prevention of ICU Syndrome," *International Journal of Nursing Studies*, 8 (February 1971), 48.

WERNER, HEINZ, "Toward a General Theory of Perception," *Psychological Review*, 59 (July 1952), 324-338.

WOODS, N. F., and S. A. FALK, "Noise Stimuli in the Acute Care Area," *Nursing Research*, 23 (1974), 144.

WORRELL, JUDITH, "Nursing Implications in Sensory Deprivation," *Advanced Concepts in Clinical Nursing*, ed. Kay Corman Kintzel, p. 130. Philadelphia: Lippincott, 1971.

13

Sensory Deprivation

BEHAVIORAL OBJECTIVES

1. Define the terms *emotional deprivation, perceptual deprivation,* and *sensory deprivation.*
2. Identify how reduction in stimulation of senses applies to the critically ill patient.
3. Describe how reduction in meaningfulness of stimulation affects the critically ill patient.
4. Describe how restriction of body movement affects the critically ill patient.
5. Identify five regulatory behaviors associated with sensory deprivation.
6. Identify five cognitive behaviors associated with sensory deprivation.
7. Describe how the nurse can reduce sensory deprivation by managing the patient's environment and maintaining meaningful stimulation.

During the past several years, more critical care nurses have become cognizant of the concept of sensory deprivation. Nurses know that an individual's sensory environment can have a profound effect upon his or her behavior. For example, polar explorers, shipwrecked sailors, and prisoners of war have experienced changes in mood, perception, and thinking. Scientists are still studying data about changes that occur in space flight.

Research in sensory deprivation has dealt with the effects of long-term sensory and/or social deprivation during development and of relatively brief deprivation with adult organisms. The first category of this research has dealt mostly with experimental treatment of subhuman species while the latter typically has involved human beings who were isolated in natural situations. According to Suedfeld (1980), sensory deprivation research was originally conceived partly to test the then-dominant theory that the initiation of behavior was generally traceable to disruptions of physiological homeostasis. A radical version of drive-reduction theory would predict that when placed in a restricted environment the individual would not be motivated toward mental or physical activity. The findings contradicted the hypothesis. There have been recent studies of boredom and vigilance, and the popularity of theories of activation and arousal has increased (Suedfeld 1969; 1980).

Traditionally, relatively healthy individuals have been used for studies of sensory deprivation. These individuals were placed in environments where they could be isolated from sensory input. What is needed today is scrutiny of the relationship between hospitalization and sensory deprivation. Studies have examined these relationships on a limited basis; scholars have looked at patients with eye surgery, with casts, and those confined to a tank respirator.

Now we need to study the relationship between the patient and the critical care environment. We must find out whether the critical care environment could cause sensory deprivation. Some people would immediately think that such an environment is much too hectic to cause sensory or technological deprivation since it is filled with tremendous sensory input, as we saw in the previous chapter. However, we must remember that while the patient may experience environmental or sensory overdose, he may simultaneously experience emotional deprivation. Moreover, if the stimulation he receives is not patterned in a meaningful way, the patient can feel sensory deprivation even while living in the hectic critical care environment. The degree and duration of deprivation vary with each patient and unit involved.

The critical care nurse needs to be aware of contributing factors that could lead to sensory deprivation. Once an awareness exists, the nurse can look to her patient's environment and discover creative ways of preventing or alleviating the potential problem. First, it would be helpful to define sensory deprivation and some of its related terms.

DEFINITION OF TERMS

How an individual responds to an altered sensory environment is influenced by his or her ability to handle the alteration and variables in the environment. It is not only the quality of stimulation that is significant for cortical arousal, but also the quantity. An altered sensory environment, then, upsets the balance of function of the reticular activating system (Aiello 1978).

Sensory deprivation goes by a variety of names: technological deprivation, perceptual deprivation, isolation, sensory restriction, and confinement. It deals with the phenomena that result from reduction in the absolute level and/or degree of structure in sensory input. We will examine emotional, perceptual, and sensory deprivation.

Emotional Deprivation

The terms *emotional deprivation* and *technological deprivation* can be used interchangeably. In a highly technical environment dominated by machines, the patient loses precedence to the machine. The patient then experiences technological deprivation. With technological deprivation comes emotional deprivation. For example, a patient in ICU may be surrounded by various pieces of equipment: a cardioscope, a chest tube and gomco suction, a CVP, an arterial line, a Swan-Ganz line, a Foley catheter, IVs, and a respirator. As the nurse comes to the patient's bed, she will first approach his equipment and only later look at the patient. This is a normal response: she must run rhythm strips, check dial settings on the respirator, check wave forms and pressure settings, check rate of IV solution, and carry out other procedures. After gathering her data, the nurse will move toward her patient and possibly even touch him, but she has given more nursing care time to the various machines than to the patient. This is not the fault of the nurse: she must fill the squares on her patient's flow sheet with numerical values and words at the designated time. Heaven help the nurse whose doctor arrives before she has properly filled all the squares. Because of her patient responsibilities, her time is limited. She must gather her data and move on to the next patient. Day nurses must gather their data before the parade of doctors and technicians begins.

Sometimes machines make the data collection too easy. The nurse may begin to rely on machines for data instead of her eyes and judgment. Reliance on machines diminishes the amount of sensory input to the patient from touch. When the nurse limits her touches to the patient's equipment, the patient experiences emotional or technological deprivation.

Perceptual Deprivation

In recent years, the labels *sensory deprivation* and *perceptual deprivation* have been used systematically in some laboratory investigations. Absence or reduction of stimulus variability is referred to as *perceptual deviation* or *perceptual isolation*. This occurs when the quality of stimulus from the environment remains constant, but when there is reduced patterning, imposed structuring, and homogeneous stimulation. Perceptual deprivation occurs in an environment in which sound is muffled, light is diffused, and bodily sensations are nondistinct (Worrell 1971). Perceptual deprivation is experimentally induced in an environment designed to produce an absence of or decrease in meaningful patterning or sensory stimuli (Bolin 1974).

Critical care units have their own unique sounds. Depending on the unit and the patient's placement within that unit, sounds can be either muffled or intense. The sounds may seem distant to the patient housed next to the sounds. The patient in hemodialysis may only hear the humming of his dialysis machine, punctuated by an occasional alarm. The respiratory care patient hears the humming, sighing, and buzzing of his volume respirator.

The isolation patient may only hear the passing of footsteps; all other sounds are distant and muffled. The coronary care patient hears the buzz of his cardioscope. The intensive care patient is surrounded by alarms or buzzes that have no meaning to the patient. Perceptual deprivation in these cases refers to reduction in the patterning or meaningfulness of stimulation.

Monotonous or varying stimuli found in critical care units are similar to conditions that lead to perceptual deprivation. Critical care units are characterized by the meaningless hum of life-supporting monitoring equipment, such as oxygen units, used to provide protection and comfort to the patient (Parent 1978).

As we move through our daily encounters, we are aware of bodily sensations, which help us to perceive our environment: the rain, the heat, the cold, the damp, and the potentially dangerous. The patient who is immobilized due to surgery, myocardial infarction, respiratory failure, or burns is unable to perceive his environment spatially. At one time he could move through space to perceive the world. Now he must depend on other sensory processes. He has reduced sensory input. Perceptual deprivation also refers to the reduction in the meaningfulness of stimulation.

Sensory Deprivation

Sensory deprivation is caused by a reduction in the amount and intensity of sensory input. It also implies a decrease in the amount and intensity of meaningful sensory input. Furthermore, deprivation can occur when the absolute level and/or degree of structure in sensory input are reduced (Bolin 1974; Linn 1979: Ballard 1981). In experimental situations, sensory deprivation is the generic term for a variety of complex conditions aimed at drastically reducing the level of variability of a person's normal stimulation from, and commerce with, his environment for a relatively prolonged period of time (Goldberger 1982).

To deprive is to take away. The sensory process is not completely taken away in an intensive care unit, and the individual is not divested of the sensory experience. The experience of sensory deprivation can be described as one in which reception or perception of stimuli is blocked or altered, or one in which the environmental stimuli themselves are blocked or altered. According to Chodil and Williams (1970),

> All cases of sensory deprivation will exhibit an alteration of sensory input in the form of sensory underload. Stimuli in the environment may be below normal level for attention purposes. Therefore the stimuli do not find the body receptors at tension or ready to respond. Repetition, lack of change, or cues of inadequate intensity exist. Poorly functioning receptors will block adequate stimuli and result in sensory underload. Perception altered by an anxiety state will not allow the body to attend to a normal stimulus received by a healthy receptor. (P. 456)

Wood (1977) defines sensory deprivation as a combination of social isolation and reduced sensory stimulation, leading to an environment providing little stimulus change. Disturbances in vision, hearing, body-touch, smell, taste, and cognition as well as noncompliant behaviors manifested by patients can be signs of sensory deprivation.

Sensory deprivation is not an isolated condition; it occurs with immobilization, confinement, and interpersonal isolation, and each condition is stressful. Sensory isolation and sensory deprivation refer to reduction in quality, with or without a change in pattern. The deprivation may be of single modality: for example, one sensory channel may be blocked due to the aging process or an injury. An individual, due to cataracts or trauma to the eyes, may lose his sight. But deprivation can also be multimodal. The three major senses—visual, auditory, and touch—can become involved.

The hospitalized patient experiences clinical sensory deprivation. Such hospitalized individuals undergo more than the average degree of reduced stimulation, social isolation, and/or physical confinement. These are the people who may suffer from eye disorders, orthopedic patients, individuals in reverse isolation, neurological disorder patients, and those undergoing long-term care. Patients in critical care units can also be included. Many of the older critically ill patients may have impaired sensory-perceptual function such as visual or hearing problems (Suedfeld 1980).

Major medical treatments sometimes necessitate immobilization. These include bedrest for a variety of illnesses and postoperative recovery from surgeries such as open heart surgery. Immobilized patients do exhibit some aversive and adverse reactions. For example, patients in bedrest situations have reported sensations in various modalities without observable concomitant external stimuli (Suedfeld 1980).

In order to evaluate a given deprivation situation, one should at the characteristics of the setting and of the person undergoing deprivation. Jackson (1971) believes important characteristics of the setting include the following:

> reduction in the amount of intensity of stimulation in each sensory modality (vision, hearing, touch, internal body sensation, taste, and smell); reduction in the patterning or meaningfulness of stimulation in each sensory modality; changes in stimulation other than decreases, such as the many new stimulations associated with hospitalization; restrictions imposed upon movements and body positions; degree of social isolation; duration of deprivation; and the realistic dangers, if any, which are present in the deprivation situation. (P. 46)

Aiello (1978) has noted that common characteristics are consistent in situations of sensory deprivation. First, there is lessened sensory input or sensory underload with repetition, lack of change, or cues of inadequate intensity. Poorly functioning receptors block adequate stimuli and result in sensory underload. A second characteristic is relevance deprivation in which there is a reduction in the patterning or meaningfulness of stimulation. Stimuli that stand out provide useful external information and become more meaningful. Third, there is alteration in the reticular activating system. In sensory deprivation cortical arousal is decreased.

It is interesting to note that there may be situations in which the results of sensory deprivation are not entirely negative. Stewart (1977) in a study of a total of 39 orthopedic patients found a decrease in negative affects including depression and anxiety, but not hostility, regardless of degree of immobilization or social isolation.

THE CONCEPT OF SENSORY DEPRIVATION APPLIED TO THE CRITICALLY ILL PATIENT

Hospitalization in a critical care unit increases the likelihood that the patient will experience sensory deprivation. The tense environment greatly alters the type of sensory input a patient receives. All familiar stimuli that help keep an individual oriented are missing.

In this section we will discuss patient behaviors caused by sensory deprivation due to reduction of stimulation in senses, reduction in meaningfulness of stimulation, removal from familiar stimulation, and restrictions imposed on bodily movements. One must remember that there are instances in which sensory deprivation and sensory overload, which were discussed in Chapter 12, resemble each other. One such instance has to do with reduction in meaningfulness of stimulation. Patients experiencing either deprivation or overload manifest similar behavioral responses.

Reduction of Stimulation of Senses

People tend to orient themselves to their environment by receiving and organizing stimuli, a process which involves the reticular activating system (RAS). It is the RAS which plays a significant role in the efficient processing and patterning of stimuli and in the resulting behavior. Both the quality and the quantity of stimulation are important for cortical arousal. The latter is reflected in stimulus variation and meaningful contact with the outside world so that behavioral efficiency can be achieved. An altered sensory environment can alter the optimal level of the RAS. When there is decreased sensory input, the RAS is no longer able to project a normal level of activation to the cortex. The stimulus-deprived person becomes more sensitive to the remaining stimulation, and, as a consequence, his thoughts and perceptions become diminished by residual stimuli. The patient may begin to hallucinate in an attempt to maintain an optimal level of arousal (Bolin 1974).

In a normal environment, the individual experiences stimulus density and stimulus variability. The patterning of environmental stimuli is of great importance to adaptive behavior. The patient in a critical care unit may be reacting to reduced intensity of some stimuli, to reduced patterning of stimuli, to increased intensity of other stimuli, to the addition of new stimuli, and to change in the meaning of stimuli. Patients in coronary care units, for example, experience unfamiliar stimuli related to the pain, fear, and discomfort induced by their condition and from dependency on the medical personnel and equipment. At the same time they experience social isolation and reduced input and motility (Suedfeld 1980).

Aiello (1978) notes that because of the often extensive, physically compromised condition of the critically ill patient, and the life-support techniques utilized to maintain the patient, normal sensory mechanisms are either blocked or at least interfered with.

Many patients experience a reduction in the amount or intensity of stimulation. Those that come to mind most vividly are the aged, tracheostomy, burn, or isolation patient. The aged patient may experience multimodal deprivation. Such patients have reduced visual, auditory, and taste sensations. To compensate for their reduction, the patient wears glasses and a hearing aid. His taste may be reduced not only from the aging process but also through the use of dentures. When an aged patient enters an intensive or coronary care unit, he may soon have to endure removal of his glasses, hearing aid, and dentures so that the staff can administer oxygen or insert an endotracheal tube. When his condition improves, the nurse may forget to give the patient back his prosthetic devices. She may find herself screaming in the patient's ear, before she remembers that his hearing aid has been neatly tucked away in the nightstand. Next, the nurse may give the patient his diet tray and leave him alone to eat. When she returns to pick up the tray, she may discover more food on the patient than in him. The patient will obviously need his glasses and dentures in order to enjoy his meal. If the nurse does not wear glasses, a hearing aid, or dentures, she may have a tendency to forget that her aged patient depends on these devices.

The patient who has had a tracheostomy experiences loss of auditory stimulation created by his own voice. Some tracheostomy patients obviously become anxious when they are unable to speak. They fail to realize that their voice has not been permanently lost. The nurse may need to deflate the cuff so that the patient can create auditory stimulation through use of his voice. Each hour, as the cuff is deflated, the patient should be encouraged to talk. The patient may become preoccupied with his illness and his inability to make auditory stimulation. He needs reassurance that as his respiratory problems stabilize, he will regain use of his voice. As Meinhart and Aspinall (1969) point out, the person whose "Physical and emotional energies are absorbed in the struggle to overcome physical illness . . . may manifest a lowered level of perception, awareness, recognition and realization" (p. 994).*

The burn patient can also experience reduction in stimulation. This is especially true if the burns involve much of the patient's body. He may have experienced burns of his face, arms, chest, and hands. His sense of hearing is not impaired, but his sense of vision, touch, and bodily sensations are reduced. The visual reduction may have begun the moment he was injured. Consequently, he is unable to perceive happenings or changes within his environment. He has no visual frame of reference or visual contact with the world around him. If he is able to see his environment momentarily, he will have a vague sense of orientation, but as the edema increases, his visual awareness and stimulation will be reduced. He hears sounds but does not know their significance or location. He may perceive them to originate from the left side of his bed only to discover they originate from the right. His internal world becomes confused. He is unable to receive visual input. He hears voices, but they have no face or form. In time he learns to recognize his nurse by her footsteps or voice.

The patient with burns on his hands as well as face experiences further communication impairment. He is unable to touch objects or people in his environment because of the pain involved. Although he is subjected to the sensation of touch, he is unable to initiate touch. Furthermore, his bodily sensations are reduced or altered due to the burns. The sensations he experiences may be reduced or intensified. The sensation of pain can be intensive. The sensation of heat versus cold can be intensified; or the patient may lose altogether the ability to sense the changes. He no longer has hair, which gave him piloerection and heat isolation. His bodily sensations may be distorted and blurred.

With reduction in intensity of stimulation, the patient experiences deprivation, and, with deprivation, he also experiences behavioral changes. Most scientists believe that the reticular activating system plays an important role in altering a patient's behavior. Its response level projects upon the cortex, where it influences perception and learning, and it probably plays a role in the control of emotions. When the reticular system is affected through reduced sensory input, the role of cortical function may become more prominent. This may explain the behavioral changes that have been observed in patients who experience sensory deprivation (Ruff 1966).

A patient in isolation may experience social isolation. Due to his infection, he is isolated from all other people with whom he has a common identity, the other patients. He is in a room by himself. People who enter his room wear masks and protective gowns. The only physical identity they present to him is a set of eyes. He hears voices and footsteps quickly passing his room, but due to their physical separateness, they do not represent meaningful stimuli. His nurses may enter his environment only to perform the necessary procedures and leave. Again, he is left alone. His senses may be intact and capable of stimulation, but his immediate environment is devoid of such stimulation.

As Suedfeld (1980) points out, it is impossible to separate the psychological effects of the isolation from those of the illness itself and from other aspects of treatments. Some of the psychological effects of sensory deprivation are depression, anxiety, irregular sleep, and psychological withdrawal.

Because of the reduction in the amount of intensity of stimulation, the patient may withdraw into sleep. It is not unusual to learn from a report that a patient spent most of his day sleeping. Most of us would say, "Great, I wish I could do the same thing." Possibly we are tired, and sleep would be appropriate, but this may not be the case for our patients. We can evaluate why the patient slept most of the day. A look at the nursing notes may reveal that he had a "good" night. Of course there are times when the patient's environment may have been overstimulating or he may himself have become more critical. Sleep in this case is the best thing. However, if these events did not occur, and if the patient still sleeps, his nurse must examine his environment and the stimulation therein. She may discover that he is bored and deprived. He may even have had episodes of hallucinations. One view suggests that isolation demonstrates how the brain itself can become a source of information. During isolation, the brain stores energy that cannot be discharged through normal somatic channels. Under these conditions, the mind projects its contents outward in the form of delusions and hallucinations. Perceptual monotony may cause the patient to become inattentive to his environment. In turn, his decreased ability to sustain attention may cause him to be unable to perceive his environment accurately (Ruff, 1966).

Reduction in Meaningfulness of Stimulation

Meaningless and unpatterned sensory input are present in the clinical setting. To the patient in the hospital, cardioscopes, ventilators, and suction machines are strange and complex gadgets. Because unit routines and technical language have little meaning, monotony and boredom can result. The technological world surrounding the critical care patient has little meaning to him. He sees strange pieces of machinery and wonders what they all do. He feels as if he is wired for sound, with all his wires and tubes connected to their appropriate machines. As his nurse moves into his technical environment, he watches her turn dials, make recordings, and adjust settings. He sees in her a sense of competency and feels comfortable in her care. The nurse seems like a master of his machine-oriented world.

But while the nurse adjusts the machine and records the data, the machine in itself is a foreign object, humming monotonously, a cacophony of mysterious technology. Without an explanation of the objects in his environment, the patient is left alone with his meaningless machines. Patients have a need to order the stimuli in their environment into a meaningful pattern. The experience of deprivation may not allow the critical care patient to derive meaning. When the deprivation barrier cannot be overcome, the unfulfilled need for sensory input leads to behavior characterized by regression, disorganization of sensory coordination, and difficulty in thinking coherently.

A patient must also be able to derive meaning from words and actions. The messages received from staff regarding the patient's illness, progress, and future must be on the level of his comprehension. Doctors or nurses who talk to each other or the patient on a technical level will only force him to withdraw. The incoming verbal stimuli have no significance. He will not understand words like hypokalemia, ischemic changes, extension of myocardial infarction, granulation, cardiac catheterization, disseminated intravascular coagulation, adult respiratory distress syndrome, and azotemia.

Instead of listening to the nurse's and doctor's discussion, he assumes they are talking in symbolic language to each other. Therefore he attempts not to eavesdrop on their conversation, even though it involves him. He simply does not understand the "big words" or technical language. Again, absence of meaningful stimulation produces the effects of sensory deprivation. According to Worrell (1971), "It appears that it may not be the quantity of changes in sensation that the brain requires for normal functioning, but a continuous, meaningful contact with the outside world" (p. 134).

Placement of the patient within a critical care unit must also have meaning. Patients in hemodialysis, CCU, and the burn unit realize why they are in such units. CCU, hemodialysis, and burn patients can look around and see other patients like themselves. They have similar needs and problems. To a certain extent, this is also true of the ICU patient. Even though their needs are more varied, there nevertheless exist common basic needs. In each setting, patients can observe the progress of their neighbors and compare it to their own progress. They can even talk with each other and compare progress. The isolation patient, on the other hand, is in a world all of his own. He experiences aloneness of isolation. He has lost his reference to models in the external world. Both sensory stimulation and social contact are required for maintaining these models and sensory deprivation disrupts the vital evaluative processes.

Removal from Familiar Stimulation

The environment of critical care has been assessed as the cause of an altered sensory experience. When he becomes ill, the patient must quickly leave his familiar settings. He is taken away from his comfortable bed and pajamas, his favorite overstuffed arm chair, and the other familiar objects—and people—of his everyday life. At home he could relax, unwind, and feel secure. He had independence and personal freedom of choice. He had a variety of stimuli around him at all times. He could increase or decrease the stimuli as he wished.

As discussed earlier, perceptual deprivation is a form of sensory deprivation. Noises and constant light are examples of perceptual deprivation. Meaningless and unpatterned input such as strange machines, technical language, strict hospital routines, and isolation from friends and family all contribute to sensory deprivation (Ballard 1981).

The actual number of stimuli in the patient's environment diminishes when he enters the hospital. He leaves behind the familiar sights, sounds, and smells, and he no longer has close tactile contact with his family. Once in the hospital, someone else assumes his decision-making responsibility. He exchanges the familiar for the unfamiliar. His personal possessions are either locked up, sent home, or neatly placed in a closet elsewhere. His familiar and comfortable pajamas give way to a loose white gown and tight, constricting pants. His comfortable king-size bed is replaced by a hard, narrow bed with side rails. His private bathroom is replaced by a urinal, bedpan, or commode, none of which ensures privacy. He is not free to walk around his immediate environment, as he would normally have done. His freedom to ambulate, and to attain environmental stimulation, is restricted. He is even restricted in his ability to sit in a chair other than a commode. His environment may be devoid of a television set or radio. His familiar dining room table and chair are replaced by a bed and overside table. This is where he now eats his meals. His familiar tasty food is replaced by bland food, which may be lacking in oral stimulation. Depending upon his problem, he may not even be allowed food; he may instead receive an IV solution or nasal-gastric tube feedings. If there is room around his bed, he can have flowers. These can at least add sensory stimulation in the form of smell and color. The rules and regulation of visiting hours may restrict the presence of his family. These factors create deprivation.

Each critical care unit imposes its own special deprivation on the patient. There are still intensive care units that do not have windows. Consequently, the patient is unable to differentiate between day and night. He misses seeing the early morning sunrise, which may have represented to him the beginning of a new day. Patients without outside stimulation from windows have a tendency to become confused and disoriented. The natural light of the sun is replaced by artificial overhead lights, which can overstimulate the patient until he finally closes them out from boredom. In some critical care units, the patient's bed is surrounded by curtains that serve to separate him from other patients. The ensure his visual privacy. Environmental sounds can still be transmitted through the curtains, but he is protected from a fishbowl effect when using the bedpan or commode. The curtains each have their own design, stained by blood and medications of previous patients.

The patient who must stay in an isolation room is prevented from both communicating and contacting organisms. His input of hospital stimuli is also limited. He does not have the auditory or visual stimulation of neighbors. If the patient is not in acute crisis, he can have all the privacy he wants. The privacy goes with the private room. Here he has his own bathroom. He may event have a television set or radio. Even though he has some degree of sensory stimulation, his routine soon becomes monotonous. He prefers the human contact of social interaction, but because of isolation precautions, visitors are often discouraged. His immediate family members may be the only ones who are brave enough to enter the unclean environment. This alone may not be enough stimulation for the patient. After all, he may see his wife twice daily and feel he has exhausted his conversation during the first visit. In his boredom, the patient may spend time counting holes in the ceiling above his bed.

Coronary care units are usually very quiet units. The floors are carpeted in an attempt to reduce stimulation. The staff talk in whispers. If the patient is going to hear what his nurses are saying, he must be adept in lip reading. The nurses' station is usually enclosed in glass. With the doors closed, patients are unable to hear what their nurses are saying. The environment is usually a relaxed one. The only major sounds are the clanking of dinner carts or the humming of machines. A dialysis patient may be in a similar environment.

The only stimulation he receives is from other patients, staff, or machines. Because of fatigue, most hemodialysis patients sleep throughout their exchange.

Like the ICU patient, the burn patient may also be in an active environment. He realizes things are happening around him but is unable to participate in those events. If his eyes were injured, he has to listen to his environment. Even if the burn patient is able to receive visual stimulation from his environment, he may not have the energy to respond.

Illness absorbs a great portion of a person's attention and available emotional energy. Because of this, he is left with fewer resources for cognitive processes, and thus his adjustment to illness becomes more difficult (Aiello 1978). It is reasonable to speculate that due to the highly stressful nature of the illness and/or hospital experience, every patient may suffer a cognitive disturbance to some degree (Meinhart and Aspinall 1969). The degree is simply magnified for the critical care patient. As illness lowers the energy level of the patient, it also reduces the patient's cognitive level. There may be events in his environment that can stimulate him, but reduced cognition limits his awareness.

Successful adjustment of the critical care patient during illness requires that he maintain an integrated, coordinated functioning. He must also be able to interpret his environment correctly. If he only sees the familiar being replaced by the unfamiliar, he will have difficulty adjusting. He may be inclined to focus upon the negative aspects of his hospital environment. For example, the patient fails to understand why he cannot wear his pajamas. At least he feels properly covered with his own pajamas. In the excitement, his nurse may have failed to explain that it is difficult to thread IV tubing through the narrow sleeve of his pajama top. Furthermore, if his top is snug it could cause pressure points where the cardioscope leads are placed. With simple explanations, the nurse can get her patient to accept the hospital gown. There is no apparent reason why he could not wear his own bottoms. They may be more comfortable than the tight-fitting ones. With each subsequent loss of familiar stimulation, the nurse needs to offer meaningful explanations in its place. Such interpretation or explanation depends upon input from the real environment. Providing appropriate input is the role of the nurse who works with patients who experience sensory or technological deprivation.

Restriction Imposed on Body Movement

Illness not only absorbs a great portion of a patient's attention and available emotional energy, but it also reduces sensory input. This is especially true where one of the special senses has been affected by illness, but it also occurs in toxic and metabolic diseases that affect the central nervous system. Treatment procedures themselves often result in a change or reduction in contact with the environment and cause consequent functional changes in behavior (Linton 1965). A patient may be immobilized by a particular illness or injury. Immobility becomes a treatment procedure, and immobilization implies confinement, which produces stresses of its own. There are patients who are immobilized due to therapeutic approach to an illness or because they have lost mobility: patients whose movements are restricted by burns; whose movements are restricted by bedrest; who are recovering from an acute myocardial infarction; who have severe respiratory insufficiency; who have spinal cord injuries; who are in traction recovering from a severe auto accident; and postoperative patients who are confined by equipment and pain.

A severely burned patient has restricted sensory input due to confinement. His environment has tremendous sensory stimulation, but his energy levels are focused upon his injury. Therefore he is unable to take in from his environment anything beyond noises and sounds. He is also in severe pain. The patient with first- and second-degree burns experiences intolerable pain when he moves. His dressings and equipment further confine or immobilize him. Both have their therapeutic purposes, but they also serve to reduce bodily movement and bodily sensations derived from movement. If the burns are extensive, the patient may be confined to his bed. As his condition stabilizes, he is taken by stretcher to the Hubbard tank. Even though he is physically moving to a new environment, his visual perception is still limited to the ceiling, walls, and faces of the staff. Furthermore, the patient is not free to touch objects or people in his environment. The attempt would be too painful. Because he is immobilized with equipment, cumbersome dressings, and severe pain, he experiences perceptual deprivation. The deprevation seems to produce further bodily discomfort and cognitive difficulties. Medication can be given to reduce the pain, but it also has a tendency to reduce sensory input and possibly to produce sensory confusion.

There are patients whose movement is restricted by bedrest. The patient is confined to a territory four feet wide. This becomes his only environmental frame of reference. He can look through the side rails and partially see other beds, patients, and staff. Like the burn patient, his nearest constant visual stimulation is the ceiling, but when all the holes are counted, it becomes less stimulating. The ceiling never changes and always remains in sight. If his curtains are partially pulled, the patient's vision of the equipment is further restricted. He is unable to get out of bed and pull his own curtains. The primary reduction in stimulation that leads to deprivation is immobility. The patient is unable to gather sensory stimulation by walking around his bed. In addition, he is limited in his ability to extend himself physically in social contact with other patients and staff. To a certain extent, he is isolated even though he is not in an isolated setting. As Ziskind (1964) points out, a patient "can be isolated without marked curtailment of sensation from the physical environment but the stimuli are then of inanimate or at least nonpersonal nature, with the whole range of sensory stimuli related to social interchange excluded" (p. 226).

The acute myocardial infarction patient is immobilized to permit his myocardium to adapt to the crisis. He is physically immobilized by illness, cardioscope leads, oxygen, and IV tubing. He is also psychologically immobilized by anxiety and fear of death. Either factor limits his sensory input.

He may be afraid to move for fear of disrupting his cardioscope pattern, pulling his IV tubing out of place, endangering his heart, or increasing his pain. To most laypersons, their heart is the center of all activity. When their heart becomes sick or injured, they become anxious and fearful that the end is near. Their anxiety creates tunnel vision and perceptual sensory deprivation. The anxiety immobilizes their physical and psychological movement. They fail to hear that their condition is stable and their myocardium is healing. Until the patient is able to increase his mobility, he experiences reduced stimulation of his senses. He is forced into a monotonous environment.

The spinal cord patient is a classic example of someone whose movement is restricted. This type of patient becomes a prisoner in his own body. Unlike the patient restricted to his bed, the spinal cord patient is limited to the confines of his body. If he is a quadriplegic, he is unable to turn himself or touch the side rails. He is unable to lift his hands in an effort to reach out and touch his world. He is unable to experience sensory stimulation from bodily sensation, as he has no sensation. A tracheostomy restricts his vocal touching of people. Indeed the patient is totally restricted to his own body. The injury, itself, not the treatment, has rendered him immobile.

The orthopedic patient in critical care is immobilized by various tractions. He is subjected to prolonged monotonous immobilization. The traction limits him to one position, his back. The type of fracture and traction he has may limit his visual awareness. All he sees is the traction.

The postoperative patient does not suffer as much as the patients discussed above, but he, too, is temporarily immobilized by pain and equipment. This is especially true of the cardiac surgical patient who is surrounded by an arterial line, chest tube, cardioscope leads, a CVP, Swan-Ganz line, a Foley catheter, IVs, and possibly a pacemaker. He experiences overstimulation of some senses and understimulation of others. Until the surgical patient begins ambulating, he is confined to his bed. According to Worrell (1971), the psychological reaction to therapeutically realistic and necessary immobility may be related to changes in body image. These changes are influenced by immobility-induced sensory deprivation as well as by the modification of body image consequent to illness or injury. Immobility therefore reduces stimulation of the senses and creates deprivation.

NURSING ASSESSMENT OF SENSORY DEPRIVATION

The nurse assesses sensory deprivation through the patient's behavioral response. The responses are categorized into regulatory behaviors and cognitive behaviors.

Regulatory Behaviors

The regulator system involves inputs, processes, effectors, and feedback loops. It involves stimuli from the external environment and from changes in the internal state of dynamic equilibrium. The regulatory behaviors are physiological responses.

In sensory deprivation the patient experiences feelings of bodily changes in sensation, function, and position. There is impaired fine or gross motor coordination. These changes may be related to the feelings of changed function. Some of the regulatory behaviors associated with sensory deprivation may be due to stress reaction. Nevertheless the following regulatory behaviors can be attributed to sensory deprivation (Jackson and Ellis 1971; Esberger 1979; Ballard 1981):

Regulatory Behaviors

Increased galvanic skin response
Minor itching
Increased catecholamines
Altered electroencephalogram patterns
Feeling warmer or colder
Muscle movement
Numbness in fingers and toes

Cognitive Behaviors

The cognator system involves inputs from internal and external stimuli which include psychological and social factors. The specific aspects of the cognator mechanism consist of perceptual/information processing, learning, judgment, and emotion. The cognitive behaviors are psychological responses.

Bolin (1974) notes that altered sensory environments have been shown to produce changes in affect, cognition, and perception. Reported affective changes have included anxiety, fear, depression, and rapid changes in mood. The intensity of the changes can vary from mild to panic. Cognitive disturbances such as difficulty in maintaining an ordinary sequence of thoughts, and unusual or unrealistic ideas, ranging from the slightly strange to the frankly bizarre, are frequently reported as occurring in altered sensory environment.

Worrell (1971) believes that the major source of subjective stress produced by sensory or perceptual deprivation appears to stem from the loss of contact with reality. The individual experiences a confusion of internal and external sensation, an increase in primary process thinking, and disorientation in space and time overwhelm him. The patient may not realize that his wires and tubes are part of him, even though they are attached to external machines. In his confusion, he accidentally pulls out his IV, Foley catheter, or CVP tubing. He may temporarily forget he is in a hospital and attempt to get out of bed. The patient has no awareness of his actions other than that they elicit a negative response from his nurse. If the patient thinks he is home, he will see his nurse as an intruder. Furthermore, he may lose track of time. To him 11:00 P.M. may seem like 11:00 A.M. The patient also develops disturbance in perception characterized by decreased attention, selection, and organization, resulting in increasing degree of deprivation. As he loses attention, he becomes bored and finally disoriented.

Behavioral changes have been found to occur in sensory deprivation. The following cognitive behaviors are attributed to sensory deprivation (Wood 1977; Linn 1979):

Cognitive Behaviors
Visual and auditory hallucinations and illusions
Temporal and spatial disorganization
Inability to think clearly or to concentrate
Anxiety
Loss of sense of time
Delusions
Restlessness
Psychotic behavior
Noncompliance behavior
Confusion

Wood (1977) points out that sensory deprivation of extended duration is often characterized by decreased cortical activity and increased autonomic activity. The following behaviors are thought to occur:

1. Negative affective tone: depression
2. Reduced ability for sustained, self-directed activity: dependency
3. Disorganization or loss of control over cognition: confusion

The bored or disoriented patient fails to realize the significance and implications of events around him. They have no relevance to him. Relevance implies that the external information have use or meaning to the individual. When the usefulness of external information is reduced by alteration of stimuli or blockage of receptors, it becomes difficult to develop a sense of relatedness to the information at hand. An irrelevant environment is a boring one.

It was mentioned earlier that the reticular activating system (RAS) is responsible for arousal and alertness. Suedfeld (1980) points out that the unit for regulating activation, alertness, or the orienting reflex is involved because it is clear that states of arousal change under REST (Restricted Environmental Stimulation Therapy) conditions. Structurally, the units involved are the reticular formation and limbic system, the nonspecific nuclei of the thalamus, the caudate nucleus, and the hippocampus. Because of the close link between the orienting reflex and memory which is ascribed to this area of the brainstem, alterations in activation are associated with memory phenomena.

When stimulation of the RAS is reduced, the resulting behaviors include boredom, inactivity, and sleep. Sleep offers its own stimulation. At least in sleep the patient can dream. Sleep also helps to pass time which, to the patient, seems to stand still. Furthermore, sleep is an acceptable way to withdraw from one's monotonous environment.

The sensorially deprived patient has difficulty paying attention or concentrating on something and difficulty in maintaining an ordinary sequence of thought (Jackson and Ellis, 1971). Some critically ill patients experience noncompliant behavior. Noncompliant behaviors consist of removing bandages, pulling out tubes, getting up while on bedrest and engaging other prohibited activities, and refusing to cope with treatment ordered by the physician (Wood 1977).

NURSING DIAGNOSIS OF SENSORY DEPRIVATION

The nursing diagnosis is a statement of the current problem. Regulatory and cognitive behaviors coupled with stressors lead the nurse to diagnose the clinical problem of sensory deprivation. Internal stressors consist of alterations in sensory processing, age, illness, and meaninglessness of the stimuli. External stimuli are primarily environmental. Environmental stimuli consist of noise from supportive devices, patients, or staff; lights; and pain.

NURSING INTERVENTIONS ASSOCIATED WITH SENSORY DEPRIVATION

In providing nursing care for the sensorially deprived critically ill patient, the nurse knows that the regulatory or cognitive behavior can be attributed to a combination of physiological, psychological, and environmental factors. Furthermore the range of stimulation that may be considered normal varies from patient to patient.

The critical care nurse can help prevent deprivation by being aware of her patient's physical environment. She can identify, for herself, things within his environment that contribute toward sensory or perceptual deprivation. The nurse accomplishes her goals through management of the patient's environment and by maintaining meaningful stimulation.

Management of Environment

To manage something successfully, the individual must be aware of factors involved in the management process. The nurse who manages her patient's environment must be aware of objects, people, and sounds within it. It is as if she enters into her patient's physical being and sees the world through his eyes. There are things within his environment that the nurse learns to turn off. The patient, if overloaded or underloaded, does not have this ability to differentiate. Instead he may tune out many stimulations and be left in a void or deprived state.

Another source of altered sensory input from the environment is fear. The unfamiliar institutional environment or crisis situation can give rise to the stress of fear. Some patients may be afraid their illness, injury, or disease will lead to their death. Furthermore the patient may associate the symptoms of altered sensory input with a worsening of his condition. In many cases the nurse can reduce the effects of altered sensory input by encouraging uninterrupted rest periods or sleep (Esberger 1979).

The nurse must create an environment that has little sensory monotony or overload in order to prevent intellectual, neurological, or physical degeneration. She begins her sensory awareness prior to her patient's arrival in the critical care unit. If the nurse knows an aged patient is to be admitted, she can assess the best placement for him. Knowing that he already has reduced sensory processes, she can attempt to place him near the nurses' station. She can also realize that the environment may be unfamiliar and confusing to him. His close proximity to her will enable the nurse to keep visual surveillance on the patient. Also she may stop and talk with him on her way to the nurses' station. Because he has auditory impairment, the noises from telephones, charts, and voices may not create sensory overload, whereas to a younger patient with excellent auditory senses, the noises would create unbearable overload.

When possible the nurse can reduce the amount of noise produced by ventilators by positioning them as far away as possible from the patient (there is a difference in sound level between the outflow valve and the opposite side of the IPPB machine) and, in the case of the MA-1 ventilator, in such a way that the bellows of the machine are not adjacent to the patient's ears (Bolin 1974).

It is difficult to remove monitoring devices from the patient's immediate environment. However, there are ways to compensate for the monotony of constant rhythmic sounds from alarms or IVAC. For example, as soon as it is realistic to do so, the patient's mobility can be increased so that his immediate visual stimuli is increased. Furthermore various wires and tubes can be removed as soon as possible.

After the patient arrives, the admission routine begins. The nurse can begin by familiarizing the patient with his immediate environment. She can explain his bed control, call light, and side rails. She can orient him to the nurses' station, the family room, other patients, the nightstand, and if he is in a private room, the bathroom. With a family member present, the nurse can explain the policy regarding visiting hours. She can also save time by explaining pieces of equipment to both the patient and the family member simultaneously. Obviously her explanation will be only a brief introduction into their purposes, because she wishes to avoid overload as well as deprivation. Having completed her explanation, she will continue with the physical admission.

Whenever possible, the patient's physical environment can contain elements of his personality. The patient who is immobilized by burns, traction, spinal cord injury, or isolation for long periods of time needs his personal belongings in close proximity: clock, glasses, toilet articles, books, cards, and pictures. If he has pictures of his dog, children, or grandchildren, the nurse can tape them to the patient's overhead heat cradle or traction. This keeps the patient in visual touch with the familiar. A clock nearby will keep the patient oriented to time. The nurse must consider what Worrell (1971) terms "the potentialities of the patient's orientation to time. The ability of the patient to estimate time intervals between events, the relationship of the past to the present and to the future, and his ability to relate the sequence of events are additional parameters to be assessed. It is often with these more subtle areas that disorientation of reality is most apparent" (p. 140). To the patient who is unable to estimate time intervals, two hours become five minutes, or five minutes become two hours. He does not understand why time seems to race by or stand still. If the patient normally wears glasses or a hearing aid, he can have these items. The hearing aid will reduce sensory overload for other patients. The nurse will not need to talk in a loud voice. The glasses permit the patient to participate visually in his environment. Even visual participation fosters stimulation.

The use of television, radios, and telephones can facilitate sensory stimulation. Patients in burn and isolation units have television sets for diversional activity. For patients who are immobilized or confined in their beds, television programs provide entertainment. In the future, all patient beds might have a slide projector to show slides of interest or current movies on the patient's ceiling. After all, the burn, spinal cord, or isolation patient may spend many hours staring at the holes in the ceiling. The patient can choose a movie of interest, insert a set of ear plugs, and quietly be entertained by the program of his choice. The device could be utilized by the burn patient when he is having his daily therapy in the Hubbard tank. It might serve to divert his attention from the painful burns to visual sensation. Intensive care, hemodialysis, and coronary care are devoid of such visual and auditory stimulation. Some units even lack radios with headsets which could keep the patient oriented to date and time.

Another stimulation often lacking in critical care units is the telephone. Patients, especially the aged, normally spend time each day in telephone conversation. The telephone keeps the individual in contact with friends. If we attempt to familiarize the patient's hospital environment and make it comparable to home, telephones must be included, but they should be used only for outgoing calls, to avoid excess outside stimulation. Naturally the nurse will make the final decision as to who will use the telephone, radio, or television. Obviously a patient who is agitated, extremely critical, or confused will have little use for these devices.

Patients receiving reduced or increased sensory input must be oriented to happenings occurring to and around them. The various sounds of voices or machinery in the patient's immediate environment can be explained. Noises that are unexplained become focal points for fantasies or hallucinations. Machines need to be explained as the patient's sense of readiness increases. If at all possible they can be kept out of view. What the patient can see are people. He needs to feel the closeness of other people. The sensorially deprived patient has a greater need than most patients for security and protection against harmful stimuli. The critical care nurse meets these needs by fostering a sense of closeness. In addition, she can encourage the closeness of his family.

Patients who experience fantasies, illusions, or hallucinations need to be oriented rapidly. If this is not done, the patient may become agitated or panicked. A simple explanation may alleviate the problem and reassure the patient. The patient may think he sees bugs crawling on the wall. For fear of being laughed at, or being labeled confused, he refrains from telling his nurse. Later, he may become confused and fall out of bed. Had the patient informed his nurse, the outcome could have been prevented. The patient may be frightened by a feeling of loss of control over events affecting him.

Maintenance of Meaningful Stimulation

According to Esberger (1979) individuals need to be able to order stimuli in their environment into a meaningful pattern or to find meaning in the environment. If this need is unfulfilled a variety of behavioral responses may occur.

The nurse can attempt to make her patient's environment meaningful. She can accomplish this through identification and limitation of the meaningless stimulation. Another avenue is through explanation of unfamiliar facets within the patient's environment. After the patient's arrival in a critical care unit, he is subjected to various procedures, rules, and regulations. The nurse can explain why each wire or tube is connected to the patient, without, however, overloading his senses, which might "turn off" the patient psychologically. Too little information oversimplifies a potentially dangerous situation and gives the patient a false sense of security. The information given can, if possible, be repeated by the patient in order to ascertain his level of comprehension.

Meaningful sensory input can be achieved in numerous ways. By spending time talking with the patient and his family, the nurse decreases sensory deprivation. Allowing the family and friends to visit provides meaningful sensory input with a time structure (Linn 1979).

The fact that a patient is immobilized from bedrest and/or machines needs to be explained. The burn, hemodialysis, spinal cord injury, or surgical patient understands his immobility. None of these patients feel like moving around in their environment. The burn patient fears the pain of movement. The spinal cord injury patient is physiologically unable to ambulate. The surgical patient is limited by pain and machines. He realizes that he will soon be ambulatory, possibly sooner than desired. The hemodialysis patient realizes he is only immobilized physically for eight hours or less. Burn, spinal cord, and surgical patients understand why they must use a urinal or bedpan, receive their meals in bed, and in general be cared for like infants. They may not like the dependence and loss of decision-making responsibility. These patients are more acutely aware of their physical limitations.

The cardiac patient in CCU probably has the greatest difficulty adjusting to the unfamiliar. He entered the unit with severe chest pain and fear that death was coming. After his crisis passed, he felt better. The only thing that reminds him of his illness are the wires and tubes. He has nothing visible like burns, loss of function, or an incision to remind him of his critical condition, and he cannot understand why he must be immobilized, why he must use a urinal and bedpan, or why his visitors are limited. He does not understand why his nurse is being so protective. His nurse can spend time explaining the reasons behind each treatment and unfamiliar aspect of his immediate world. Explanations replace the unfamiliar and meaningless. If she fails to explain, she forces her patient to withdraw into a world of reduced stimulation.

Bolin (1974) points out that the nurse can be cognizant that perceptual monotony can be produced by a long period of hospitalization. Meaningful diversion can be encouraged by placing the patient near a window so that he can see more than the sky. Furthermore the patient can be allowed to sit at the nurses' station and observe their activity.

As the patient's condition improves, the nurse can involve him in decision-making processes. This will serve to increase his stimulation through participation in his care. In the process of enhancing his involvement, the nurse helps her patient cope with his illness. She accomplishes this by increasing his awareness of his feelings, needs, and fears. The nurse who is aware of the inherent dangers from the physical and social environment can mobilize her resources toward making the sensory input meaningful to the patient. Reassurance is also a vital necessity in avoiding deprivation. According to Worrell (1971), "Reassuring the patient enables him to cope. The patient is reassured by trust, and by having appropriate limits set for him. The patient is reassured when he finds that he is respected and understood by the nurse who cares for him. It is the development of the patient's own resources that restores the necessary confidence in himself and improves his self-esteem" (p. 140).

In sensory deprivation the patient may be experiencing slowness or disorganization of his thought processes. The critical care nurse can help the patient focus his thoughts on meaningful topics and stimulate his cognitive functioning by conversing with him regarding topics such as hobbies, family, or current events (Esberger 1979).

The nurse creates internal stimulation by use of energy mobilization. The patient has energy, but he has turned it inward toward the illness or injury. The nurse needs to make use of that energy in order to move her patient along the continuum toward wellness. He can use overt or covert activity, in attending and thinking as well as in movement and manipulation. The extent of energy release is determined by the degree of effort required by the patient. If he sees the situation as requiring too much effort, he will not utilize his energy. The nurse must formulate meaningful tasks that initially require little energy. Energy that creates movement toward a goal also stimulates his senses.

NURSING EVALUATION

The nurse evaluates the effectiveness of various interventions by assessing whether or not the behaviors associated with sensory deprivation are present or absent. The nurse designs nursing care to manage the patient's immediate environment so as to control the level of cortical arousal. The goal is to reduce technological deprivation and provide more human contact. In addition the nurse attempts to maintain meaningful stimulation so that the patient feels a bond with his environment and the people therein.

SUMMARY

The nurse can attempt to create an optimal physical environment for her patient, one in which there is freedom from sensory overload and sensory deprivation. The task is obviously a very difficult one, but it is possible to create an environment that resembles the familiar and restores meaningful stimulation to the patient. This is possible only when we begin thinking of the individual as a human being and not simply an entity.

REFERENCES

ADAMS, HENRY, "Sensory Deprivation and Personality Change," *Journal of Nervous and Mental Disease*, 143, no. 3 (1966), 256-265.

AIELLO, JUDY, "The Concept of Sensory Deprivation," *Australian Nurses Journal*, 7, (May 1978), 38-40.

ASHWORTH, PAT, "Sensory Deprivation 2: The Acutely Ill," *Nursing Times*, February 15, 1979, pp. 290-294.

BALLARD, KAREN, "Identification of Environmental Stresses for Patients in a Surgical Intensive Care Unit," *Issues in Mental Health Nursing*, 3, (1981), 89-108.

BOLIN, ROSE, "Sensory Deprivation: An Overview," *Nursing Forum*, 13, no. 3 (1974), 241-258.

BURTON, ARTHUR, "The Touching of the Body," *Psychoanalytical Review*, 57 (1964), 122-134.

CHODIL, JUDITH, and BARBARA WILLIAMS, "The Concept of Sensory Deprivation," *Nursing Clinics of North America*, 5, no. 3 (September 1970), p. 456.

DOWNS, F. J., "Bedrest and Sensory Disturbance," *American Journal of Nursing*, 74, (1974), 434-438.

DUFFY, ELIZABETH, "The Concept of Energy Mobilization," *Psychological Review*, 58 (1951), 30-39.

ESBERGER, KAREN, "The Significance of Altered Sensory Input," *Baylor Nursing Education*, 1, no. 1 (1979), 24-28.

GOLDBERGER, LEO, "Sensory Deprivation and Overload," in *Handbook of Stress: Theoretical and Clinical Aspects*, ed. Leo Goldberger and Shlomo Breznitz, pp. 410-417. New York: Free Press, 1982.

JACKSON, C. WESLEY, and ROSEMARY ELLIS, "Sensory Deprivation As a Field of Study," *Nursing Research*, 20, no. 1 (January-February 1971), 46-54.

KONCELIK, JOSEPH, "Compensating for Sensory Deprivation," *American Health Care Association*, 4 (July 1978), 5-18.

KUBIE, LAWRENCE, "Theoretical Aspects of Sensory Deprivation," in *Sensory Deprivation*, pp. 208-220. Cambridge, Mass.: Harvard University Press, 1965.

LINN, LAVRA, "Psychosocial Needs of Patients with Acute Respiratory Failure," *Critical Care Quarterly*, (March 1979), 65-73.

LINTON, PATRICK, "Sensory Deprivation in Hospitalized Patients," *Alabama Journal of Medical Sciences*, 2, no. 3 (July 1965), 257.

MEINHART, NOREEN, and MARY JO ASPINALL, "Nursing Intervention in Hypovigilence," *American Journal of Nursing*, 69, no. 5 (May 1969), 994.

PARENT, LILLIAN, "Effects of a Low-Stimulus Environment on Behavior," *The American Journal of Occupational Therapy*, 32, no. 1 (January 1978), 19-25.

PARKER, DONALD, "Delirium in a Coronary Care Unit," *Journal of the American Medical Association*, 201, no. 9 (August 28, 1967), 132-133.

RUFF, G., "Isolation and Sensory Deprivation," in *American Handbook of Psychiatry*, vol. 2, ed. Silvano Arieti, p. 371. New York: Basic Books, 1959-66.

SCHAEFER, KARL, "The Effect of Restricted Manipulative Experience in Problem Solving," *The American Journal of Occupational Therapy*, 32, no. 3 (March 1978), 165-170.

SCHULTZ, DUANE, *Sensory Restriction Effect on Behavior*. New York: Academic Press, 1965.

SNYDER, LORRAINE, "Environmental Changes for Socialization," *Journal of Nursing Administration*, (January 1978), 44-50.

STEWART, N. J., "Psychological Effect of Immobilization and Social Isolation on Hospitalized Orthopedic Patients." Unpublished master's thesis, University of Saskatchewan, 1977.

SUEDFELD, PETER, "Introduction and Historical Background," in *Sensory Deprivation: Fifteen Years of Research*, ed. John Zubek, pp. 3-15. New York: Appleton-Century-Crofts, 1969.

____, *Restricted Environmental Stimulation*. New York: John Wiley, 1980.

THOMPLEINS, EMILY, "Effect of Restricted Mobility and Dominance on Perceived Duration," *Nursing Research*, 29, no. 6 (November-December 1980), 333-338.

WOOD, MARILYNN, "Clinical Sensory Deprivation: A Comparative Study of Patients in Single Care and Two-Bed Rooms," *Journal of Nursing Administration*, 7, no. 10, (December 1977), 28-32.

WORRELL, JUDITH, "Nursing Implications in the Care of the Patient Experiencing Sensory Deprivation," in *Advanced Concepts in Clinical Nursing*, ed. Kay Corman Kintzel, pp. 618-638. Philadelphia: Lippincott, 1971.

ZISKIND, EUGENE, "A Second Look at Sensory Deprivation," *Journal of Nervous Mental Diseases*, 138, no. 3 (March 1964), 226.

14

Body Image and Self-Concept

BEHAVIORAL OBJECTIVES

1. Define the terms *self-concept* and *body image.*
2. Describe how Lee's four phases apply to the critically ill patient.
3. Identify four regulatory behaviors associated with body image alterations.
4. Identify five cognitive behaviors associated with body image alterations.
5. Design a nursing care plan around Lee's four phases.

The body of an individual is a source for both external and internal perception. To touch and perceive its surface elicits two different kinds of sensations, namely, of the interior and of the exterior, which separates the body from the external world. Therefore body-self is an entity with a surface and a mental projection of that surface. The boundaries of the body image enclose a narrower conceptual area than do the boundaries of the self. However when the body image expands, the self is likewise expanded (Hagglund and Piha 1980).

The concepts of body image and self have found application in various disciplines. One finds reference to these concepts in studies of psychiatric and neurological problems, hypnotic phenomena, drug effects, psychotherapy results, and psychosomatic illness. Each expert handles these concepts differently. Neurologists confront them in terms of distorted attitudes of patients who have brain damage. Other professionals approach them according to their own specialties. Consequently, these concepts have not been examined or applied in a holistic way in literature. According to Norris (1978), many theorists have been unable to integrate the concept of the individual's body into the collection of personality concepts referred to as psychodynamic theory. The theory of body image consists of a series of measures designed to relate body type to personality type or other body-personality correlations, and studies that explain the behavior of individuals whose body structure becomes distorted.

Body image or the mental picture of the body's appearance changes constantly. There is often a time lag in bringing our body concept up to date. In other words a biological crisis occurs and the patient requires time to incorporate any physical alterations. The mental picture of the self may not be consonant with the actual body structure (Bille 1977).

Nurses are becoming increasingly more aware of the body image concept. They realize that any individual, no matter what his level of wellness, cherishes and guards his wholeness. Our culture is based upon wholeness. It is the whole body that represents beauty and the achievement of beauty. Television commercials foster this image. There are commercials for every aspect of the body—teeth, hair, stomach, legs, and other parts. In an average evening of television viewing, one might see a beautiful girl walking through a dense forest discussing her form-fitting bra or panty hose, a handsome man lying in bed telling the public that he might not use his deodorant today, a lovely woman showing how easily a certain product removes hair from her legs, a beautiful 40-year-old woman telling how a moisturizer keeps her young, and two elderly men or women walking through a park discussing what they do for constipation. How does a young woman who has lost a breast identify with the commercial for a form-fitting bra? A person who has recently experienced facial and chest burns can hardly identify with the handsome model, who reminds him of his own loss or alteration in body image. Cardiac or hemodialysis patients may wish they could walk through a park and discuss a curable problem such as constipation, but their energy and pain level may not permit them the luxury. Whether or not the individual can identify with various commercials, he is still a whole being. The individual's "wholeness must depend not only on the private resources of his own body but equally on the interaction in which he unceasingly is engaged with his environment" (Levine 1969, p. 98).*

The human body image develops through sensory messages from inside the body and from the surrounding environment. There are several kinds of sensation that a person receives as he takes inventory, experiments with, and manipulates the body and the environment. They may be tactile, thermal, or painful. Sensation comes from the muscles, organs, and nerves of the body in response to inner functioning or contact of the body with the environment (Norris 1978). The individual feels free to move through his environment without restrictions, but injury, illness, or disfigurement can restrict his sense of freedom. He may no longer feel a sense of uniqueness, and his ability to make choices and decisions may also be altered. He may be forced to assume new social roles, one of which could be temporary or permanent dependency on things or people outside himself.

DEFINITION OF TERMS

A person's body, as he perceives or evaluates it, plays a significant role in determining his security and sense of self-esteem. The body concept includes all of his perceptions and knowledge concerning his own body—appearance, boundaries, limits, and inner structure. One's concept of self or body image may be accurate or inaccurate. Body image and self-concept are concepts that are closely related.

Self-Concept

Self implies a unique personality we wish to single out from the rest of humankind. Concepts of self vary in clarity. The self is the individual's basic frame of reference. Turner (1982) considers the conception of self an object that emerges out of distinctively human reflexive process—an object which has no existence apart from the conceptions and attitudes by which one constitutes it. In his view, the self-conception identifies a person in qualitative and locational terms, not merely in evaluative ones such as self-esteem. The self is an object in relation to other objects all of which are modified in dynamic interrelationships.

In the view of Wells and Marwell (1976), the self is some specialized cognitive or behavioral subject of the personality. The self represents that part of the personality which is phenomenal and more specifically reflexive— the perceiver and the perceived are the same organism. It is the individual's experiences that constitute the self, not the person or the person's body.

Each individual has numerous perceptions of self during his or her lifetime. The concept of self is an organization of how the person sees himself, principles that the individual regards as part, or characteristic, of his being. They include all perceptions of what the individual calls "I" or "me." Combs and Snygg (1959) have described three basic characteristics of the phenomenal self: clarity and centrality of self-perception, consistency, and stability.

The individual does not always perceive himself with clarity. Like all other perceptions, the phenomenal self feels real to the individual. His perceived self seems truly to be himself. It is probably not possible, however, for the individual to perceive the total organization of his self clearly at any one moment. Rather, he perceives aspects or concepts of self that merge from time to time. Sometimes he discovers inconsistencies between his phenomenal self and the environment. Placed in an environment that he does not and cannot understand, the individual has to create an understandable world in which he can put faith. Patients who are unable to cope with their environment create a substitute one through fantasies. A person's self-made scheme of life is his only guarantee of security, and its preservation soon becomes a goal in itself. He seeks the type of experience that conforms and supports the unified attitude.

Any alteration in the body is a disturbance of integrity, a threat to self. How an individual copes with the threat to self depends on how he has coped with stress during his lifetime. The capacity to cope is dependent upon the individual's educational background, work patterns, family, and values (Motta 1981). Possessing values implies phenomenal self which involves perceptual and/or experimental information.

The phenomenal self has a high degree of stability. With the self-concept at its core, it represents our fundamental frame of reference, our anchor to reality; and even an unsatisfactory self-organization is likely to prove highly stable and resistant to change. Once the phenomenal self has become established, it interprets all experience in terms of that self. Thus the perceptions that are meaningful to the individual derive their meaning from their relation to the existing phenomenal self. The latter characteristic makes the phenomenal self less likely to change (Combs and Snygg 1959).

In addition, one's concept of self is related to one's self-esteem. Self-esteem refers to whether one accepts oneself, respects oneself, and considers oneself a person of worth (Rosenberg and Kaplan 1982). It is a more or less phenomenal process in which the individual perceives characteristics of himself and reacts to them emotionally or behaviorally. Self-esteem is a reflexive term meaning that the object perceived and the perceiver are the same. In other words, it results from an evaluation of the self by the self (Wells and Marwell 1976; Greenleaf 1978).

Body Image

Body image is the interaction between physical and emotional stimuli. It is formed by the interaction between the perceptual pool and the experiential pool. An individual's body image including physical appearance, bodily sensations, beliefs, and emotions about the body makes up part of his self-concept. The significance of body image within the self-concept will vary mainly according to the nature and intensity of values and emotions invested in it (Becken 1978; Esberger 1978).

Norris (1978) has defined body image as follows:

> Body image is the constantly changing total of conscious and unconscious information, feelings, and perceptions about one's body in space as different and apart from all others. It is a social creation, developed through the reflected perception about the surfaces of one's body and responses to sensations originating from the inner regions of the body as the individual copes with a kaleidoscopic variety of living activities. The body image is basic to identity and has been referred to as the somatic ego. (P. 5)

Body image is the way we see our body. A person perceives himself to be tall, short, thin, or fat. His image may be 50 pounds lighter than what others see. Fisher (1968), an expert in the study of body image, believes that the term refers to the body as a psychological experience and to the individual's feelings and attitudes toward his own body. As each individual develops, he has the difficult task of meaningfully organizing his bodily sensations, which are among the most important and complex phenomena in his total perceptual field.

According to Esberger (1978) body image has four characteristics. First, the phenomenon of body image can be said to be the totality of perceptions regarding one's own body and its performance. The way in which other individuals perceive a person will be influenced by both the image he really projects and the images perceived by others whose perceptions are influenced by their own body images. Second, body image serves some definite function for each person which influences most aspects of his activities of daily living. Furthermore, elements of his body image can be identified as his values, attitudes, and feelings. Third, body image is dynamic. A person's body image is constantly changing and never static. The dynamic feature can be seen in response to a threat to one's body image. The dynamics are related to one's adaptation to a coping with a threat such as myocardial infarction, coronary artery bypass graft, acute renal failure, or adult respiratory distress syndrome. Fourth, body image includes elements of both reality and identity. An individual may incorporate so much of the ideal into his body image that he may be surprised when confronted by the reality of a mirror.

Body image involves a number of things. It represents a unity between temporal, environmental, and interpersonal factors. The term also implies an interpersonal experience between the individual's feelings and attitudes and his body. For example, a woman may wear a size 18 dress. She decides to diet, and her dress size goes from size 18 to 14. Her body image, however, may still be a size 18. As she approaches a dress rack, she may inadvertently look at the larger sizes. She has not yet assimilated her new image. Another person may feel inferior or unattractive because of a large nose. He has the size of his nose altered but finds that his old feelings still exist. These feelings regarding image have been internalized over a span of several years. Consequently it takes time to change the concept one holds of his body image. The cardiac patient's image of himself may have been an athletic and energetic one. It will be difficult for him to alter his life-style and concept of self to incorporate the new image. Much of the editing of the experiences that go into making and modifying the body image is not conscious, and no one can describe his own total body image.

Each individual has a mental image of his own appearance. This image may or may not be consistent with his actual body structure. The body image, as an entity, derives itself from past and current experiences. It has been defined as a psychological variable, formed gradually in the course of a learning process in which the individual experiences his body in manifold situations and also notes the reactions of others to it. The individual may or may not be conscious about the image he projects. By and large a person's body, as he perceives it and evaluates it, plays an important role in determining his security and his sense of self-esteem.

THE CONCEPT OF BODY IMAGE AND SELF-CONCEPT ALTERATION APPLIED TO THE CRITICALLY ILL PATIENT

Today medical and technological advancement has led to invasive procedures, replacement of body parts, and reconstructive surgery. In the future, kidney, heart, and liver transplants will be a common occurrence. Regardless of the surgical intervention, the individual experiences some degree of body image and/or self-concept alteration.

Alterations in the body image of the critical care patient will be examined according to the four phases described by Lee (1970) through which each individual must pass after an illness or injury: impact, retreat, acknowledgment, and reconstruction. The patient's perception of his body contains the preinjury or preillness image. His medical crisis forces him to change the concept of his body. Lee points out that the transition does not occur at the time of injury or illness but is a lengthy process in which the injury or illness is one event. The patient must then assimilate the event into his body image and self-concept.

Impact Phase

Adaptation to alteration in the body's function and structure depends upon the nature of the threat, its meaning to the critically ill patient, his coping ability, the response from others significant to him, and the assistance available to him and his family as changes occur. With the occurrence of an injury or illness, the individual finds himself thrown into experiences that force him to alter his concept of self and body image. The event may or may not have given the critical care patient prior warnings.

The patient first experiences shock as the impact takes its toll. This initial emotional reaction may occur at the time of the injury and/or illness or whenever the individual becomes consciously aware of his problem.

> A crisis such as a physical trauma generates a series of phenomena geared for the return to the preexisting state of affairs. When in the life experience of a person a crisis occurs that changes the appearance of his body the event is recognized by everyone in his social milieu. The recognition of the change prevents the return to the previous state of affairs and demands a process of adjustment. The person must find a new way of approaching personal, interpersonal, and social aspects of living. (Lee 1970, p. 577-578)

The following are examples of patients who experienced various degrees of loss of function, loss of a bodily part, or loss in terms of disfigurement. Mr. J. and Mr. P. are examples of patients who experienced the impact of loss of function. Mr. J. was a 33-year-old patient in coronary care with arrhythmias. This was Mr. J.'s first admission into the hospital. Prior to this time he was active in his law practice, family, sports, and community service. He had never to his knowledge been told that he had coronary artery disease. Mr. J.'s arrhythmias ranged from first- to second-degree block. Due to the threat of complete heart block, his doctors decided to insert a temporary external pacemaker. Several days later, it became apparent that Mr. J. would need a permanent pacemaker. Since no other viable alternatives were available, Mr. J. agreed to the procedure. The procedure was carried out without any complications, and the threat of a fatal arrhythmia was overcome. Everyone thought that Mr. J., even though he was relatively young to have a permanent pacemaker, should be happy over the positive outcome. Despite the positive preventive outcome, Mr. J. became quiet and seemed to withdraw into himself.

Mr. P. was a patient frequently hospitalized for respiratory failure due to longstanding emphysema. He was 50 years old and during the course of one year had been admitted into ICU three times. Mr. P. and his respiratory problems were well known to the ICU health team. With each hospitalization his condition became more critical. In addition, each pulmonary crisis led to more loss in his pulmonary reserve. Weaning off the volume respirator became more difficult with each subsequent admission. Between hospitalizations Mr. P. utilized the efforts of other supportive systems, particularly the respiratory therapist in his hospital's pulmonary rehabilitation program. Mr. P. became discouraged, because he was unable to see any stability in his limited future. Needless to say Mr. P.'s doctors were concerned about his deteriorating physical status. They realized that a permanent tracheostomy would be necessary.

Mr. J. and Mr. P. both experienced loss of function: loss of cardiac function with dependency on a pacemaker in one case, and loss of pulmonary function with ultimate dependency on a tracheostomy in the other case. Loss of body function has overwhelming implications to critical care patients. An individual's body image matures over a span of many years. This image is anchored to his need for self-esteem. Any body alteration disturbs his integrity and appears to be a movement down the negative continuum toward death.

Severyn (1969) notes that body image "refers to the picture of our body that we form in our mind or the way that the body appears to ourselves. The image has both a psychological and a physiological foundation since it is based on the senses and involves the sense of posture, optic image and sensory perception" (p. 234). Both of our patient examples had active images of themselves. Now Mr. J. feels he will be less than what he was prior to the pacemaker implantation. He is afraid of being inactive and as a result withdraws from other people. During the impact phase, he even rejects explanations about his possible future activities. Mr. P. realizes his loss on a daily basis. As his pulmonary status becomes more critical, he finds that his shortness of breath and reduced energy curtail any activity. Each additional loss of pulmonary function and loss of movement adds to his discouragement.

The meaning the loss has for the patient is dependent upon his body perception. Body perception refers to the direct mental experience of the physical appearance of the body. It encompasses surface, depth, and mental pictures of the body and is measured by observational method. Perceived body space is the amount of space individuals perceive their bodies to occupy and indicates perception of the limits of body boundaries. In contrast to body perception, body attitude encompasses a broad spectrum of feelings, attitudes, and emotional reactions toward the body (Fawcett and Frye 1980).

Mr. B., Mrs. L., and Mr. V. are examples of critical care patients who experienced loss of parts and disfigurement. Mr. B. was a 45-year-old oil worker. Like Mr. J., he was married and had a family. He loved his work at an oil refinery. The job provided him with a degree of freedom and responsibility, but it was sometimes quite hazardous. One day while Mr. B. was making his routine survey of the valves and pressures gauges in the pump house, an unexpected explosion occurred. Mr. B. was knocked unconscious. When he awoke, he found himself surrounded by strangers in white gowns and masks. As his perceptual awareness increased, he realized he was in a new environment. Furthermore he became increasingly aware of his bodily sensations. His chest, face, and arms were extremely painful. It was at this time he learned of the explosion and fire in the refinery's pump house. As a result of the fire, he received first- and second-degree burns over 30 percent of his body. The work he once loved had pointed its deadly finger at him. The entire episode of injury and disfigurement overwhelmed him and pushed him into temporary despair.

Mrs. L. was a young mother with a history of chronic glomerulonephritis. Throughout the past year she had attempted to regulate her activity and diet in order to stabilize her nitrogenous level. It soon became apparent, however, that her kidneys were creating an overload of toxins. She had to submit to bilateral nephrectomy. Mrs. L. realized besides the immediate necessity of surgery, she must spend the rest of her life dependent on a hemodialysis machine. To the patient, the thought of surgery is a threat in itself, but the additional financial threat of hemodialysis is even more threatening and frightening.

Mr. V. was a 68-year-old veteran who was hospitalized for peripheral vascular disease and diabetes. He had experienced intermittent claudication and color changes predominately in his right leg and foot. Contrary to his doctor's instructions, Mr. V. had attempted to clip his own toenails, and he had cut his great toe. As the weeks progressed, it became evident to Mr. V. that the discoloration and pain were more prominent than ever before. At this point Mr. V. entered the hospital for treatment. His doctors attempted conservative treatments; however, they failed to rectify the situation. For fear of gangrene, the doctors scheduled surgery. The surgery would involve amputation of Mr. V.'s right leg below the kneee. The potential threat of loss caused Mr. V. to become less active and less involved in his own care. He passively accepted what happened around him and submitted to the wishes of others.

Mrs. L., Mr. V., and Mr. B. all shared the common experience of loss of a part. Mrs. L.'s loss is not immediately obvious to others, but as she begins using the hemodialysis machine, the loss will become apparent. Mr. V. and

Mr. B. experienced immediate and obvious loss of parts. The focus in their care is upon the missing parts of the body. As Spiegel (1964) points out, the person who is injured or ill becomes the center of group concern. There are people who are concerned and want to help. When Mr. B. awakened, he saw not one but several masked faces peering at him. The staff may have been intent upon doing the technical things necessary to ensure him safety, but they placed him at center stage at a time when he wanted to remain invisible. The same was true of Mr. V. The hospital staff focused upon his loss by checking the dressing, the color, and signs of bleeding or edema, and they limited their inspection to the site of amputation rather than continuing to include his remaining whole. Both Mr. V. and Mr. P. are constantly aware of their losses—and continued focus on their losses by the staff may only serve to frighten them.

Their losses also create internal feelings of shame because of their disfigurement. In these cases, both patients may feel shame for the causes of their losses. Each may feel that his own neglect precipitated the biological crisis. Mr. V. may have been warned about potential complications from failure to care adequately for his extremities, and Mr. B. may have been worried about the potential hazard in altering the various pressure gauges in the pump house. Regardless of the crisis origin, each patient may view his own crisis as shameful. According to Lange (1970), "The diagnosis, the medical treatment, the body changes, the reactions of family and friends, hospitalization, and the many contacts during nursing care all may precipitate feelings that range from social discomfort to embarrassment to abject humiliation" (p. 68). Focus upon each patient's loss by nurses and staff members makes the patient more cognizant of his disfigurement. As Rubin (1968) notes, such disfigurement or loss is a severe threat to the patient's sense of self:

> To lose or be threatened the loss of a complex, coordinated, and controlled functional activity which has been achieved and integrated into the personal system is to lose or be threatened with the loss of self. Psychosocially, the loss, or threat of loss, of self is equivalent to loss of life. Emotional responses serve as warning signals of the extent of danger, and we immediately mobilize energies for self-protection and self-preservation. (P. 20-23)

Each organ has a function, a movement, a purpose. Movement is essential for the individual's sense of well-being. But the individual must be able to control these qualities, and illness or injury signals a loss of control.

Mr. B. and Mr. V. also experienced the horror of physical disfigurement. Disfigurement brings unique changes in body image. One can begin to integrate loss of some function, especially if the loss is not externally obvious. The cardiac patient's loss of myocardium is not obvious, and the subtle injury of one's back, the loss of a breast, or the loss of a uterus is not publicly visible, although each loss has special significance to the individual. This is especially true for a patient who experiences loss of function of a sexual organ, or loss of the organ itself. Such a loss has very special and sensitive implications to the individual and his family. The loss makes the individual feel less than complete. Such patients may fear they will be failing their sexual partners. Thus the individual may move into conflict with his or her phenomenal self.

When the physical loss is obvious, the individual has a much more difficult adjustment. The adjustments to a disfigured body arouse feelings of threats. The individual may desire to abandon his body because he feels a loss of wholeness. The way each patient adapts to his environment determines whether or not he perceives a threat to the body image. The illnesses of Mr. B. and Mr. V. carried with them the prospect of further loss, causing a mobilization of anxiety. Mr. V. realizes the possibility of developing severe peripheral vascular insufficiency in the remaining leg. He may learn from other patients about the possibility of infection in his stump, necessitating further amputation. The fear of additional loss is constantly on his mind. Mr. B. worries about whether or not his skin grafts will take. He knows there is the possibility of infection, which could cause his grafts to fail. Like Mr. V., he also feels the threat of additional loss. Mrs. L. has already lost both kidneys—she has nothing else to lose. Mr. J. has lost the normal electrical activity of his heart, but an electrical pacemaker has taken over the lost function. His only fear would be loss of myocardial function due to further coronary artery insufficiency. During the initial impact phase, though, he focused all his attention on his immediate concerns. The anxiety of most patients at the moment of crisis creates tunnel vision; they see or hear nothing else at the time. The sudden or expected change in body image also produces a distortion of the self.

The critical care patient may experience behavioral changes associated with his loss. Critical care nurses and other members of the health team must be cognizant of behavioral clues given by the patient. During the impact phase the nurse may assess a wide range of behavior such as despair, discouragement, passive acceptance, anger, and hostility. Despair results when the critically ill patient's change in body image makes him feel less than complete. His despair reaches out to encompass his family, showing concern for their future as well as his own. The patient may despair because he realizes the financial implications of his illness. Such is the case of the patient entering a critical care unit for the third time in one year, the burn patient who needs long-term critical care, or the hemodialysis patient. Discouragement and passive acceptance result because the patient cannot see beyond his immediate loss, surgery, or disfigurement. Mr. B. and Mr. V. focused upon their disfigurement. The burn patient may feel a greater degree of disfigurement. He lives in the here and now, and it is difficult for him to see improvement in his own condition. His care team seems to focus its attention on therapy, healing stages, grafting, and rehabilitation. The end result of all these endeavors is in the very distant future, a future that the burn patient has difficulty visualizing. Seeing only the obvious changes in his body image, he becomes discouraged and passively accepts events within his environment.

The critical care nurse may assess that most of her patients in the impact phase manifest despair, discouragement, and passive acceptance. Their energies have been turned inward as they attempt to cope with changes in their body image. Suddenly the nurse may detect anger and hostility, manifested verbally in statements such as, "What is the use?" "You know it won't do any good," or "You have come to see the freak." The patient has turned his energies outside himself. He may blame others for alterations in his body image. Patients like Mr. V. may blame the health team for failure to teach him adequate foot care. Mr. B. may blame his company for the explosion and fire that led to his loss. Mr. J., Mr. P., and Mrs. L. are angry at themselves for becoming ill. Their behavior is simply a projection onto others for the guilt or shame they feel for themselves. Each may feel a sense of failure in his or her own body.

Whatever the meaning, each patient does react behaviorally to the impact phase, often without fully comprehending the significance of his injury, illness, or disfigurement. Each critically ill patient experiences some degree of loss, whether it be loss of function, loss of part, or disfigurement. He may also experience psychological and social loss. The critically ill patient may not be cognizant of the latter two loses during the impact phase of his illness, but when his sensations expand beyond himself and into his environment, he moves into the next phase, retreat.

Retreat Phase

The retreat phase begins when a patient suddenly becomes aware of his injury or illness. The shock or impact phase allowed him to dissociate his body from the event, but as the shock and threat of death subside, he can see the reality of his problem. With his sudden realization comes a new array of feelings. His immediate reaction is to run. The immobilization created by his injury or illness does not permit him to do so. Instead, he can only retreat emotionally from the problem he must inevitably face. When he looks at himself, he perceives someone else's body. The normal body image processes have been interrupted. The retreat phase allows the critically ill patient to rally his resources so he can deal with the event's implications. At this time, he becomes aware of his own strengths that assist him eventually to acknowledge what has transpired. The retreat phase also gives the patient an opportunity to mourn his loss. He needs time to reflect upon the meaning of the lost part and its implications for his future.

Body image isn't simply what we think about our appearance. It also includes our perception of our function, sensation, and mobility. Our perception of our physical self shapes what we feel about ourselves as a person. Basically there are two types of boundary disturbances in hospitalized patients. The first comes when, through an accident or surgery, the body wall changes but the patient keeps the old body boundary. This is the experience of the amputee patient with a phantom limb. The second type of disturbance occurs when the patient changes a body boundary even though his body remains intact. An example is the patient who has sustained a stroke. The stroke patient may be unaware that half his body is paralyzed and he remains unaware despite efforts to make him conscious of it (McCloskey 1976).

The patient may perceive the situation to be far worse than it is. Mr. J. may feel his active days are over. Like most cardiac patients, he fails to realize that he can still lead a productive life, even though he may have some limitations. Some cardiac patients, rather than fighting the battle, choose to become cardiac cripples and spend most of their waking hours sitting in overstuffed chairs. Such unnecessarily restricted activity does in fact restrict their lives. Mr. B., like most burn patients, fears his physical injuries will isolate him socially. In time, with corrective surgery and skin grafts, the injury may not be as obvious. Nevertheless, his once-perfect body has been rendered imperfect. Burn patients have difficulty seeing their progress. All they see are the ugly burns, which serve as a constant reminder of their imperfection. This is why it becomes easy to retreat into denying the potential threat of the situation. Mrs. L. can continue to retreat into denial during the early stages of her dialysis. She is still hospitalized and is the responsibility of someone else. In time she will be assuming the responsibility of coming to the hemodialysis unit for her exchanges. Until that time, she can deny her involvement with the hemodialysis machine.

Each patient feels a degree of threat, one which, according to Norms of being discovered or found inadequate. Mr. J.'s pacemaker may be hidden from the public's eye. If he so desires, he can keep his inadequacy a secret. Possibly someone can learn that Mrs. L. is missing both kidneys. Close friends might be able to see that Mr. V. is wearing a prosthetic leg; for the public, however, his trousers hide his secret. Mr. P. and Mr. B. are unable to hide alteration in their body image. Mr. P.'s physical appearance changes as his emphysema becomes more serious. He must assume a position that facilitates breathing. His skin, once pink, now becomes dusky ashen; his broad chest now assumes a barrel shape; his lips are now puckered; and his once-muscular body now becomes thin and frail. Mr. B.'s physical appearance changes in an obvious fashion. Outsiders can quickly identify his problem or injury.

Each patient feels a degree of threat one which, according to Norms (1978),

> is also related to the extent to which the individual's patterns of adaptation are interrupted. Each person develops patterns of behavior that meet his needs for security and does this within the framework of the requirements of his environment. These habits or patterns may depend heavily on certain organs of the body. If these organs become diseased or have to be removed the threat is greater than if an organ unimportant to the patient is affected. (P. 29)

Whether the loss is internal or external, the individual's appearance or physique changes. The patient has experienced a loss and must inevitably deal with its implications to his life.

Medical and nursing activities can appear as potentially threatening to the patient. Shortly after his arrival in a critical care unit, the patient must submit to intrusive procedures, many of which must be done immediately. Consequently, he has little or no time to recover from each intrusion. He may have an arterial line, CVP, intravenous therapy, an oxygen mask, a chest tube, a pacemaker, a cardioscope, a tracheostomy, or a volume respirator. Each intrusion reminds him of how critical he really is. The illness or injury itself, coupled with new intrusive procedure, threatens the patient.

Threats may force the patient to avoid reality by retreating into peripheral areas, topics of thought or discussion that focus on something or someone other than the patient himself. An aged patient may talk at great length about her pet or her flowers. She may describe in detail all of her cat's daily activities, and she may even compare her current cat with previous cats. This patient does not want to face reality, because reality may mean living in a convalescent home away from her cat and her flowers. A businessman may spend his time discussing various business deals that he must handle as soon as he is discharged. He talks of his company—its products, employees, liabilities, and assets. He concentrates his energies upon his business, and he may become annoyed when he is refused a telephone to make additional business transactions. The patient fails to see how his current bleeding ulcer, hypertension, or myocardial infarction is anything to be alarmed about. After all, "The doctors will fix everything and I'll be as good as new." Another patient may talk about his grandchildren or children. He may show his nurse countless pictures of the family. He always keeps the conversation on his family, home, or children rather than himself and the fears he must experience. Peripheral topics become safety valves for the release of energy. They give the patient an opportunity to focus on nonthreatening areas, and this diverts energy away from himself. These conversations may also be subtle questions. The elderly patient may want to know if she will see her cat or rose garden before she dies; the businessman is really asking if he can eventually return to work; and the patient who always talks about his family may be asking if he will see his children or grandchildren again. The retreat phase allows the mobilization of energy necessary to acknowledge that an illness or injury has occurred.

Burn patients experience tremendous alteration in body image. In a study of such patients by Bowden et al. (1980), 85 percent of the respondents had adequate to high self-esteem. Although the size of the burn and part of the body burned did not seem to significantly affect self-esteem, age when burned and time since burn did. Respondents with low self-esteem spent twice as many days in bed and missed considerably more days of work in the year prior to the study than did those with moderate or high self-esteem. In summary, the study indicated that the majority of burned people make a successful adjustment following even large and disfiguring injuries and that successful rehabilitation is long-term and episodic in nature.

Facts about the self that the patient is unable to accept into awareness cannot be assimilated. If the facts are not part of the perceptual field, they do not affect behavior. Mrs. L. may not be ready to accept strict diet changes, even though her diet was limited prior to surgery. Mr. P. may find it initially difficult to accept a less active life, although his pulmonary problem dictates such a life. As during the impact phase, the critically ill patient in the retreat phase also manifests behavioral responses. The major behavioral response during the retreat phase is denial. The patient may choose to deny in a number of ways, but the critical care nurse can usually assess that the overall behavior is due to denial. Behavioral manifestations of denial, for example, may include refusal to learn how to transfer from bed to chair; to use a prosthetic device; to learn how to take one's pulse in detecting possible pacemaker failure; to regulate fluids, salt, potassium, calories, and protein in diet; and to learn and practice breathing exercises. The patient falsely believes that if he ignores certain treatments, the problem will disappear. Other patients may be quite euphoric about alterations in their body image. One patient who had a leg amputation below the knee made open jest of his appearance. He told his nurse, "I am going to get a peg leg, put a ring in my ear, wear a scarf around my head, and chase women." He saw himself something like Captain Cook. He was making himself into a clown—something or someone to laugh at, but he was also asking if he would still be appealing to women even though he would be missing a part of his body. Even the jokes a patient makes relate, whether consciously or unconsciously, to his new image.

The hemodialysis patient may talk to his dialysis machine: "Come on, George, do your thing so I can get out of here." George is the nickname he has given his dialysis machine. The patient attributes certain powers to the machine so that he can quickly retreat from the hospital to his day-to-day existence. The cardiac patient who wears a pacemaker may also refer to it by nickname. In addition he may make fun of what he views as his new image. We overheard one patient saying, "I feel like the $400 man with my new battery. I wonder if it is a Diehard battery. Just think! When my battery runs down, I need only plug into a socket and become recharged." His jest serves to cover his true feelings and even fears: "I wonder if it is a Diehard battery?" A burn patient disfigured by scars said, "Well, I can always get a job in the circus side show. People enjoy laughing at a freak." His statement revealed how he felt others viewed him—as a freak.

The clues that lead critical care nurses to assess denial as a behavioral problem are a refusal to accept or participate in rehabilitation and the use of symbolism when referring to the self or to a supportive device in the environment. Each clue reflects varying degrees of denial in the retreat phase. The patient retreats behind his refusal to participate in his rehabilitation and his symbolic statements. By refusing to participate in his care, the critical care patient attempts to retreat into denying a problem exists. Other patients retreat into symbolism. Through symbolism the critical care patient can make fun of himself or of his life-supporting devices. His symbolism may temporarily allow him to retreat into jest and humor. How the patient refers to himself and how he refers to supportive devices—"George"—give the critical care nurse insight into the patient's concept of himself and his body image.

Acknowledgment Phase

Realization that something is wrong with one's body may arouse tension and stress. This is especially true for the patient experiencing a myocardial infarction. Such an individual will behave in such a way as to attempt to reduce his tension. One tension-reducing mechanism may be learning about the disease, injury, or illness (Bille 1977).

The critical care patient has often suffered an injury or illness that has resulted in a change in his physical appearance. He must face the reality of such a change if he is to continue daily existence. The task in the adjustment phase is to help the patient and his family acknowledge the alteration, which he equates with loss of his body image. Family reactions can influence and be influenced by patient reactions. In this phase, the patient mourns his loss, which he must acknowledge, regardless of its degree of severity. He realizes he no longer can hide or retreat. He perceives that he must fight the battle before he can hopefully win the war. The loss of his image influences his individuality and uniqueness. In illness a wide array of messages about the body constantly bombard the system, which either receives them for interpretation and integration into the self or rejects them. As Corbeil (1971) notes, the process of integration is often subject to disturbance:

> The sequence that is necessary for the normal relation between the perception of events and the formation of body image, i.e., meaningful organization of sensations, may be disturbed. This disturbance may stem from either physical, psychologic, or emotional aggression; the quality of disturbance is much more related to the individual's perception of it than to the actual fact. (P. 156-157.)

According to Bille (1977), a patient who has recently suffered a myocardial infarction may be instructed to adjust his life-style to meet the limitations imposed upon him by his condition. If the patient has not yet been able to intellectualize the fact that his heart is damaged, he may also reject information given him to help him adjust his life-style to accommodate for his condition.

The critically ill patient, no matter what his physical problem, acknowledges alteration in his uniqueness. Atrophy usually accompanies failure of a body part to function if the failure lasted for a considerable length of time or is permanent. The patient who has a myocardial infarction, pulmonary disease, acute tubular necrosis, minor burns, or staphylococcus infection of an incisional wound would not lose body function. He has suffered a temporary insult, but in time the adaptative processes take over, and stability results. Only a portion of the whole has been lost, not the whole. Words such as *heart, lung,* or *kidney* conjur up images of their own. Therefore, according to Norris (1978), "The symbolism of [disease related to these organs] in terms of life and death may cause distorted notions concerning structure, function, or significance. The organ may have a special image, even to the point of being independent of the body" (p. 11). Such independence is evident when patients give their prosthetic devices nicknames. Patients may find it difficult to refer to these objects by their proper names. The disfigurement from a burn or loss of limb forces the patient to lose his uniqueness and possibly his social freedom. The patient who must undergo isolation because he has an incisional staphylococcus infection receives the communication that his body is unacceptable and undesirable. The loss of function or part, or disfigurement, creates a lowered self-esteem. A patient feels that his value as a human being has diminished.

During the acknowledgment phase, the patient will discuss the details or events that led to his hospitalization. He symbolically goes through the day's experiences, including activity, sleep pattern, or diet, trying to find that the cause of his injury or illness was external to himself, rather than an internal dysfunction. The burn patient may retrace every detail in the pump house in an attempt to learn if he was at fault. According to Combs and Snygg (1959), such events, or the patient's analysis of the events "acquire their meaning from the relations we perceive between them and our phenomenal selves. The perceptions we hold about self determine the meaning of our experiences. Generally speaking, the more closely related an experience is perceived to the phenomenal self, the greater will be its effect upon behavior" (p. 149). The patient goes over causative events in an attempt to prevent them from recurring in the future. The patient may be in need of reassurance or support regarding his future. Because of the complexity of the situation, he may feel a future is beyond his reach. He needs reassurance from his nurse and family that a future can and does exist.

As Norris (1978) notes, patients with third-degree burns over a large portion of their bodies can be saved. Nevertheless the resulting disfigurement can be terrible. Only slightly less appalling is the pain suffered from the burn and from innumerable plastic surgeries. The face is a major vehicle of communication. People respond to each other according to nonverbal facial cues. Therefore facial disfigurement produces a large number of emotional responses from other people.

The family needs help in acknowledging the patient's illness or injury. They may try to protect the patient by refusing to talk about his problem. Like the patient, they will focus on peripheral topics. Instead of asking the patient how he feels, what type of day he had, or what the doctors said, the family will elicit such information from the nurse. If the family has never seen a loved one in a critical care unit, they may remain in the impact phase and never progress to acknowledgment. The noises and strange attachments of the machines are all frightening. Besides the environmental impact, there is the emotional impact of physical disfigurement. Their loved one, once seen as a whole, has suffered a loss. The burned patient may be covered with ointment, gauze, or grafts. Instead of focusing upon him as a father or husband, the family focuses on the horror of his disfigurement. To the family, even though the words are unsaid, the patient is repulsive. Even though the words are not expressed verbally, the patient can read the words of repulsion on the faces of his family. To the wife of a patient like Mr. V., his loss of limb may be difficult to acknowledge. But eventually acknowledgment does take place. The nurse assesses her patient's acknowledgment when he asks such questions as, "How long does a pacemaker last?" "How long does it take before my grafts take?" "How long do I need to remain in bed?" or "How many days a week will I be in dialysis?" Each statement gives the critical care nurse clues about her patient's acknowledgment. Once the patient has verbally acknowledged his loss through these questions, he is ready to move into the rebuilding, or reconstruction, phase.

Reconstruction Phase

Levine (1969) provides a valuable clue for nursing care during the pathophysiologic process that causes loss of function or part or disfigurement:

> The discrete interaction may be disrupted because the individual organs or systems are incapable of performing their required interacting role. But even in the presence of disease, the organism responds wholly to the environmental interaction in which it is involved, and a considerable element of nursing care is devoted to restoring the symmetry of response—symmetry that is essential to the well-being of the organism. (P. 98)*

Reconstruction occurs in varying degrees, and it does not imply perfection. The disfigured patient may intellectually realize that the disfigurement was inevitable. The amputee patient can depend on his prosthetic device; the cardiac patient on his pacemaker; the emphysema patient on his tracheostomy; and the dialysis patient on her dialysis machine. The burn patient may need further constructive surgery to minimize any physical limitations. Regardless of the degree of construction, one should encourage the individual to try new approaches to life. During the retreat phase, he mourned his loss. During the reconstruction phase, he tries to adapt to changes in his body image. He has survived the physical loss, and now he must resolve the psychological and social loss. In doing so, he may discover things about himself never before known. With the help of other supportive systems such as the social worker, minister, psychiatrist, nurse, doctor, and family, he realizes his own strength. Throughout the crisis these supportive systems serve as an external source of energy, strength, and motivation. The patient and his family have realized that a crisis has occurred and that adaptative changes must be made.

The hemodialysis patient is reminded of his altered body image each time he is placed on the dialysis machine. Such patients must live with the continuous evidence of the existence of disease by maintaining a patent vascular access. Furthermore the patient's skin becomes jaundiced or assumes an ashen hue. Significant weight loss and neuropathy can occur with the latter causing mobility limitations. The dialysis machine reinforces the illness process. Visible circulation of blood outside the body makes the facts of treatment unavoidably apparent. Some patients may become confused as to whether their body is the machine or the machine is part of their body (Hutchful 1980).

The goal of the patient and members of his supportive systems is to help him achieve the highest level of reconstruction possible. The cardiac patient should reorganize his style of living to incorporate his new image. He will accept his pacemaker and feel fortunate that such a mechanical device was developed. Otherwise he would surely have died. The patient may assume a more positive attitude toward living his life to the fullest. He feels that he has been given a second chance. He may pay more attention to his new image in terms of activity, rest, and diet. Furthermore, he will have a new appreciation of his family. The surgical patient who lost a limb is thankful that he only lost one limb. He also appreciates the staff that gave him support and reassurance as he attempted to use a prostehtic device. The hemodialysis patient is thankful for the existence of a machine that will prolong her life, giving her the hope of seeing her children grow and develop—a hope that would have been unrealistic several years ago. The burn patient has hopes that therapy and grafting will minimize his disfigurement. He realizes that he alone can help himself through his determination to achieve a new level of wholeness.

Above all the reconstruction phase involves interaction and integration of the patient with other patients and with members of his family. Each interaction becomes an experience in social encounter. How the patient succeeds or fails will determine how he will react to new social interaction in his not-so-immediate environment. As Combs and Snygg (1959) point out, the individual's self "is essentially a social product arising out of experience with people. Although some of the individual's experience of self may be achieved in isolation from other people, by far the greater portion of his self arises out of his relationship with others" (p. 134).

NURSING ASSESSMENT OF BODY IMAGE DISTURBANCE

The critical care nurse assesses body image disturbance through the patient's behavioral response. The responses can be categorized into regulatory behaviors and cognitive behaviors.

Regulatory Behaviors

The regulator system involves inputs, processes, effectors, and feedback loops. It involves stimuli from the external environment and from changes in the internal state of dynamic equilibrium. The phenomena of body image can be said to be the totality of perceptions regarding one's own body and its performance. An individual receives stimuli relative to his body from many sources, both internal and external. Examples of internal stimuli affecting body image include hormonal influences, distention of gastro-intestinal tract, and retention of fluids. Stimuli from external sources, such as light or seeing oneself in the mirror, bring about inner reactions which affect the individual's perception of his body image (Esberger 1978).

The regulatory behaviors or physiological responses associated with body image disturbance consist of the following:

Regulatory Behaviors

Anorexia
Weight loss
Numbness of body part
Hypertension
Tachycardia
Tachypnea

Cognitive Behaviors

The cognator system involves inputs from internal and external stimuli which include psychological and social factors. The specific aspects of the cognator mechanisms consist of perceptual/information processing, learn-ing, judgment, and emotion. According to Norris (1978), cognitive and affective input about one's body boundaries, body competence, physical disability, and body worries over a lifetime require complex integration and interpretation by the cerebral cortex.

The cognitive behaviors or psychosocial responses associated with body image disturbance consist of the following:

Cognitive Behaviors

Anger
Hostility
Withdrawal
Hopelessness
Restlessness
Depression
Inability to focus on topic
Apathy

NURSING DIAGNOSIS OF BODY IMAGE DISTURBANCE

The nursing diagnosis is a statement of the current problem. Regulatory and cognitive behaviors coupled with stressors causing the problem combine to facilitate a diagnosis of body image disturbance. Internal stressors can be either physiological or psychological alterations. For example, biological illness, injury, or disease may cause a psychological response due to tumors, surgical removal of a body part, edema, or color changes. Psychologically the individual may need to change his perception of himself, which can lead to role disturbance. External stressors involve people's reaction to a change in physical appearance, life-style changes, or changes in values, beliefs, and attitudes.

NURSING INTERVENTIONS SUPPORTIVE OF ALTERED BODY IMAGE

The critical care nurse can attempt to support her patient as he moves through the various phases involved in his altered body image. The nurse and other members of the health team help the patient accept and adapt to changes in his body image. Each supportive member does this through his or her sensitivity to the patient's needs and anxieties expressed in each adaptive phase.

Impact Phase

The nurse keeps in mind that for a critically ill patient the impact phase can determine whether or not he progresses to the reconstruction phase. As Becken (1978) points out, the impact phase can cause psychological shock, especially when physical input from all body parts or boundaries has become altered, reduced, or eliminated. This is especially true for the stroke patient. Physical input contributes to body image formation through the central and peripheral nervous system. The nerve tracts that innervate skeletal muscles control both motor movement and muscle tone. Messages from the dorsal roots of the spinal end provide sensory input indicating the individual's body position. This is significant nervous input for the development of body image. It tells the individual where his body is and what it is doing. Furthermore it is vital in pathology, since, without this input the individual loses all of this stimuli and subsequently loses contact with portion of the body.

The responsibilities of admitting a patient at first submerge the intensive care nurse. These responsibilities include life-saving treatments and procedures. The nurse must assist in numerous activities that intrude upon the patient: the application of cardioscope wires, CVP, IV, a Foley catheter, or an oxygen mask. The pulmonary patient's status may warrant a tracheostomy or endotracheal tube connected to a volume respirator. Another patient may need an arterial line, Swan-Ganz line, or chest tube. Regardless of the patient's illness or injury, he is subjected to the intrusion of needles. Depending upon the patient's problem, he may need additional laboratory blood work to confirm a diagnosis. It is just as well the patient is in psychological shock: the threat of each intrusion may thus be less intense. At this time the nurse has to look beyond the scope of her procedures. She must realize that her interventions may create psychological stress, and she cannot give all her energies to the physical aspects of illness. She can learn the patient's perception of what happened to him and what will happen to him, in order to help her and the health team to anticipate potential behavioral responses. The patient who experiences guilt over his illness or injury may later despair; the patient who projects his crisis as originating outside himself may later express anger or hostility.

During the impact phase, according to Becken (1978), the predominant emotional alteration due to body image disturbance involves feelings of forced dependency due to reliance upon strangers, frustration over immobility, denial, situational depression directly related to the extent of the injury, the need to attract attention to oneself, the need for significant others to communicate openly, and uncertainty toward the future. For the stroke patient, the impact phase is associated with changes in perception of body space, posture, movement, somatic bulk and size, and continuity.

During the initial stages of the impact phase, the patient may be in psychological shock. The nurse can intervene continually to define for the patient his physical location and, if necessary, the location of his illness or injury. It may be necessary to tell a burn patient, like Mr. B., the location of his burns. In addition he will want to know about his accident, the extent of his injuries, and the nature of his hospitalization. The nurse can answer to the best of her ability and, because the patient's own anxiety state may not permit his intake of too many details, she can provide simple and direct answers. As he begins to move into the acknowledgment phase, the patient may demand more lengthy and complex answers, but in the initial phase the nurse can spend more of her teaching time with family members. Like the patient, they also experience psychological shock, but their psychological shock is not, like the patient's, compounded with a physiological crisis. Therefore the family becomes ready much earlier for supportive systems other than those offered by the nurse. Not all patients and their families will need outside supportive systems such as social workers or psychiatrists, but when such help is needed, it can be introduced during the impact phase.

Another duty of the critical care nurse during the impact phase is to assess the patient's behavioral changes and respond to them accordingly. If her patient despairs for too long, he may become so discouraged that he passively accepts death. Therefore, she and other members of the health team work together to identify the origin of their patient's despair. They can be mindful that his despair and discouragement may necessitate the support of others, such as a psychiatrist or a minister, but even with various supportive systems in operation, the patient will move into the retreat phase and subsequent denial.

The nurse can also keep in mind that sudden and traumatic injuries tend to result in more severe reactions because the individual has not had a gradual opportunity to begin incorporating the alterations into his life-style and his body image (Becken 1978).

Retreat Phase

As discussed above, it is during the retreat phase of alteration in image that the patient may choose to deny. His denial takes the form of refusing to participate in his care and of using symbolism when referring to himself or his supportive devices. The nurse can intervene to discover why her patient may not want to participate. The following dialogue illustrates how a nurse can persuade an amputee patient to practice his transfer techniques. Rather than forcing him to participate or allowing him to avoid participation, the nurse involves herself in discovering why he refuses.

NURSE: Mr. B., you haven't been practicing your transfer exercises.

MR. B.: I don't need to. I can do it when the time comes.

NURSE: The time is now.

MR. B.: No. I want to rest a little longer.

NURSE: Mr. B., it takes practice to transfer safely. If you begin now, you can independently transfer into a chair.

MR. B.: No I really don't want to. I like it here in bed.

NURSE: Why?

MR. B.: I just do, that's why.

NURSE: Is that your only reason? Wouldn't you like to visit your friends?

MR. B.: No, I don't want them to see my leg. In bed I can keep it covered.

NURSE: I see, Mr. B. What if I pulled the curtains around you while you practice transferring? Then no one can see you. Once in your chair, I'll cover your legs.

MR. B.: I might try that.

NURSE: Great!

The critical care nurse can remember that the patient may want to hide his disfigurement. In order to encourage his involvement, the nurse can intervene to protect him from disclosure of the disfigurement. She will realize that as the patient adequately mourns his loss, he will independently share his disfigurement with others. In the situation illustrated in the dialogue, the nurse successfully intervened to protect her patient's image by closing his curtains and covering both legs. Had she not pursued his reason for not getting out of bed, she would not have discovered his own concept of his altered body image.

The patient who uses symbolism may be seeking reassurance or validation from his nurse. The nurse can respond with concern; laughter would only validate the patient's negative body image. Instead the nurse responds by reacting to the patient's symbolism. The following is an example of a nurse's response to patient symbolism:

PATIENT:	You know, Alice, I have been thinking about a future job.
NURSE:	Oh? Tell me about it.
PATIENT:	Well, I decided I can always get a job in a circus side show. (*Silence.*)
NURSE:	Why a circus?
PATIENT:	Everyone loves to laugh at the freaks in a circus.
NURSE:	Is that how you see yourself?
PATIENT:	Well isn't that how everyone sees me?
NURSE:	No, and you didn't answer my question. Do you see yourself as a freak?
PATIENT:	I guess so.
NURSE:	But you are not sure.
PATIENT:	Yes. I am afraid I'll be completely disfigured, so no one will look at me without laughing.
NURSE:	First of all, you will not be completely disfigured. It is too early to tell. Later, corrective surgery can be done. Let's look at the positive changes.

The nurse can then focus on the positive aspects of the patient's body image. She may realize that this patient needs a great deal of reassurance, and she will therefore organize a team conference designed to create a plan of affirmative input for his changing body image. The entire team can establish a framework in which the patient is helped to view himself as a person. The objective is to help the patient identify positive changes in his progress.

The nurse and other members of the health team can assess the patient's reason for refusal to participate in his own care. Next she can listen for evidence of symbolism, whether projected toward himself or toward supportive devices. In hemodialysis the team may even encourage naming of the dialysis machine. The nurse can learn the patient's feelings by his references to the dialysis machine. For example, one patient said, "Well, how is George today?" Later during his hospitalization, the same patient referred to George as "my friend." The dialysis nurse realized that the patient saw his machine as his friend. He had acknowledged his dependency upon it. Of course, not all patients will view life-supportive devices with such affection.

Acknowledgment Phase

The nurse and others in the health team help the patient acknowledge alteration in body image through their own involvement. Involvement allows the nurse to become knowledgeable about the patient's particular needs. He may need affection, control, or perhaps inclusion in planning his care. Such knowledge helps the nurse look at the patient in light of the alteration of his body image. During the acknowledgment phase, she can learn about the patient's feelings of self-esteem and security as well as his ability to cope.

This knowledge becomes helpful in identifying actual or potential problems. Through discussions while bathing the patient, changing his dressing, observing his dialysis exchange, obtaining culture of a wound, checking his pacemaker, or simply sitting at his bedside, the nurse learns a great deal regarding her patient's self-concept. Furthermore, the nurse who works with patients who have experienced alteration of body image can recognize, as Norris (1978) points out, that body image attack involves "problems of altered appearance, discomfort, dependence, stigma, social isolation, action and movement limitation, vocational threat, deformity, and loss of control" (p. 34).

It should be noted that many burned people who have lost hair, nose, eyes, ears, and chin have also lost fingers, toes, and feet. These people often express the desire to die. They cannot integrate so much destruction into their body schema or face the prospect of living as a cripple (Norris 1978). In addition, the changing of the body's appearance surgically can be emotionally devastating to the person's self-esteem. Realizing that a loss of health or alteration in body image can threaten an individual's ability to cope, as well as his feelings of usefulness, is imperative in understanding people. Angry reactions may occur against feelings of helplessness (Motta 1981).

The acknowledgment phase may be a difficult one for the patient. It is at this time that the patient comprehends his altered body image. Norris (1978) provides valuable clues for nursing care at this stage:

> In relation to a patient's body image, the nurse can look for indication that his life roles are challenged, threatened, or are meaningless; that the patient is questioning who he is; that he is experiencing strange bodily sensations, loss of feeling or contact, detachment or depersonalization, as if he were observing what is happening to him instead of experiencing it. (P. 34).

To reinforce the patient's realistic acknowledgment of his altered body image, the nurse can encourage him to interact with other patients who have a similar problem. The critical care nurse can intervene to establish one-to-one or group encounter sessions. A dialysis group, for example, can have a mix of men and women and both experienced and new dialysis patients. Members within the group could support one another and share any concerns they might have. Such group encounters can be encouraging to new dialysis patients like Mrs. L. The more experienced dialysis patients can provide helpful hints to new dialysis patients. A nurse and psychiatrist can attend some of the meetings to provide professional input. Similar groups can be organized for cardiac and burn patients. Group or encounter sessions can originate in the hospital and can continue once the patient leaves the hospital. Family members can be encouraged to attend the group sessions or to originate their own group sessions.

The critical care nurse will realize that when her patient arrives at the acknowledgment phase of his adaptation, he has a partial picture of his own image. She can discover what the picture is and help the patient complete his drawing, realistically enhancing his self-esteem by identifying his positive attributes and actively reinforcing his accomplishments. She can determine her patient's point of readiness and initiate steps for his future, which is the focus of the reconstruction phase.

Reconstruction Phase

The critical care nurse knows that a person's self-esteem will greatly influence how the patient adapts to body image alterations during the reconstruction phase. High self-esteem expresses the feeling that one is good enough. The individual simply feels that he is a person of worth; he respects himself for what he is. On the other hand, low self-esteem implies self-rejection, self-dissatisfaction, and a poor self-concept (Wells and Marwell 1976).

All the nurse's original interventions eventually lead the patient to this final phase, so reconstruction really begins during the impact phase. The critical care nurse can attempt to reconstruct the patient's body image as soon as possible: the patient will need constant realistic encouragement that his recovery is progressing. A disfigurement like scars from burns or loss of a limb may create internal feelings of worthlessness, and the nurse must be aware of such feelings and help the patient to feel significant during the crisis. She can draw upon the patient's internal and external strengths. The amount of internal strength depends upon the patient's concept of self, body image, or self-esteem prior to the injury. If he has a well-defined image, the nurse will have a much easier time moving her patient along the health continuum. But if he had a poor body image or self-concept, her task will be difficult. She must carefully assess his strengths, no matter what they might be, and capitalize upon them.

Most of the actual reconstruction takes place between the patient and his family. The adaptive changes made to alteration in body image depend upon the family and patient. Each is aware of the physical, psychological, or social loss, and each is aware of the gains in terms of new approaches to their future and new strengths.

NURSING EVALUATION

Evaluation of the patient's problem and nursing care is an ongoing process. The critical care nurse assesses regulatory and cognitive behaviors supporting the diagnosis of body image disturbance. Interventions designed to minimize body image disturbances are evaluated for their effectiveness. The behaviors may not be totally removed until the patient is returned to a familiar environment. Depending upon the type and degree of body image alterations, the patient may require follow-up care to facilitate continued adaptation.

SUMMARY

The nurse's involvement with the critical care patient's body image and self-concept begins by her active and quiet role at the onset of his hospitalization. While caring for him, she gains knowledge about his concept of self and body image. On the basis of this knowledge, she assists him in planning for the future. A significant part of the future includes his family, so the nurse helps her patient and family reorganize his altered body image into something meaningful and worthwhile.

REFERENCES

BECKEN, JANICE, "Body Image Changes in Plegia," *The American Associate of Neurological Nurses*, 19 (March 1978), 20-23.

BELAIEF, LYNNE, "Self-Esteem and Human Equality," *Nursing Digest*, 6, no. 1 (Fall 1978), 59-67.

BILLE, DONALD, "The Role of Body Image in Patient Compliance and Education," *Heart and Lung*, 6, no. 1 (January-February 1977), 143-148.

BOWDEN, LEORA, IRVING FELLER, DAN THOLEN, TERRANCE DAVIDSON, and MICHAEL JAMES, "Self-Esteem of Severely Burned Patients," *Archives of Physical Medicine Rehabilitation*, 61, (October 1980), 449-452.

BREZNITZ, SHLOMO, *The Denial of Illness.* New York: International Universities Press, 1983.

COMBS, ARTHUR W., and DONALD SNYGG, "Development of Phenomenal Self," in *Individual Behavior*, rev. ed., p. 122. New York: Harper & Row, 1959.

CORBEIL, MADELEINE, "Nursing Process for a Patient with a Body Image Disturbance," *Nursing Clinics of North America*, 6, no. 1 (March 1971), 156-157.

DIXON, J. C., "The Relation between Perceived Change in Self and in Others," *Journal of General Psychology*, 73, (1965), 137-142.

ESBERGER, KAREN, "Body Image," *Journal of Gerontological Nursing*, 4, no. 4, (July-August 1978), 35-38.

FAWCETT, JACQUELINE, and SUSAN FRYE, "An Exploratory Study of Body Usage Dimensionality," *Nursing Research*, 29, no. 5 (September-October 1980), 324-327.

FISHER, SEYMOUR, and SIDNEY CLEVELAND, *Body Image and Personality*. New York: Dover Publications, Inc. 1968.

GORDON, CHAD, "Self Conceptions: Configurations of Content," in *Social Psychology of the Self-Concept*, ed. Morris Rosenberg and Howard Kaplan, Arlington Heights, Ill.: Harlan Davidson, 1982, pp. 13-23.

GREENLEAF, NANCY, "The Politics of Self-Esteem," *Nursing Digest*, 6 (Fall 1978), 1-7.

HAGGLUND, TOR-BJONN, and HEIKKA PIHA, "In Inner Space of the Body Image," *Psychoanalytic Quarterly*, 49 (1980), 256-283.

HENDERSON, LYNDA, and C. J. GANTLAND, "Testing Disorders of Body Schema in Stroke Rehabilitation," *Physiotherapy Canada*, 30 (July-August 1978), 192-194.

HUTCHFUL, CONNIE, "Psycho-Social Stresses on Adults in Hemodialysis," *Nephrology Nurse*, 2 (September-October 1980), 31-50.

JOURARD, SIDNEY, *Personal Adjustment*. New York: Macmillan, 1963.

KOLB, LAWRENCE, "Disturbances of the Body Image," in *American Handbook of Psychiatry*, vol. 1, ed. Silvano Arieti, pp. 750-768. New York: Basic Books, 1959.

LANGE, SILVIA, "Shame," *Behavioral Concepts and Nursing Interventions*, coord. Carolyn E. Carlson, pp. 51-71. Philadelphia: Lippincott, 1970.

LEE, JANE M., "Emotional Reaction to Trauma," *Nursing Clinics of North America*, 5, no. 4 (December 1970), p. 578.

LEVINE, MYRA E., "Pursuit of Wholeness," *American Journal of Nursing*, 69, no. 1 (January 1969), 98.

McCLOSKEY, JOANNE COMI, "How to Make the Most of Body Image Theory in Nursing Practice," *Nursing '76*, May 1976, pp. 68-72.

McGUIRE, WILLIAM, and ALICE SINGEN-PADAWER, "Trait Salience in the Spontaneous Self-Concept," in *Social Psychology of the Self-Concept*, ed. Morris Rosenberg and Howard Kaplan, pp. 24-37. Arlington Heights, Ill.: Harlan Davidson, 1982.

MARKUS, HAZEL, "Self-Schemata and Processing Information about the Self," in *Social Psychology of the Self-Concept*, ed. Morris Rosenberg and Howard Kaplan, pp. 50-66. Arlington Heights, Ill.: Harlan Davidson, 1982.

MARLEN, LUCY, "Self-Care Nursing Model for Patients Experiencing Radical Change in Body Image," *Journal of Gynecological Nursing*, 7, no. 6 (November–December 1978), 9-13.

MOTTA, GLENDA, "Stress and the Elderly: Coping with a Change in Body Image," *Journal of Enterostomal Therapy*, 8 (January–February 1981), 21-22.

MURRAY, RUTH, "Body Image Development in Adulthood," *Nursing Clinics of North America*, 7, no. 4 (December 1972), 617-30.

NORRIS, CATHERINE, "The Professional Nurse and Body-Image," *Behavioral Concepts and Nursing Interventions*, coord. Carolyn E. Carlson, pp. 5-36. Philadelphia: Lippincott, 1978.

ROSENBERG, MORRIS, and HOWARD KAPLAN, eds. *Social Psychology of the Self-Concept*, Arlington Heights, Ill.: Harlan Davidson, 1982.

RUBIN, REVA, "Body Image and Self-Esteem," *Nursing Outlook*, June 1968, pp. 20-23.

SEVERYN, BETTY, "Nursing Implications with a Loss of Body Function," in *ANA Clinical Sessions*, p. 234. New York: Appleton-Century-Crofts, 1969.

FISHER, SEYMOUR, *Body Image and Personality*. New York: Dover, 1968.

SMITH, CATHERINE, "Body Image Changes after Myocardial Infarction," *Nursing Clinics of North America*, 7, no. 4 (December 1972), 663-668.

SPIEGEL, J. P., "Attitudes toward Death and Disease," in *The Threat of Impending Disaster*, ed. Grosser, Wechsler, and Greenblatt, p. 296. Cambridge, Mass.: M.I.T. Press, 1964.

TURNER, RALPH, "The Real Self: From Institution to Impulse," in *Social Psychology of the Self-Concept*, ed. Morris Rosenberg and Howard Kaylan, pp. 79-87. Arlington Heights, Ill.: Harlan Davidson, 1982.

WAGNER, SEYMOUR, *The Body Percept*. New York: Random House, 1965.

Webster's New Collegiate Dictionary, Springfield, Mass.: Merriam, 1974.

WELLS, EDWARD, and GERALD MARWELL, *Self-Esteem: Its Conceptualization and Measurement*. Beverly Hills, Calif.: Sage Publications, 1976.

15

Stress

BEHAVIORAL OBJECTIVES

1. Define the terms *stress* and *stressors*.
2. Identify the stages of stress.
3. Describe how the degree and duration of stress apply to the critically ill patient.
4. Identify how physiological stress applies to the critically ill patient.
5. State how previous experience regarding stress applies to the critically ill patient.
6. Describe how internal and external resources apply to the critically ill patient.
7. Identify five regulatory behaviors associated with stress.
8. Identify seven cognitive behaviors associated with stress.
9. Design a nursing care plan using the stress framework.

Stress has become a part of the twentieth-century person. Our daily lives are filled with various levels or degrees of stress. No age, economic, or cultural group is free from the effects of stress. There are individuals who experience daily stress because of their occupation, geographic location, or health status. Haan (1982) has indicated some of the many facets of stress:

> Stress is either a bad event or a good event that did not come about; its meanings are commonly understood even though some people's histories may be especially vulnerable to certain kinds of stress. Contrasting values about the best way to live—invulnerability or reactivity—permeate stress research. Finally, stress does not invariably lead to deterioration. It may facilitate growth by tempering arrogance and by enhancing our tenderness toward ourselves and others. (P. 254)

In many instances, stress involves a number of factors which can operate simultaneously or separately. Stress can originate from the individual's internal or external environment. Whatever the influencing factors, they tend to alter the individual's stable equilibrium.

Furthermore, the factors that constitute stress are not perceived in the same way by all persons. Two individuals confronted with the same task or situation may react with varying degrees of stress. What is perceived to be stressful by one individual is not by another. The individual's perception of stress is most significant. According to Cox (1978), the person's perception of the demand and of his own ability to cope affect his stress level. Stress may be said to arise when there is an imbalance between the perceived demand and the person's perception of his capability to meet that demand. An individual cognitively appraises a stressful situation and ability to cope. If a situation demands too much, he may not have realized his limitations. Yet the person will work on the situation without being stressed until it becomes obvious he cannot cope. The perceptual factor permits a balance between the situation and coping skills. Regardless of how others view the situation, for the individual experiencing stress, it is real, and causes him to respond behaviorally. One's response may be viewed as inappropriate by those not directly involved in the stress situation. However, to the involved individual, the response is appropriate.

Stress takes place when individuals or larger social systems are confronted with an environmental demand that exceeds their response capability. The consequences of not adapting to stress become significant to the critically ill patient. An environmental demand leads to stress only if individuals anticipate that they will not be able to cope with the demand and only if the consequences of failure to cope are perceived as signficant (Garbin 1979).

It is interesting to note that throughout his or her life, an individual learns various ways of coping or adapting to a stressful state. Exposure to actual stress or what is perceived as actual stress for long periods of time can endanger or even shorten an individual's life. According to Selye (1950), "Anything that causes stress endangers life, unless it is met by adequate adaptive responses; conversely, anything that endangers life causes stress and adaptive responses. Adaptability and resistance to stress are fundamental prerequisites for life, and every vital organ and function participates in them" (p. 4667).

Each individual perceives and adapts to stress in a unique way. This means that everyone has the potential or ability to realize their limits within a stressful situation or to destroy themselves through failure to recognize these limits. It should be pointed out that, as with anxiety, some stress is necessary to mobilize the individual into action; however, beyond this point, stress becomes a concern for all members of the health team.

The health team is becoming more cognizant of the interrelationship between stress and disease. There is interest in understanding the mechanisms which maintain health and those which cause disease. Obviously there is a delicate balance between health and disease. According to Selye (1982), the adaptive response can break down or go wrong because of innate defects, understress, overstress, or psychological mismanagement. When this happens, the most common stress diseases or diseases of adaptation consist of ulcers, hypertension, heart attacks, or nervous disturbances. Besides the physical stress of illness itself, hospitalization leads to changes in daily life and activities which can result in psychologic stress (Volicer and Burns 1977).

Stress is a growing concern for critical care nurses who provide care for multiproblematical patients. Important terms relating to stress will be defined before we discuss how the concept applies to the critically ill.

DEFINITION OF TERMS

The terms to be defined are *stress, stressors,* and the *stages of stress* as identified by Selye (1977).

Stress

Stress is defined as an intense exertion being experienced by the individual in response to a stimulus. Stress is an essential body response to environmental stimuli. However, stimuli that create extreme levels of stress cause responses that are inappropriate and are considered to be *negative stressors* (Hanebuth 1980). Stress arises from a transaction between the individual and the environment when the individual views stimuli as damaging, threatening, or challenging. In general, stress situations involve awareness of demands that exceed the available resources of the individual (Scott, Oberst, and Dropkin 1980).

Stress seems to represent a variety of responses manifested as anxiety, emotional tension or frustration, anger, inability to adjust to a situation, or difficulty with judgment and decision-making processes. Stress as an experience can be temporary, recurrent, or continual. Recurrent or continual stress can cause physiological and psychological exhaustion.

It is difficult to assess how much stress any one individual can endure. Measurements of stress tolerance have been accomplished inside a well-defined and structured experimental setting, but not in a nonexperimental setting. Therefore, when an individual is confronted with a stressful situation no one, including the individual, knows how he will respond. One can frequently hear a spectator of someone else's stress say, "I wouldn't react that way if I were him." Unless the spectator has experienced the same stressful situation or crisis, this statement is unjustified. There are times when members of the health team make the same or similar judgments. Regardless of whether the stress is real to the spectator, it is real to the individual involved.

There are many definitions of stress as it relates to events within the individual's internal and external environment. Many individuals define a stressful event as a threatening encounter, one that causes the individual to become insecure with himself or herself and the immediate environment.

Each individual needs to feel secure with himself, if not with the environment. If a stressful event causes the individual to react in ways unlike normal behavior, he or she becomes self-threatened. After a crisis has occured in which an individual responds in a totally unique way, he or she may be heard to say, "I even scared myself," or "I didn't know I was capable of acting that way."

Stress is conceptualized as a universal phenomenon in which the individual perceives environmental stimuli that tax the physiological, psychological, or sociological systems. Therefore stress is the physiological reaction of the body to an increase of demands made upon it. The overall response can be adaptive or maladaptive (Claus and Bailey 1980; Greiner 1981).

Selye, who has done vast research in the area of stress, provides one of its most practical definitions:

> We can look upon stress as the rate of wear and tear in the body. When so defined, the close relationship between aging and stress becomes particularly evident. Stress is the sum of all the wear and tear caused by any kind of vital reaction throughout the body at any one time. That is why it can act as a common denomination of all the biological changes which go on in the body; it is a kind of speedometer of life. (1956, p. 274)

In some regions of the world, a significant number of people live beyond the age of 100. In examining their culture, one notes a marked reduction in stressful situations; life seems to be tranquil and slow paced. In Western civilization, on the other hand, people are continually exposed to numerous daily stresses, including the growing stress of illness and disease. Stress, then, is the overall wear and tear on an individual's physiological and psychological being. Adaptive processes usually allow the individual to cope with stress. However, with prolonged stress even the adaptive process can become depleted and eventually fail. Nurses working with patients in critical care can assess potential stressful situations and the patient's stress response.

Stressors

Each individual, at some point, is confronted with stressors. *Stressors* are defined by Luckmann and Sorensen (1974) "as agents or factors that challenge the adaptive capacities of an individual, thereby placing a strain upon that person which may result in stress and disease" (p. 41). Lawrence and Lawrence (1979) note that any agent of harm that challenges our adaptive capabilities can be considered a stressor. Although stressors affect each individual in different ways, there is nevertheless a predictable similarity among people. For some individuals the stressor is minor and can be controlled. More frequently, however, stress is prolonged and of high intensity, requiring a series of behavior changes before adaptation can occur.

External stressors are effective to the extent that they are perceived as dangerous or threatening, that is, to the extent that they are cognitively interpreted as inimical. Thus, a situation is stressful if and when the interpretive cognitive activities of the organism transform the input in such a way that a perceptible internal change results (Selye, 1982; Mandler 1982).

The stressors or stimuli that produce stress diffuse in quality and intensity for each individual, and they may act together to augment, intensify, or reduce the total effect. It should be noted that both the pattern and time required to adapt to stress are affected to a great extent by the illness, injury, or disease necessitating hospitalization (Scott, Oberst, and Dropkin 1980); Lawrence and Lawrence 1979).

Stages of Stress

Selye (1977) has identified three stages of stress. The first stage is the alarm reaction. During the alarm reaction, the adrenal cortex discharges into the bloodstream. Eventually the gland can be depleted of its stores. At the alarm stage of disease, illness, or injury there is a fight to maintain the homeostatic balance of the individual tissues when they are damaged. Critically ill patients cannot exist in a state of constant alarm. Any agent so damaging that continuous exposure to it is incompatible with life causes death within hours or days of the alarm reaction (Selye 1979).

The second stage of adaptation or resistance is characterized by the lessening of the initial symptom associated with the alarm reaction. The individual's body is achieving optimal adaptation. During the resistance stage an abundant reserve of secretory granules accumulates in the cortex. It is as if the individual's body is getting ready for the next crisis (Selye 1979).

If the individual is exposed to prolonged stressors, the acquired adaptation may be lost. The overall result is the third stage of stress, namely, that of exhaustion. The adaptative energy or adaptability of an individual is finite. When the body is exposed to a noxious stimuli for a prolonged period of time, the individual loses its acquired ability to resist and enters into the stage of exhaustion. This final stage occurs as long as the stress is severe enough and applied long enough because adaptability has its own limits (Selye 1979).

THE CONCEPT OF STRESS
APPLIED TO THE CRITICALLY ILL PATIENT

Stress affects all critically ill patients. The very idea of being hospitalized and separated from the familiar and secure is stressful. When one is hospitalized, one relinquishes one's being to the control of others who manipulate the body in ways that are perceived to be intrusive. Of course loss of control depends upon the severity of the illness, injury, or disease process, and the causes and effects of psychological stress can vary.

The critically ill patient who is experiencing a biophysiological illness can also experience a number of psychological stresses. Some of the stressors consist of loss of presence of familiar persons, loss of identity as a person, loss of familiar surroundings and activities, and loss of self-actualization (Hanebuth 1980).

In order for the critical care team to assist its patients in coping with stress, a systematic means or tool of assessment is necessary. For the purposes of stress assessment, the tool will be referred to as a *stress framework*. The stress framework, consisting of three components, is a way of assessing the severity of a patient's stress experience. The three components are degree and/or duration of stress, the individual's previous experience with stress, and his available resources.

Degree and Duration of Stress

The degree and duration of stress can be further divided into two categories: psychological and biological. Both categories are affected by the severity of the illness, injury, or disease. The resulting stress can cause the individual to behave in psychologically predictable ways. Likewise, the individual's body must adapt to acute or chronic biological changes. With acute biological changes, the individual experiences short-term stress of tremendous magnitude. Because the stress is hopefully short term, adaptive responses will only be temporarily weakened and not depleted. However, chronic biological changes of a long-term nature can cause the individual's adaptive processes to become depleted. Such an individual may be unable to cope with even the simplest additional stress.

Psychological Stress. Janis (1974) has identified three phases of psychological stress: the threat phase, the danger impact phase, and the post-impact victimization phase.

Threat Phase. During the threat phase, the patient anticipates an on-coming danger. Of significance is the degree of danger anticipated. This is also referred to as the severity of stress, which Coleman (1973) defines as follows:

> Severity of stress refers to the degree of disruption in the system that will occur if the individual fails to cope with the adjustive demands. The severity of stress is, in turn, determined primarily by three factors; the characteristics of the adjustive demand, the characteristics of the individual, and the external resources and supports available to him. (P. 170)

The patient entering critical care is usually subjected to an unfamiliar, frightening, and stressful experience. For example, the coronary artery by-pass graft (CABG) patient may see the surgery as a devastating blow to himself and to his family. The patient is usually informed of the surgical procedures and postoperative course including the use of various intrusive and/or supportive devices. In some instances the patient may tour the surgical intensive care unit to see where he will spend a few postoperative days and to meet the staff who will be providing his care. For CABG patients the preoperative period is normally a stressful anxiety-ridden time when the activities of the nurse may be particularly significant in providing support and comfort as well as the routine physical ministrations required (Rakoczy 1977).

The patient may be confronted with both external and internal stresses, both implying a psychological traumatization for the individual. This is particularly significant if something of value is lost. External stresses are those associated with losses such as an important job, social role, values, or a loved one. Internal stresses are usually related to biological alteration in integrity. Biological alteration can also have a psychological effect upon the individual's self-concept and body image. Even though both types of stress imply a tremendous demand and can simultaneously affect the same individual, the nurse's intervention focuses more closely on the patient's internal stresses.

Hay and Oken (1979) point out that a stranger entering a critical care unit is bombarded with a massive array of sensory stimuli, some emotionally neutral but many highly charged. Initially, the great impact comes from the intricate machinery, with its flashing lights, buzzing and beeping monitors, gurgling suction pumps, and whooshing respirators.

The patient entering the emergency department is also confronted with numerous stressful stimuli. In a study by Jalowiec and Powers (1980), life stress and coping behavior were examined in emergency room patients with nonserious acute illness and in hypertensive patients. The researchers compared the number and types of stressful life events (SLE) reported by persons with acute illness and by persons with chronic illnesses for a one-year period prior to illness onset. They identified methods used by the two groups in coping with stress, and explored the relationship between selected coping styles, level of stress, and health status. The results were as follows: ER patients reported significantly more SLEs for the one year preceding illness onset, although more hypertensives subjectively rated their stress levels as high; ER patients experienced significantly more SLEs in personal and social, home and family, and financial categories; hypertensives experienced significantly more health-related SLEs; and hypertensive patients used significantly more problem-oriented coping methods than did ER patients.

It is hard for the nurse to assess what factors determine how a patient will psychologically cope with illness, injury, or disease. The factors may be highly individualized for the particular patient, usually focusing on the significance, duration, and variation of the adjustive demands during the threat phase. As Coleman (1973) points out, the timing of stress events is also significant:

> The importance, duration, and multiplicity of demands are some of the key characteristics of the stress situation that determine its severity. The longer the stress operates the more severe it is likely to become. Similarly a number of stresses operating at the same time or in a sequence that keeps the individual off balance are more stressful than if these events occurred separately. (P. 170)

Therefore, if the patient anticipates a continued exposure to a threat over a prolonged period of time, that patient will undoubtedly experience psychological stress.

Danger Impact Phase. The danger impact phase is the time during which the patient realizes that the illness or disease is at hand. The patient is environmentally surrounded by evidence of an altered biological being. Such evidence may take the form of supportive devices that are attached to the body. It is at this time that the patient further realizes that success depends greatly upon the protective actions of his own biological adaptive system and the support of the health team in the immediate environment. The degree of stress associated with the danger impact phase may depend upon the specific biological system involved. To many patients, their health represents life and the essence of their biological being. Therefore, any threat to this system is a threat to life itself. Likewise many patients fear renal problems or complication that might lead to dependency on a hemodialysis machine. A simple urinary tract infection may become a source of monumental stress for such a patient.

The patient who enters a critical care unit in the process of dealing with another stressor (e.g., unemployment or divorce) may need additional help. The burden of coping with additional stress such as illness, disease, or injury coupled with complications can be more than the patient is capable of tolerating (Bilodeau 1981). When confronted with stress, the individual uses his self-regulatory biochemical and psychosocial mechanisms to restore and maintain optimum functioning of the life-support processes. If the patient experiences a prolonged stress, the stressors act as a strain on the adaptive mechanisms (Lawrence and Lawrence 1979).

During the danger impact phase, the individual realizes the seriousness of his illness or injury. How the individual survives this phase is sometimes dependent upon the assessment of his capability for survival. This implies the notion that, "I survived in the past; I will survive in the future."

Patients may also experience stress if they are frequently hospitalized for the same biological problem. The patient with chronic obstructive pulmonary disease feels threatened with each recurrent respiratory infection. Each breath is exhausting and brings the patient closer to the things causing fear: dependency on a ventilator and dependence on others to help him continue breathing. Both threats of potential dependency cause psychological stress.

Within the danger impact phase, the patient behaviorally reacts in a unique way, directly associated with the degree and duration of stress. As stress increases, the patient experiences changes in cognitive functioning, including a reduction in objective thinking and adaptive efficiency. While experiencing stress, the individual also experiences a degree of emotional arousal. However, as the stress situation remains intense, the individual's emotional response may be inappropriate. These variables influence adjustment to stress and contribute to behavioral response. They include fear of loss to body integrity through damage and externalized anger. The patient manifests fear of altered body image through apprehension, nervousness, and attempts to protect the weakening biological being. The patient may manifest protective behavior by refusing intrusive procedures or treatments.

Externalized anger may be directly expressed toward members of the health team. The anger may be behaviorally manifested through resentment. As the illness, injury, or disease process becomes more of a reality during the danger impact phase, the patient resents forced dependency, especially if it becomes dependency without dignity. Throughout adult life the individual has moved independently, made decisions, formulated alternative plans, and in general recognized himself as a controlling force over internal and external elements in life surroundings. Suddenly the patient is confronted with the reality of illness or injury only to realize that there is a loss of control of the being. The patient fears that total control may never be completely restored. Therefore, the expressed resentment or anger at others is really misplaced.

In reality the patient is angry at his or her own body or the situation that led to hospitalization. It is far easier and safer to express anger toward strangers than toward oneself or one's family. Thus, externalized anger as behaviorally manifested through resentment is to be expected during the danger impact phase. The difficulty lies in assessing the behavioral response, as it may be latent or disguised as sarcasm, negativism, or inappropriate humor.

Postimpact Victimization Phase. The postimpact victimization phase is the time when the patient perceives losses. The battle has ended and the casualties need to be assessed. In assessing the sustained losses, the patient may experience deprivation. Depending upon the illness, injury, or disease, the loss may involve only a temporary loss of function or a permanent loss of part or whole.

Take, for example, the cardiac patient whose loss may be minor since only a small loss of myocardial function results from a myocardial infarction. Such a patient is free of complications and with proper supportive care can return to a moderately curtailed life-style. For the cardiac patient whose loss is major, complications such as congestive heart failure or cardiogenic shock may severely limit the patient's future. Each complication may signify a poor prognosis because loss of a part exists. Therefore, the biological and psychological losses are great.

Patients can experience loss of the whole. For the burn patient the loss involves large parts of skin, extremities, or fingers and toes. According to Brodland and Andreason (1979), patients who have been severely burned experience an intense and varied trauma. The trauma involves catastrophic injury, severe pain, possible cosmetic or functional deformities, and a threat to their sense of identity and value. The burn patient and his family seem to go through an adjustment process. The first stage is the acute shock and grief when both are confronted with acute physical and emotional trauma. During the second or convalescent stage, the patient and family begin to accept the event and work towards recovery. This latter stage is comparable to the postimpact victimization phase. The patient is able to look at the injury or trauma, realize his losses, and, with support, design a new future.

Another example of loss of the whole is the diabetic ketoacidosis patient who enters the hospital with a thrombophlebitis. The thrombophlebitis has severely diminished peripheral perfusion, thus causing the loss of the leg. Each individual experiences a loss of varying magnitude. The loss, especially that consisting of a part or whole, leads to deprivation. The cardiac patient may be deprived of an active life. For patients with an amputated body part, the deprivation focuses on altered body image and fear of future loss. As the newness and strangeness of the environment wears off, each of the above patients become aware of several perceptions that have specific stressful emotional significance.

Realization of loss, together with various biological and/or psychological deprivations, causes the patient to experience frustration. Frustration arising from altered or unfulfilled goals leads to psychological stress. The individual's frustration can compound an existing clinical problem, thus increasing stress related or induced illness. As psychological stress increases, biological process can break down. This can lead to biological and psychological disease.

Physiological Stress. Physiological stress is the second component to be assessed within the degree and duration component of the stress frame-work. Ironically, physiological illness or disease can be the result of psychological stress. According to Kral (1967), "It seems possible that under the impact of multiple severe stresses acting over a considerable length of time not only one, but all parts of the stress resistance mechanisms might suffer longlasting and even irreparable damage, although perhaps to a different degree" (p. 180).

Illness and disease cause the patient to feel as though he has an unknown thing inside his body. It becomes an entity with an existence of its own. Depending upon the severity of the illness, injury, or disease, the "thing" may render the patient a helpless victim. The nurse must keep in mind that stress affects people in different ways and, as Luckmann and Sorensen (1974) point out, that prolonged stress has its own dangers:

> A very stressful situation that is short lived is often better tolerated by an individual than a less stressful situation that tends to be chronic. This is because chronic stress demands continuous adaptive efforts. Eventually, because of constant wear and tear of a chronic nature, the individual actually changes physically and psychologically, becoming more vulnerable to other stressors. (P. 41)

Such is the case with patients who have pain. A few examples are patients with angina, peripheral neuropathy, pancreatitis, or incisional pain. The pain focuses the patient's attention on the affected body part. Likewise, after the patient has experienced an illness, there is a reduction in the adaptive capacity of the involved organ or system, although the same individual may be healthy in all other areas. An exception occurs when the individual strains the already altered organ beyond its capacity. When this occurs, other systems seem to become involved. The cardiac patient who sustains repeated myocardial infarction leading to a marked reduction in myocardial reserve and adaptable capacity further experiences other biological changes. The patient experiences pulmonary edema and possible hepatocongestion and acute tubular necrosis due to perfusion deficit.

Another example is the patient with mitral insufficiency due to rheumatic heart disease or papillary muscle dysfunction from myocardial infarction. If the patient's mitral insufficiency is due to rheumatic heart disease, the limitations are gradual and may not manifest themselves for years. Such individuals carry the potential threat with them for years and learn to adapt to its existence. Papillary muscle dysfunction may occur suddenly, thus minimizing the individual's ability to adequately adapt. The former condition is an example of long-term duration with less stressful significance. The latter, however, represents intense stress with short-term duration. Engel (1960) summarizes the concept of physiological and psychological stress as follows: "A person may satisfy all the criteria of health at any point in time simply because the adaptive capacity of a defective system—be it biochemical, physiological, or psychological—has not been exceeded . . . it may be a matter of time; eventually the system will break down under the impact of accumulated and repeated small stress" (p. 469).

Previous Experience

The critically ill patient's previous experience with hospitalization focuses upon two characteristics. These are stress tolerance and perception of stressful events.

Stress Tolerance. Stress tolerance refers to the degree of stress the individual can tolerate before becoming disorganized or decompensated. Each patient has a unique level of stress tolerance which depends on genetic and constitutional make-up, past experiences, or self-concept. Patients who have experienced continued biological crisis over a prolonged period of time seem to have a higher level of stress tolerance than others. Such is the case with critical care patients with chronic illness such as chronic obstructive pulmonary disease, congestive heart failure, or chronic renal failure. The patient has had to learn to adapt to continued stress. In other cases, the critical care team may not see the stresses in the patient's life or environment that contribute to the illness, injury, or disease process. The nurse may assess the situation to be tolerable; however, the patient's assessment is different.

Stress tolerance also involves the presence of stress coping. Coping with stress represents a gradual movement toward specified goals and is a necessary characteristic of growth. Coping strategies consist of the neurocognitive, affective, and physiologic responses to a stress situation and may be observed in the behavioral response dimension (Scott, Oberst, and Dropkin 1980). Guzzetta (1979) points out that if stress is manifested by high levels of psychophysiological anxiety, the patient may not be capable of attaining the desired goals of energy conservation, integrity, or effective function. Instead, the critical care patient may be in a maladaptive or ineffective state of learning. Therefore, when the patient is exposed to a new situation, he attempts to adjust in a variety of ways such as fighting or fleeing.

Stress tolerance also refers to the limitations and potentialities of the patient for dealing with stress. These factors are often dependent upon peer adaptation to stressful situations. Illness may be a new experience. Consequently, the individual has little previous experience with adapting to biological crisis. Stress tolerance is also influenced by the type of crisis involved. In other words, certain stresses have more significance and meaning to some individuals than others. The loss of a job may be less stressful to one individual than another. The fear of cancer may be more stressful to the individual who has a strong family history of cancer. Another individual may fear cardiac, pulmonary, or renal disease more than cancer itself. No one can predetermine what illness, injury, or disease will have the greatest degree of stress for a particular individual or that person's ability to tolerate the stress. The patient strives to maintain a balance or to reestablish a balance. According to Martin (1962) "Meeting his needs and adapting to the stress which confronts him in life, the individual, including his body, resorts to various measures—physiological, psychological, social—which tend to maintain a relatively stable balance between and among the various systemic parts" (p. 238).

Perception of Stressful Events. The second factor in previous experience deals with the patient's perception of the clinical problem. The patient's response to a situation is affected by a variety of factors. Previous experience, physical and psychological state, and his perception of the situation are all likely to affect an individual's response. How the patient views himself in a situation can determine his perception of the situation. When the patient receives inadequate explanations, he may attempt to develop one based upon his own perception (Errico 1977).

For critical care patients the severity of the perceived stress is dependent upon interpretation of the clinical problem. For example, a patient may enter the hospital complaining of abdominal pain, distention, and constipation and in that patient's mind a tentative diagnosis is formulated. Diagnostic studies and X-rays confirm what the patient fears; an abdominal tumor. The patient's doctor, in explaining the diagnosis, treatment, and prognosis, may outline the possibilities of the tumor being benign or malignant. In all probability the patient's attention focuses on the term *malignant*. For this patient, life has ceased with the diagnosis. Possibly he has known someone with a similar clinical problem who, in fact, did have a malignant tumor. Thus, the severity of perceived stress is tremendous. Unless the patient shares these fears and anxieties no one will realize the magnitude of the stress. Patients receiving a new diagnosis need time to think through their clinical problem and supportive assistance in asking the question that could alleviate some of their perceived stress. The questions and answers need to be provided in a definitive manner. Helberg (1972) points out the particular influence of stress on the patient's ability to understand and problem-solve:

People under stress seem less able to cope with ambiguous or unresolved problems. They feel a need to have things definite, sure and in clear figure, even though this may mean sacrificing accuracy. As a result of "tunnel vision," the individual becomes incapable of focusing on the total perceptual field. This results in a drastic reduction in the number of acceptable solutions. (P. 48)

The perception of stress is significant in determining whether a stressor will have negative or positive effects. Perception encompasses reception and cognitive appraisal of information. The individual is uncertain about the nature of a stimulus which encourages the arousal of the protective physiological mechanism of the body. Perception becomes a key to the internal and external conditioning factors that determine how a stimulus is evaluated by an individual (Claus and Bailey 1980).

It is interesting to note that the patient may distort perception of the stressful event in an attempt to reduce experienced threat. A major surgical operation such as a coronary artery bypass or the reconstructive surgery necessary after severe trauma constitutes a stress situation. These stress situations can be perceived as a catastrophe or disaster in which the patient feels like a victim. In seeing himself as a victim, the patient faces a combination of three major forms of danger—pain, body mutilation, and death. Furthermore, the once-independent individual is now a dependent patient. The patient in the prime of life is found in a critical care setting dominated by a sometimes impersonal health team. The patient perceives the health team as being unable to satisfy needs for pain relief and meaningful stimulation. Janis (1974) has graphically described what such a patient may experience:

Caretakers repeatedly demand submission to painful, disagreeable, and embarrassing manipulation. Needles are jabbed into the patient's arms; probes, swabs, or drainage tubes are poked into sensitive wounds; stomach tubes are inserted through the nose and down into the throat; evil-tasting medicine is poured into his mouth; bedpans are shoved under his buttocks and belatedly removed—these and a variety of other disagreeable demands and indignities are imposed upon him at a time when he is already in a state of general malaise, beset by incisional pain, backaches, sore muscles, distended bowels, constipation, and perhaps a generous spread of angrily itching skin. (P. 215)

Resources

Within the stress framework, resources are assessed according to their external or internal availability.

Internal Resources. Depending upon the severity and duration of the patient's illness, injury, or disease, biological resources may or may not be bountiful. One patient may have a greater host of internal biological defenses available than does another patient. Illness and disease involve an internal battle between the pathogen and the diseased organ. In most cases the latter defends itself against the catalyst of disease by an adaptive phenomenon. The patient may have a weakened or depleted adaptive protective membrane.

Therefore, a particular system or the entire body succumbs to the stress of illness and disease.

The range of stress-producing stimuli confronting the critically ill patient is extensive. The diversity of the individual's prior experiences and intellectual resources affect the capability of stimuli to produce stress. The stimuli that produce threat or nonthreat reactions are cues which inform the patient that a situation is good or it is bad (Errico 1977). For some critical care patients, their internal physiological or psychological resources may be depleted.

An example is the patient with chronic obstructive pulmonary disease or emphysema. The pulmonary system has attempted to adapt to the stress of continued changes in lung tissues and alterations in pulmonary function. For this patient a simple cold is a nightmare because of the potential consequences: pneumonia and/or the additional loss of pulmonary reserve. The patient fears the ultimate will happen: a tracheostomy, dependency on a volume respirator, extensive hospitalization in an expensive respiratory care unit, and inevitable death. As the biological condition worsens, stress is placed upon other biological systems. The patient develops cor pulmonale or right-sided ventricular failure due to pulmonary hypertension. This may even lead to hepatocongestion. Eventually, the status worsens, every breath becomes a struggle to the point where the patient refuses to eat. In this example, the pulmonary system tried first to adapt to the biological stress; when it failed to do so, other biological systems were called into action. Eventually healthy organs became weakened due to the continued role they had to play in adapting to a biological crisis, resulting in decompensation.

Stress also has its effect upon the patient's psychological reserve. The patient's psychological adaptation to stress can be affected in different ways. Coleman (1973) points out that "Under severe stress there is a lowering of adaptive efficiency—a narrowing of the perceptual field and an increased rigidity of cognitive processes so that it becomes difficult for the individual to evaluate the situation or perceive more effective coping responses than the ones he is using" (p. 173). On the other hand, the patient may realize that he has adapted to stressful events in the past and therefore can accomplish the same or similar goals in the future. The patient is then motivated by internal goals, desires, values, and ideas. As a result of stressful events, patients often gain confidence in themselves and develop new potentials. In other words, they have confronted a stressful situation and adapted to it.

External Resources. External resources consist of the patient's family, friends, and members of the health team. The younger patient's family resources may be more extensive than those of the aged critically ill patient. The latter may have outlived his or her own family. The nurse must assess the significance of the family's resources. The patient's wife, for example, may have limited abilities of her own for adapting to a crisis. Therefore, if her reserve becomes depleted the nurse has two people in need of supportive input. Like the patient, the spouse may demonstrate behavioral responses indicative of reduced stress tolerance. For example, a wife may become angry when her husband's dinner tray arrives without milk. This is a seemingly insignificant omission to the nurse; however, to the wife it becomes an outlet for her own accumulated stresses and anxieties.

There are times in critical care when stressed relatives misinterpret a situation. Furthermore, if they feel that their loved one is getting inadequate care they may become verbally abusive (Hay and Oken 1979). It should also be pointed out that different families may experience several of the same problems in dealing with value issues. In addition the family is concerned with financial concerns. The family may want the patient helped but view the care as dehumanizing. Therefore what the family desires and what is realistically possible may be in conflict.

Friends are another significant external resource to the patient. This is especially true for the older critically ill patient. If the family support systems are diminished or absent, there is more reliance upon friends. Friends can be encouraged to visit the patient when feasible. They become one of the last contacts with the nonhospital community. They keep the patient informed about social, church, or business events.

Members of the health team can become a source of external support to the patient but they can also become a source of additional stress. The patient may perceive staff members to be the source of stress. Therefore, the patient may direct anger toward them rather than utilizing them as a source of strength. Likewise, the staff may become upset with the patient, thus contributing to the stress. Needless to say, the patient's perception needs to be assessed and clarified so that his recovery will be expedited rather than extended.

NURSING ASSESSMENT OF STRESS

Stress is a nonspecific response, both physiological and psychological, to any disruption of one's homeostasis or equilibrium. Psychological stress affects physiologic variables such as blood pressure, pulse rate, secretion of adrenalin, and excretion of catecholamines and corticosteroids; it has also been suggested as an etiologic factor in thyroid disorders, cardiac pathology, essential hypertension, and gastrointestinal dysfunction (Lippincott 1979; Volicer and Burns 1977).

The nurse assesses stress through the patient's behavioral responses. The responses are categorized into regulatory and cognitive behaviors.

Regulatory Behaviors

The regulator system involves inputs, processes, effectors, and feedback loops. It involves stimuli from the external environment and from changes in the internal state of dynamic equilibrium. The regulatory behaviors are physiological responses.

When a sudden injury or acute illness occurs, the afferent impulses lead to activation of the sympathetic/adrenal medullary system through the centers in the hypothalamus and hindbrain. Stress creates several physiological behaviors which can be categorized as follows (S. Williams 1979; Guzzetta and Forsyth, 1979):

Regulatory Behaviors
Increased heart rate
Increased myocardial contraction
Increased coronary vasoconstriction
Increased vasoconstriction
Increased blood pressure
Pupil dilatation
Increased serum glucose
Bronchiolar dilatation
Increased cardiac output
Decreased urinary output

Other physiological responses include increased serum glucose, increased free fatty and amino acids, increased sodium and chloride reabsorption, and increased potassium and hydrogen excretion.

Physiological stress causes hormonal and neural reactions. These events help the body adapt to its physical and emotional environment. As discussed earlier, when the body is under stress it responds with a unified defense mechanism. During the alarm stage, the nervous and endocrine system produces chemicals necessary to deal with the stresses. Adrenocorticotropic hormone (ACTH) is secreted, which in turn stimulates the secretion of cortisone and aldosterone from the adrenal cortex (Slay 1976).

Some stress is useful for the critically ill patient. However, when physiological and/or psychological stress is prolonged, the result can be harmful for the patient with cardiac dysfunction such as myocardial infarction, cardiogenic shock, or congestive heart failure. The sympathetic nervous system releases norepinephrine. This leads to tachycardia, increased atrial and ventricular contractility, increased myocardial oxygen consumption, and decreased coronary venous oxygen saturation due to coronary vasoconstriction. Peripheral vascular resistance is increased, thereby increasing blood pressure. Lastly, vasoconstriction of most blood vessels, especially those of the abdominal viscera and extremities, occurs (Guzzetta and Forsyth 1979).

Cognitive Behaviors

The cognator system involves inputs from internal and external stimuli which include psychological and social factors. The specific aspects of the cognator mechanism consist of perceptual/information processing, learning, judgment, and emotion. The cognitive behaviors are psychological responses.

The amount of stress and the patient's ability to handle it determine whether a specific stimulus constitutes a psychological stressor. For example, the stress potential found in the dehumanization aspects of life-support technology may lead to disruption of psychological equilibrium. The use of endotracheal tubes, respirators, monitors, intravenous and intraarterial lines all serve both to heighten tension and to separate the critical care team from the patient (Lippincott 1979; Hanebuth 1980).

The cognitive behaviors associated with stress consist of the following (Guzzetta and Forsyth 1979; Lippincott 1979; Hanebuth 1980):

Cognitive Behaviors
Anxiety
Fear
Increased mental activity
Abnormal head movement
Dyspnea
Shortness of breath
Hyperventilation
Irrelevant or constant conversation
Gastric discomfort
Hand tremors
Muscle tension
Diaphoresis
Restlessness
Palpitation
Agitation
Fatigue
Increase in errors

Some behaviors may actually signify the fight or flight stress response. The fight response is manifested by irritability, argumentativeness, anger, or explosiveness. On the other hand, flight stress response consist of depression, withdrawal, distance, and quietness.

NURSING DIAGNOSIS OF STRESS

The process of nursing diagnosis involves placing a patient in a diagnostic category for the primary purpose of identifying and directing appropriate nursing management (Guzzetta and Forsyth 1979). The nursing diagnosis is a statement of the current problem. The regulatory and cognitive behaviors help the critical care nurse make her diagnosis. For example, one of the major diagnostic indicators of a stress response syndrome, the neurotic response to personal injury or loss, is the experience of recurrent, intrusive episodes of thought and emotion (Krupnick and Horowitz 1981). The overall problem diagnosed by the nurse is stress.

NURSING INTERVENTION TO REDUCE STRESS

Facilitating the patient's adaptation to illness, injury, or disease and progression toward self-dependency involves a series of goal-directed nursing activities. The activities begin with the formulation of a therapeutic relationship where the nurse and patient work toward mutually acceptable goals. Nursing interventions focus on the three phases within the stress framework. These include the degree and duration of stress, the previous experience with stress, and the resources available to alleviate stress.

Degree and Duration of Stress

The nurse assesses both psychological and physiological components relating to the degree and duration of stress as it pertains to the patient's illness, injury, or disease process.

Psychologial Stress. Communication is a major factor in lessening the psychological intensity and duration of stress. The critically ill patient needs to communicate fears and anxieties related to his illness or disease. Prolonged illness may deplete financial reserve, thus creating additional stress that may be more overwhelming than the illness itself. The illness, injury, or disease may cause the patient to lose a job and/or social status. For example, the male patient may have experienced repeated renal infection to the point where he is now dependent upon a hemodialysis machine. His illness and dependency upon the dialysis machine may also lead to role changes. Now his wife must assume the financial responsibilities of the household. Such role changes associated with financial concerns can represent an additional source of stress. Therefore, the nurse needs to assess the degree of stress experienced by the patient prior to behavioral manifestations. The nurse realizes that illness itself causes stress of varying magnitude. Once the nurse assesses what is believed to be the potential source of stress, she validates her assessment with the patient. As emphasized before, each individual may have a different definition and perception of what is a stressful event. Talking about stressful events gives the nurse insight into the patient's ability to adapt to stress and to formulate alternative plans designed to incorporate the stressful event. In addition, it gives the nurse the opportunity to assess the patient's openness to external resources. There are patients who desire total independence in handling their own problems, including biological ones.

The physical environment of critical care presents the patient with obstacles to functioning well. Distracting noises emanate from the unit's complex supportive devices, from patients who are confused or in pain, and from the critical care team. The nurse helps the patient identify meaningful stimuli from the multitude of existing stimuli. Explaining the significance of supportive devices or treatment procedures also helps to minimize psychological stress. As she explains, the nurse helps the patient to assess the illness and therapy objectively. This involves a systematic teaching program that includes information designed to help the patient at various stages of the illness.

In a study by Volicer and Burns (1977), the question was raised whether high life stress patients have high hospital stress regardless of the severity of the diagnosis. Their findings suggest that life stress has both psychological and physical effects. Patients who have experienced high stress prior to hospitalization perceive themselves as experiencing higher stress because of the hospitalization, itself, when compared to patients who have experienced low prehospital stress. The investigation sought to identify predictors of the level of hospital stress according to the hospitalization stress rating scale (HSRS). Several variables were identified to determine which could be used as predictors of hospital stress. The finding revealed that age and life stress were predictors of hospital stress. For medical patients the recency of previous hospitalization was a significant predictor of hospital stress whereas surgical patients with serious illness reported more stress. In addition, women reported more stress than men. Therefore it is possible that preexisting correlates of hospital stress can be identified at the time of hospital admission.

Sometimes older critically ill patients have their own unique set of problems. Due to their particular illness or debilitating disease, they may be unable to adequately care for themselves. Normally after discharge from the hospital, the patient returns to the security of familiar territory, usually the home. However, the aged patient may, out of necessity, be discharged into a convalescent home. The time spent in the new surroundings recovering from illness or disability is dependent upon the severity of the clinical problem.

The degree and duration of psychological stress can be reduced by assessing the origin of the patient's stress. If feelings of abandonment and separation anxiety are the sources of stress, longer visiting hours may be encouraged between family and patient. If financial concern is the source of stress, a social worker or financial consultant may talk with the patient. The nurse, then, is able to intervene in a variety of different ways, each dependent upon the source of clinical stress.

Physiological Stress. Alleviating the degree and duration of physiological stress may be a more difficult task for the nurse. Greiner (1981) points out that managing the physiological manifestations of stress is a significant nursing intervention. On many occasions, by the time the patient is ready for cognitive identification of and planning in regard to their stressors, a transfer to a less intense level of care in the hospital is also in order.

The critical care nurse diagnoses the specific nature of the stressor producing the stress response. Furthermore the nurse assesses physiological parameters to determine whether or not the patient is stressed. For example, the coronary care patient's cardiac rate can signify a regulatory manifestation of psychophysiological stress. The specific characteristics that would define the limits of heart rate might include a rate greater than 100 beats per minute. When the patient's rate increases to this rate, independent of arrhythmias or other physiological variables affecting heart rate, the nurse can suspect stress as the cause.

Physiological stress as a result of illness, injury, or disease cannot be completely alleviated. In this area, the nurse again assesses the intensity or severity of the physiological problem. The nurse's interventions are designed to help the patient establish a physiological balance or stability. The nurse supports the patient through stressful diagnostic tests. Part of the supportive care is to explain the purpose of each test. The patient and the family have a right to know the results of each test beyond the simplistic statement that, "Your BUN is slightly elevated." If the patient doesn't understand the meaning of BUN, he fails to relate it to a renal function or dysfunction. The nurse also intervenes to teach the patient about diet, medications, and discharge activities. In this way the nurse helps to lessen the stress associated with transition from hospital to home. The patient is given a set of realistic guidelines which will hopefully facilitate recovery.

Previous Experience

The patient's previous experience with illness and hospitalization contributes to stress tolerance and perception of stress. The critical care patient is in need of a supportive system that will raise his stress tolerance and foster a positive perception of bodily changes. In a highly technical environment, it is easy for the nurse to provide more supportive care to the equipment than to the patient. In so doing the nurse may not be aware of stress signals by the patient indicating his inability to tolerate stress. While her activities may seem like a natural coping mechanism to the nurse, they can make the patient feel more dehumanized. Therefore the nurse attempts to manage her own individual stress level and that of the patient in an attempt to raise the tolerance of both to stressors.

The critically ill patient has many responsibilities. He is responsible for his family, children, and job. Illness, injury, or disease threatens the individual's continued performance in fulfilling these responsibilities. Furthermore, a threat to body integrity also becomes a threat to ego strength. Hopefully, both are temporary problems. However, once the illness has stabilized there can be residual emotional effects, such as lowered self-esteem. This can lead the patient to have reduced stress tolerance to further crisis, such as complications.

The nurse assesses the patient's previous experience with illness and hospitalization. In doing so, the nurse assesses how each was tolerated by the patient and family. From this, the nurse learns things about the patient's ability to cope with stress and the patient's likes or dislikes. The nurse's primary intervention consists of enhancing the patient's ability to tolerate stress and clarifying any misperception regarding care and progress.

The critical care environment is perceived as highly stressful. In approaching stress from the patient's point of view, several ideas about structuring the physical environment of the critical care unit, with consideration of lighting, privacy and more control, have been examined (Greiner 1981).

Bilodeau (1981) points out that whatever is perceived as stressful by the individual evokes a physiological and psychological response. Furthermore a patient's perception can be altered through education. Perception is a cognitive process and is amenable to educational use. Educating patients about how to manage stress in the environment is cognitively oriented. Individuals can be taught to become aware of the stimuli that trigger defensive reactions and to develop appropriate coping strategies (Claus and Bailey 1980).

Resources

The nurse assesses both internal and external resources available to the patient. Internal resources are of physiological and psychological nature. Physiological resources may be absent, limited, or vast. Psychological resources involve the patient's internal strength, values, ideas, and goals. Illness, injury, or disease may temporarily interfere with the patient's life goals or values. Often the patient must be encouraged to temper or relinquish certain goals and values because of the nature of his illness and the fact that they may conflict with his care. Such conflict needs to be assessed and decreased. If ignored it will only serve to increase the stress experienced by the patient. The patient may not agree that the illness or disease warrants immobilization and/or dependency upon others. The patient feels threatened because there is no longer a sense of security within his body. He fears that a similar physiological crisis will occur and won't be noticed. Therefore, the nurse needs to facilitate the patient's sense of security in the external world and the internal being. As the physiological problem stabilizes, the patient turns attention toward the future.

Internal resources can be augmented through relaxation training and biofeedback, which emphasize modification or physiological responses, or through other means, such as the self-statements approach and imagery techniques, which focus on cognitive changes (Stoyva and Anderson 1982). Relaxation procedures counteract the physiological effects of stressors and can be useful in diminishing stress-related symptoms such as chronic anxiety, tension headache, and localized muscular tensions. They do this by reducing the patient's heart rate, lowering the metabolism, and decreasing the respiratory rate. All these responses can have a beneficial effect upon an already overcompromised cardiac or pulmonary system (Bilodeau, 1981). The methods of relaxation have many features in common. There is usually some emphasis on muscular relaxation; the individual is encouraged to use relaxation in everyday stressful situations; and the individual is given some cognitive procedures for producing mental quieting (Stoyva and Anderson 1982). Biofeedback, a technique using instrumentation to give a person immediate and continuing information of specific bodily functions of which he is unaware, has been used to teach patients greater awareness of mind-body correlates and conscious control of certain body functions (Bilodeau 1981).

External resources can help the patient realize a future. For most families, having a family member in critical care is a stressor. A brief application of the process used by the patient to identify stressors can be helpful to the family. It is imperative that the nurse try to listen to the family express their distress. The family can become a tremendous supportive system for the patient. Together they can make realistic plans for the present and future. They need to communicate any stresses regarding potential role changes or financial crisis. If there are children involved, they can be encouraged to communicate with the hospitalized parent. This can be accomplished through telephone calls, drawings, letters, or cards. Friends can be encouraged to communicate in a similar manner. If a telephone is not available in the room, one can be plugged into it. Lastly, the nurse herself becomes an important external resource, assessing the level of stress, intervening to alleviate or minimize stressful events, and evaluating the effects. The nurse realizes that individuals relate better if they are able to express their own threats, fear, and anxieties to others. The nurse accepts her patient's feelings and encourages his expressions of stress.

NURSING EVALUATION

Evaluation of the patient's problem and nursing care is an ongoing process. The nurse assesses regulatory and cognitive behaviors supporting the diagnosis of stress. Interventions designed to minimize stress are evaluated for their effectiveness. All stress cannot be totally eliminated; however, it can be identified and reduced. Therefore effectiveness is measured by a reduction in both regulatory or cognitive behaviors that indicate stress.

SUMMARY

In summary, the nurse assesses the patient's stress according to the stress framework. The nurse realizes that illness together with hospitalization constitutes stress for the patient. In assessing the level of stress, the nurse takes into consideration the degree and duration of stress, the patient's previous experience with stressful events, and the resources available to the patient which will alleviate stress.

REFERENCES

ANDREWS, GAVIN, CHRISTOPHER TENNART, DAPHNE HEWSON, and GEORGE VAILLANT, "Life Event Stress, Social Support, Coping Style, and Risk of Psychological Impairment," *Journal of Nervous and Mental Disease*, 166, no. 5 (May 1978), 307–316.
BAILEY, JUNE, "Stress and Stress Management: An Overview," *Journal of Nursing Education*, 19, no. 6 (June 1980), 5–7.

BILODEAU, CAROLYN BASCOM, *"Psychological Aspects," Critical Care Nursing: Body-Mind-Spirt,* ed. Cornelia Kenner, Cathie Couzzetta, and Barbara Dossey, pp. 171-196. Boston: Little, Brown, 1981.

BIRLEY, J. L., "Stress and Disease," *Journal of Psychosomatic Research*, 16 (1972), 235-240.

BROCKWAY, BARBARA, ORA PLUMMER, and BARBARA LOUIE, "Effect of Nursing Reassurance on Patient Vocal Stress Levels," *Nursing Research*, 25, no. 6 (November-December 1976), 440-446.

BRODLAND, GARE, and J. C. ANDREASEN, "Adjustment Problems of the Family of the Burn Patient," in *Stress and Survival the Emotional Realities of Life-Threatening Illness,* ed. Charles Garfield, pp. 230-235. St. Louis: C. V. Mosby, 1979.

CASSEM, NED, and THOMAS HACKETT, "Stress on the Nurse and Therapist in the Intensive and Coronary Care Unit," *Nursing Digest,* Fall 1976, pp. 76-79.

CLAUS, KAREN, and JUNE BAILEY, *Living With Stress and Promoting Well Being.* St. Louis: C. V. Mosby Co., 1980.

COFER, C. N., and M. H. APPLEY, *Motivation: Theory and Research.* New York: John Wiley, 1964.

COLEMAN, JAMES, "Life Stress and Maladaptive Behavior," *The American Journal of Occupational Therapy,* May-June 1973, p. 172.

COX, TOM, *Stress.* Baltimore: University Park Press, 1978.

DAVIDHIZAR, RUTH, "Stress Patient: A New Dimension in Psychiatric Nursing Education," *British Journal of Clinical Psychology,* 12 (1973), 130-136.

DOHRENWEND, BARBARA, and BRUCE DOHRENWEND, *Stressful Life Events: Their Nature and Effects.* New York: John Wiley, 1974.

ELIOT, ROBERT, *Stress and the Heart.* New York: Futura Publishing Company, 1974.

ENGEL, GEORGE, "A Unified Concept of Health and Disease," *Perspectives in Biology and Medicine,* 3 (Spring 1960), 469.

ERRICO, ELIZABETH, "Effect of Cardiac Monitoring on Blood Pressure, Apical Rate and Respiration with and without Information Feedback," *International Journal of Nursing Studies,* 14 (1977), 77-90.

FINESILVER, CYNTHIA, "Reducing Stress in Patients Having Cardiac Catheterization," *American Journal of Nursing,* October 1980, pp. 1805-1807.

FOSTER, SUE, "Behavior Following Acute Myocardial Infarction," *American Journal of Nursing,* November 1970, pp. 2344-2348.

GARBIN, Margery, "ANS Open Forum," *Advances in Nursing Science,* 1 (July 1979), 101-106.

GARDNER, DANIEL, ZNE PARZEN, and NANCY STEWART, "The Nurse Dilemma: Mediating Stress in Critical Care Units," *Heart and Lung,* 9, no. 1 (January-February 1980), 103-106.

GREENBERG, SHELDON, and PETER VALLETULTI, *Stress and the Helping Professions.* Baltimore: Paul H. Brookes, Publishers, 1980.

GREINER, DORIS, "Anxiety, Stress and Crisis," in *AACN's Clinical Reference for Critical Care Nursing,* ed. Marguerite Kinney, Cynthia Dear, Donna Packa, and Dorothy Voorman, pp. 323-330. New York: McGraw-Hill, 1981.

GROUT, JAMES, SUSAN STEFFEN, and JUNE BAILEY, "The Stresses and the Satisfiers of the Intensive Care Unit: A Survey," *Critical Care Quarterly,* 3 (March 1981), 35-45.

GUZZETTA, CATHIE, "Relationship between Stress and Learning," *Advances in Nursing Science,* 1 (1979), 35-49.

_____, and GARYFALLIA FORSYTH, "Nursing Diagnostic Pilot Study: Psychophysiologic Stress," *Advances in Nursing Science*, 1 (1979), 27–44.

HAAN, NORMA, "The Assessment of Coping, Defense and Stress," in *Handbook of Stress: Theoretical and Clinical Aspects*, ed. Leo Goldberger and Shlomo Breznitz, pp. 254-269. New York: Free Press, 1982.

HANEBUTH, L., "Behavioral Responses to Stress," *Journal of Nursing Care*, 13 (September 1980), 17-19.

HARTL, DAVID, "Stress Management and the Nurse," *Advances in Nursing Science*, 1, (July 1979), 91–100.

HAY, DONALD, and DONALD OKEN, "The Psychological Stresses of Intensive Care Unit Nursing," in *Stress and Survival the Emotional Realities of Life-Threatening Illness*, ed. Charles A. Garfield), pp. 121-130. St. Louis: C. V. Mosby, 1979.

HELBERG, DONALD, "Communicating under Stress," *Association of Operating Room Nurses Journal*, November 1972, p. 48.

HOFFER, WILLIE, "Notes on the Theory of Defense," *Psychoanalytic Study of the Child*, 23 (1968) 178-188.

HUCKABAY, LOUCINE, and BETTY JAGLA, "Nurses' Stress Factors in the Intensive Care Unit," *Journal of Nursing Administration*, February 1979, pp. 21-26.

JALOWIEC, ANNE, and MARGORIE POWERS, "Stress and Coping in Hypertensive and Emergency Room Patients," *Nursing Research*, 30, no. 1 (January-February 1981), 10-15.

JANIS, IRVING, *Psychological Stress*. New York: Academic Press, 1974.

KACKETT, THOMAS, "The Coronary Care Unit: An Appraisal of Its Psychological Hazards," *The New England Journal of Medicine*, 279 (December 19, 1968), 1365-1370.

KRAL, V. A., "Long-Term Effects of a Prolonged Stress Experience," *Canadian Psychiatric Association Journal*, 12 (1967), 180.

KRUPNICK, JANICE, and MANDI HOROWITZ, "Stress Response Syndrome," *Archives of General Psychiatry*, 38 (April 1981), 428-435.

LAWRENCE, SALLY, and RENA LAWRENCE, "A Model of Adaptation to the Stress of Chronic Illness," *Nursing Forum*, 18, no 1 (1979), 32-42.

LEE, DOUGLAS, "The Role of Attitude in Response to Environmental Stress," *Journal of Social Issues*, 22 (1966), 83-91.

LEVINE, SEYMOUR, "Stress and Behavior," *Scientific American*, 224 (January 1971), 26-31.

LIPPINCOTT, RICHARD, "Psychological Stress Factors in Decision Making," *Heart and Lung*, 8, no. 6 (November–December 1979), 1093-1097.

LUCKMANN, JOAN, and KAREN SORENSEN, "Stress and Disease: Major Causative Factors," in *Medical-Surgical Nursing: A Psychophysiologic Approach*, pp. 41-47. Philadelphia: Saunders, 1974.

MANDLER, GEORGE, "Stress and Thought Process," in *Handbook of Stress: Theoretical and Clinical Aspects*, ed. Leo Goldberger and Shlomo Breznitz, pp. 88-104. New York: Free Press, 1982.

MARTIN, HARRY, "Human Adaptation: A Conceptual Approach to Understanding Patients," *The Canadian Nurse*, 58 (March 1962), p. 237.

MENDENHALL, JOYCE, "Factors Affecting Job Satisfaction/Dissatisfaction among Critical Care Nurses," *Focus*, October-November 1982, pp. 14-18.

MENNINGER, KARL, "Regulatory Devices of the Ego Under Major Stress," *International Journal of Psycho-Analysis*, 35 (1954), 412-420.

MILLER, STUART, "Ego-Autonomy in Sensory Deprivation, Isolation, and Stress," *International Journal of Psycho-Analysis*, 43 (1962), 1-20.

O'FLYNN-COMISKY, ALICE, "Stress: The Type A Individual," *American Journal of Nursing*, November 1979, pp. 1956-1959.

OSKINS, SUSAN, "Identification of Situational Stressors and Coping Methods by Intensive Care Nurses," *Heart and Lung*, 8, no. 5 (September-October 1979), pp. 953-960.

PEPLAU, HILDEGARD, "Interpersonal Relations and the Process of Adaptation," *Nursing Science*, October-November 1963, pp. 272-279.

RAKOCZY, MARY, "The Thought and Feelings of Patients in the Waiting Period prior to Cardiac Surgery: A Descriptive Study," *Heart and Lung*, 6, no. 2 (March-April 1977), 280-287.

ROMIROWSKY, SAMUEL, "Psychological Adaptation Patterns in Response to Cardiac Surgery," *Journal of Rehabilitation*, May-June-July 1980, pp. 50-52.

SCHAFER, WALT, *Stress, Distress and Growth*. Davis, Calif.: Dialogue Books, 1978.

SCOTT, DIANE, MARILYN OBERST, and MARY DROPKCIN, "A Stress-Coping Model," *Advances in Nursing Science*, 3, no. 1 (October 1980), 9-23.

SELYE, HANS, "Stress and the General Adaptation Syndrome," *British Medical Journal*, June 17, 1950, pp. 4667.

——, *The Stress of Life*. New York: McGraw-Hill, 1956.

——, "A Code for Coping with Stress," *AORN Journal*, 25, no. 1 (January 1977), 35-42.

——, "Stress Without Distress," in *Stress and Survival*, ed. Charles Garfield, pp. 11-16. St. Louis: C. V. Mosby, 1979.

——, "History and Present Status of the Stress Concept," in *Handbook of Stress: Theoretical and Clinical Aspects*, ed. Leo Goldberger and Shlomo Breznitz, pp. 7-17. New York: Free Press, 1982.

SHUVAL, JUDITH, "Migration and Stress," in *Handbook of Stress: Theoretical and Clinical Aspects*, ed. Leo Goldberger and Shlomo Breznitz, pp. 677-691. New York: Free Press, 1982.

SLAY, CONNIE, "Myocardial Infarction and Stress," *Nursing Clinics of North America*, 11, no. 2 (June 1976), 329-338.

SMITH, MARCY, and HANS SELYE, "Reducing the Negative Effects of Stress," *American Journal of Nursing*, November 1979, pp. 1953-1955.

STEHLE, JOAN, "Critical Care Nursing Stress: The Findings Revisited," *Nursing Research*, 30, no. 3 (May-June 1981), 182-186.

STOYVA, JOHANN, and CATHY ANDERSON, "A Coping-REST Model of Relaxation and Stress Management," in *Handbook of Stress: Theoretical and Clinical Aspects*, ed. Leo Goldberger and Shlomo Breznitz, pp. 745-763. New York: Free Press, 1982.

VANSON, SISTER RITA, BARRY KATZ, and SISTER KATHLEEN KREKELER, "Stress Effects on Patients in Critical Care Units from Procedures Performed on Others," *Heart and Lung*, 9, no. 3 (May-June 1980), 494-497.

VOLICER, BEVERLY, "Perceived Stress Levels of Event Associated with the Experience of Hospitalization," *Nursing Research*, 22, no. 6 (November-December 1977), 491-497.

——, and MARY BURNS, "Pre-existing Correlates of Hospital Stress," *Nursing Research*, 26, no. 6 (November-December 1977), 408-415.

WILLIAMS, MARTHA, "Crisis Intervention: A Social Work Method," *Social Work in Health Care*, 5, no. 1 (Fall 1979), 23-31.

WILLIAMS, STEPHANIE, "Physiological Aspects of Stress," *The Australian Nurses Journal*, 9 (July 1979), 44-48.

WOLFF, SULA, *Children under Stress*. Baltimore: Penguin Press, 1969.

16
Family In Crisis

BEHAVIORAL OBJECTIVES

1. Describe the functions of the family.
2. State how the stress of illness affects the family of a critically ill patient.
3. State how the stress of social loss affects the family of the critically ill patient.
4. Identify four cognitive behaviors associated with family in crisis.
5. Describe how fostering family support will help the family in crisis.
6. Describe how facilitating family education can help the family in crisis.
7. Discuss how fostering acceptance of the temporarily dismembered family systems will help the family unit.

When the patient is suddenly thrust into a critical care unit where the focus is on life and death, the family's homeostasis is altered. Responsibilities once mastered by the patient will now be added to the responsibilities of others, thereby requiring a sometimes drastic change in their schedules and activities (Busch 1982). Normally in critical care, the patient becomes the primary focus of the nurse's attention. This is understandable because the patient enters a critical care unit in biological crisis. His problems demand her full attention. To ensure that the nurse is able to focus her total attention on her critically ill patient, the family members are kept within a boundary labeled "Family Room." If family members should venture outside their well-defined boundaries and beyond the clearly labeled double doors of critical care, they will be immediately approached by the unit greeter. In most instances, the unit greeter is the unit clerk. The clerk may answer the family's questions or refer them to another nurse who may be unfamiliar with the new patient. Naturally, the nurse who best knows the patient is busily involved in his immediate care. In fear, confusion, or frustration, family members retreat into their boundaries and begin their long vigil.

The critical care nurse must focus her attention on the biological well-being of her patient. As Craven (1972) points out, however, "if the nurse expands her concept of the patient from that of an individual in a bed to that of a participating member of a family, then she will expand her role to assist relatives to cope with the patient's illness while simultaneously maintaining the family function" (p. 191). Ackerman (1958) describes the importance of the family as follows:

> None of us lives his life alone. Those who try are foredoomed; they disintegrate as human beings. Some aspects of life experience are, to be sure, more individual than social, others more social than individual; but life is nonetheless a shared and a sharing experience. In the early years, this sharing occurs almost exclusively with members of our family. The family is the basic unit of growth and experience, fulfillment or failure. (P. 15)

A critically ill patient may need his family more than ever. He is able to derive strength from his family to sustain him through his biological crisis. Critical care nurses must become more actively aware of their patient's position within the family and whether the family has strength needed by the patient. Unfortunately, the family may realize during a crisis that the sick member was the one responsible for the family's strength; they have no resources on which he can draw. He must rely on his own internal strength. This implies that the family members themselves have limited internal coping mechanisms.

As Craven (1972) has noted, the reduction in internal coping mechanisms may be the result of modernization in family living:

> Because of the very nature of the modern urban family, the resources it possesses to cope with the impact of illness are relatively weak. This weakness is partly because of the size of the nuclear family and partly because of the high emotional demands placed on it. As a result of the reduced size of the family, there is the definite probability that its members will overreact to illness, further intensify the stress loss for the sick individual as well as other family members. (P. 188)

Families may overreact to illness either by using the sick member as a scapegoat or by being too permissive with him. The family of a critically ill patient needs to be studied in more detail. No one really knows the fears and frustrations experienced by the family. In some instances, we can only speculate through clinical experiences about the family's inner feelings. Needless to say, more research needs to be done in this area.

The family has many functions and purposes. In illness, the temporarily separated individual realizes the significance of his family; similarly, the family realizes the significance of the sick member. Prior to this time, each may have taken the other for granted. Before discussing the family's response to critical illness, we will briefly explore some of the basic functions of the family.

FUNCTIONS OF THE FAMILY

According to Stern and Pascale (1979), the family constitutes perhaps the most significant social context in which illness occurs and is hopefully resolved. The family serves the function of defining whether a family member is termed sick or not, the type of care chosen, and the degree of compliance with the recommended medical regimen.

The family functions as an interacting and transacting organization, and, moreover, as Ackerman (1958) points out, has done so in all historical periods and cultures:

> The family is a designation for an institution as old as the human species itself. The family is a paradoxical and elusive entity. It assumes many guises. It is the same everywhere; yet it is not the same anywhere. Throughout time, it has remained the same; yet it has never remained the same. On the contemporary scene, the family is changing its pattern at a remarkedly rapid rate; it is accommodating in a striking way to the social crisis which is the mark of our period in history. There is nothing fixed or immutable about family, except that it is always with us. (P. 15)

A family functions in the capacity of supporting and protecting its members, both individually and collectively. When a threat to the family structure occurs, the members close their ranks in an attempt to protect themselves. Illness or injury to one member places other members in a state of readiness. If possible, the healthy members assume the roles of the sick member. Hill (1949) believes that "when family status is threatened from outside, there is a rallying of forces to meet the challenge, bringing sometimes a realignment of roles, but oftener reinforcing the original patterns" (p. 3).

Families have been described in terms of their functions as a small group or an open system. Hill (1949), for example, describes the family's internal relations in terms of paired roles:

> Family sociologists have come to view the family as a small group, intricately organized internally into paired positions of husband-father, wife-mother, son-brother, and daughter-sister. Norms prescribing the appropriate role behavior for each of these positions specify how reciprocal relations are to be maintained as well as how role behaviors may change with changing ages of the occupants of these positions. (Pp. 32-33)

Therefore, because each person within the small group has a role, illness disrupts the normal activity of the family. When a member becomes sick, other members must assume his or her role. This can place tremendous stress upon the remaining family members, who are already experiencing stress. Hopefully, family members apply their own sense of checks and balances to assure that no one member is assuming more than his share of the responsibility. In this respect, the family functions as an open system. As an open system, the family is capable of intake and output from the environment. In addition, it maintains control through self-regulation. Families attempt to maintain a steady state. There are obviously times such as in illness when the family cannot function as a steady state. The input in terms of stresses or crisis may create a temporary imbalance, but over a period of time, the stability returns to a more normal level.

If the family has a high degree of integration, role flexibility and predictive empathy, the patient will feel secure. In addition, the patient will be able to make the necessary adjustments required to assure an optimal recovery (Stern and Pascale 1979).

Families of patients hospitalized in a critical care unit attempt to continue in a steady state. They accomplish this goal either by minimizing the significance of the patient's illness, or by being overprotective of him. In either instance, the family may not realize the implications of their actions. The critically ill patient enters the hospital in biological crisis. Unlike the patient, the family enters the same hospital, or critical care unit, in psychological crisis. The patient has a better awareness of what is happening to him than does the family. After all, he lives with the minute-to-minute changes in his cardioscope pattern, CVP, urine output, arterial pressure, blood gases, and BUN level. He experiences first-hand the fluctuations or stability in his biological status. His family, on the other hand, must live in blind suspense. It is not unusual for the remaining family members to fantasize all types of unrealistic problems that could be happening to their loved ones. Needless to say, the family experiences its own personal and unique crisis.

THE FAMILY OF THE CRITICALLY
ILL PATIENT IN CRISIS

A crisis affecting any family member can have an effect upon all members. The crisis will produce shifts in the family equilibrium. It should be noted that crisis is not an isolated event. What affects the individual also affects the system of which he is a part (Cronin-Stubbs 1978).

Crisis has been defined by Hill (1949) "in terms of its effect upon families as those situations which create a sense of sharpened insecurity or which block the usual pattern of action and call for new ones" (p. 9). Parad (1959) further defines crisis as a "period of disequilibrium overpowering the individual's homeostatic mechanisms. During a crisis, a person is faced by a problem which, on the one hand, is of basic importance to him because it is linked with his fundamental instinctual needs and, on the other hand, cannot be solved quickly by means of his normal range of problem-solving mechanisms" (p. 56). A crisis occurs when an event happens that cannot be solved through usual means of problem solving. The individual or family must formulate alternative approaches to their problems. If the family has had to cope with crisis in the past, it may be better equipped to handle current crisis. There are families for whom illness or injury is a totally new experience. They lack previous experiences from which to draw new means of coping. Instead of effectively coping, the family may be disorganized by the crisis. When the initial impact of illness subsides, the family may collectively strive toward reorganization. Things may go smoothly until the sick member experiences a biological complication. Suddenly the family is once again thrust into disorganization. This fluctuation in the family's coping ability is characteristic of an open system. Miller (1965) has described the coping patterns utilized by the family as an open system as follows: ". . . as stress increases, the functioning of systems at first improves and then gradually worsens. This has been observed in families coping with a crisis. Initially, families function more efficiently, but as the stress continues, the family system may gradually disintegrate" (pp. 380–381). Hopefully, the disorganization is only temporary. If the family feels it has the support of the health team, it can better cope with the crisis.

According to Braulin, Rook, and Sills (1982), the impact of physical trauma is devastating not only for the patient but also for the family. The traumatic event and subsequent hospitalization in a critical care setting frequently result in a crisis within the family unit.

Each family reacts in its own particular way to crisis situations. As Hill (1949) points out, the degree of hardship experienced by the family is a significant element in its response to crisis:

> No crisis precipitating event is the same for any given family; its impact ranges according to the several hardships that may accompany it. Since no stress or event is uniformly the same for all families, but varies in striking power by the hardships that accompany it, the concept of hardship itself requires some additional attention. Hardships may be defined as those complications in a crisis-precipitating event which demand competencies from the family which the event itself may have temporarily paralyzed or made unavailable. (P. 35)

The sick member represents a subsystem within the whole system called family. As the stress resulting from illness increases, all subsystems within the family become involved. The immediate family may try to keep the crisis contained within its own boundaries. Likewise, the extended family (e.g., grandparents) may try to keep their children from worrying and becoming involved. In time, both family systems learn of each other's crisis and become involved.

Pollitt (1977) suggests that there are two major types of stress that result in symptoms. The first is *acute stress*, which involves a sudden change created from within the individual such as illness, injury, or disease. The second is *chronic stress*, which arises from a conflict or fear of loss of something valuable including changes in life-style or roles. The family in crisis will be examined according to events impinging on the family in terms of the stress of illness and the stress of social loss. Even though the two categories will be discussed as separate entities, they are interrelated.

Stress of Illness

In traumatic injury the losses are sudden, unexpected, and multiple. The family may be ill prepared to deal with the anxiety and tension created by the stressful event. Initially, family members may be immobilized by feelings of fear, shock, and disbelief. The family has lost the predictable function of the injured relative. Consequently the family's concerns are frequently focused on how they will manage to fill the functions now lost to them due to the injury (Braulin, Rook, and Sills 1982).

Crisis or stresses differ in origin. Some come from events outside the family, such as war, depression, or natural disasters. Other stresses develop within the family; illness is one such source of stress. The crisis begins for the patient the moment he understands his illness, injury, or disfigurement. The family experiences a similar state of crisis. The major difference is that the patient or sick member is centrally involved in the crisis; the family, though equally involved, must remain on the periphery. While remaining on the periphery, the family quietly experiences its own special stress, the sources of which have to do with the illness itself and the threats it implies. The threats include the critical care environment, with all its strange machines, smells, and sounds, and the frustration of being forced to remain outside the unit in a small territory designated for critical care families.

As Braulin, Rook, and Sills (1982) point out, the family spends much of its time in a family waiting area where members are separated from their sick relative. The family may respond with feelings of isolation and mistrust. In addition, the family may withdraw from the situation and attempt to minimize the importance of the stressful event.

Therefore when a traumatic injury occurs, the family is confronted with several stressors which include the following: sudden onset without warning; the foreign aspect of critical care, including unfamiliar staff; separation from significant others; an uncertain prognosis; and a potential financial crisis (Silverberg 1982).

A family member may learn of a husband's, wife's, mother's, or father's illness, injury, or disfigurement by telephone. For example, a man might have been playing golf, conducting a business conference, or driving his car when he suddenly became ill or injured. The wife, receiving the phone call, may be told that her husband had a coronary. She quickly makes plans for someone to watch her children while she desperately rushes to the hospital. In between receiving the tragic phone call and her arrival at the hospital, the wife has probably worked herself into an acute anxiety state. Meanwhile, the husband has been transferred from the emergency room into the appropriate critical care unit. There are times when the family has been instructed to meet a family member in the emergency room only to discover that he has been moved. The family may become further alarmed when the staff has difficulty remembering who this person is and where he has been transferred. After what must seem like an eternity, the family finds the location of their spouse or parent. Depending upon the type and severity of her husband's illness, the wife in our example may not be allowed direct admission into the unit. Instead she is greeted by the unit clerk or a nurse, who gives her a skeletal overview of her husband's status. The wife then retreats into the lonely family room to await further progress reports of her husband's condition. If all her husband's admission papers have not been filled out, she may be directed to the admission office in order to expedite the process. Family members may spend their first hour in the hospital locating the sick member, filling out numerous papers, and finally waiting to gain admission into the critical care unit.

The next source of crisis for the family occurs when it learns the diagnosis. The doctor enters the family's territory and informs them that the patient suffers from acute myocardial infarction with multifocal premature ectopic beats, acute tubular necrosis necessitating peritoneal dialysis, or some other strange sounding and frightening ailment. Even if the nurse or doctor translates the problem into a language understood by the family members, they still may not comprehend the significance. To them, the fact that the patient needs critical care is overwhelmingly enough. In their attempt to maintain a steady state, family members may not be ready to hear these explanations. All they want to do is see the sick member and be reassured that he will survive the biological crisis.

Finally, they can enter the critical care unit and see the sick member. It is not unusual to have families react with fear to the critical care environment; critical illness may be a new experience for family members, and they do not know what to expect. The last time they saw their ailing relative, he was leaving the house for work. At that point, he appeared healthy and free from injury. Now they see strange looking supportive devices. They may be so preoccupied with not disturbing the various wires and tubes that they remain at the foot of the bed. If they are brave enough to approach the side of the bed, they remain at arm's length. In this uncomfortable setting, the family and the patient may make superficial conversation. Each is afraid of frightening the other. Both subsystems are attempting to maintain some type of steady state.

Family units while helpful may have a stressful effect upon the patient. In a study by Brown (1976), it was hypothesized that family visits could be considered as a type of stress-producing activity and that the measurement of changes during such visits would give some indicator of the patient's physiologic response to this psychosocial interaction. The findings revealed that visiting periods of ten minutes every hour create a stressful effect on the blood pressure and heart rate of cardiac patients in CCU. The fact that cardiac patients may be subject to fatigue in the early stages of the illness may help account for this finding.

In time, the stability will increase as the stresses decrease. The family members and sick member will then become aware of the effects illness has on them. But until then, the patient is encouraged to rest. Each critical illness has its own effects on the family. The situation may be more crucial when the sick member is severely burned: the family must confront not only various supportive devices but also the sight of their disfigured spouse and his similarly disfigured colleagues in the burn unit. The family can be prepared for what it will see and hear.

We can also examine the stress of illness according to its effects on family configuration. Hill (1949) points out that illnesses, as stresses, do not result in "dismemberment in the sense of a change in the plurality patterns of the family, but do bring marked changes in the family configuration. Those family situations where roles are involuntarily vacated through illness are examples. Families experience significant strains when members become ill. A critical illness requires a reallocation of a patient's role to others in the family" (pp. 37–38). As family members realize the void created by temporary loss of the sick member, their ability to cope with the stresses decreases. The family and sick member may no longer be able to maintain the steady state. While initially caught up in the impact of illness and socialization process, the members of each subsystem attempt to continue in their respective roles. The husband continues to make both household and business decisions. The wife, if hospitalized, gives instruction regarding the household responsibilities, location of various items, schedule of children's activities, and general care of the children. Neither subsystem wants to admit illness and relinquish their roles. However, as the stresses increase, the steady state of the system becomes imbalanced. Consequently, the healthy family member assumes the sick member's role.

The period of dismemberment is a difficult time for the entire family. The crisis causes a temporary cessation of all extrafamilial activities. All energies are directed toward the sick member and toward intrafamily restructuring. Even though the family is an open system, it sometimes gives the appearance of a closed system. This is especially true when the family is trying to reorganize and restructure itself. In order to understand better the critical care family, we will look at two types of families affected by illness—*expanding* and *contracting* families. The first signifies a young family with small children. The latter signifies an older family whose nest is emptying, or empty.

The J. family is an example of an expanding family. The family consists of both parents and two children, whose ages are 10 and 14. The parents themselves are in their mid-30s. The family system is a close one in which the members know and experience the others' love. Except for financial problems or childhood illnesses such as chicken pox, or measles, the family has been free from crisis. Mr. J., who worked as a manager of a large department store, had been complaining of abdominal pain. He attributed the pain to poor lunch habits and pressures of his work. Therefore, he negated its significance and continued his hectic pace. Within the last year, Mr. J.'s responsibility had grown to encompass managerial duties at four major stores. This involved dividing his time among the four stores. He was under great pressure making multiple decisions, commuting between the stores, and spending less time at home relaxing with his family. As his pressures increased, so did his abdominal pain. A conservative treatment of diet and antacids did not relieve the pain, mainly because he could not be consistent with the treatment.

One day, he no longer could minimize or rationalize the pain. While getting ready for work, he experienced an episode of nausea, vomiting, dizziness, diaphoresis, and bloody stools. The symptoms frightened the entire family, who convinced him to see his doctor. The doctor ordered him hospitalized for diagnostic studies. An upper bowel series revealed a bleeding duodenal ulcer, and the doctor thought conservative treatment might stabilize the problem. However, Mr. J.'s pain continued, and he became febrile. This new sign alarmed Mr. J.'s physicians and caused them to think he had a possible perforated bowel. It became more obvious that surgery must take place. Naturally, he and his family were quite apprehensive. Illness, especially critical illness, was unknown to them.

In the interim between hospitalization and surgery, Mr. J. tried to continue making business decisions. Even though his involvement was peripheral, he nevertheless did not want to relinquish his managerial role. After all, he had worked hard to obtain his current business status. In addition, he also attempted to continue in his household decision-making responsibilities. Throughout their marriage, his wife had depended on him for certain duties. Therefore, he felt compelled to continue with his role. To the J. family surgery was an inconvenience, but hopefully only a temporary one.

Mr. J. entered surgery for an exploratory laparotomy. Mrs. J. entered the family room to begin her lonely wait. Surgeons performed a partial bowel resection, which was successful, but Mr. J. experienced hypotension during and after the operation. Doctors ordered his transfer to intensive care. Medications helped raise his blood pressure. Meanwhile, Mrs. J. was extremely fearful. To her, intensive care was synonymous with major biological crisis and potential death. She was afraid of losing her husband. She attempted to maintain an attitude of optimism, but her behavior was primarily for her husband's and children's benefit. Mr. J.'s condition seemed to stabilize. The only problem that remained was a reduction in his urinary output and an increase in his BUN levels. The doctors decided to keep Mr. J. in intensive care for a few more days. Mrs. J. believed that her husband's condition was improving to the point of eventual transfer. However, she learned from her husband that he must remain a few more days. During the next three days, Mr. J.'s BUN and creatinine levels increased to the point of being unsafe. The doctors felt it necessary to begin hemodialysis. It was hoped the hemodialysis would rectify the problem. The doctors decided to inform Mrs. J. of her husband's current biological crisis. They found her quietly sitting in the family room.

DR. T.: Mrs. J., I am Dr. T. We have met a few times in the past. I am sorry for all the inconvenience.

MRS. J.: Yes. How is my husband doing?

DR. T.: That's what I want to discuss with you.

MRS. J.: Now what's the problem?

DR. T.: You know we have been quite concerned with your husband's kidney problem.

MRS. J.: Yes. I don't understand why.

DR. T.: You remember that your husband experienced an episode of postoperative hypotension. That's why I had him moved to ICU.

MRS. J.: Yes, but what does that have to do with his current problems?

DR. T.: I am afraid your husband sustained kidney problems at that time. This resulted in acute renal failure.

MRS. J.: I am not sure I fully understand. Why didn't you stop the problem before it happened? (*She beings to cry.*)

DR. T.: These things sometimes happen after major surgery. The hypotension caused renal insufficiency. This means a reduced blood flow.

MRS. J.: Will his kidneys be normal again?

DR. T.: That's what we are hoping. The problem is that his kidneys are not getting rid of toxic products. That is what I really want to discuss with you.

MRS. J.: What else! (*Bitterly.*)

DR. T.: I want to try hemodialysis. This procedure will help eliminate the toxic products I mentioned earlier.

MRS. J.: It is all confusing, but if you feel it will help. Please just help him. I don't know how much I can hold together.

DR. T.: We will try, Mrs. J. You try and take care of yourself. I'll talk with you soon after we start the treatment. (*He leaves Mrs. J. alone.*)

Out of desperation and loneliness, Mrs. J. finally asked her mother and mother-in-law to join her. She had not called upon the extended family for help because they lived in another state. Furthermore, she was afraid that the sight of them would unnecessarily alarm her husband. However, Mrs. J. was no longer able to cope with all the additional stresses. She needed extra family support. The children had been most supportive, but she felt guilty for spending so much time at the hospital just waiting for answers. She felt alone and helpless as she continued her lengthy vigil in the family room. Mrs. J. was only allowed to see her husband for short periods of time. Visits were limited to five minutes each hour. Five minutes sitting alone seemed like two hours. Five minutes with her husband passed much too quickly.

Mr. J. had two hemodialysis treatments. Mrs. J. felt that no one was keeping her informed of her husband's progress. It was difficult for her to time her visits with those of his doctor. In despair, she ran from nurse to nurse seeking information. Once informed of his progress, she would ask another nurse the same questions. It was as if Mrs. J. did not hear what was being said. The nurses tried to be consistent in their answers and reassurances. They realized that, as Davidson (1973) has noted, "the acute anxiety the family experiences often is manifested by the family's short attention span, difficulty with listening, jumping to conclusions, and running from staff member to staff member with the same questions" (p. 374). After two weeks of hemodialysis, Mrs. J. finally had the answers to her questions. Mr. J.'s kidneys had not responded as expected. Therefore, the hemodialysis would be permanent. Both Mr. and Mrs. J. knew the answer to their questions. Hemodialysis was not the answer they desired, but it was far better than death.

Mr. and Mrs. S. represent a contracting family. Both are 75 years old and have been married to each other for 45 years. Their marriage resulted in no children. All they had was each other. Mr. S. had worked for over 45 years for the same company. Finally, their dream had come true. Mr. S. had retired less than a year before. Retirement was something both individuals had anticipated with great expectation for several years. They had wanted to spend their time traveling, camping, fishing, golfing, and visiting friends. Mr. and Mrs. S. had so many plans that neither one knew how they would find all the time. Their retirement seemed to be going well until one day when Mr. S. was mowing the lawn. He suddenly grabbed his chest and screamed for his wife. He then collapsed on the front lawn. Neighbors quickly called the paramedics, who immediately took unconscious Mr. S. to the nearest emergency room for emergency procedures and treatments. Meanwhile, Mrs. S. impatiently paced back and forth in the waiting room.

One hour after Mr. S.'s arrival in the emergency room, he was transferred to coronary care. The doctors informed Mrs. S. that her husband had sustained a massive myocardial infarction. She was told to wait in the family room, and once her husband was admitted, she could see him. Like Mrs. J., Mrs. S. began her sleepless and lonely wait. The next several days were critical for Mr. S. He experienced cardiogenic shock, pain, and arrhythmias. During the acute phase of her husband's illness, Mrs. S. suffered intense emotional pain. Her husband had been the focal point of her life for 45 years. Now, when he had just retired, a biological crisis occurred. As the days progressed, the staff noted Mrs. S.'s fatigue and nervousness. She spent very little time at home. Most of her time was spent sitting in the family room, or at her husband's bedside. It is understandable that Mrs. S. would be tense and nervous. As Croog (1968) has noted, "in the typically small family there is high level of emotional intensity and, consequently, the illness of a single member produces a higher degree of shock than a larger family system" (p. 135). Knowing this, the nurses allowed Mrs. S. to remain at her husband's bedside. Even then, she couldn't completely relax. Every time a nurse approached Mr. S.'s bed, the wife would immediately jump out of her chair. The nurses all tried to help Mrs. S. relax, but they could not succeed. One afternoon, as Mr. S. slept, a coronary care nurse discovered Mrs. S. crying.

NURSE: What's wrong, Mrs. S.?

MRS. S.: Oh, nothing. (*She continues to cry.*)

NURSE: Something must be wrong. (*The nurse pulls Mrs. S. away from her husband's bed.*)

MRS. S.: I feel so afraid.

NURSE: What makes you feel afraid?

MRS. S.: The fact that I might lose my husband. We have been together for 45 years.

NURSE: That's a long time to spend together. I can see where you would miss him.

MRS. S.: Yes, I can't imagine living without him. The house seems so empty, and I feel so alone.

NURSE: I am sure you do. Your husband's condition is improving.

MRS. S.: He has been so sick.

NURSE: Yes, he has, but he is doing better each day.

MRS. S.: I hope so, I just couldn't go on without him. You know we don't have any children. We only have each other. We had so many plans.

NURSE: You had better take care of yourself so the two of you can continue with your plans.

The S. family consisted of two subsystems. Mrs. S. as an open subsystem reached her limit in terms of input from the environment. She could no longer cope independently with the stress of illness. Her husband seemed to cope with the crisis much better than she. As Miller (1965) notes, "varying levels of stress may be tolerated by members of the same unit. Intolerable stress for one member of a family may be moderate stress for the others of the unit. Both subsystems try to protect each other until one system can no longer maintain a steady state. The family member, like Mrs. S., copes by admitting the nurse into her intrafamily system. Her behavioral output system took control. The output system permitted her to share tears and concerns with the nurse. Not all family systems are like Mrs. S. Many would not express or expose themselves in such display of emotion. They become closed systems to extrafamily support and comfort. Some family members feel it is a sign of weakness to need help from others. Such feelings may only exist as the family attempts to maintain a relatively steady state. However, as they live with the effects of illness in their family configuration, they realize the need for supportive assistance.

Mrs. J. and Mrs. S. represented different types of family configuration—one expanding, and the other contracting. Nevertheless, each experienced the stress associated with serious illness and its effects upon family configuration. These families, though presented as unique experiences, typify experiences of other families. No matter which critical care unit contains their sick member, families react in similar ways to the threat of serious illness. Because they are under tremendous stress, they do not always hear explanations. If they do hear the diagnosis, or if they see the sick member in his environment, they do not understand its meaning. It is quite understandable to have family members run from nurse to nurse asking the same questions and receiving the same answers. Such behavior is normal in times of stress. As Miller (1965) points out, "information transfer is affected by stress. As stress increases, relief of that stress is determined by the way information is interpreted. For example, periods of increased stress to the system are somewhat relieved when stress-reducing messages are given priority over neutral or stress-producing messages" (p. 403). Family members may run from nurse to nurse in order to obtain the information they want to hear. Like the sick member, the family initially denies the threats or implications of illness. To them, a biological threat has occurred but can be cured. This may be an attempt on the family's part of relieving its stress. The sick member feels guilty for becoming ill. The family feels guilty for not being more aware of the other's biological well-being. Both subsystems temporarily rationalize the stressor event, so that neither one feels totally responsible for the problem.

The family fearing the loss of a loved one is confronted by the stress-provoking critical care environment. Many times the unexpected death of a close relative renders an individual's present coping mechanism inadequate or useless. While anticipating possible death, the family makes frequent inquiries regarding the patient's condition. Such inquiries indicate that the family members are attempting to seek support and reassurance that the patient is receiving the best care. Research is needed to explore the needs of families during the crisis of critical illness (Cronin-Stubbs 1978; Potter 1979).

No matter why someone is in a critical care unit, the family has tremendous influence over the sick member's immediate and long-term recovery. If the family system has been a strong, supportive one, the members can survive the crisis. The sick member who survives the first hurdle, the biological crisis, looks forward to his next hurdle, his long-term recovery. The family plays a major role in helping the sick member make appropriate adjustments. It is understandable that this phase, called stress of social loss, may be most difficult. All subsystems have virtually depleted their energy systems. Family members have had to assume more than their normal share of responsibilities. For some, the responsibility is assumed by the only surviving member (e.g., Mrs. S.). In some families the role changes will be permanent. Such was the case with Mr. J. The family of any critically ill patient must restructure or reorganize their ranks and assign new roles to the sick member.

Stress of Social Loss

An acute illness that occurs in the midst of other changes may necessitate family restructuring. The restructuring can impose additonal stress and anxiety in an already stressed system. When the nurse assesses the family's adaptation, it is important to assess the reallocation of roles in the family as the stress of acute illness progresses. As Dashiff and Biddle (1981) point out, knowledge of the family's prior illness experiences will assist the nurse in anticipating the nature of stresses.

Dashiff and Biddle also note that age is an important variable in assessing the stress of social loss. The age of the critically ill person has an important effect upon the expectations of the individual and others regarding the sick role. The older person may be less inclined to view the sick role as a temporary state that he has some responsibility for ending.

The stress of social loss, or reorganization, affects all families. The larger immediate family has more members to assume additional responsibilities and from which to draw strength. The remaining subsystems must assume all the responsibility. In such cases, dismemberment through illness or injury is immediately felt.

Changes in family status often include financial alteration or loss. The degree of loss may depend upon the amount of financial status enjoyed by the family. Illness, injury, or disfigurement affects all people, no matter what their financial status. It is understandable that the more wealthy patients and families can afford costly care and specialists. The majority of critical care patients and their families have moderate incomes. To them, illness necessitating critical care or long-term therapy, such as dialysis, can be catastrophic. Unfortunately, there are patients in critical care who do not have health insurance. One illness can totally wipe out the family's savings. Even if the family is covered with insurance, hospitalization in critical care can deplete at least a portion of their savings. If the primary provider is ill, injured, or disfigured, the family experiences financial hardships. The financial hardship may affect the critical care patient's recovery process. According to Croog (1968), "The impact of medical care costs upon families, and the ways in which these affect long-term planning of individual members, may possibly relate to the kinds of adjustments made by patients" (p. 140). Families of critical care patients are no exception. Their medical expenses can be overwhelming. The family of a hemodialysis patient, for example, will experience tremendous financial hardships.

Such is the case with the J. family. Mr. J. will no longer be able to work his previous long hours. His reduced energy level and frequent visits to the hemodialysis unit will not permit it. The cardiac patient may no longer be able to work in areas of intense stress and pressure such as business, or in areas of heavy physical labor such as construction work. The patient with respiratory problems will be discouraged from future work that might further damage his debilitated lungs. Regardless of the biological crisis, the patient and his family experience social loss in terms of their financial status. Financial problems are not the only ones created by illness. The family also experiences conflict among themselves as they assume new roles.

A family who has been coping adequately with unemployment may not be able to deal with the added stress of a critically ill family member. What may appear to be a family's overreaction to a small stress may be explained by the fact that that stress is the last straw in a long series of stresses. The family may not be able to adequately handle the additional stress (Busch 1982).

Illness creates either temporary or permanent family dismemberment. Both involve role changes within the intrafamily structure. If temporary dismemberment occurs, the sick member returns to the family. His illness may have been severe enough to warrant restructuring of family roles. The sick member who experienced biological loss through illness, injury, or disfigurement may not be able to assume his previous role. Therefore, he returns home to a reorganized and restructured family. The transition between hospital and home can greatly influence the sick member's recovery process. Family members unsure of their new roles unintentionally create confusion. According to Hill (1949), "Most crises of crippling illness, sooner or later, involve demoralization since the family's role patterns are always sharply disturbed. It may involve a situation in which the patient's roles must be reallocated, and a period of confusion-delay ensues while the members of the family cast learn their new lines" (p. 38). As Hill also points out, the strength of the family system as a whole determines how well the independent subsystems do in the adjustment period:

> Adjustment to a crisis that threatens the family depends upon the adequacy of role performance of family members. The family consists of a number of members interacting with one another, and each member is ascribed roles to play within the family. The individual functions as a member of the family largely in terms of the expectations that other members place upon him; the family succeeds as a family largely in terms of the adequacy of role performances of its members. One major effect of crisis is to cause changes in these role patterns. Expectations shift, and the family finds it necessary to work out different patterns. (P. 45)

Hopefully, the family members will be capable of substituting for or assuming the role of the sick member.

A study by Stern and Pascale (1979) examined the major causes of concern in spouses of men who had sustained a myocardial infarction. For the postmyocardial infarction patient, posthospitalization can be a difficult period. Loss of direct medical supervision, forced inactivity, and a feeling of physical weakness cause many patients to experience anxiety and inner conflict. The family frequently experiences dysfunction, disorganization, or disequilibrium. Three major concerns were identified. First, the spouses were preoccupied with their husbands' health. The wives were afraid that a wrong word would lead to another infarction. Second, many spouses felt that the family equilibrium was disturbed. Prior to hospitalization the spouses felt they could share problems with the patient. However, after the illness had occurred, the spouses felt they had to handle the problem on their own. Third, a small group of spouses became anxious or depressed when confronted with external threats beyond their control. A principle finding in the study was that, whereas many of the sympathetic spouses had had marital difficulties prior to the infarct, most claimed worsened difficulties in the postinfarct period. A desire to avoid communication that might disturb the patient led to further marital stress.

A family that depends on the sick member instead of having a system of mutual interdependence will have difficulty restructuring and adjusting to new responsibilities. Furthermore, the degree of role change depends on which family member is ill. For example, Parson (1960) describes the special problems resulting from a mother's illness:

> Illness of the mother herself is clearly the most disturbing of all—and this may well be the nub of the whole matter. For, in the normal course of events, the mother is the primary agent of supportive strength for the entire family unit. Her illness, therefore, subjects husband and children alike to a condition of undersupport, at a time when they are suddenly being asked to meet unexpected demands of major proportions. (P. 353)

The husband must now assume not only his normal responsibilities, but also those of his wife. He must minister to the needs of his children. If he is fortunate to have access to an extended family, he can utilize its services. Families in which children are older can better distribute the mother's role. Remaining family members sometimes come in conflict with one another. The conflict is a result of their adjustment to new roles. Initial adjustment to new roles is confusing. As mentioned previously, the new roles may become permanent.

Take for example, the mother who has serious cardiac disease, severely compensated pulmonary system, or renal pathology necessitating hemodialysis. Not only is she biologically unable to perform her household chores, but she may be too much in need of emotional support to be able to give supportive assistance. A small family is not always able to assimilate all the new changes and roles. Here is where extrafamily members such as parents, grandparents, aunts, uncles, or close friends can be of assistance. If financially possible, the family should incorporate other types of extrafamily systems, including housekeepers and gardeners. A family system that has been basically dependent upon its own members to accomplish the tasks of daily living has difficulty adjusting to role changes and integrating extrafamily strangers.

Like the illness of the mother, illness of the husband-father creates intrafamily conflicts. Normally, the father functions as a provider, disciplinarian, and maker of decisions. Parsons (1960) describes the effect on the family when these responsibilities have to be temporarily or permanently assumed by the wife:

> Although the exemption from adult masculine responsibilities granted him by the sick role worsens the position of the family and makes its adaptive problems more difficult, it is the husband-father's claim to be taken care of which has the more immediately disruptive impact of the family's internal situation. The wife, of course, is the primary sick room attendant. The most obvious consequence of her ministrations is the withdrawal of her full quota of attention for the children. (P. 353)

Some of the wife-mother's intrafamily responsibilities can be assumed by other family members or strangers. These primarily include management of the household. When the father is the sick member, the problem is not as easily solved. Because extrafamily members usually cannot assume the financial responsibility or role of provider, these must be assumed by someone within the immediate family structure. A husband's illness or injury may necessitate that the wife obtain permanent employment. It is quite possible that she has never worked prior to this time. Therefore, her adjustment period is more difficult than that of the individual who has worked in the past. Furthermore, the wife's skills may be such that she cannot financially provide for her family on the same level as did her husband. Members of the family system are forced to alter some of their social habits. They must adjust to a reduced financial income while simultaneously experiencing increased financial output. Fortunately, the family system as a whole and its subsystems have the potential for growth. Growth, in turn, as Miller (1965) points out, often involves a process of differentiation: "As a family grows emotionally, it moves toward increased differentiation of its members, more obvious boundaries between its members, and more dispersed decision-making" (p. 411).

Serious illness does bring about stresses of social loss both in financial matters and in role changes. Emotionally and financially, members are bound together by their mutual interdependence for satisfaction or provision of mutual needs. The critical care nurse's responsibility extends beyond caring for the sick member. Instead, she must also provide supportive care for the family. The nurse becomes the only constant, informative individual directly accessible to the family. Therefore, she sometimes becomes the family's sounding board against which anxieties and feelings of anger can be expressed. By understanding the behavior of family members, the critical care nurse can better support them in coping with the initial illness crisis and early recovery process.

NURSING ASSESSMENT OF THE FAMILY IN CRISIS

The critical care nurse assesses the family for excess stress and need for crisis intervention. The family's response will take the form of cognitive behaviors. The nursing problem is to assess the immediate events causing the disruption and then to help the family assign priorities to their needs in an attempt to help them act appropriately.

Cognitive Behaviors

The cognator system involves inputs from internal and external stimuli which include psychological and social factors. Cognitive mechanisms include how the individual processes information, learns, and makes decisions. The cognitive behaviors are psychological responses. Family members may react to the stress of illness, injury, or disease in any of the several ways listed below:

Cognitive Behaviors
Helplessness
Decreased problem-solving ability
Fear
Anxiety
Panic
Withdrawal
Crying

As families attempt to maintain balance in the face of change, they may be maintaining maladaptive or ineffective behaviors within the family. In general, the critical care nurse may observe behaviors which indicate emotions signifying helplessness and urgency. An inability to make decisions and mobilize resources can be noted. A sense of fear and panic pervades. In addition, irrational acts, demanding behavior, withdrawal, preservation, and fainting all have been observed (Busch 1982).

Braulin, Rook, and Sills (1982) note that the circumstances surrounding the injury may contribute to feelings of anger and guilt expressed by family members. In response to the suddenness and unexpectedness of the event, family members often seek ways to express their anger and perhaps guilt in an effort to begin to cope with the strangeness or uniqueness of the experience.

NURSING DIAGNOSIS OF THE FAMILY IN CRISIS

The nursing diagnosis is a statement of the current problem. Various cognitive behaviors manifested by the family help the nurse make her diagnosis of family in crisis. Stressors contributing to the crisis situation can be categorized as internal or external. Internal stressors depend upon the strength of the family unit, its communication patterns, its ability to handle crisis, the degree of role disruption, and the maturational level of the family. External stressors can be caused by the illness itself and/or the need for hospitalization. These include possible loss of employment, forced retirement, financial loss, or changes in values.

NURSING INTERVENTIONS
TO FACILITATE FAMILY INVOLVEMENT

Family members need to be prepared for their experience in critical care. The patient's condition, alertness, and physical appearance can be described in understandable terms. When possible, supportive devices or intrusive instrumentation can be explained to the family before they actually see the patient. Once at the bedside the family may require additional explanations (Busch 1982).

While the critical care nurse is in a position to assist both the patient and his family, the patient is the primary focus of the nurse's attention. This may be due in part to the abrupt onset of the biological injury such as myocardial infarction which precludes sufficient preparation of the family for the crisis (Bedsworth and Molen 1982). The nurse intervenes to minimize or eliminate as many of the demands and stresses on the critically ill patient as is realistic. Supporting the family is an area in which the nurse can facilitate stress reduction (Fuller and Foster 1982).

The critical care nurse is the primary provider of health care in the family's world, in the sense that she spends more direct time with the critically ill patient than any other member of the health team. The family turns to the nurse for support and for answers to their numerous questions. The nurse tries to facilitate family involvement by accomplishing three major goals: fostering family support, facilitating family education, and fostering acceptance of the temporarily dismembered family subsystems.

Fostering Family Support

Fostering family support is one of the most important nursing interventions. Crises or stresses on the family make them feel suddenly lonely and alone. To the family, a significant member is ill, injured, or disfigured. In addition, his place in critical care makes him inaccessible. At a time when the family and sick member need each other's emotional support, the hospital restricts the length of time they can spend with one another. Therefore, the amount and degree of support is limited. The nurse must convey and provide support for both the larger family and for the sick family member. When providing supportive care for the family, the nurse should be alert to other stresses it may be experiencing. As Craven (1972) points out, "The obvious facet for the nurse to recognize is that illness is a stress or crisis to the family. However, what we may lose sight of, is that illness is only one of probably many stresses on this family at any given time" (p. 189).

The nurse provides individualized and supportive care by identifying and acknowledging the family's needs. In a study by Potter (1979), a questionnaire was developed to generate findings about four stress categories. The categories delineated major sources of stress: environmental stimuli, information and visitation, family responsibilities and roles, and patient's body image. The findings revealed two items that had statistical significance. Family members viewed the lack of privacy within the critical care unit as a source of concern. In addition, failure on the part of nurses to assist families in finding useful tasks to perform for patients was perceived as a potential source of stress.

One area of support includes the preparation of the family for what it will see in critical care. As Wallace (1971) points out, "There is a need to prepare relatives of patients in the intensive care unit beforehand for what they will encounter. As most people have never before set foot in such a specialized and mechanized area of the hospital, the equipment alone overwhelms them" (p. 33). It is not unusual for family members to begin crying at the sight of their loved one. This is especially true if the individual sustained injuries in an automobile accident or fire. The sight of physical disfigurement is overwhelming. In addition, the patient's immediate environment may be filled with various supportive devices. Each device has its own unique flashing light and buzzing alarm. It is a foreign environment to the family members. Initially, they feel as though they have entered forbidden territory. The critical care nurse can attempt to make the family feel comfortable in the strange territory. The family should know that the treatment plan, including various pieces of equipment, is normal for the patient and his particular problems. The nurse can give brief explanations regarding their normalcy. The nurse must realize that the family is experiencing tremendous stress and will hear only fragments of her explanations. But family members will hear the word "normal." A supportive critical care nurse can remain with the family throughout their initial visits. The family feels secure in her presence. Should one of the machine's alarms buzz in their presence she will know what to do. In addition, the nurse's presence communicates her caring.

The critical care nurse can foster support and stress reduction by providing information, answering and reanswering questions, and preparing the family for their initial visit. Furthermore, the nurse fosters feelings of hope and hopefulness by maintaining the individuality of the patient as a person and member of a family through meaningful communications. It is also helpful to help the family become actively involved in caring for the injured patient. Helping the family become involved with the patient seems to focus their energy on a particular goal. In addition the involved family member feels helpful in a technical world that is otherwise foreign to herself and the patient. Lastly, the nurse can help the family to network with other families who have experienced or are experiencing a similar crisis (Braulin, Rook, and Sills 1982).

The family must be prepared for what it is to see in the patient's environment, and it can be prepared for unusual behavior manifested by the sick member. During the impact phase of illness, the sick member may not be aware of his own behavior. The family may wrongfully assume the patient has sustained neurological damage or some other problem. According to Davidson (1973), "As families see the symptoms of regression in their loved one, they often become embarrassed by his childish, demanding behavior. Or, they are frightened when he becomes verbally threatening with them. Families need a great deal of support from the staff. One of the most effective means is to teach them about the situation" (p. 374). Just as the nurse explained equipment in terms of its normalcy, she can explain the patient's behavior in the same manner. Any negative behavior expressed by the patient and directed toward the family needs to be explained.

Problem solving is a tool designed to help the family clearly state their perception of the immediate problem. The acute crisis causes the family to feel overwhelmed and immobilized. According to Busch (1982), helping the family formulate the problem allows them to achieve cognitive mastery. Simply stating the problem tends to reduce anxiety by helping the family to feel that they have achieved some sort of understanding of what is happening. When the family is able to state the problem, they can also be helped to identify choices or alternatives designed to help them achieve an element of control over the situation or their lives. The family can then formulate goals which will help them through the immediate crisis and the early postdischarge phase when support systems are reduced.

The critical care nurse becomes a communication link between the family and the sick member. Such communication can extend beyond the walls of the hospital. It is not unusual to give the unit's phone number to intrafamily members and encourage them to call the unit before retiring or upon rising. Such intervention personalizes the family's care. The phone call can have two purposes: the nurse can give the family members a current report of the sick member's progress, while simultaneously giving the sick member the latest report regarding his family. In time, the sick member can make his own phone calls. The nurse fosters communication between family and sick member by increasing the visiting hours or time. A family member can often be permitted to remain quietly at the patient's bedside for periods longer than the alloted five minutes. This exception is not applicable to all patients. The continual presence of some family members only serves to make the sick member more anxious. The exception applies to those sick members whose biological status is terminal and to those families who demonstrate supportive strength. In the latter case the nurse can perceive a type of mutual interdependence between family and sick member. Flexibility in visiting hours facilitates the family as the primary adjustment support system in the sick member's life. Naturally, the critical care nurse wants to continue to keep the support system functioning. This implies that the critical care nurse must "recognize the importance of the patient and family interrelationship as well as energetic encouragements to stimulate the family members' active involvement whenever possible are concrete actions that can be taken by the nurse to assist the family in keeping close and strong ties during an illness" (Craven 1972, p. 193).

Regardless of the specific type of family support offered, the critical care nurse's caring attitude about relatives and their reactions decreases their feelings of neglect or of jealousy about the care or attention the patient is receiving.

Facilitating Family Education

The second goal of the critical care nurse is to facilitate family education. As soon as is realistic the family is educated to the geography and procedures of the critical care unit. The educational process can include explanation of the physical status of the patient, including supportive devices or lines; identification of the health care team; and orientation of the family to the organization of the critical care unit (Braulin, Rook, and Sills 1982).

Barden (1972) points out the importance of teaching programs for patients and their families:

> The patient has a right to information that will enable him to return to a normal way of living and the professional nurse has an obligation to provide this information. Patients and their families can live better lives through education. Teaching can begin in the acute phase and be continued throughout convalescence, and families must be included in teaching programs. (Pp. 570-571)

Such programs are particularly important for families of cardiac and hemodialysis patients. A family that lacks knowledge regarding the patient's problem is unable to provide support. This is especially true for cardiac and hemodialysis patients. The nurse can educate the family by starting with the illness. Teaching can begin in the acute phase, and the nurse can remember to keep things simple. Like the sick member, the family also has a tendency to hear and learn selectively. Once the critical phase has subsided, the family can begin a more detailed educational program. Such a program includes both family and patient. Each needs to learn expectations of the other. The critical care nurse constantly keeps in mind that a necessary part of a patient's care and rehabilitation is the education of his family so that they can be a help rather than a detriment to him. The family of the patient plays a significant role in determining whether or not the patient accepts his problems. In addition the family assists the critical care patient in modifying his life-style.

In a study by Doerr and Jones (1979), it was hypothesized that family members who receive pre-CCU preparation would transmit less family-to-patient anxiety than would family members who did receive such preparation. The findings of the study revealed that patients whose family members were prepared for the visitation showed a mean decrease of 1.67 points on the State Anxiety Scale while the patients exposed to nonprepared family members showed a mean increase of 3.13 points. It was concluded that family preparation significantly reduced the amount of anxiety transferred from the family members to the CCU patient.

Many times family members are reluctant to approach or touch a critically ill patient. When the nurse takes the relative to the patient's bedside, she can encourage them to touch or talk to the patient.

Family-centered care and teaching involves assisting the family in group education. The nurse will begin to educate the cardiac patient and his family in the critical care unit and will continue in the intermediate care unit. If the unit has a clinical specialist, the specialist can conduct the program. Group education includes the total family and/or other cardiac patients and their families. Hemodialysis patients and their families can be educated in the hemodialysis unit. Hopefully, both spouses participate in the education program. There are instances in which the husband or wife cannot accompany the sick member to the hemodialysis unit, for example, when the healthy member is forced to assume financial responsibility for the entire family. Therefore, group teaching is not always possible.

Education programs can be initiated by any critical care unit. They require that the nurse take time to assess the family's readiness for learning. In situations where the illness becomes chronic, such as hemodialysis and respiratory care, the family can use group conference to verbalize their feelings and frustrations. According to Craven (1972), "By giving family members the opportunity to express their feelings, the nurse can contribute to the therapeutic role while providing the same function for the patient who, aware of the additional pressures on his family, does not want to further burden them" (p. 131).

Fostering Acceptance

The third and last major goal of the critical care nurse is to foster acceptance of the temporarily dismembered family subsystem. This seems like a simple task, but it may be a trying time for the entire family. The nurse keeps in mind that both the family and sick member have experienced many stresses. These stresses do not cease the minute a sick member is discharged from the hospital. Instead, new stresses can inhibit the sick member's recovery process and the family adjustment as a whole.

Before the family can accept the possible loss of a loved one or the alteration in life-style, they go through the grieving process. Since the traumatic injury represents both crisis and loss to the family, it is also useful to understand the grieving process. All stages of the grieving process can be facilitated when the family is encouraged to ventilate their feelings. The nurse can also facilitate the grieving process by providing time to meet with the family and providing an atmosphere conducive to the expression of feelings (Braulin, Rook, and Sills 1982).

When a temporarily dismembered individual who sustained a disabling illness or injury returns home, he finds a newly organized family structure. Members within the family system have assumed his previously assumed roles. The sick member may already feel a social loss in terms of finances. The new roles at home further enhance this feeling. The degree of loss experienced by the sick member depends on the severity of his illness. As the sick member watches his family assume new roles, he feels guilty. He may feel particularly guilty when his wife is forced to seek employment, and he feels a sense of personal failure. The strong family system supports and assists the sick member to accept his current limitations and to assume new roles. These include roles that are significant within the intrafamily structure. The nurse works together with family and sick member in anticipating potential changes in roles that might create early adjustment problems. In this respect, the entire family is prepared for those problems experienced by other families in similar situations. If the nurse has maintained a close personal relationship with the family and sick member, she may encourage them to call the unit with their questions and concerns. Again, this communicates a genuine interest on the nurse's part. The family views her as a warm, helpful person.

Families who avoid crisis by successfully meeting the demands of change are most often well-integrated systems in which individual members are committed to the group and its collective goals (Cronin-Stubbs 1978).

Although the critical care nurse works primarily with the sick member, she often comes in contact with anxious family members who have many questions and concerns. The nurse can utilize her time with the family to make it a meaningful input session of support and education. The family can become involved only in what it understands. All else is meaningless or frightening. Therefore, the nurse has the responsibility of educating not only the patient but the family as well. Consequently, the family will have a better understanding of his care, treatment program, and future restrictions. The nurse must remember that her time with the family is sometimes limited in comparison to the amount spent with the sick member. Therefore, a program needs to be quickly established for the family to assure their needs and expectations are being fulfilled.

NURSING EVALUATION

The nurse assesses the crisis situation, its significance to the family, and cognitive behaviors manifested by the family. An assessment of these factors assists the nurse in diagnosing a family in crisis. The nurse knows that many of the family problems may not be resolved until the sick member has returned home or to work. It is possible that the needs of the family require ongoing counseling. Therefore the nurse can refer the family to the appropriate support system.

SUMMARY

The family is an open system. Families of critical care patients experience crisis and stress as they relate to illness and social loss. Stress of illness includes the family's response to the news of illness, the critical care unit itself, and the realization of dismemberment. Stress of social loss revolves around finances and role changes. Each family will respond to crisis in its own unique way—a way based upon previous coping patterns. Understanding families of critical care patients is an area in which more research can be done.

REFERENCES

ACKERMAN, NATHAN, *The Psychodynamic of Family Life*. New York: Basic Books, 1958.

BARDEN, CATHERINE A., "Teaching the Coronary Patient and His Family," *Nursing Clinics of North America*, 7, no. 3 (September 1972), 570-71.

BEARD, MILDRED, "The Impact of Hemodialysis and Transplantation on the Family," *Critical Care Quarterly*, 1 (September 1978), 87-91.

BEDSWORTH, JOYCE, and MARILYN MOLEN, "Psychological Stress in Spouses of Patients with Myocardial Infarction," *Heart and Lung*, 11, no. 5 (September-October 1982), 450-456.

BILODEAU, CAROLYN, "Psychological Aspects," *Critical Care Nursing: Body-Mind-Spirit,* ed. Cornelia Kenner, Cathie Guzzetta, and Barbara Dossey, pp. 171-196. Boston: Little, Brown, 1981.

BRAULIN, JERI, JANICE ROOK, and GRAYCE SILLS, "Families in Crisis: The Impact of Trauma," *Critical Care Quarterly*, 5, no. 3 (December 1982), 38-46.

BROWN, AGNES, "Effect of Family Visits on the Blood Pressure and Heart Rate of Patients in the Coronary Care Unit," *Heart and Lung*, 5, no. 2 (March-April 1976), 291-295.

BUSCH, KAREN, "Families in Crisis," in *Critical Care Nursing*, ed. Carolyn Hudak, Thelma Kohr, and Barbara Gallo, pp. 29-35. Philadelphia: Lippincott, 1982.

CHATHAM, M. A., "The Effect of Family Involvement on Patient's Manifestations of Postcardiotomy Psychosis," *Heart and Lung*, 7 (1978), 995.

CROOG, SYDNEY, "The Heart Patient and the Recovery Process," *Social Science and Medicine*, 2 (1968), 136.

CRAVEN, RUTH, "The Effects of Illness on Family Function," *Nursing Forum*, 11, no. 2 (1972), 191.

CRONIN-STUBBS, DIANE, "Family Crisis Intervention: A Study," *JPN and Mental Services*, 16, no. 1 (January 1978), 36-44.

CUMMINGS, JONATHAN, "Hemodialysis—Feelings, Facts, Fantasies," *American Journal of Nursing*, 70, no. 1 (January 1970), 76.

DASHIFF, CAROL, and SUSAN BIDDLE, "Psychosocial Assessment of the Patient and Family," *AACN's Clinical Reference for Critical Care Nursing*, ed. M. Kinney, C. Dear, D. Paclca, and D. Voorman, pp. 349-359. New York: McGraw-Hill, 1981.

DAVIDSON, S. B., "Nursing Management of Emotional Reactions of Severly Burned Patients during Acute Phase," *Heart and Lung*, 2, no. 3 (May-June 1973), p. 374.

DOERR, BARBARA, and JOHN JONES, "Effect of Family Preparation on the State Anxiety Level of the CCU Patient," *Nursing Research*, 28, no. 5 (September-October 1979), 315-316.

DUNKEL, J., and S. F. EISENDROTH, "Families in the Intensive Care Unit: Their Effect on Staff," *Heart and Lung*, 12 (1983), 258.

EICHEL, ELLEN, "Assessment with a Family Focus," *JPN and Mental Health Services*, (January 1978), 11-14.

FULLER, BARBARA, and GALE FOSTER, "The Effects of Family/Friend Visits vs. Staff Interaction on Stress/Arousal of Surgical Intensive Care Patients," *Heart and Lung*, 11, no. 5 (September-October 1982), 457-463.

GARDNER, KATHRYN, "Supportive Nursing: A Critical Review of the Literature," *JPN and Mental Health Services*, 17, no. 10 (October 1979), 10-16.

HASSETT, MAJORIE, "Teaching Hemodialysis to the Family Unit," *Nursing Clinics of North America*, 7, no. 3 (June 1972), 349.

HILL, REUBEN, *Families Under Stress*. New York: Harper & Row, 1949.

HOLUB, NANCY, PATRICIA EKLUND, and PATRICIA KEENAN, "Family Conferences as an Adjunct to Total Coronary Care," *Heart and Lung*, 4, no. 5 (September-October 1975), 767-769.

HOSKINS, CAROL, "Level of Activation, Body Temperature, and Interpersonal Conflict in Family Relationships," *Nursing Research*, 28, no. 3 (May-June 1979), 154-160.

KIRCHHOFF, K. T., "Visiting Policies for Patients with Myocardial Infarction: A National Survey," *Heart and Lung*, 11 (1982), 571.

MAYOU, RICHARD, ANN FOSTER, and BARBARA WILLIAMSON, "The Psychological and Social Effects of Myocardial Infarction on Wives," *British Medical Journal*, March 18, 1978, p. 699.

MCCLELLON, MURIEL, "Crisis Groups in Special Care Areas," *Nursing Clinics of North America*, 7, no. 3 (June 1972), 363-364.

MILLER, JAMES, "Living Systems: Cross Level of Hypothesis," *Behavioral Science*, 10 (1965), 380-411.

NADELSON, THEODORE, "The Psychiatrist in the Surgical Intensive Care Unit," *Archives Survery*, 3 (February 1976), 113-117.

PARAD, HOWARD, "A Framework for Studying Families in Crisis," in *Crisis Intervention*, ed. H. Parad, pp. 53-72. New York: Family Service Association, 1965.

PARSONS, TALCOTT, "Illness, Therapy, and the Modern Urban American Family," in *A Modern Introduction to the Family*, p. 353. New York: Free Press, 1960.

POLLITT, J., "Symptoms of Stress," *Nursing Mirror*, 44, no. 24 (June 16, 1977), p. 14.

POTTER, PATRICIA, "Stress and the Intensive Care Unit: The Family's Perception," *Missouri Nurse*, 40 (July 1979), 5-8.

RICHTER, JUDITH, "Physical Symptom: A Signal of Distress in the Family System," *Topics in Clinical Nursing*, 1 (October 1979), 31-40.

SILVERBERG, E., "Cancer Statistics," *Cancer*, 32, no. 1 (1982), 15-31.

SILVERSTONE, BARBARA, "The Family Is Here to Stay," *Journal of Nursing Administration*, May 1978, pp. 47-51.

SMILEY, OLGA, "The Family-Centered Approach—A Challenge to Public Health Nurses," *Canadian Journal of Public Health*, 63, no. 5 (September-October 1972), 424-426.

STERN, MELVIN, and LINDA PASCALE, "Psychosocial Adaptation Post-Myocardial Infarction: The Spouse's Dilemma," *Journal of Psychosomatic Research*, 23 (1979), 83-87.

STRAUSS, ANSELM, "The Intensive Care Unit: Its Characteristics and Social Relationships," *Nursing Clinics of North America*, 3, no. 1 (March 1968), 7-15.

WALLACE, PAT, "Relatives Should Be Told About Intensive Care But How Much and by Whom?" *Canadian Nurse*, 67, no. 6 (June 1971), 33.

17

Depression

BEHAVIORAL OBJECTIVES

1. Define the term *depression.*
2. State the three stages identified by Kanfer as they relate to his general model of self-regulation.
3. Apply the three stages and their component parts to the critically ill patient.
4. Identify six regulatory behaviors associated with depression.
5. Identify seven cognitive behaviors associated with depression.
6. Describe how fostering cognitive reappraisal will reduce feelings of depression.
7. Describe how facilitating realistic independence will reduce feelings of depression.

Each individual experiences feelings of depression at some point in his or her life. For some the feelings are transient or momentary. For others the feelings are deeper and may last for longer periods of time. Deeper and longer-lasting depression occurs when individuals are confronted with a major loss. In such cases depression results when the feelings associated with the major loss have broken through the individual's own defenses.

Authier, Authier, and Lutey (1979) point out that the depressed individual is well known to the health care delivery system, since 10 percent of the general population presents for treatment due to depression. Moreover, people who become sick experience feelings of depersonalization, powerlessness, and hopelessness, which often result in depressive symptomatology.

When a major loss, illness, or injury occurs, the critically ill patient and his family can experience tremendous feelings of helplessness and depression. It is hoped that the depression will not become all-consuming to the point that it hinders physiological processes.

DEFINITION OF DEPRESSION

Depression is one of the products of learned helplessness. As Kallio (1982) notes, because of its adverse effects on the patient's readiness to learn and general sense of well-being, depression becomes a major obstacle to health. Before applying the concept of depression to the critically ill, various definitions of depression will be reviewed.

Schneider (1980) observes that depression is generally seen as a clinical syndrome characterized by negativism, helplessness, lowered mood, and reduced self-esteem. Depression often occurs in response to a narcissistic injury, a blow to the image of oneself as whole, intact, and independent.

According to Seligman (1974), depression is defined as a manifestation of felt hopelessness regarding the attainment of goals when responsibility for the hopelessness is attributed to one's personal deficit. In this context hope is conceived to be a function of the perceived probability of success with respect to goal attainment. When the achievement of personal goals is obstructed, the individual experiences feelings of sadness, of being down or even depressed. The individual may be so focused on the loss that he or she is unable to identify alternative ways of achieving the same or similar goals.

Jasmin and Trygstad (1979) view depression as a specific collection of thoughts, feelings, bodily responses, and actions. This syndrome has a cluster of identifying characteristics. The core characteristics are low self-esteem, feelings of sadness, despondency, helplessness, hopelessness, altered bodily functions, and diminished social functioning. Any or all of these characteristics may be present in depression; no one is essential.

Depression is also described as a syndrome much like adult respiratory distress syndrome or disseminated intravascular coagulation, and not really a specific diagnosis. Instead it may be considered a feeling state like sadness unaccompanied by the other classic signs and symptoms (Drucker, Heefner, and Wilder 1980). An obvious aspect of depression is a marked reduction in the frequency of certain kinds of activity and an increase in the frequency of others, usually avoidance and escape.

Finally depression has been characterized as a specific alteration in mood in which tension and anxiety are expressed in the form of isolation and withdrawal from activity with the outside world, self-depreciation, and cognitive disturbances. In summary, depression has been characterized as a feeling, a reaction, a syndrome, and an illness. Depression as a feeling is known to everyone under ordinary conditions of life and loss, and is a component in the symptom complex of most, if not all, illnesses (Schwartzman 1976).

THE CONCEPT OF DEPRESSION
APPLIED TO THE CRITICALLY ILL PATIENT

A model of depression which views it in terms of a self-regulation dysfunction incorporates aspects of the other behavioral models along with inclusion of cognitive components and self-punitive dimensions. The concept of self-regulation deals with the processes by which an individual alters or maintains his behavior in the absence of immediate environment support. Self-regulation occurs within the individual and often is a completely private experience (Mathews 1977).

Kanfer (1970) has developed a general model of self-regulation which involves three stages: self-monitoring, self-evaluation, and self-reinforcement. Each stage will be discussed as it applies to various critically ill patients.

Self-Monitoring Stage

In the instances when a behavior chain does not complete smoothly, self-monitoring is hypothesized to go into operation. With information from the environment and response-produced feedback obtained in self-monitoring, the individual engages in self-evaluation. According to Mathews (1977), within the self-monitoring stage, the role of response-produced feedback largely depends upon the individual's learning history and individual patterns of interpreting proprioceptive, sensory, and affective feedback (Mathews 1977).

As it applies to depression, the self-monitoring stage involves two components: perception of the loss and perception of life stressors.

Perception of the Loss. The loss that is perceived may be loss in general, potential loss, or actual loss. The issue in any depression is some type of loss. The loss produces feelings of loneliness, inadequacy, and sadness. These general feelings can come under the heading of mourning.

For example, Mr. J., a 45-year-old executive with a construction company, entered coronary care complaining of chest discomfort. His tentative diagnosis suggested evaluative studies be conducted to rule out myocardial infarction. Because of a family history of cardiac disease and stresses in his life, Mr. J. was admitted for these evaluative studies. While undergoing various laboratory studies and diagnostic tests, Mr. J. began to focus on the threat to his existence and earning power. According to Swanson (1975) a loss or failure in adult life, real or perceived, inflicts a wound to any human being, but the depth of reaction differs according to one's self-view. While waiting for the results of his diagnostic studies, Mr. J. expressed his sadness over the hospitalization and his desire to be discharged. Fortunately the various evaluative tests were negative for a myocardial infarction. Nevertheless Mr. J. was instructed to reduce the cholesterol in his diet, lose weight, stop smoking, exercise, and develop a hobby. Since Mr. J. is at risk for developing cardiac disease, failure to comply with the above suggestions could eventually lead to myocardial loss or more importantly a threat to his life.

For Mr. J. a loss whether it be temporary removal from work or home and loss of life-style usually can be accepted as a legitimate reason to be depressed.

It should be noted that in depressive reactions there may or may not be an immediate precipitating loss. When losses are noted and seen as related to his emotional state, the depressed individual is likely to consider the loss as deserved or as punishment for some real or assumed transgression. The myocardial infarction or diabetic ketoacidotic patient who chooses not to comply with medical therapy may actually feel the outcome is not worth the effort. Some patients feel the quality of their life has already been reduced by the illness or disease process. Therefore they resist further restriction in their life-style. Any reminder of the biological loss contributes to further feelings of depression. It is possible that the depressed cardiac or diabetic patient sees the loss as confirming that they are bad, that they deserve what has happened, that fate is against them, and that they are indeed worthless. Some patients use the loss to prove a negative self-image. Therefore the critically ill patient who enters the hospital with a poor self-concept before the loss is more vulnerable to depression as a reaction to loss (Schneider 1980). It is important for the critical care nurse to monitor signs and symptoms of illness after a loss in order to prevent complications, including the psychological complication of depression.

For the critically ill patient, potential loss can also be perceived as loss. The coronary artery bypass and trauma patient are two examples of individuals who experience potential loss. Mr. L., a 52-year-old man, was playing golf with his friends when he began experiencing chest pain. Mr. L. attributed the pain to indigestion and continued playing. While sitting in the club house Mr. L.'s chest pain increased in intensity. Furthermore his golfing partner observed that Mr. L. was diaphoretic, pale, and rubbing his chest. After validating his observations, Mr. L.'s friend took him to an emergency department. There an EKG revealed ST segment changes. Mr. L. was quickly scheduled for a cardiac catheterization which revealed significant stenosis of the major arteries. Within less than seven hours after the initial pain experience, Mr. L. was undergoing coronary artery bypass surgery. Needless to say Mr. L. had very little time to assimilate the surgical intervention or the postoperative changes in his life. In addition, Mrs. L. was unable to spend significant preoperative time with her husband. Mrs. L.'s immediate postoperative course was uneventful without biological complication. However, the reality of the event and its potential severity began to affect Mr. L. As he thought about the potential loss or what could have happened and what did happen, he experienced feelings of depression. It has been noted that depression is apt to be felt as the danger of the acute stage decreases. It occurs toward the end of the patient's stay in the unit or shortly after being transferred to an intermediate care unit.

Depression affects the outcome of any illness. The rapid recovery from disease and disability is related to lack of depression. The preoperative coronary artery bypass graft (CABG) patient who experiences hopelessness or depression may have a difficult postoperative course (Jasmin and Trygstad

1979). The CABG patient can experience feelings of depression simply thinking about a potential loss whether it be a loss of function or a loss associated with a change in life-style. To many patients, their heart is the focus of their being or even a symbol of youth. Cardiac disease is associated with the aged. Therefore a threat to one's heart such as myocardial infarction or coronary artery bypass surgery make the patient feel old. Feelings of depression can occur over the potential loss of the individual's youthful mental image. According to Hackett and Cassem (1979), degression focuses on concerns about reduced earning power, restrictions of activity, sexual dysfunction, premature old age, and recurrence of illness.

The trauma patient is also confronted with the threat of potential loss. As with the coronary artery bypass patient, the loss may occur suddenly without prior warning. The trauma patient experiences two traumas: the initial trauma and the trauma of admission into the hospital through an emergency department or designated trauma center. Mrs. P. is an example of such a patient.

Mrs. P. was driving home from work on a freeway when a car suddenly swerved in front of her, setting off a chain of accidents. Mrs. P.'s car was pinned between two other cars. After the impact, she temporarily lost consciousness. Her head and chest had impacted on the steering wheel. Fortunately several people were able to safely remove Mrs. P. from her car before the fuel tank ignited. Because she was unconscious, they were careful to support her neck. Mrs. P. was aware of the initial injury but vaguely aware of events immediately thereafter. Once the paramedics arrived, Mrs. P. became more aware of her surroundings and her own discomfort. She was aware of the pain in her chest, shortness of breath, pain in her right leg and left arm, and headache. In the trauma unit, Mrs. P. became acutely aware of the potential loss of her life. The trauma team rapidly assessed Mrs. P.'s condition. Various laboratory and diagnostic studies were quickly done to determine the severity of Mrs. P.'s injuries. The initial diagnoses were pneumothorax, fractured and lacerated right leg, facial lacerations, severely contused left arm, and possible concussion. Supportive procedures were immediately implemented. The entire trauma team including the orthopedic surgeon and neurologist worked together to stabilize Mrs. P.'s physiological status thereby reducing the potential for loss of life. Mrs. P. survived the physiological crisis without complications. However, as the awareness of the initial and post-trauma event was assimilated, she expressed feelings of sadness or depression. Mrs. P. began questioning whether or not she could have prevented the accident, whether her insurance would cover the costs of the hospitalization, whether she would lose her job, and whether she could afford a new car. All these factors preoccupied Mrs. P.'s thoughts to the exclusion of participating in therapy designed to enhance her physiological progress. Authorities point out that as the traumatized person reflects about adverse events, he wonders what it tells him about himself. The tendency to extract personality-relevant meanings from unpleasant situations is particularly characteristic of the depression-prone individual.

The critically ill patient continually monitors himself. The patient looks for signs of progress or reversal as indicators of his rate of recovery. Therefore, when complications occur they need to be explained in the context of the illness, injury, or disease. Some complications are anticipated or expected by the critical care team and therefore do not come as a shock. However each reversal reinforces the patient's perception of himself as being unworthy of complete, uncomplicated recovery. In other words, the individual sees a psychological deficit in himself. According to Beck (1974), when the patient erroneously explains reversals as due to a deficit in himself, he produces additional undesirable effects. His awareness of the presumed defect become so intense that it infiltrates every thought about himself.

In addition to perception of a potential loss, the patient can perceive an actual loss. An actual loss involves the loss of some function, part, or whole. For example, the stroke, burn, or renal patient each experiences an actual loss.

Mr. V., a 52-year-old construction worker, complained of severe headache one morning while at work. He simply associated the symptoms with fatigue and overwork, not to his history of hypertension. Several hours later Mr. V. collapsed after having told his partner that the headache was more severe. Mr. V. was quickly taken, by paramedics, to a local hospital. While he was being evaluated by the emergency department team, it became apparent that Mr. V. had suffered a stroke. He demonstrated left-sided weakness and slight confusion. Once the evaluative studies were completed, Mr. V. was transferred to intensive care for continued observation and supportive interventions. Throughout the next several days Mr. V. was tearful and expressed a deep sadness over the actual loss. He kept rubbing his left arm hoping it had simply gone to sleep and would eventually respond. When Mr. V.'s nurse entered the room the following dialogue took place:

MR. V.: Why doesn't my arm and leg wake up?
NURSE: Wake up?
MR. V.: Yes. It feels like it is asleep. You know, numb.
NURSE: Mr. V., your stroke has affected the left side of your body.
MR. V.: (*With tears in his eyes*) When will the feeling return?
NURSE: That we don't know right now. It is too early to determine. The staff is monitoring your condition.
MR. V.: Do people like me recover?
NURSE: What do you mean by recover?
MR. V.: Get the feeling back in my leg and arm. I depend on them for my income.
NURSE: With recovery some function can return. It is really too early to determine. I am going to talk with your physician and together maybe we can answer all your questions.

The nurse at this point is simply answering questions without offering false hope or hopelessness. The entire critical care health team needs to be alerted to Mr. V.'s questions and expression of sadness. According to Schwartzman (1976), the loss of body function through hemiplegia raises feelings of loss that are consistent with mourning experience; the patient expresses feelings of helplessness, shame, unworthiness, guilt, and hopelessness which may be contributing to a depressive reaction.

Like the stroke patient, the patient with burns also experiences an actual loss. The loss can involve facial disfigurement, scars, loss of hair, or loss of body parts such as digits or extremities. Regardless of the loss, the experience of being burned is extremely threatening, as are the subsequent long-term medical and surgical interventions. The burn patient's depression can be attributed to the physical alteration caused by the burn and the eventual reaction of strangers to any resulting disfigurement. In addition, both patients experience immobility caused by their illness or injury. McCann (1979) points out that the person who is severely immobilized is one who is confined to a bed or small area. His visual range of ambulation and means of locomotion have been greatly restricted, either temporarily or permanently, and he may possess concomitant disability with respect to the movement of his upper extremities.

The renal patient's perceived actual loss can be complete loss of renal function necessitating dependency upon hemodialysis treatments. This can come as a complete shock to the critically ill patient who is hospitalized for a biological problem unrelated to renal dysfunction. However hemodynamic alterations, complications, or high doses of nephrotoxic drugs can cause secondary renal dysfunction. The loss of renal function can sometimes be more traumatic to the patient than the primary physiological problem. Needless to say such patients can experience feelings of depression. The actual loss of renal function and subsequent dependency upon hemodialysis can psychologically immobilize the patient. McCann (1979) notes that immobility restricts the way in which a human being is able to interact with his environment. The usual way in which he has done this over the years have been altered and often are no longer effective. He finds that he is suddenly unable to fulfill his own basic needs and that he must rely upon others to do this for him.

Perception of Life Stresses. Critically ill patients may perceive stressors in their life as contributing to the current illness, injury, or disease. According to Jacobson (1980), life stresses have been correlated with psychological illness including depression. These stressors are usually discrete life events which often involve a loss of something valuable or a threat to one's self-image. Depression may occur when the individual believes that he or she has little control over the various stressors. For example, it may be perceived as more stressful to terminate a relationship that is nonproductive, to terminate a business venture, or, to seek a change in employment. The individual believes that the loss of the relationship, venture, or job would bring about additional stresses. For such individuals, life stressors become problematical and undesirable circumstances over a long period of time and are possibly tied to a social role. The greater the number of stressors, the greater are the symptoms of depression (Jacobson 1980).

Loss is a stress event in anyone's life. Individuals are vulnerable physically and psychologically, after the loss. This is especially significant when the individual did not have a choice over the loss. When an illness or injury occurs, choices are now placed in the hands of strangers. Furthermore, a decision regarding termination of a relationship, business venture, or job may now be forced upon the individual. Instead of facing a wide range of alternatives, the patient perceives his choices to be restricted or vastly limited.

Self-monitoring requires the patient to examine all aspects of the loss, including the immediate event and future outcomes. In so doing, the patient perceives the loss's significance to him, whether it be potential or actual, and perceives the life stressors contributing to the loss. Once self-monitoring has taken place, the patient begins the second stage of self-regulation, namely self-evaluation.

Self-Evaluation Stage

Self-perception, the individual's recall of his past performance, may have an effect on both the self-evaluation phase and the self-monitoring phase. Evaluative statements may come to acquire secondary positive or negative reinforcement value as they, too, serve as discrimination stimuli for reinforcement. The self-evaluation stage relates most obviously to the cognitive distortions of depression (Mathews 1977).

Self-evaluation encompasses a cognitive triad developed by Rush and Beck (1976). The cognitive triad consists of the following: negative view of self, negative view of experiences, and negative view of future.

Negative View of Self. Cognitive disturbances of the depressed person which relate to self-evaluation are details of body image and ideas of deprivation. The depressed individual is likely to assign the cause of an adverse event to some shortcoming in himself. Once the initial crisis has subsided, the patient begins to evaluate his losses. Such was the case with Mr. L., Mrs. P., and Mr. V. Each had experienced a potential, actual, subtle, or obvious loss. Mr. L. experienced a psychological loss that involved a change in his mental image of himself. Mr. L. evaluated himself to be less youthful because of various changes in his life-style that had to be made. Mrs. P. and Mr. V. both experienced more obvious losses in the form of facial laceration, fracture, and hemiplegia. Of the three patients, Mr. V.'s losses may be perceived to be the greatest. Regardless of the loss, each individual experiences a negative self-evaluation in the form of low self-regard. According to Mathews (1977) low self-regard and feelings of inferiority and guilt easily follow from a failure of an individual to meet his or her standards, whether or not those standards are realistic.

The negative view of self contribute to feelings of depression. The burn or hemodialysis patient may feel that his illness or injury has made him a less significant member of society. His life goals and desires are no longer possible. Rush and Beck (1976) note that such patients see themselves as defective, inadequate, and unworthy. They tend to attribute their unpleasant experiences to physical defect in themselves. The patient believes he is undesirable and worthless because of his presumed defects.

The burn or hemodialysis patient or the patient like Mr. V. with hemiplegia are forced into a dependent role. For the more active individual, dependency upon others or supportive devices can be just as threatening as the initial loss. Because the individual sees himself as inept and undesirable, the depressed person unrealistically overestimates the difficulty of normal tasks and expects things to turn out badly. The patient tends to seek help and reassurance from others whom he considers more competent and capable (Rush and Beck 1976).

The critically ill patient may compare himself to other patients with similar problems. If another coronary artery bypass patient has complications, the patient is positive the same complication will occur to him. The trauma, burn, stroke, or renal patient may compare his physiological problem and loss to those of other patients in the unit. The tendency to make comparisons with other people further lowers the individual's self-esteem. Every encounter with another person may be turned into some negative evaluation of himself. To cope with self-negation, the patient may avoid interacting with the nurse, family, or other patients. According to Ferster (1973), the depressed person engages in a high frequency of avoidance and escape from aversive stimuli, usually in the form of complaints or requests for help, along with the reduced frequency of positively reinforced behavior. Besides maintaining a negative self-view, the critical care patient may maintain a negative view of experiences.

Negative View of Experiences. The depressed critically ill patient has a tendency to interpret his ongoing experiences in a negative way. He views the intrusive procedures, supportive devices, and diagnostic procedures as an invasion of his privacy. For some patients the various treatment modalities are viewed as contributing to further losses. Furthermore, the patient does not always understand the technical language used by members of the critical care health team. The patient may actually misinterpret what is being said and evaluate his illness, injury, or disease as more serious than necessary. Rush and Beck (1976) point out that the patient tends to misinterpret his interaction with the world around him in such a way as to provide evidence for defect or deprivation. The nurse knows that negative misinterpretation is taking place when she observes that the patient negatively construes situations even when less negative, more plausible, alternative interpretation are available.

The burn, trauma, renal, or stroke patient evaluates any small reversals in his condition as indicators of further physiological defects. A small reversal may involve alterations in electrolytes or blood gases. The changes may necessitate a change in medication, electrolyte replacement, or a temporary increase in ventilatory support. In terms of the patient's overall physiological losses, the changes are viewed by the staff as small. However the patient distorts their significance. According to Ferster (1974), the depressed person's perception of his own activities and those of people around him may be grossly distorted by extreme feelings of self-blame or incompetence and indifference to and rejection by those around him.

There are times when the depressed patient completely distorts the immediate environment. Environmental distortion is characteristic of the depressed person's repertoire. Furthermore his distorted, incomplete, and misleading view of the environment may include distortion of body image and physical appearance, distortion of his competence, exaggeration of errors, complete inability to evaluate the way other people see him, a tendency to take blame for events for which there is really no responsibility, and a limited and unhopeful view of the world (Ferster 1974).

Negative View of the Future. The last component of the cognitive triad is a negative view of the future. Mr. V. is an example of a patient who maintained a negative view of his future. Until his stroke and subsequent left-side hemiplegia, Mr. V. had maintained an active life based upon physical mobility. His construction job and physical dexterity were the focal point of his life. The work provided income for his family and a sense of self-esteem for himself. The stroke threatened his future and forced upon him changes in his life-style. When confronted with possible forced changes, the patient can become depressed. According to Rush and Beck (1976), as the depressed patient looks ahead, he anticipates that his current difficulties or suffering will continue indefinitely. He expects hardships, frustrations, and deprivation.

Likewise the renal, trauma, or burn patient can also experience similar feelings. The illness, injury, or disease has created a potential or actual loss which reduces future alternatives. The individual may be forced into retirement that was neither anticipated or desired. This represents a drastic change in performance for the individual. The patient may believe he no longer has a significant role in the future. Furthermore he may believe his physiological loss will be negatively received by others. This is especially true for the burn or stroke patient whose losses are visible. Nevertheless during the evaluative stage the patient examines himself, his environment, and his future. Next the patient focuses on the final stage of self-regulation, namely, self-reinforcement.

Self-Reinforcement Stage

Depending on the outcome of self-evaluation, the depressed patient may provide self-reinforcement. According to Mathews (1977), the execution of a response which matches the criterion as a discriminative stimulus may acquire reinforcing value and become the reinforcing event itself. The patient's standards are realistic but prior reinforcement experiences may distort his perception of his behavior.

The patient's prior experience with illness or disease can influence current self-reinforcement. If previous hospitalizations were negative—that is, if they included physiological complications, intrusive procedures and supportive devices, and psychological trauma—the patient may not be motivated to expect a successful outcome from the current hospitalization. If the depressed burn, renal, or stroke patient believes that he will not be able to master a serious problem, to reach his goals, or to forestall a loss, he tends to downgrade his assets. The individual comes to the conclusion that he cannot get satisfaction out of life and that all he can expect is pain and suffering. The depressed patient proceeds from disappointment to self-blame to pessimism (Beck 1974).

The critically ill patient who is depressed sometimes has a tendency to regard the future as an extension of the present. The depressed patient expects a loss, deprivation, or defect to continue permanently. For the renal, burn, or stroke patient the losses are permanent. They begin to wonder what additional losses the future holds for them. They fail to see any possible internal or external gains from the event. On the other hand, patients may discover internal strengths which were previously hidden. In addition, the patient may discover sources of external strength such as friends or family.

It should also be noted that negative expectations involve more than the illness experience; they can also encompass how the patient makes decisions. Mathews (1977) gives the following specific examples of how negative expectations may operate in a depressed person: passiveness, indecisiveness, anticipation of making an incorrect decision, anticipation of failure, and belief that the problems are overwhelming. A patient with a recurring illness requiring frequent readmission into critical care may question his decision-making ability. For example, a cardiac patient may be told that he will be at risk of further myocardial damage if he does not comply with various treatment modalities. His decision to continue smoking and eating foods high in salt and cholesterol content, and not to exercise can eventually contribute to a myocardial infarction. Therefore when the chest pain begins, the patient is confronted with the outcome of his incorrect decisions and anticipation of further biological failure.

Mathews (1977) points out that self-criticism, self-punitive thoughts and behavior, as well as escape and avoidance ideation and behavior are related to the self-reinforcement stage. When the critically ill patient has thoughts of self-criticism, he is involved in negative self-reinforcement. The negative self-reinforcement can have a variety of effects on the individual which are consistent with eventual depression.

During the self-reinforcement stage, the depressed critically ill patient may demonstrate avoidance behavior. Such a patient avoids entering into interpersonal relationships with either his family or nurse. Furthermore, he may avoid participating in his care or seeking information which would enhance his knowledge of illness or treatment events. The patient utilizes escape ideation by either focusing on nonillness topics, sleeping, or watching TV.

The more active trauma, burn, renal, or stroke patient can experience negative self-reinforcement when faced with forced dependency. Some patients have difficulty depending upon others for their physical needs to be met. Furthermore, depending upon supportive devices can also be threatening to the individual. This may be especially true for the renal patient who is dependent upon hemodialysis to sustain his life. Forced dependency may also contribute to the avoidance of meaningful social contact. According to Mathews (1977), depressed individuals are observed both to be dependent upon others and to avoid social contact. In relation to self-reinforcement the dependency could be considered a means of obtaining external positive reinforcement to compensate for negative self-views. It is thought that a series of minor events or a major crisis in an individual predisposed to depression creates a condition of decreased external positive reinforcement.

NURSING ASSESSMENT OF DEPRESSION

When depression is subtle, one's own feelings may provide an important clue that the other person is depressed. As Swanson (1975) points out, the communication of a depressed individual is excellent in one sense; namely, the efficiency with which messages of dejection, hopelessness, or underlying anger get through to another.

The nurse assess depression through the patient's behavioral responses. The responses are categorized into regulatory behaviors and cognitive behaviors.

Regulatory Behaviors

The regulator system involves inputs, processes, effectors, and feedback loops. It involves stimuli from the external environment and from changes in the internal state of dynamic equilibrium. The regulatory behaviors are physiological responses and, in cases of depression, consist of the following:

Regulatory Behaviors
Anorexia
Weight loss
Insomnia
Diurnal variations
Constipation
Diarrhea
Ulcers
Menstrual changes
Headaches
Tightness in chest
Tachycardia
Fatigue

For the depressed patient, changes in appetite are common and vary from anorexia to increased appetite. In general, weight loss in depression should not exceed one pound per week depending upon the duration of the illness. Gastrointestinal complaints are common, including a tendency towards constipation, dry mouth, indigestion, diarrhea, abdominal pain, and unusual taste (Drucker, Heefner, and Wilder 1980).

Depression can also contribute to alteration in the patient's sleep pattern. Insomnia is the most common alteration; however, hypersomnia may also occur. Depressed individuals have a marked decrease in REM cycle sleep, which is associated with dreaming. Nonspecific symptoms consist of loss of energy, fatigability, tiredness, headache, tension, and neck pain (Drucker, Heefner, and Wilder 1980).

Cognitive Behaviors

The cognator system involves inputs from internal and external stimuli which include psychological and social factors. The specific aspects of the cognator mechanism consist of perceptual/information processing, learning, judgment, and emotion. The cognitive behaviors are psychological responses which, in cases of depression, consist of the following:

Cognitive Behaviors
Sadness
Crying easily
Sleep disturbances
Social withdrawal
Loss of feeling
Boredom
Indifference
Lack of interest
Self-criticism
Avoidance
Hopelessness
Confusion
Emptiness
Irritability

Depression can be secondary to many organic illnesses. Sometimes the depression is such a marked presenting feature that the underlying organic pathology is missed. Furthermore the patient with congestive heart failure may present with symptoms such as fatigue, insomnia, and marked depression. Reserpine causes profound depression as do steroids (Cline 1977).

According to Drucker, Heefner, and Wilder (1980), various cognitive manifestations occur in depressed patients. There may be complaint of inability to remember events and a slowing down with decreased quality or spontaneity of the thinking process. Other signs of depression are a saddened face, disinterestedness, listlessness, slowness of speech, or weeping.

As the critically ill patient becomes more aware of the reality of his situation, he may become withdrawn, listless, apathetic, and pessimistic; show retarded speech and motor activity; and express feelings of hopelessness (Bilodeau 1981).

NURSING DIAGNOSIS OF DEPRESSION

The nursing diagnosis is a statement of the current problem. Regulatory and cognitive behaviors coupled with stressors causing the problem help the nurse make her diagnosis. The current problem is depression. The cause of the problem may be aggression turned inward, learned helplessness, insufficient positive reinforcement, or biochemical changes (Jasmin and Trygstad 1979). Internal stresses involve age; illness, injury, or disease; anxiety; and medical or chemical alterations. External stresses can be attributed to the environmental noises, the critical care team, and supportive devices.

NURSING INTERVENTIONS TO REDUCE
FEELINGS OF DEPRESSION

The health status of the patient influences the course and expression of depression in a circular process. First, a decreased level of health may initially lead to depression. An illness, injury, or disease resulting in loss of health—from simple urinary or respiratory tract infection to acute problems such as adult respiratory distress syndrome—affects functioning.

Depression subsides when goals are within reach or goals are relinquished or modified to become attainable. Therefore the nurse's interventions are divided into two categories, namely, fostering cognitive reappraisal and facilitating realistic independence.

Fostering Cognitive Reappraisal

Seligman (1974) believes that successful manipulations change the negative cognitive set to a more positive one. He argues that the primary task of the health team is to change, if possible, the negative expectation of the depressed patient to a more optimistic one whereby the patient comes to believe that his responses will produce the outcomes he wants. Interventions designed to foster cognitive reappraisal consist of providing meaningful communication, increasing self-esteem, and incorporating a teaching-learning framework that will help the patient monitor his own feeling of depression.

The critical care nurse encourages the depressed patient to ventilate his concerns and listens to his discussion of the illness, injury, or disease process. Only when the patient is encouraged to ventilate his depressed feelings can acceptance begin. When the patient feels that someone is listening, he is able to accept reassurance, engage in realistic appraisal of strengths and assets, and pursue new endeavors.

As the nurse listens to the depressed patient, she focuses on the thoughts and thinking pattern of the person. A significant intervention is to focus on the patient's ability to determine reasonable, realistic goals and solutions. Judgment and thinking must be retrained and reformulated so that it becomes reasonable and realistic.

Encouraging the burn, renal, stroke, or trauma patient to share his fears, concerns, thoughts, and reasons for depression involves the skillful use of empathy. Empathy skills help to establish the role of the nurse as a helping professional and communicate the impression that the nurse subjectively understands how the patient is really feeling (Authiers, Authiers, and Lutey 1979). The patient may need permission or encouragement to express the painful feelings associated with depression. The use of empathy skills will provide such permission. The critical care nurse is most effective when she provides a supportive atmosphere wherein all emotions can be expressed. Focusing on depressive feelings and discussion of those feelings can be painful. Nevertheless, expression of depressive feelings is a significant way of working through and experiencing relief from them (Jasmin and Trygstad 1979).

While it is important for the critically ill patient to express his feelings, the nature of the illness or injury may temporarily postpone this goal. The use of an endotracheal tube, tracheostomy, volume respirator, or other supportive devices may limit the patient's ability to communicate his depressive feelings. Furthermore the patient may be too fatigued from the illness or injury, lack of sleep, medications, electrolytes imbalance, anemia, or depression to deal with the reality of his current experience. Therefore, as Authiers, Authiers, and Lutey (1979) note, sometimes the depressed individual will avoid dealing openly and honestly with his feelings, despite the nurse's appropriate and skillful use of the empathy skills.

Besides the use of empathy skills, the nurse provides the patient with meaningful feedback. The critically ill patient needs feedback regarding his physiological and psychological status. The patient sees laboratory tests or diagnostic procedures being done but many times receives little, if any, feedback regarding the outcome of those tests. Therefore, when it is realistic to do so, the nurse can provide laboratory, treatment, or physiological feedback as it relates to the illness, injury, or disease. According to Authiers et al. (1979), feedback can be used to communicate positive feelings as well, and is in fact one of the most effective means of providing encouragement and support to the patient.

The second component in fostering cognitive reappraisal is to increase the patient's self-esteem or self-concept. This is especially important for the critically ill patient who has sustained an obvious or visible alteration in his physical appearance. For example, a stroke patient like Mr. V. may have visible evidence of his illness or injury. If the individual's self-concept was based upon his external physical appearance, any alteration in physical appearance will have a negative effect. A depressed patient who had a low self-esteem before the physiological crisis will in all probability have his low self-esteem reinforced. Therefore it is helpful to look for ways to increase the patient's self-esteem.

Raising the patient's self-esteem or self-concept involves identifying positive gains in his physiological status. When the nurse does this, the depressed patient is able to see progress. Progress can only be found when the knowledgeable provider of his care identifies positive changes. The nurse helps the patient to focus on small aspects of his illness and care rather than on the entire illness or injury event. Focusing totally on the latter will only overwhelm or discourage the patient. This is why it is so important to provide the patient with feedback regarding his status and future progress. It may be extremely significant to Mrs. P. to know that her facial lacerations are healing normally. Therefore a nursing intervention is to provide immediate positive feedback. Throughout this intervention, the nurse also positively reinforces the thoughts and feelings that signal relief from the depressive feelings (Jasmin and Trygstad 1979).

The critical care nurse's attitude is also significant in raising the patient's self-concept. If the nurse maintains a positive attitude toward the patient, he begins to believe that he is a valuable person. According to Authiers et al. (1979), the depressed individual tends to interpret the nurse's attitude as impersonal and uncaring and then to see this attitude as a confirmation of his own existing low self-image. The environment is perceived by the patient as even more hopeless when a professional who is supposed to care seems not to.

Therefore depression requires cognitive reappraisal or altering the patient's overwhelming feelings of helplessness, hopelessness, dejection, and meaninglessness of his illness, injury, or disease.

The final component of cognitive reappraisal consists of developing a teaching-learning framework that will help the patient monitor his own feelings of depression. Within the self-regulation model, the nurse teaches the patient new patterns of coping with the illness, injury, or disease. According to Jasmin and Trygstad (1979), intervention to alter or change the actions of depression includes the use of teaching and positive reinforcement. Initially, positive reinforcement is provided for behavior signaling movement away from the depression. The patient soon learns that responding and reward are connected. In this way the patient is able to see the results of his behavior.

The nurse also teaches the patient how to make accurate self-evaluation. The patient is taught to evaluate himself and the illness situation. The patient may not have been responsible for the illness or injury. Mrs. P., while she blamed herself for the accident, was not responsible for the crisis event. Likewise a patient who is burned by the action of another need not enter into self-blame. Finally the nurse helps the patient evaluate the illness or injury in relationship to treatment modalities. He needs to understand the reasons behind various supportive devices or diagnostic procedures as they correlate to his particular physiological problem.

Next the nurse helps the patient establish realistic goals. The stroke patient's mental image of himself may be the same as his preillness or pre-injury image. Therefore the patient will need to make adjustment or modification in his internal mental image. Failure to make adjustments may cause the patient to have unrealistic expectations or goals. Therefore the nurse listens to the patient's expectations or goals. She then helps the patient make a realistic appraisal of them in relationship to his particular strengths and weakness. It is important to incorporate the family in this phase of the teaching-learning program. Unrealistic family goals may only serve to frustrate the patient, thereby contributing to feelings of depression.

Finally, when it is realistic, the nurse can provide success experiences. This implies that the nurse will assess what the patient can accomplish. For the stroke patient, it may be the successful transfer from his bed to a commode or chair. Even this small accomplishment in physical activity may serve as a motivator. For the cardiac patient success may be a positive change in serial EKG, absence of arrhythmias, or decreased serum enzyme levels. Each successful event makes the patient believe in himself more again and in a possible future.

Facilitating Realistic Independence

The second way in which the nurse can reduce feelings of depression is by facilitating realistic independence. Helping the critically ill patient achieve independence is accomplished through physical mobilization and encouragement of decision-making ability.

Many critically ill patients are immobilized by their illnesses or injury and supportive devices. When such patients have limited mobility they tend to become depressed. Sometimes the nurse becomes so concerned with the completion of procedures or treatments that she forgets the more simple intervention of position changes. McCann (1979) points out that mobilization, however, should be more than getting a person up in a chair at the side of the bed, or placing a patient in a wheelchair out in the hallway where he can only stare at the opposite wall. The stroke patient may prefer immobility to mobility. When he is forced to get out of bed, he becomes acutely aware of his limitations. Nevertheless the nurse continues to encourage mobilization. Each successful attempt at mobilization can motivate the patient to achieve more.

Fostering mobilization also enhances the patient's perception of his environment. As the patient is able to sit in a chair and look at his environment, the environment should contain some familiar items. Naturally the space in his immediate environment may be too small to contain many personal possessions, but it can include drawings, pictures, glasses, and a clock. Such possessions can have special significance to the patient. Drawings from children or grandchildren can have a positive influence on the removal of depressive feelings. The patient may become more motivated to participate in all aspects of his care. The motivator is the thought of being reunited with the family. There are times when it may be necessary to allow the grandchildren to physically see the patient. Hospital policy may not allow such an intervention. However, if it decreases feelings of depression then the intervention should be temporarily implemented.

Another way to facilitate realistic independence is to encourage decision making. When realistic, the patient needs to participate in all aspects of his care. Participation implies that the patient is included in decisions concerning his care. When the patient is encouraged to make decisions, he feels that his opinion is respected and valued. Maintaining a patient's ability to make his own decisions regarding his care is of paramount importance if prevention of depression is a goal (McCann, 1979).

As discussed previously, depressive feelings can be reduced when the patient is physically active. Physical mobility also plays a role in decision making. According to McCann (1979) an immobilized patient's lack of decision-making power within a hospital setting can further contribute to his feeling of helplessness and depression. Decreased decision making can overwhelm him and reduce his capacity to cope effectively with environmental and physical stresses.

In summary, when the patient is encouraged to increase his physical mobility and decision-making ability, feelings of depression can be reduced.

NURSING EVALUATION

Evaluation of the patient's problem and nursing care is an ongoing process. The nurse assesses regulatory and cognitive behaviors supporting the diagnosis of depression. Interventions designed to minimize depression are evaluated for their effectiveness. Effectiveness is measured by the control, reduction, or elimination of depression. The behaviors suggesting depression may not totally disappear until the patient is transferred from critical care or discharged.

SUMMARY

The illness, injury, or disease process can contribute to the critically ill patient's feeling of depression. The critical care nurse intervenes, first, by fostering cognitive reappraisal. Cognitive reappraisal is achieved when the nurse provides meaningful communication, increases self-concept, and incorporates a teaching program that helps the patient reduce feelings of depression. Second, the nurse facilitates realistic independence through encouraging physical mobility and decision-making abilities. It is hoped that as the physiological crisis subsides the patient will find meaning in his life.

REFERENCES

AUTHIER, JERRY, KAREN AUTHIER, and BARBARA LUTEY, "Clinical Management of the Tearfully Depressed Patient: Communication Skills for the Nurse Practitioner," *JPN and Mental Health Services*, 17, no. 2 (February 1979), 36-41.

BECK, AARON, "The Development of Depression: A Cognitive Model," in *The Psychology of Depression: Contemporary Theory and Research*, ed. Raymond Friedman and Martin Katz, pp. 3-19. New York: John Wiley, 1974.

BILODEAU, CAROLYN BASCOM, "Psychological Aspects," *Critical Care Nursing: Body-Mind-Spirit*, ed. C. Kenner, C. Guzzetta, and B. Dossey, pp. 171-196. Boston: Little, Brown and Co., 1981.

BURNS, WILLIAM, and PATRICIA IANNETTA, "Attacking Boredom and Depression," *American Health Care Association Journal*, 3 (May 1977), 34-38.

CLINE, FOSTER, "Dealing with Depression," *Nurse Practitioner*, 2 (January-February 1977), 21-24.

DRUCKER, JOHN, JOHN HEEFNER, and RUSSELL WILDER, "Depression in a Medical Setting," *Minnesota Medicine*, 63, no. 6 (June 1980), 399-404.

FERSTER, CHARLES, "A Functional Analysis of Depression," *American Psychologist*, October 1973, pp. 857-869.

_____ , "Behavioral Approaches to Depression," in *The Psychology of Depression: Contemporary Theory and Research*, ed. Raymond Friedman and Martin Katz, pp. 29-45. New York: John Wiley, 1974.

FROESE, ARTHUR, THOMAS HACKETT, NED CASSEM, and ELIZABETH SILVERBERG, "Trajectories of Anxiety and Depression in Denying and Nondenying Acute Myocardial Infarction Patients during Hospitalization," *Journal of Psychosomatic Research*, 18, (1974), 413-420.

JACOBSON, ANN, "Melancholy in the 20th Century: Causes and Prevention," *JPN and Mental Health Services*, 78, no. 7 (July 1980), 11-21.

JASMIN, SYLVIA, and LOUISE TRYGSTAD, *Behavioral Concepts and the Nursing Process*. St. Louis, C. V. Mosby, 1979.

KALLIO, JOHN, "Reduction of Depression: Three Simple Interventions," *Focus*, August-September 1982, p. 6.

KANFER, F. H., "Self-Monitoring: Methodological Limitations and Clinical Applications," *Journal of Consulting and Clinical Psychology*, 35 (1970), 148-152.

KICEY, CAROLYN, "Catecholamines and Depression: A Physiological Theory of Depression," *American Journal of Nursing*, November 1974, pp. 2018-2020.

LAZARUS, ARNOLD, "Learning Theory and the Treatment of Depression," *Behavioral Research and Therapy*, 6 (1968), 83-89.

LEHMANN, HEINZ, "Classification of Depressive States," *Canadian Psychiatric Association Journal*, 22, no. 7 (November 1977), 381-390.

LIBERMAN, ROBERT, and DAVID RASKIN, "Depression: A Behavioral Formulation," *Archives of General Psychiatry*, 24 (June 1971), 515-523.

MATHEWS, CHRISTINE, "A Review of Behavioral Theories of Depression and a Self-Regulation Model for Depression," *Psychotherapy: Theory, Research and Practice*, 14, no. 1 (Spring 1977), 70-85.

MCCANN, VALERIE, "The Prevention of Depression in the Immobilized Patient," *ONA Journal*, 6 (November 1979), 433-438.

MILLER, WILLIAM, and MARTIN SELIGMAN, "Depression and Learned Helplessness in Man," *Journal of Abnormal Psychology*, 84, no. 3 (1975), 228-238.

ROBERSON, DIANE, "Post-Surgical Depression: The Medical Assistant's Role," *The Professional Medical Assistant*, 12 (January-February 1979), 12-14.

RUSH, JOHN, and AARON BECK, "Cognitive Therapy of Depression and Suicide," *American Journal of Psychotherapy*, 32, no. 2 (April 1976), 201-219.

SCHNEIDER, JOHN, "Clinically Significant Differences between Grief, Pathological Grief, and Depression," *Patient Counseling and Health Education*, 2 (1980), 161-169.

SCHWARTZMAN, SYLVIA, "Anxiety and Depression in the Stroke Patient: A Nursing Challenge," *JPN and Mental Health Services*, 14, no. 7 (July 1976), 13-17.

SELIGMAN, MARTIN, "Depression and Learned Helplessness, in *The Psychology of Depression: Contemporary Theory and Research*, ed. Raymond Friedman and Martin Katz, pp. 83-107. New York: John Wiley, 1974.

——, LYN ABRAMSON, and AMY SEMMEL, "Depressive Attributional Style," *Journal of Abnormal Psychology*, 88, no. 3 (1979), 242-247.

STAFFORD, LINDA, "Depression and Self-Destructive Behavior," *JPN and Mental Health Services*, 14, no. 8 (August 1976), 37-40.

STOREY, PETER, "Depression after Strokes," *Chest, Heart and Stroke Journal*, 1 (September 1976), 14-17.

SWANSON, ARDIS, "Communicating with Depressed Persons," *Perspectives in Psychiatric Care*, 13, no. 2 (1975), 63-67.

WESTLAKE, ROBERT, "Life-Stress and Depression Symposium," *Rhode Island Medical Journal*, 63, no. 4 (1980), 97-114.

18
Loss

BEHAVIORAL OBJECTIVES

1. Define the following terms: *loss, dying, death, mourning,* and *grief.*
2. State the stages of loss.
3. State how concern for biological survival applies to the critically ill patient experiencing a loss.
4. State how competent behavior as it relates to coping applies to the critically ill patient experiencing a loss.
5. Identify four regulatory behaviors associated with loss.
6. Identify five cognitive behaviors associated with loss.
7. Design a nursing care plan that will assist the patient to cope with a loss.

We live in a technological era devoted to youth; exploration of space seeking new life; aerobic exercising and dieting designed to prolong life; and lotions, creams, or ointments advertised to prevent wrinkling and balding. It is indeed a time for youth. Yet the same youth seems to seek a life-style that flirts with the threat of loss and death through alcohol and drug abuse. In addition, our communication system makes us cognizant of senseless bombings, killings, and accidents. According to Shneidman (1970), life is viewed in a two-fold fashion. It is very precious and very cheap. One's life can be taken by another or by oneself. The Western world seems to be more death-oriented than ever before.

Human beings realize that death is inevitable. It is a phenomenon associated with life itself. What one doesn't know is when or how one's own death will occur. Many individuals intellectualize death as it pertains to another, not to themselves. This is because people are basically future-oriented, planning the future as if they will live forever. While one is free of illness and the threat of a limited future, such behavior is normal. It does not imply denial. However, as loss moves beyond the boundaries of loss of function or part only, death and denial sometimes become fused together. Denial for many individuals is a coping mechanism, one that enables them to guard against the threat of death or dying.

The forms of loss include loss of function, part, or whole. Loss can also take the form of death and dying. The purpose of focusing on loss in any one of its forms is to help those who must cope with their own loss. In addition, it provides help for members of the health team who care for the dying. The goal of the latter is to help the individual attain what Weisman (1972) refers to as significant survival, which implies achieving a purposeful death: "Significant survival is a quality of life that means much more than simply not to die. Purposeful death also means more than dying; it includes a measure of fulfillment, quiescence, resolution, and even traces of personal development" (pp. 33–34).

Many people die each year of acute illness, injury, or disease. Prior to their death many of these individuals are hospitalized in a critical care unit. Therefore there is a growing awareness of the dying process which has led critical care nurses to identify behavioral stages of loss or dying. Even though there is a growing body of literature on the patient's behavioral reaction to the dying process, many agencies fail to utilize the various theories.

DEFINITION OF TERMS

The terms to be defined can be categorized as components of loss and the stages of loss.

Components of Loss

The components of loss to be defined are *loss, dying, death, mourning,* and *grief.* The latter two are behavioral responses to death and dying, encompassing the overall stages of death and dying.

Loss. Loss is defined as any changes in the individual's situation that decreases the probability of achieving implicit or explicit goals. It is believed that an individual's goals, hopes, or desires exist to satisfy his or her needs. The blockage of hopes or goals seem to be inherent in most events or situations involving losses. A body part or function may be missed because certain outcomes are no longer attainable when the object or function is gone (Carlson 1978).

Loss includes both biological and psychological loss. Biological loss includes loss of function, part, or whole. Illness necessitating hospitalization causes biological changes ranging from temporary alteration of a system's function to complete removal or loss of that system. Take for example the patient who develops a renal infection. The inflammatory process may lead to chronic renal failure and ultimately loss of both kidneys. Similarly such loss can involve the myocardial, pulmonary, endocrine, and neurological systems. Losses within these biological systems can cause further impairment of mobility, speech, or hearing. Psychosocial losses are equally significant. They can occur simultaneously with biological loss or as independent problems. Such losses include loss of employment, family member, or status. Some losses are externally visible whereas others are known only to the individual. Regardless of the degree of loss or its implications, the individual involved can experience grief and mourning.

Therefore loss is the deprivation of an object, person, possession, or ideal that was considered valuable and had an investment of self. It maybe actual, potential, or symbolic (Dracup and Breu 1978).

Dying. For many, the dying process pertains only to the aged and terminally ill. Terminal illness does not apply only to those individuals dying from various forms of cancer. It also applies to noncancerous patients whose biological system progressively deteriorates toward total failure. The dying process is longer for some patients than for others. As Sudnow (1967) observes, it also has important social implications:

> Dying becomes an important, noticeable process insofar as it serves to provide others, as well as the patient, with a way to orient to the future, to organize activities around the expectability of death, to prepare for it. The notion of dying appears to be a distinctly social one, for its central relevance is provided for by the fact that it establishes a way of attending a person. (P. 68)

Just as the dying process makes the individual cognizant of a limited future, it also has the similar effect upon those providing care as well as family members. The dying process seems to serve the function of putting into perspective roles, values, and expectations of each of those involved. This is one of the ways in which the dying process becomes social. Some family members temporarily abandon their own personal needs and attend to the immediate needs of the dying individual. Likewise, the health team can attend to more than the physical needs of the dying patient. In selected settings in which dying is the anticipated outcome, the staff may be better equipped emotionally to handle its behavior by offering both patient and family the emotional support needed to eventually orient themselves to the expectation of death. Needless to say, this process does not take place immediately but occurs in various stages. The individual at each stage will present certain behaviors. These behaviors may range from initial fear and panic to quiet withdrawal. As Weisman (1972) notes, "Fear of dying is a state of episodic alarm, panic, and turmoil. It is associated with excessive autonomic symptoms, and usually conveys a preemptive conviction that collapse is at hand. When the fear of dying is intense, reality testing abandons the hopeless victim (p. 14).

Death. For many people death represents finality, the end of one's biological being, while for others it represents a spiritual beginning. At some point in time the patient's fear of dying evolves into fear of death. According to Weisman (1972), "Fear of death is not an immediate event, but rather a reflection about man's helplessness. . . . As a rule, fears about death are much stronger than the evidence produced by actual disease and invalidism" (p. 15). Those who remain after the patient has died go through the process of mourning. Those remaining are usually the members of the family and health team. Each has become involved with the dying patient in varying degrees. Like the dying process, the mourning process can be painful.

Mourning. Mourning takes place when those who remain realize the loss of a loved one. Bowlby (1961) describes mourning as the psychological processes that follow a loss (or the anticipation of loss) of a significant or valued object. These processes usually culminate in giving up the lost object.

Grief. Not only does the dying individual mourn actual physical, psychological, or social loss, he or she also grieves the potential loss, which involves anticipatory grief. According to Torpie (1974), "The anticipatory grief of the dying patient is a total response to the realization of future total loss, it is characterized by absolute finality. It is felt before the actual fact of loss and yet may never be experienced since, in a philosophic sense, death presumes the end of all experience" (p. 120). Anticipatory grief implies the internal changes experienced by the significant others who must watch the dying patient. It occurs prior to the actual grief process which occurs when loss is associated with death. Therefore, actual grief occurs after the real loss whereas anticipatory grief is associated with potential loss. Torpie notes further that anticipatory grief is affected by the patient's history:

> Anticipatory grief must be compared, interpreted, and magnified by the patient's sense of past loss and grief and past premonition of threat of loss. This anticipation, therefore, consists of elements of fantasy which have a realistic basis, but which also may be colored quite unrealistically by weakness, fear, isolation, feelings of inadequacy, and loss of control. (P. 120)

Grief, whether it is anticipatory or normal, consists of a culmination of behavioral responses. Some of the behavioral responses are hopelessness, loneliness, powerlessness, depression, anger, hostility, and guilt. The various behavioral responses can be found within the different stages of the grief and mourning process.

Stages of Loss

Kübler-Ross (1975) has identified five phases of dying: denial and isolation, anger, bargaining, depression, and acceptance. Therefore, the nurse can be aware when she assesses a particular behavioral response in a patient that it may represent a particular phase or stage in the grieving process.

Lipowski (1969) has identified four stages associated with loss through which an individual may progress. The stages have subjective meaning for symptoms and disability of the patient. According to Lipowski, evaluation begins first with the perception of a pathological process or injury and continues throughout the course of illness. The actual meaning is the patient's psychological response to his disease. The four stages to be discussed are threat, loss, gain (relief), and insignificance.

Threat. The first stage is referred to as threat. Threat implies anticipation of an event over which the individual may feel there is no control. If the event leads to personal physical or emotional suffering, it becomes all the more threatening. Anticipation of a threatening event may result from perception of bodily changes that signal potential loss or disability. Again the loss may be loss of physiological function or of social status. Loss need not always be associated with dying and death. Even the slightest biological change (toothache) can be threatening with the perceived threat ranging from a simple filling to complete removal of the tooth. Threat then causes anxiety. Anxiety in turn causes behavioral responses designed to avoid, reduce, or work with the anticipated threat, all of which help the patient to eliminate the unpleasant experience of anxiety. The dying patient utilizes defense mechanisms which help him cope with the future.

Loss. Loss is the second stage. As previously discussed, loss encompasses many facets ranging from simple loss of a fingernail to the more complex loss associated with death and dying. According to Lipowski (1969), the stage of loss "refers not just to body parts and functions actually lost but also to deprivations of personally significant needs and values. The latter are related chiefly to self-esteem, security, and satisfaction. The emotional response to each anticipated loss, whether concrete or symbolic, takes the form of a grief reaction" (p. 1199).

Gain. For some critically ill patients, their loss represents gains or relief. The patient who has sustained a myocardial infarction involving loss of myocardial tissue and temporary loss of social mobility may have certain unconscious dependency needs fulfilled. In this respect, illness has a secondary gain. Through the illness, the sick individual is able to control others either directly or indirectly. The patient can control family members or staff directly by giving orders and indirectly by inflicting guilt feelings. "On the whole, when subjective gains derived from illness, disability, and so forth, outweigh the losses, the patient is likely to cling to his sickness and develop an emotional disturbance when recovery occurs" (Lipowski 1969, p. 1200).

Insignificance. The last stage is insignificance. The patient who is dying should be permitted to approach death with dignity. Even though the individual has sustained or is in the process of sustaining a biopsychosocial loss, that patient needs to feel significant. However, there are times when the loss makes the patient feel insignificant as a human being. Insignificance associated with loss has two meanings for the patient. First the patient attaches insignificance to the illness, injury, or impending loss. Initially, the loss may be perceived as insignificant if the patient denies any threat. The second implication of insignificance involves others' perception of the individual. There are times when the chronically disabled patient is made to feel less significant than the more healthy patients around him. Possibly the patient experiencing loss perceives that more time is spent caring for patients with less complicated and disabling problems. A dying patient makes members of the health team cognizant of their own vulnerability and inevitable death. This is particularly true of younger patients. In addition, death or dying implies failure to alter a potentially fatal process. It must be kept in mind that loss, no matter what the cause or degree of severity, need not be perceived as a failure. Instead the loss can be approached in a more positive manner. Even though the patient is unable to reestablish a previous level of mobility, that patient can still be a significant member of the family unit. To further this feeling, the health team needs to maintain a sense of hopefulness in the patient's emotional contributions.

Regardless of the stages or phases, each patient who experiences a loss manifests a unique behavioral response. Loss has a different meaning for each patient. Furthermore, it is possible that one patient may bypass a particular stage or phase as one adapts to the immediate or impending loss.

THE CONCEPT OF LOSS APPLIED
TO THE CRITICALLY ILL PATIENT

The process of hospitalization and the loss of control over one's wishes and needs often lead the patient to gradually adopt the self-image of an ill, deviant, unworthy person. For the critically ill patient, serious life-threatening illness will exacerbate deviant reality and severely alter his life-style (Hamilton 1977).

It must be remembered that regardless of its cause, severity, or duration, illness implies a loss. The loss involved can range from temporary loss of function to loss of life. Regardless of the duration or severity, loss has significance for all involved, including the patient, family, and members of the health team. Loss occurs in many patients. It can affect the lives of many people. Each individual, depending on his location on the continuum of growth and development, reacts differently to the loss experience. Depending upon the type of patient, the nurse is confronted with different behavioral manifestations of inner feelings.

Carlson (1978) points out that a large percentage of individuals who require hospitalization and nursing care have experienced or are anticipating losses of body parts or functions. Physical alterations or possible limitations can be very disturbing since the body with its parts and functions are tied to objects in the environment, social interaction, and one's psychological self.

Shusterman (1973) describes the range of behaviors that may be exhibited in the face of death as follows:

Some persons withdraw from the threat of death into a life pattern of hopelessness and lose personal control; others regress in their behavior to an immature level of self-centeredness, psychosomatic complaints, and bitterness at being dependent on others. Awareness of impending death may also be minimized or eliminated by such defense mechanisms as repression, rationalization, devaluation, or obsessive-compulsive ritual. (P. 366)

Needless to say, complex losses such as those associated with complete dysfunction of a biological system or impending loss of life are the most difficult with which to cope. Each individual has a unique way of coping with loss. Loss has different significance for each critically ill patient. Hopefully, the way each patient copes will not be maladaptive.

Loss or the threat of loss can be a new experience for the critically ill patient. The loss can be the result of acute illness, chronic disability, or terminal process. Regardless of the cause, the patient may be unable to fulfill psychological or physiological needs. Illness is an inconvenience for the patient who must temporarily submit ownership of his body to others. The patient depends upon the nurse to feed, bathe, turn, or assist him to the bathroom. As the illness or disease process increases in severity or chronicity, the patient may become totally dependent upon others. As Weisman (1972) notes, "For most people, sickness is uncomfortable, inconvenient, temporary, but rarely a menace. Then, if sickness persists, enduring beyond the healing effects of treatment and time, the personal dimensions of being sick gradually become more conspicuous" (p. 52). In discussing the critically ill patient, two factors are of significance. First is the concern for biological survival. Second is the competent behavior utilized as each copes or adapts to their biological threat.

Concern for Biological Survival

The threat of illness precipitates the coping behaviors associated with loss. For some patients it is an adaptation to dying; for others it is the loss of health or loss of a limb, a blow to their self-concept, or the necessity to change their life-style (Busch and Gallo 1982). Furthermore loss or the threat of loss can be a new experience for the patient. The loss can be the result of acute illness, injury, or disease. Regardless of the cause, the patient may be unable to fulfill psychological or physiological needs. Illness is an inconvenience for the patient who must temporarily submit ownership of his body to others (Roberts 1980).

Acute or prolonged illness involves primary loss in bodily functions or organs. Myocardial infarction, chronic obstructive pulmonary disease, or renal failure causes loss in function, part, or whole, or of a particular system. The patient with acute renal failure is threatened by the possibility of total loss in renal function resulting in ultimate dependency upon hemodialysis. When a biological crisis occurs, the individual is removed from the familiar territory and rushed to a nearby hospital. While the sirens scream, the individual has thoughts of final separation from family and life itself. These feelings intensify as the patient becomes quickly absorbed into a rapidly changing environment. In all probability these fears will continue throughout the initial days of biological crisis. The fears and anxieties may be even more intense if the patient is hospitalized several times for the same problem.

One would think that repeated admission into a critical care unit would prepare the individual for future losses—that is, that anticipation of loss would allow for preparation, or that prior experience with loss would help prepare one for later losses. According to Carlson (1978), however, it seems that preparation for the loss does not tend to occur and past experience with loss has variable effect.

Each patient in biological crisis seeks the same goal of biological survival. Depending upon the patient's particular problem, biological survival has different meanings. For the patient with a myocardial infarction, it means surviving the initial crisis and threat of death. To the patient with chronic emphysema or renal failure, biological survival means pain relief, decrease in suffering, physical stability, and adaptation to reduced stamina. A diagnosis such as myocardial infarction or renal insufficiency is not as threatening as that of cancer. Although patients can survive any of the above biological problems, cancer is still synonymous with death. In addition, cancer is associated with extended illness and hospitalization. Weisman (1972) describes how such illness may affect the patient:

> The meaning of illness becomes more pertinent when sickness is extended and involves helplessness and the threat of death. Survival itself may be uncertain. Effective performance within a familiar orbit of activity is drastically, and perhaps permanently compromised. The affected patient must, therefore, assess his place in the world. He asks himself what has happened, where he is going, what he can expect, and what it all means. (Pp. 95-96)

The critical care nurse needs to assess the impact of past experiences with loss events. It should be noted that past experience is not a simple variable but rather it involves many factors. For example, the type of loss involved, the age at which the event took place, and the number of such events experienced are three such variables. Furthermore the nurse assesses the relationship of the individual to the lost object as it applies to goal achievement. The more significant the object, the greater the subjective loss as well as the subsequent grief are likely to be (Carlson 1978).

The type of biological loss or injury has tremendous significance for some patients. For example the trauma or burn patient who has sustained facial injuries can experience tremendous losses. For most individuals the face is significant in almost all face-to-face interactions with people. Any or all of these interactions may be altered or terminated by visible scars and deformities of the face; therefore any goals involving other people may be less attainable (Carlson 1978).

Regardless of the biological or psychological problem, most patients desire to live. The nurse must recognize, however, that there are patients who, because of chronic debilitating illnesses, enter the hospital without the desire, will, or motivation to live. The nurse may hear the patient say, "Please let me die in peace." When she encounters such a patient, the nurse will attempt to instill the desire to live, even though the patient has already willed the self to death. Positive peripheral factors such as spouse or a family to support the desire to live, or meaningful social activities may not be operating in this group.

On the other hand, there are times when it seems that medical technology is more concerned with prolonging death than life. The patient is almost inevitably confronted with the issue of prolongation of life. This is particularly applicable to the critically ill patient. It must be pointed out that there are many patients with acute or chronic biological problems who maintain an active desire and motivation to live as long as possible. They are usually people who have been relatively healthy all their lives and for whom illness is simply an inconvenience or waste of valuable time. Such patients are eager to return to their homes, families, social activities, and pets. There are several positive peripheral factors in their lives which motivate them to return to a level of health. One may be the fact that they have been free from repeated, debilitating illness. Another significant factor may be that the patient realizes that a spouse is home waiting for his return. Because such patients in acute or chronic care facilities have a strong motivation to live, their wishes should be acknowledged and respected. The patient's desire to live causes him to behave in certain ways.

Competent Behavior

The concept of competent behavior implies that an individual who is ill can choose the manner in which to solve or cope with biopsychosocial losses. The way chosen will depend upon the direct or potential loss involved and how it interferes with life goals. A patient may choose to deny severity of his condition and possible loss of life, to bargain with significant others for the loss's removal, to develop an awareness of the loss's relatedness to physical being, or to resolve or accept the loss.

During times of acute exacerbations or the raising of expectations or during any significant change, the initial response will be to regress to an earlier emotional position of safety. Weaning from a respirator, removal of monitor leads, or increased activity and reduction in medication often triggers anxiety and regression (Busch and Gallo 1982).

The patient uses negation as a process through which the individual responds to something perceived to be a threat. Negation behaviorally manifested as denial is a defense behind which the patient, family member, or nurse can retreat. If one denies the loss, then its meaning or future implication cannot be emotionally assessed. Sometimes it is difficult for the nurse to assess whether or not the patient is denying. The nurse may falsely assume that, since the patient does not discuss the loss, it has been both assimilated and accepted. Therefore, signs of denying and denial are missed. The nurse's assessment can include how and when denial seems to occur. Weisman (1972) has identified three degrees or orders of denial which he terms first-order denial, second-order denial, and third-order denial. Although he relates these orders to death, they can also be applied to patients experiencing other significant losses.

First-Order Denial. First-order denial deals with the period of time in which an individual realizes that something is wrong. This period of time involves two phases. The first is the initial impact of a biological crisis such as myocardial infarction, respiratory failure, or sudden abdominal pain. The symptoms tell the individual a potential problem exists. The person may choose to acknowledge the presence of the pain or symptom and seek professional help. On the other hand, he may intellectualize the magnitude or etiology of the problem through self-diagnosis and self-treatment. Take for example the hard-driving young male executive who experiences chest pain while conducting a business meeting. He has experienced a similar pain on previous occasions. With each new occurrence, he rationalizes or intellectualizes its significance and origin. He attributes the pain to indigestion and prescribes antacids. Therefore, through self-diagnosis and self-treatment, he denies the threat of a biological crisis. He continues to deny until the time when the symptoms can no longer be hidden behind denial. For some, unfortunately, this time of awareness is at death.

The second phase begins when the individual's problem is professionally labeled or diagnosed. At this point fears are confirmed. During this time, the patient fails to comprehend and experience the emotional impact and meaning of the diagnosis. Because the diagnosis has no emotional meaning, the patient sometimes fails to cooperate with preventative measures (Busch and Gallo 1982). Shock usually accompanies this phase. It follows the perception of an event that seriously disrupts a person's actual or potential goal attainment whether or not there was a warning (Carlson 1978).

Denial begins at either phase and it is interesting to note that the patient does not realize the denial. Besides sheltering the patient from reality, denial also allows the patient to maintain and present a positive self-image. American society places great emphasis upon youth and life. Therefore, a person who is experiencing several biological losses resulting in a premature dependency, disability, or death begins to view himself as one of life's mistakes. To avoid such feelings of worthlessness, the patient will attempt to deny the seriousness of the biological loss or potential death. Weisman (1972) describes the connection between denial and self-esteem as follows:

> Patients who deny a great deal seem to do so in order to preserve a high level of self-esteem. For this reason, they need to preserve contact and stabilize their relationship with someone essential to self-esteem. Even when there seems to be no one in particular who threatens or could be threatened by a patient's illness, deterioration, or death, the patient himself may deny because he wants to maintain the status quo of already existing relationships. (P. 64)

According to Busch and Gallo (1982), while denying illness can prevent adaptation at a new level, denial also has its advantages. High deniers with a myocardial infarction have been shown to have a higher survival rate than moderate or low deniers. Furthermore, high deniers often return to work sooner and reach higher levels of rehabilitation.

The patient is expected to present courageous behavior even when death approaches. Such notions require that the patient maintain relative composure and cheerfulness or, at the very least, that death should be faced with dignity. They dictate that the patient should not cut himself off from the world, nor turn his back on the living; if he has a family, he should continue to be a good family member. The patient should "be nice" to other patients, as well, and should cooperate with the staff members who provide care, and avoid distressing them.

In critical care units, nurses frequently hear family members say, particularly to aged patients, "Now, Papa, be nice to the little nurse. Do what she says and don't complain." It may be, however, that complaining or arguing with the nurse is the only control he feels he has over the situation; he may be physically too weak to fight, so his control takes the form of verbal abuse. The nurse may be controlling him through a pacemaker, dialysis machine, or intravenous therapy; he is controlling his nurse through yelling or pushing his light frequently. Critical care units in any hospital, with their atmosphere of heroic measures aimed at recovery, are geared toward prolonging life at almost any cost. Equipment is clustered near every bed, so that prolonging life may be just a matter of leaning over and "hooking the patient up." The atmosphere in such units counters the staff's attempts to make the patient comfortable and to let him die. As Fletcher (1960) has beautifully expressed it, "It is the living that fear death, not the dying" (p. 139).

Just as the patient or the family experiences first-order denial, the health team may not realize that they also deny the reality of a serious or terminal illness. Some doctors feel that a patient's death puts their professional competence, rather than the state of medical knowledge, generally in question, and as a consequence they will not relinquish the recovery goal until they feel assured that their own skills are not at issue. A favorite rationale of doctors who persist in the ideal of indefinitely prolonging life is the assertion that they are simply an instrument of society. They feel that society has vested in them the duty of sustaining life, and that they are therefore obligated to abdicate personal responsibility for judging whether a particular life should or should not be prolonged (Glaser and Strauss 1965).

With first-order denial, the patient attempts to minimize the illness or disease. Minimization may continue even when the illness recurs. When pain is involved, the patient is unable to deny its existence, and may instead deny its significance. A tumor that is cancerous and malignant may be emotionally treated as though it is benign. Such behavior indicates second-order denial.

Second-Order Denial. During second-order denial, the critically ill patient develops an awareness of the loss or threat of loss. A loss of sufficient magnitude to produce a grief reaction can cause anxiety of panic proportions when awareness comes (Carlson 1978). Furthermore, guilt feelings around one's own illness are difficult to understand unless one examines the basic dynamism of guilt. Guilt arises when there is a decrease in the feelings of self-worth or when the self-concept has been violated (Busch and Gallo 1982).

Biologically, second-order denial refers to the phase of more extensive losses associated with illness or disease. During this phase, the patient emotionally may or may not see the extension and overall implications of the illness or disease. It will be remembered that first-order denial revolves around the patient's first reaction to the diagnosis. However, once the patient accepts the fact that he is ill, there is an inability to comprehend the implications and severity of the loss.

For example, the patient with acute renal failure may deny the probability of the illness evolving into chronic renal failure which would require dependency upon a supportive device such as hemodialysis. The cardiac patient experiencing myocardial infarction associated with congestive heart failure for the second time in six months may choose to deny the severity of the loss. This patient wants to believe that his loss is only temporary. The nurse realizes that the loss is more extensive even to the point of death. Likewise, the patient with a malignant disease may deny the extensiveness of the illness. Such behavior represents the patient's coping mechanism. The nurse may assess that the patient, at this phase, is only able to take in and assimilate small aspects of the illness.

Another manifestation of second-order denial, according to Weisman (1972), is fractionation of the illness: "Denial of implications often takes place when a patient fractionates his illness and persistent symptoms into many, minor complaints, each of which can then be handled separately. As a result, the total illness cannot amount to much" (p. 71). Patients engaging in this type of denial often refuse to adhere to an overall restrictive treatment program. Each may follow one aspect yet refuse to follow another equally significant aspect. The patient with myocardial infarction may refuse to remain in bed even after having been instructed of the dangers of early mobilization. The patient with renal failure may fail to follow a proper diet, eating food high in protein and potassium content. Likewise, the patient with pulmonary edema who refuses to restrict fluid intake only contributes to the biological crisis. Regardless of the biological or psychological problem, each patient has a unique reason for refusing to adhere to a particular treatment procedure. The patient, through assimilation, finally reaches the transitional stage in which he becomes aware of his possible extinction. The nurse assesses that such behavior is reflective of third-order denial.

Third-Order Denial. Third-order denial deals with the patient's acceptance of loss, various hazards, or complications. The critical care patient adapts himself to his new image. He spends time going over significant memories about the loss. Behaviors in this stage include the verbalization of fears regarding the future. At this time the patient may question his ability to reassume specific roles. For example, after severe trauma resulting in scarring or removal of a body part or loss of sensation, the patient may question his sexual adequacy and the future response of his spouse to the changed body (Busch and Gallo 1982).

Resolution of the loss is another characteristic of third-order denial. At this time the individual may detail the traumatized part such as a stoma, prothesis, scar, or paralyzed limb by naming it and referring to it in a simultaneously alienated and affectionate way. In time the patient moves towards identifying himself as an individual who has certain limitations due to the illness, injury, or disease rather than as a cripple. When this happens, the critical care patient no longer uses his deficit as the basis of his identity (Busch and Gallo 1982).

The patient whose loss results in denying and death becomes aware of a limited future sooner than the family or sometimes the health team. After all, the patient is living within the body that is experiencing a biological or emotional loss. Elmore (1967) points out that, "To the extent that the individual perceives and interprets the nature of the internal messages and is consequently able to plot the rate of decline, and to extend this declining curve from the present into the future to a terminal point—to this extent we can speak of a premonition of death" (p. 36). The internal messages received by the patient are constant. They keep the patient continuously informed about biological stability or decline. No matter how hard a patient may try to deny, he cannot avoid the close monitoring of biological events with the body. Therefore, the internal messages contribute to awareness. As the messages become more intense, the patient begins to accept the reality of his death.

The nurse can realize that it is possible for the patient to acknowledge his own loss and its finality sooner than the nurse or health team is able to do so. Some family members request heroic measures even when the patient's losses are so extensive that only death will be prolonged, not life itself. The nursing and medical staff may need to go along with the family until the family can understand that such measures may not be the wisest choice. If the patient is being kept alive by equipment, the doctor has greater control over life than in the case of natural prolonging of life. The doctor also has more time to plan, to calculate risks, and to negotiate with the family and nurses.

Although the medical ideal of prolonging life at all costs and with all possible facilities conflicts with the awareness that prolonging life may be useless and unduly expensive, the ideal often wins out. According to one physician, "There are too many instances . . . in which patients in such a situation are kept alive indefinitely by means of tubes inserted into their stomachs, or into their veins, or into their bladder, or into their rectums— and the whole sad scene thus created is encompassed with a cocoon of oxygen which is the next thing to a shroud" (quoted in Glaser and Strauss 1965, p. 202).

Not all patients respond to a loss in the same manner. A patient's response may be dependent upon age, previous experiences with loss, or severity of the loss. Nevertheless, there are stages, previously mentioned, through which each individual moves. The nurse assesses the patient's behavioral response in an attempt to assist in coping with the loss. In addition, the nurse simultaneously helps the patient's family cope with their feelings. The nurse keeps in mind that each individual, family, or patient is unique and that some move toward acceptance faster than others. To effectively assist the patient, the nurse assesses and utilizes various influencing factors or variables as they specifically apply to the individual.

NURSING ASSESSMENT OF LOSS

The nurse assesses loss through the patient's behavioral response. The responses can be categorized into regulatory behaviors and cognitive behaviors. Recognition of specific behaviors that are commonly exhibited at various stages of grief can be an aid to nursing assessment as long as the nurse realizes that behaviors seldom match phases perfectly (Carlson 1978). In terms of loss, the primary behaviors are cognitive in nature.

Regulatory Behaviors

The regulator system involves input, processes, effectors, and feedback loops. It involves stimuli from the external environment and from changes in the internal state of dynamic equilibrium. The regulatory behaviors in situations of loss are physiological responses and consist of the following:

Regulatory Behaviors
Increased heart rate
Increased blood pressure
Increased respiratory rate
Nausea
Abdominal cramps

Depending upon the type of loss involved, the regulatory behaviors may be attributed to the illness, injury, or disease process.

Cognitive Behaviors

The cognator system involves inputs from internal and external stimuli which include psychological and social factors. The specific aspects of the cognator mechanism consist of perceptual/information processing, learning, judgment, and emotion. The cognitive behaviors are psychological responses. Some of the behaviors in situations of loss are the following:

Cognitive Behaviors
Crying
Trembling
Fighting
Screaming
Attacking
Moaning
Sighing

As discussed earlier, competent behavior exhibited by the critically ill patient focused on first-, second-, and third-order denial. It might be inferred that the patient is angry or anxious, that he is denying reality or is feeling loss of self-esteem, helplessness, or frustration. Other competent behaviors associated with loss include expressions of hopelessness, depression, fear, and finally an awareness of the loss. The severity of a patient's loss influences the degree of depression and hopelessness. A more serious biological illness, possibly resulting in death, causes the patient to feel less hopeful about the future. As Verwoerdt (1967) notes, instead of looking forward to an expansive future, the patient becomes depressed thinking of a constricting one:

> Loss of hopeful prospects in fatally ill patients is associated with a turning away from the future. A certain amount of satisfaction with the past is associated with a more hopeful outlook and with looking forward into the more distant future. The degree of disability for current life activities shows a significant relationship to loss of hope and to constriction of future. (P. 16)

Normally an individual looks forward to the future, anticipating positive accomplishments. One dreams of how leisure time will be spent in the pursuit of yet unmet goals. The individual, together with the family, plans for the future because there is hope in its existence. Hope is a future-oriented concept. Loss resulting in a constricted future removes the patient's sense of hope and replaces it with the feeling of hopelessness and depression. To protect himself from the hopeless feelings of his finality, the patient may avoid any reference to the future. The family or nurse attempts to offer the patient a sense of hope by focusing upon positive aspects of the present and future. Such an approach may eventually have a positive effect on patients with biological losses leading to disability rather than immediate or impending death. Chronic pulmonary patients and dialysis patients need an element of hope in order to cope with their constricted future. Their attention may focus only on the present state of biological loss. Each patient needs to find hope in the present so that, in case of survival, a future, no matter how limited, still exists. The terminally ill patient focuses on the past and present because the future is too painful. Therefore, the patient recoils into events of the past that represent pleasure.

Feelings of hopelessness and depression are normal adaptive behavioral responses to a loss. Maladaptive behavior occurs when a patient whose loss only means temporary obstruction of future goals continues to feel hopeless and depressed. The nurse may assess that the loss was a greater threat to emotional integrity than anticipated or realized. The biological crisis may reach stability; however, the patient's emotional equilibrium may remain unstable. Free from diagnostic studies and treatments, the patient has time to think about the loss. It may be at this point in the hospitalization that the patient requires a greater degree of attention from the nurse. Unfortunately, this is also the time when members of the health team shift their attention to someone else in more acute biological crisis. As a result, the patient is left alone with unresolved conflicts and unanswered questions; consequently, fears remain and sometimes become intensified.

Initially, the patient with a biological loss experiences fear of dying or death. It is natural that fears are dependent upon the nature and severity of the loss. The biological insult may not be as threatening as the diagnosis itself. For example, a 34-year-old woman had recently passed her yearly physical examination with flying colors. Two months later she began complaining of nonspecific symptoms such as generalized aches and tiredness. Shortly thereafter she developed some rectal bleeding. Still unconcerned about her symptoms, she nevertheless entered the hospital for diagnostic studies. To everyone's amazement the studies revealed what was not anticipated: leukemia. What two months earlier was assumed to be perfect health and an expanding future, the diagnosis of leukemia revealed as terminal disease with constricted future (3 to 12 months). For this patient and others like her the fear of dying and death become a reality. The fear of dying and death may be experienced during the early stages of a terminal illness. As the disease progresses, the patient, more so than the family, becomes more accepting of the losses. Consequently, as death approaches, the patient's fears may be subsiding. Instead, the awareness of his own biological finality has made the patient more accepting of it. The nurse can keep in mind that the absence of fear does not always imply denial. It may imply that awareness has led the patient into the last stage of mourning: acceptance.

NURSING DIAGNOSIS OF LOSS

The nursing diagnosis is a statement of the current problem. Regulatory and cognitive behaviors coupled with stressors causing the problem combine to help the nurse make her diagnosis. The problem is loss. Stressors contributing to loss can be categorized as internal or external. The internal and external stressors or variables will be examined under the section on nursing interventions.

NURSING INTERVENTIONS TO ASSIST
THE PATIENT IN COPING WITH LOSS

Facilitation of adaptation or restoration of equilibrium following a loss great enough to disrupt equilibrium involves determining ways to help the individual find new methods to reach goals and new goals that, when attained, will be approximately as satisfying as prior goals. Personal variables both internal and external that may influence the nature and course of grief are numerous (Carlson 1978).

The nurse needs to assist the patient in adapting to the loss. The nurse realizes that the loss implied by a threatening fatal disease can lead to a diminished sense of self-worth in the patient. As Weisman (1972) points out about such a patient, "The healing effect of treatment and time are not his. Therefore, as his illness progresses, he is forced to settle for less and less, to compromise his expectations, and to become less than what he had been or might be. Finally, survival becomes and end in itself" (p. 57). To help the patient accomplish his goals, the nurse assesses both internal and external influencing factors or variables. Once these are assessed, the nurse intervenes to alter, maintain, or strengthen the variables.

Internal Variables

Internal variables are concerned with the pathological processes; psychological processes such as self-esteem and personality variables; age; prior experiences; beliefs and values; and anxiety and other behaviors.

The nurse accepts and recognizes the critically ill patient's pathophysiological process by watching supportive devices or interpreting hemodynamic parameters. The nurse assesses the loss according to its nature, extent, rate of progression, degree, and reversibility of the reduced function. These are the biological variables through which the nurse and other members of the health team intervene. Take, for example, Mr. J., an aggressive 39-year-old who maintained his own construction business. He was married and the father of three children. His job involved both physical and emotional pressures. Throughout his life he has enjoyed relatively good health. However, one morning while jogging, he experienced severe chest pain. He was quickly admitted to a nearby coronary care unit. A social history revealed that he smoked two to three packs of cigarettes per day, drank, and maintained late hours. An emergency cardiac catheterization revealed 95 percent occlusion of both his right and left coronary arteries. The patient's cardiologists felt surgery was mandatory; otherwise his preinfarction status could lead to severe myocardial damage or death. Mr. J. submitted to the surgery. Needless to say, his family was quite concerned. Because Mr. J.'s symptoms, diagnostic evaluation, and surgery all took place in the same day, he had difficulty relating to his own loss. Postoperatively he minimized the entire event as if it had never happened. He felt that in a few weeks he would resume his previous life-style. The surgery saved his life; however, Mr. J. never completely internalized that his life was in danger. Mr. J.'s image of himself was that of "one of the group at the construction site." He wanted to continue his active life, including smoking, drinking, and keeping long difficult hours. Any discussion to the contrary was avoided by the patient. He denied that any change in his future life-style was necessary.

In the above situation, the nurse and health team intervened to alter those behaviors that led to the biological crisis to maintain those factors which would reduce its extension or promote stability, and to strengthen already stabilized processes. When a patient like Mr. J. denies behaviors contributing to his illness, it becomes difficult for his nurse to alter those behaviors. The nurse can allow the patient to deny a loss; however, the nurse does not support him in his denial. The patient's denial is important in attempting to continue presenting a positive image. The nurse keeps in mind that, regardless of the patient or the loss, "The greater the value and psychodynamic significance the body part or function affected by disease has for the patient, the more intense this psychological reaction is likely to be" (Lipowski 1969, p. 1201).

Recognizing the patient's need to present a positive physical body image, the nurse helps the patient realize that there are other aspects of the physical being and personality which permit the patient to continue a positive self-image. In other words, the patient need not depend on what he thinks are the behaviors of "the construction gang," such as drinking, smoking, and physical labor. Once the illness has stabilized and the loss has been realized, the patient can be helped to look at contributing behaviors which led to the biological crisis. These behaviors can then be altered. All treatments or activities designed to stabilize the biological loss should be maintained. Last, those factors which strengthen the patient's adaptation to the loss and eventual recovery can be encouraged.

Regardless of the biological loss, it is important to remember that patients who set a high value on their physical well-being, including the ability to physically move through their environment, are threatened when faced with an illness or pathological process. Different parts of the body have different significance for each individual. Therefore, the part of the body that is affected becomes an important variable. According to Lipowski (1969), "Different organs and functions may have different value and psychological significance for different persons. These values often have little to do with biological factors related to survival. An injury to the nose or amputation of a breast may have greater psychological impact on a person than, for example, hepatic disease directly threatening his life" (p. 1202). Pathological processes can and do lead to psychological changes, which become the second internal variable.

Psychological processes involve self-esteem and personality variables. The nurse intervenes to support the patient's basic sense of self-worth and to encourage the expression of direct anger. The overall goal is to help the critically ill patient attach a sense of self-esteem to his altered identity. The patient is helped to find the degree of dependence that he needs and can accept (Busch and Gallo 1982).

Many times the patient is cognitive of a potential problem prior to its confirmation by a professional. Likewise, the patient remains aware of his body's altered state throughout the illness or disease process. It is because of the patient's body perceptions that he is able to assess the seriousness of the illness or disease. This is a significant variable for the nurse to utilize when intervening to assist the patient and family through a difficult time.

While the patient is accepting the loss, the nurse can have the patient consider meeting someone who has adapted to a similar trauma or illness. The intervention provides the patient with a role model when he goes through the sometimes difficult task of acquiring a new identity (Busch and Gallo 1982).

According to Carlson (1978), personality variables include such things as coping style, motivation, assertiveness, conceptual style, attitudes, and communication style. Any of these characteristics that tend to facilitate the reestablishment of meaningful goals or the development of new methods to achieve goals that have become unachievable because of the loss event are expected to decrease the intensity and duration of grief.

Age is another internal variable. Age is significant because of developmental tasks that occur at a particular stage of life. It is possible that the dominant task of that stage will influence which events are perceived as losses as well as the nature of the brief that follows a major loss event. The more tasks one has managed successfully, the more equipped one is to progress through grief without serious complications (Carlson 1978).

Knowledge is derived from prior experiences. It is uncertain whether prior experiences strengthens one's ability to cope or hampers coping. The kind, severity, and number of loss events that lead to coping are yet to be determined. Nevertheless the interpretation of stimuli from the body is known to be influenced a great deal by past experiences and interactions with others (Carlson 1978).

A person's goals and values can be critical to his perception of a loss. Furthermore they reflect his beliefs about himself. If an individual believes that the environment is a hostile place over which he has little control, he will feel a sense of helplessness. However if the individual views the environment as supportive, he will feel a sense of power or control.

Lastly the nurse knows that certain behavioral responses such as anxiety, depression, anger, avoidance, or denial are normal. The same behaviors become abnormal if the patient remains depressed, anxious, angry, or fails to seek and follow medical advice. Regardless of the specific behavioral response, it begins the moment an individual perceives a change in the body. The patient is the first to realize that a biological change is taking place. For example, the hypertensive patient complains of severe headaches. The cardiac patient compains of tiredness and minor chest pain which is attributed to indigestion. The patient's perception is then confirmed by diagnostic studies, laboratory tests, and finally by a physician's diagnosis.

The nurse attempts to reduce anxiety. As anxiety increases, the perceptual field narrows and only a limited amount of information can be processed. The nurse may facilitate information processing and anxiety reduction by giving instructions rather than requiring decision making at this time. Furthermore the nurse can limit the number of anxiety-provoking factors impinging on the person by monitoring the number of people in his immediate environment, decreasing environmental stimuli, and mobilizing comforting family members around the patient (Carlson 1978).

There are times when the family requests that the patient not be informed of the seriousness of an illness or disease. The patient realizes the illness or disease is serious but wants to protect the family from the pain of potential or eventual death. Therefore, the loss is avoided through jovial behavior. As previously pointed out, the patient wants to maintain a positive self-image. Likewise, the family, thinking it is protecting the patient, avoids discussion of the loss and threat of further loss. Both are aware of the loss, but each avoids open discussion. Each thinks it is protecting the other. The nurse assesses the readiness of each to begin sharing its support with the other. The nurse encourages the patient and the family to openly acknowledge the loss and its implications. Together they can begin resolving it.

Within the resolving phase of an individual's loss, one may manifest behavior previously referred to as anxiety, depression, anger, avoidance, or denial. Such responses are considered coping behaviors. The nurse intervenes to channel the patient's behavior in an adaptive direction by aiding behavior recognition. However, there are times when this becomes a difficult task. With a serious loss leading to eventual death, the nurse assesses that the patient seems to withdraw. The patient pulls away from significant others. The avoidance may be wrongly assessed as self-preoccupation when it is really self-preservation. The patient withdraws internally in an attempt to hold together. This usually occurs as death approaches.

The behavioral response of anger and withdrawal may be seen more frequently with the young adult patient who becomes angry, frustrated, and anxious about a constricted future. The young married patient worries about his family. The patient becomes anxious upon realizing that he can only enjoy the family's existence to a certain point. The aged patient, on the other hand, becomes less anxious and depressed over a loss since there may no longer be family responsibilities. Therefore the concern focuses on self. The nurse remembers that the psychological variable that leads to behavioral changes is a result of the patient's inability to cope with the loss. This is particularly significant for the dying patient.

The nurse assesses the pathological variable in terms of the degree of temporary or permanent loss and the meaning it has for the individual. The nurse realizes that its meaning relates to its attachments to the patient's ego. Other variables are assessed in terms of the patient's behavioral response to the illness. The behavioral response can take many forms such as anxiety, depression, denial, avoidance, and anger. Each behavior becomes a component of the grieving process. Once the nurse assesses internal variables, she then assesses external variables influencing the patient.

External Variables

External variables or influencing factors involve the hospitalization experience or critical care environment, social cultural factors or situation, and available support systems including family, critical care team, and friends.

Hospitalization may be a new experience for the patient. The individual who has maintained total control over his being becomes threatened when faced with forced dependence upon strangers in a sometimes highly technical world. Depending upon the patient's biological problem, the environment is which he is hospitalized can be emotionally threatening. Take the patient who enters the hospital's emergency room complaining of chest pain. Even though the patient realizes that the biological crisis is serious, he rationalizes it as indigestion. The patient soon finds himself hospitalized in a critical care unit. He next relinquishes his body to various pieces of supportive equipment and strangers who poke, probe, and percuss. The patient does not know what to expect nor what is expected of him. The nurse intervenes to create a nonthreatening environment. This goal is accomplished by explaining the various supportive devices as they relate to a particular problem. In this way she helps the patient to know what is expected of him.

Illness or disease as a recurring problem can be even more threatening to the patient. Due to previous experience, the patient has knowledge of the hospital's environment, intrusive diagnostic procedures, and various supportive devices. The patient also has knowledge of his or her own biological frailty. The patient realizes that with each subsequent hospitalization he experiences greater loss. The nurse recognizes that the patient, alone, perceives biological changes which could result in further disability or even death. Depending upon the biological loss, each hospitalization brings the patient closer to the thing feared: death. Since hospitalization is not a new experience, the patient needs less environmental support and more emotional support. Instead of discussing external environmental events, the nurse focuses on the patient's external feelings. The nurse encourages expression of internal feelings and supports the fearful patient.

The second external variable or influencing factor is the patient's social value or situation. Social value is assessed in terms of age, wealth, education, profession, and appearance. Patients with the highest social value seem to receive the greatest degree of attention. A patient with high social status in the community may receive special care in addition to administrative concern. A room is quickly made available. This patient receives diagnostic studies and laboratory tests at the prescribed time and may even receive special privileges given only to high-status people. On the other hand, another patient may lose certain privileges because of a low social status. Regardless of his position in the community, each should receive the same degree of concern and attention. This means that the nurse will assess the patient's social status as it relates the education, occupation, and previous illness experience. These social variables become significant to the nurse as she formulates a teaching plan designed to raise the patient's level of understanding. Furthermore, it enables the nurse to more fully understand the patient's potential for coping with a crisis situation.

The social resources available to a person who has experienced a significant loss are likely to be critical to the nature of the recovery. Following a major loss of a person, body part, or something else, the individual is often stigmatized (Carlson 1978).

Illness or disease resulting in loss has no age boundaries. It affects each individual at some point in life. Regardless of the age involved, the nurse recognizes that for the patient and the family the loss is significant. The various elements of social value, including age, occupation, education, and wealth, all become variables to be utilized by the nurse.

Finally, the support systems available to the patient can assist him through the loss experience. The support systems consist of family, health team, and friends. A patient's family can be a supportive asset throughout the illness or disease process. The patient can draw upon the family's strength. The family, in turn, can help the patient cope with a difficult situation. The nurse realizes that, as Lipowski (1972) points out, "The response of the family and other meaningful people to the patient's illness or disability, to his communications of distress, and to his mobility to perform the usual social roles may spell the difference between optimal recovery or psychological invalidism" (p. 1200). The nurse should also keep in mind that the family itself can become emotionally depleted. Therefore, it becomes important to offer the family as much assistance as is offered the patient. The family needs to be continually appraised of the patient's biological status. If not appropriately apprised, the family develops unrealistic expectations that the patient's loss is not serious but temporary. In the latter instance, the family may request heroic measures even when they will not alter the disease process. The family fails to realize that they are only prolonging the dying rather than the living process.

According to Ransohoff (1978), the management of the family and their response to acute neurosurgical catastrophe, whether iatrogenic or as a result of external forces, requires great sensitivity on the part of the nurse. Furthermore, goals are significant for the critically ill patient. Goal achievement usually requires persons or things external to the patient. The patient needs feedback from both the family and the critical care team. Feedback is needed to develop one's body image, self-concept, and roles. This is particularly important for the trauma or severely burned patient.

When everyone, especially the family, is aware that there is "nothing more to do," the goal of recovery has, in effect, been changed to a goal of comfort. This seems to be the ideal time for ceasing to prolong the dying patient's life. Of course, in critical care the means by which the patient is allowed to die depends on whether life is being prolonged naturally or by equipment. When families request unrealistic heroics, the health team has a tremendous responsibility to aid the family in understanding the hopelessness of the situation. The nurse can convey to the family how the person is progressing. By keeping family or significant others continually informed of the acuteness of the situation, the nurse also psychologically prepares the family for the eventual death of the patient.

It is at this time that the nurse can be an attentive listener to family members. Many times a member of the family will want to share with the nurse memories of their loved one. Allowing the family to discuss pleasant memories and to reminisce will help the family accept termination with the dying patient. This is part of facilitating their awareness of the patient's potential death; it initiates some of the grief work and perhaps makes it easier when the time comes to cease heroic measures.

The family often seeks reassurance that everything that can be done is currently being done for the patient. The nurse can reinforce their feelings that, yes, everything is or has been done. Such feedback assists the family not to request heroics based on their own guilt feelings. Families who react, instead of act, because of feelings of having not done more for a spouse often drain their financial resources. Hospitalization in critical care is expensive enough and the expense of various pieces of equipment used to prolong death can be astronomical. In some instances families may incur tremendous financial burden for having tried to assuage guilt.

The family may put the nurse on the defense by asking if an aged parent is, or will get better. Many times, if it is hard for the nurse to respond honestly, she will resort to trite cliches such as, "You never know about these things," or "Why don't you ask your doctor?" Unfortunately the family rarely sees the physician, because the physician may have given up on the patient, realizing that the prognosis is terminal.

The family may be caught in a double bind of wanting to what is best, but not realizing what is best for the patient. As the family begins to understand that their loved one is being kept alive by equipment, they may ask the staff to stop treatments that result in the useless prolonging of life. When the family or the doctor decides to turn off the pacemaker or respirator, the family can be present either in the waiting room or in the patient's room. If the family is at home when the doctors make their decision to turn off life-prolonging equipment, the family may have guilt feelings about a loved one dying alone, surrounded by unyielding pieces of equipment. It is important for the family and physician to discuss the possibility of terminating life-prolonging equipment before the termination becomes a necessity. In this way guilt feelings are alleviated. More importantly the family needs to be consulted before life-prolonging supportive devices be used. Many times the family knows the patient and what his decision would be if he could participate in his own care.

NURSING EVALUATION

Evaluation of the patient's problem and nursing care is an ongoing process. The nurse assesses regulatory and cognitive behaviors supporting the diagnosis of loss. An evaluation of nursing interventions is designed to determine their effectiveness in lessening the loss or grief experience. The nurse knows that the stress of loss, mourning, or grief will not be immediately eliminated. The feelings will continue after discharge from the unit and hospital.

SUMMARY

There is a need for ministers, physicians, and nurses to discuss the concept of loss and the issue of prolonging versus not prolonging death. As openness toward the once-taboo topic of loss including death increases, nurses, physicians, and ministers may be able to decide under what conditions the termination of life-prolonging techniques and procedures is appropriate for the patient, and they may also feel better about the decisions they have shared in and carried out.

REFERENCES

BECKER, ERNEST, *The Denial of Death.* New York: Macmillan, 1973.

BOWLBY, JOHN, "Processes of Mourning," *International Journal Psychoanalysis,* 42 (1961), 317-340.

BUSCH, KAREN, and BARBARA GALLO, "Emotional Responses to Illness," in *Critical Care Nursing,* ed. Carolyn Hudak, Thelma Lohr, and Barbara Gallo, pp. 17-27. Philadelphia: Lippincott, 1982.

CARLSON, CAROLYN, "Loss," in Chapter 4, *Behavioral Concepts and Nursing Intervention,* ed. Carolyn Carlson and Betty Blackwell, pp. 72-86. Philadelphia: Lippincott, 1978.

CAUTHORNE, CATHERINE, "Coping with Death in Emergency Department," *Journal of Emergency Nursing,* 1 (November-December 1975), 24-26.

DAVIDSON, GLEN, "In Search of Models of Care," *Death Education,* 2 (Spring-Summer 1978), 145-161.

DRACUP, KATHLEEN, and CHRISTINE BREU, "Using Nursing Research Findings to Meet the Needs of Grieving Spouses," *Nursing Research,* 27, no. 4 (July-August 1978), 212-216.

ELMORE, JAMES, "Psychological Reactions to Impending Death," *Hospital Topics,* November 1967, p. 36.

FEIFEL, HERMAN, "Attitudes toward Death in Some Normal and Mentally Ill Populations," in *The Meaning of Death,* pp. 114-130. New York: McGraw-Hill, 1959.

FLETCHER, JOSEPH, "The Patient's Right to Die," *Harpers Magazine,* October 1960, p. 139.

FREIHOFER, PATRICIA, and GERALDENE FELTON, "Nursing Behaviors in Bereavement: An Exploratory Study," *Nursing Research,* 25, no. 5 (September–October 1976), 332-337.

GLASER, BARNEY, and ANSELM STRAUSS, *Awareness of Dying.* Chicago: Aldine, 1965.

HAMILTON, JAMES, "The Significance of Object Loss in Individual Response to Accidental Trauma," *Comprehensive Psychiatry,* 18, no. 2 (1977), 189-199.

JONES, WILLIAM, "Emergency Room Sudden Death: What Can be Done for the Survivors?" *Death Education*, 2 (1978), 231–245.

KÜBLER-ROSS, ELISABETH, *Death: The Final Stage of Growth*. Englewood Cliffs, N.J.: Prentice-Hall, 1975.

LAUBE, JERRI, "Death and Dying Workshop for Nurses: Its Effect on Their Death Anxiety Level," *International Journal Nursing Studies*, 4 (1977), 111–120.

LIPOWSKI, Z. J., "Psychosocial Aspects of Disease," *Annals of Internal Medicine,* 70 (December 1969), 1198–1202.

MAGUINE, DANIEL, *Death By Choice*. New York: Doubleday, 1974.

MARTIN, HARRY, "The Stages of Illness—Psychosocial Approach," *Nursing Outlook*, March 1962, pp. 168–171.

MAYOU, RICHARD, ANN FOSTER, and BARBARA WILLIAMSON, "The Psychological and Social Effects of Myocardial Infarction Wives," *British Medical Journal*, 1 (1978), 699–701.

PINE, VANDERLYN, "A Socio-Historical Portrait of Death Education," *Death Education*, 1 (1977), 57–84.

RANSOHOFF, JOSEPH, "Death, Dying and the Neurosurgical Patient," *The American Association of Neurosurgical Nurses*, 10 (December 1978), 198–201.

REDDING, RALPH, "Doctors, Dyscommunication, and Death," *Death Education*, 3, (1980), 371–385.

ROBERTS, SHARON, "To Die or Not to Die: Plight of the Aged Patient in the Critical Care Unit," in *Psychosocial Nursing Care of the Aged*, ed. Irene Burnside, pp. 221–224. New York: McGraw-Hill, 1980.

SEGAL, RABBI KENNETH, "Moral and Legal Aspects of Respiratory Care," *Respiratory Care*, 24, no. 9 (September 1979), 850–862.

SHERIZEN, SANFORD, and LESTER PAUL, "Dying in a Hospital Intensive Care Unit: The Social Significance for the Family of the Patient," *Omega*, 8, no. 1 (1977), 29–40.

SHNEIDMAN, EDWIN, "The Enemy," *Psychology Today*, August 1970, p. 37.

SHUSTERMAN, LISA ROSEMAN, "Death and Dying: A Critical Review of the Literature," *Nursing Outlook*, 21 (June 1973), 366.

SODERBERG-JOHNSON, SHERRY, "Grief Themes," *Advances in Nursing Science*, 3, (July 1981), 15–26.

SUDNOW, DAVID, *Passing on the Social Organization of Dying*. Englewood, Cliffs, N.J.: Prentice-Hall, 1967.

TORPIE, RICHARD, "The Patient and Prolonged Terminal Malignant Disease: Experience from a Radiation Therapy Center," in *Anticipatory Grief*, ed. B. Schoenberg, et. al., p. 120. New York: Columbia University Press, 1974.

VERWOERDT, ADRIAAN, "Psychological Reactions in Fatal Illness, The Prospects of Impending Death," *Journal of the American Geriatrics Society,* 15 (1967), p. 16.

WEISMAN, AVERY, *On Dying and Denying*. New York: Behavioral Publications, 1972.

19
Pain

BEHAVIORAL OBJECTIVES

1. Define the concept *pain*.
2. Explain the four major theories associated with pain.
3. Describe how the physiological and psychological components of pain apply to the critically ill patient.
4. Identify five regulatory behaviors associated with pain.
5. Identify six cognitive behaviors associated with pain.
6. Design a nursing care plan around the framework of prepain experience, actual pain experience, and postpain experience.

Pain is an individualized experience, yet for all people the experience has two components: the perception of pain and the response to pain. Furthermore pain is a complex, mysterious phenomenon which is neither simple, nor completely understood (McCauley and Polomano 1980; Ellis 1978). Most people have had some experience with pain. Pain knows no gender or cultural boundaries. Pain is expressed in various forms, several of which are not physically or bodily related. It surrounds us as the emotional and cultural entity of poverty, death, war, starvation, disasters, suicides, violence, and illness. Pain then, is a multidimensional concept. Melzack (1973) summarizes some of the current thinking on pain as follows:

> Pain, we now believe, refers to a category of complex experiences, not to a specific sensation that varies only along a single intensity dimension. The word "pain" in

this formulation, is a linguistic label that categorizes an endless variety of qualities. There are the pains of a scalded hand, a stomach ulcer, or sprained ankle; there are headaches and toothaches. Each is characterized by unique qualities. (P. 41)

Bresler (1979) notes that pain is more than a sensation of something. To some extent, it may be a perception, like vision and audition. The way we perceive pain is known to be affected by a myriad of influences—including early learning experiences.

As Melzack (1973) points out, pain has different implications and significance to each individual:

> Pain is a perceptual experience whose quality and intensity are influenced by the unique past history of the individual, by the meaning he gives to the pain-producing situation, and by his "state of mind" at the moment. We believe that all these factors play a role in determining the actual pattern of nerve impulses that ascend from the body to the brain and travel within the brain itself. In this way pain becomes a function of the whole individual, including his present thoughts and fears as well as his hopes for the future. (P. 49)

As an experience, pain incorporates the total individual.

Pain occurs throughout the body, from peripheral receptors to the higher cortex of the brain. The pain experience is composed of sensory, emotional-motivational, cultural, and cognitive factors, which interact on an individual basis, with many degrees of relative importance (Armstrong 1980). The critical care patient who has suffered severe trauma or chronic disability knows the all-encompassing world of pain. Because of its many facets, vast amounts of research have been devoted to the relief of pain. Pain clinics exist which have been established for the sole purpose of directly treating the pain or helping the individual learn to cope with it.

For some individuals experiencing pain, the pain itself becomes a way of existence. The outer world becomes monitored by internal pain experiences. LeShan (1964) describes pain-centered existence as follows:

> Pain permits personal existence to continue with little assistance from our usual orientations, defenses, safeguards, and associations. It attenuates our relationships with the outer world at the same time that it weakens the inner structure. In painless consciousness, we are filled with images, associations, and thoughts. In the loud loneliness of pain, only our existence is real. We float alone in space, conscious only of the suffering. (P. 121)

The individual in pain reaches out to those people in the external world who he feels can help him cope with the pain. He places hope in their ability to lessen fears and anxieties regarding pain. The health team realizes that fear and anxiety increase the individual's pain and that the mere anticipation of pain can magnify it.

Unfortunately, pain is primarily a patient experience rather than a dual experience shared by both the patient and members of the health team. The staff has a tendency to treat an individual's pain rather than assessing the various aspects of pain such as its duration, intensity, location, meaning, and description, as well as the patient's previous experience with pain. These are areas in which the health team must make pertinent assessments.

DEFINITION OF TERMS

Before applying the concept of pain to critical care, it would be beneficial to first define pain and then briefly examine theories related to pain.

Pain

Pain is a difficult concept to define because of its multidimensional aspects. It becomes whatever the individual says it is and what is experienced at the time. The diversity of pain experience makes it almost impossible to obtain a definition which members of the critical care team can apply. According to Kim (1980), pain is defined as an abstract construct which refers to a personal experience of hurt whose quality and intensity are known to be influenced by both psychological and sociocultural variables. Pain is not a single event which can be specified in terms of defined stimulus conditions. Rather, as Melzack (1973) has described it, pain is a complex perceptual experience that has many causes, all of which are equally significant. Wolf (1980) points out that pain is currently viewed as a complex phenomenon composed of sensory dimensions, including time, space, and intensity, and emotional, cognitive, and motivational dimensions.

Pain represents a number of experiences, each of which can be categorized and represented by unique events for each individual. In other words, what is perceived as pain by one individual is not perceived in the same manner by another. Pain, according to Melzack (1973), can then be defined "in terms of a multidimensional space comprising several sensory and affective dimensions. The space comprises those subjective experiences which have both somatosensory and negative-affective components and that elicit behavior aimed at stopping the conditions that produce them" (p. 46). Pain is not purely a stimulus response. Other factors must be taken into consideration. Physical pain involves a noxious stimulus of varying degree in intensity and duration. Psychological pain is more of a perceptual experience. Physical and psychological pain are closely interrelated. As has been noted in the various definitions, pain involves both physical and psychological experiences of the individual. According to Lesle (1972), "It is a psychological experience of events occurring within the patient's body, always unpleasant and associated with the impression of damage to the tissues. This blend of physiological and psychological events has to pass through the patient's powers of expression and speech before being described and made comprehensible to a nurse or doctor" (p. 890).

Finally pain is a protective mechanism that plays an important role in the protection of the individual from harm, in the development of personality, and in the appreciation of reality. The entire pain experience is comprehensive—involving perception, physiology, and emotions. Pain can be separated into the following components: reception, perception, and reactions. Reception includes the reception of the pain stimulus by the pain receptors and the conduction of the pain impulses by the nerves. Perception of pain involves the higher centers of the brain, namely, the thalamus and cerebral cortex. Reaction to pain is physical, emotional, and physiologic in nature (Ellis 1978).

Pain Theories

There are several different theories regarding the evolution of pain. Each attempts to explain pain in terms of its origin and the individual's physiological and/or psychological response. The four major theories are affect theory, specificity theory, pattern theory, and gate-control theory. The first three theories are traditional and fail to provide a comprehensive account of pain phenomena. The gate-control theory attempts to integrate understanding derived from the three traditional theories on the basis of new clinical evidence and assumptions (Kim 1980).

Affect Theory. Affect theory implies that pain has more than only a sensory quality. Instead it also has a negative affective quality. This quality drives an individual into activity. An individual is compelled to do something about a negative situation and will take the most effective course of action to stop the event. Therefore, the behavior is in the realm of motivation. Affect theory then, has to do with emotion and behavior.

Affect theory considers pain to be an emotion rather than a sensation. The theory views pain as an emotional quality that colors all sensory events. It fails to provide a systematic description and explanation of why pain is an emotion, but it suggests a significant yet long-neglected affective dimension of pain (Kim 1980).

Pattern Theory. Pain is considered to result from intense peripheral stimulation that produces a pattern of nerve impulses which are interpreted centrally as pain. Pattern theory proposes the existence of a rapidly conducting fiber system, which inhibits synaptic transmission in a more slowly conducting system that carries the signal for pain. The theory contributes to the understanding of delays, temporal and spatial summation, and many other properties of pathological pain but fails to provide an adequate account of the psychological dimension of pain (Wolf 1980; Kim 1980).

Melzack (1973) describes pattern theory as follows:

> Goldsheider's pattern, or summation, theory proposes that the particular patterns of nerve impulses that evoke pain are produced by the summation of the skin sensory input at the dorsal horn cells. According to this concept, pain results when the total output of the cells exceeds a critical level as a result of either excessive stimulation of receptors that are normally fired by nonnoxious thermal or tactile stimuli, or pathological conditions that enhance the summation of impulses produced by normally nonnoxious stimuli. (P. 140)

Specificity Theory. Specificity theory suggests that specific pain receptors in the skin project impulses via pain fibers and pathways to a pain center in the brain. The theory has contributed to identifying a basic physiological mechanism such as receptors and fibers of the skin sensory system which exhibit a high degree of specialization of function. Furthermore, specificity theory attempts to explain selected surgical procedures aimed at relieving severe, intractable pain. These surgical interventions include cordotomy and bulbar tractotomy as well as ablation of portions of the intralaminar nuclei in the thalamus. The specificity theory fails to provide any explanation of the psychological process of pain perception and response (Wolf 1980; Kim 1980).

Specificity theory indicates that there are special nerve fibers that respond to different stimuli. These stimuli can be pain, temperature changes, touch, or even position changes. Each stimulus is transmitted through different nerve fibers. Take for example an individual who, while running, steps on a nail. The pain in her foot tells her immediately that a problem exists. In this respect, the pain has a specific origin, the foot. The stimulus from the nail travels up nerve fibers in the foot, leg, back, and finally into the head where an alarm system is triggered. The individual feels pain and responds by ceasing further running. The overall result is that the person feels pain and responds to it.

Gate-Control Theory. The last theory is the most recent and possibly the most popular of all theories. In addition, it has the greatest significance to members of the health team. The gate-control theory was proposed by Melzack and Wall. The most significant difference, according to Siegele (1974), between gate-control theory and specificity theory

> . . . is that pain impulses transmitted from nerve receptors through the spinal cord to the brain can be modulated or altered in the spinal cord, brainstem, and cerebral cortex. The potential blocking ability of certain cells along the transmission route can result in little or no pain perception regardless of the intensity of the noxious stimulus. The gate-control theory also helps explain the influence of psychological factors on the pain experience, including perception and interpretation. (P. 499)

Gate-control theory proposes that stimulation in the peripheral area such as the skin evokes nerve impulses that are transmitted to three spinal cord systems. The first involves the densely packed cells called substantia gelatenosa (SG) in the dorsal horn. The SG extends the length of the spinal cord and becomes the site of a transmission-blocking action that closes the gate to entering impulses. There, SG functions as the gate-control system that modulates the flow of nerve impulses. The second spinal cord system involves the dorsal column fibers. The dorsal column fibers activate selective brain processes (central control system) which influence the modulating mechanism of the gate-control system. When the gate opens, sensory input is allowed to reach the transmission cells in the dorsal horn of the spinal cord. Third, there are central transmission cells (T cells) in the dorsal horn. The T cells activate neural mechanisms (action system) which are responsible for response to and perception of pain (Kim 1980).

Gate-control theory explains how the intensity of painful stimuli can be decreased at perceptual levels through a gating effect at the spinal segmental level (Wolf 1980). According to Siegele (1974), "The gate-control theory supports the hypothesis that pain is a complex perceptual experience in which sensory input is altered by a distinctive but interacting neural system before that input evokes pain perception and response" (p. 501).

The gate-control theory consists of three components: gate-control system, central control system, and action system. The gate-control theory proposes that the primary function of the substantia gelatenosa (SG) as a mechanism is to inhibit the flow of nerve impulses. This inhibiting effect of the SG is increased by activity in large fibers (L fibers) and decreased by activity in small fibers (S fibers). The L fibers inhibit the flow of impulses by activitating the inhibitory function of the SG (closing the gate), while S fibers inhibit the inhibitory function of the SG (opening the gate). The activity between these fibers from the peripheral area plus descending influences from the central control system determine the degree to which the gate opens and closes and in turn increases or decreases sensory input to the T cells (Kim 1980; Wolf 1980).

The central control system activates selective brain processes. Two subsystems in the brain are activated: the brainstem reticular formation and the cortex. The reticular formation exerts a powerful inhibitory control over information projected by the gate-control system. It includes somatic, visual, and auditory processes. The cortex, which involves cognitive processes such as past experiences and attention, also has an influence on the gate-control system (Kim 1980).

Lastly, the action system is activated only when the output of the T cells exceeds a certain level. In addition it is controlled by the central system. When the output reaches or exceeds a critical point, the T cells are transmitted to the reticular and cortical projection subsystem. Activation of these subsystems motivate the individual into action toward escape or attack (Wolf 1980; Kim 1980).

In summary, the gate-control theory provides a more comprehensive understanding about the pain mechanism that any traditional pain theories. The theory describes the following (Kim 1980):

1. How a neurophysiological system operates
2. How the input nerve impulses are transmitted and modulated by the spinal gating mechanism
3. How the central control system influences the descending nerve impulse
4. How transmission cells activate the action system

THE CONCEPT OF PAIN
APPLIED TO THE CRITICALLY ILL PATIENT

The critical care patient may or may not be experiencing pain upon entering the hospital. Due to the nature and severity of the illness, pain may become the presenting complaint. Other patients who originally enter the hospital free of pain may at some point in time develop it. For some patients, experiencing acute pain is only a temporary way of life. *Acute pain* refers to discomfort of a relatively short duration. This type of pain usually serves a useful purpose, such as providing information relative to location and type of pathology or injury (Armstrong 1980). The burn, trauma, coronary artery bypass, acute pancreatitis, or myocardial infarction patient may experience episodes of acute pain. Sometimes in critical care settings the relief of pain is not always the primary concern of the nurse. The staff in a critical care unit or emergency room may be more interested in diagnostic and emergency care than the patient's pain. Furthermore, the individual's pain may be a result of actions of the critical care team. Unfortunately, pain becomes a byproduct of various diagnostic studies, intrusive treatments, or surgical procedures. The accompanying pain is not intentional; it is simply a byproduct.

Pain as it applies to the critical care patient will be discussed according to two categories or components, physiological and psychological. Each component will be further categorized into manifestations or behavioral responses and influencing factors.

Physiological Component

The patient's physiological response to pain involves his pain threshold, pain tolerance, and pain reaction. *Pain threshold* refers to the beginning awareness of the presence of pain and is generally the same for most individuals. *Pain tolerance* describes the point at which an individual feels that the pain can no longer be tolerated. The severity and duration of the pain necessary to reach tolerance can vary from patient to patient. A patient's tolerance may be decreased by such variables as anxiety, fatigue, anger, stress, and boredom. *Pain reaction* refers to the psychological, motivational, and cognitive response to pain. This requires that the patient be conscious with involvement of the limbic brain structure and the cerebral cortex (Armstrong 1980).

Melzack (1973) considers two terms to be significant in the attempt to understand the physiology of pain. These terms are *specificity* and *specialization*. *Specificity* implies that a receptor, fiber, or other component of a sensory system subserves only a single specific modality (or quality) of experience. *Specialization*, on the other hand, implies that the components of a sensory system are highly specialized so that particular types and ranges of physical energy evoke characteristic patterns of neural signals, and that these patterns can be modulated by other sensory inputs or by cognitive processes to produce more than one quality of experience or none at all. The entire brain is considered to be the pain center. It seems that the thalamus, hypothalamus, brainstem, reticular formation, limbic system, parietal cortex, and frontal cortex are all involved in pain perception. A stimulus produces neural signals that travel through an active nervous system. In the adult, the neurological system is a combination of past experiences, culture, anticipation, and anxiety. These brain processes play a vital role in the selection, abstraction, and synthesis of data from the overall sensory input.

Pain perceived as overwhelming demands the individual's immediate attention because it disrupts ongoing behavior and thought. Pain serves as a motivating force that drives the person into activity aimed at stopping it. In this respect, pain becomes more than a sensory response and acquires motivational-affective properties. Physiologically there are central cells that monitor the input of stimuli for long periods of time. Intense stimuli can prolong neural activity which persists long after stimulation ceases. This process plays an important role in the pain process. Physiological or bodily pain is a signal to the individual of physical harm. It tells the individual that a breach in his or her protective barrier has taken place. Pain serves a purpose as a protective mechanism. The individual experiences pain whenever any tissue is being damaged and it causes the person, by reflex, to remove himself or herself from the pain stimuli.

Guyton (1981) gives the example of sitting for a long time on the ischia which can cause tissue destruction because of lack of blood flow to the skin where the skin is compressed by the body's weight. When the skin becomes painful as a result of the ischemia, the person shifts the weight unconsciously. The critically ill patient, due to paralysis, severe injury, or supportive devices, may be immobilized and unable to change position. Likewise the aged CVA or comatose patient is unable to independently change position. Each patient, particularly one who is paralyzed or comatose, depends upon the nurse to provide a protective environment in which the protective barrier—the skin—is maintained by turning. Patients who have lost their sense of pain due to spinal cord injury become a unique problem for nurses. Their inability to feel the pain due to ischemia and to respond by moving leads to ulceration at the area of the pressure.

Guyton (1981) has proposed a threefold classification of pain based on whether it is perceived as pricking, burning, or aching. A description of each is important for the nurse who attempts to assess the type of pain a patient is experiencing. A *pricking pain* is felt when a needle is stuck into the skin or when the skin is cut. It is also felt when a widespread area of the skin is strongly irritated. *Burning pain* is the type of pain felt when the skin is burned and can be the most severe in terms of suffering. *Aching pain* is not usually felt in the surface of the body. Instead it is a deep pain with varying degrees of intensity.

Physiologically, pain can originate from a noxious stimulus within the patient's body. Tissue damage can cause pain. Guyton (1981) has divided the origin of tissue damage resulting in pain into two further categories. First, he feels that bradykinin and histamine function to stimulate pain endings, thus contributing to pain experience. The exact mechanism is not known; however, it is believed that bradykinin may be the principle substance that stimulates pain endings. Cell damage releases proteolytic enzymes that almost immediately split bradykinin and other similar substances from the globulins in the interstitial fluid. In addition, damaged cells also release histamine in lesser amounts. Like bradykinin, it can also elicit a pain response.

The second origin of physiological pain involves tissue ischemia and muscle spasm. When blood flow to the tissue ceases, the tissue itself becomes painful. The greater the rate of metabolism of the tissue involved (such as the arm), the more rapidly will pain appear. The cause of pain in ischemia is not completely understood. It is believed that pain might be due to accumulation of lactic acid in the tissues. Lactic acid forms as a consequence of the anaerobic metabolism (metabolism without oxygen) that occurs during ischemia. Muscle spasm is also a cause of pain. The contracting muscle compresses intramuscular blood vessels and either reduces or cuts off blood flow. Next, muscle contraction increases the rate of metabolism of the muscle. Consequently, muscle spasm causes a degree of muscle ischemia which results in ischemic pain.

There are many stimuli to an individual's body that pose threats to its tissue integrity. These stimuli are called *noxious stimuli.* They can originate externally or internally to the body. External stimuli may take the form of a blow from a blunt object, cut, or prick. Internal noxious stimuli arise from within the body itself. They may result from tissue ischemia caused by a myocardial infarction; inflammation from abscess in a finger or deep within the pleural or visceral cavity; or from muscle spasms such as cramp or renal colic. Of significance to the nurse working with hospitalized patients is visceral pain from various organs. The viscera have sensory receptors for no other modalities of sensation besides pain. The specific areas of significance to nurses are cardiac, esophageal, gastric, biliary, pancreatic, renal, and uterine pain. The patient in describing and locating a pain may think the pain is epigastric when it is really cardiac in origin. An understanding of the various visceral pains helps the critical care nurse to locate the pain more accurately.

Besides having knowledge of the physiological origin of pain, the nurse must also recognize factors or variables that influence a patient's pain response or experience. McCaffery (1972) has identified physiological and physical factors influencing the individual pain experience. These include the following variables or influencing factors: the neurophysiological processes underlying the sensation of pain; duration and intensity of pain; alterations in the level of consciousness; cutaneous versus visceral sites of pain; environmental conditions; sensory restriction; and physical strain and fatigue. Neurophysiological processes underlying pain and visceral sites of pain have already been discussed.

The duration and intensity of pain work together and have a direct effect upon the patient. Intense pain can lead to activation of the sympathetic nervous system. If the pain continues, adaptation followed by stress reactions can occur. Furthermore, pain of long duration can establish pain memories in the nervous system which contribute to the persistence of pain after the noxious stimuli are removed. The patient may view encounters with pain of any intensity as an isolated event. After the painful experience of diagnostic testing or intrusive procedures is completed, the pain receives little attention. Instead the individual transfers the focus of attention toward something else. On the other hand, the patient in critical care with chronic pain experiences more diffuse pain. Chronic pain is not localized to one area of the body. Arthritic pain, for example, consumes the entire body. The individual focuses his attention on the pain to the exclusions of everything else. The pain becomes all-consuming to the point of physical and emotional exhaustion. Consequently, the patient's body movements and verbal communications decrease in intensity and frequency. He begins to ask why the pain occurred to him and what its effect upon his future will be.

The patient's level of consciousness can influence reactions to pain. Level of consciousness can be altered to the point where the patient is insensitive to pain. Factors contributing to reduced sensitivity are head injury; infections of the central nervous system such as meningitis or encephalitis; sedation; narcotics; and conditions that reduce oxygenation of the brain. The patient who is unconscious obviously will not respond to painful stimuli. Response to pain may be a significant diagnostic test for the neurological patient. The nurse may assess a patient's decreasing level of consciousness by his growing inability to respond to pain. Patients unable to verbalize pain may be analogous to those who overreact to pain.

The patient's immediate environment can be an influencing factor. The nurse can be aware of temperature changes in the patient's hospital environment. The critical care patient with musculoskeletal problems, such as arthritis, experience pain in a cold environment. The cold leads to muscle tension followed by pain. Similarly, patients with arteriosclerosis or peripheral vascular insufficiency may not tolerate a cool environment. The nurse may need to place a small heater by the patient's bed or place additional blankets on the bed. Lights may be a painful environmental stimulus to the patient with glaucoma or cataracts. Therefore, the nurse needs to darken the patient's environment by dimming the lights and closing the blinds. Excessive noise might be a source of pain for those individuals accustomed to silence.

Sensory restriction occurs in an environment in which the stimulus is not adequate to maintain an optimal level of cortical arousal in the patient. The stimuli may be of insufficient amount, pattern, or variation, causing the hospitalized patient to experience sensory deprivation and perceptual monotony. To counteract a situation of sensory restriction, the centrally regulated threshold for sensation is lowered. Thus, the amount of sensory input required to achieve optimal cortical arousal is reduced. As a result, the individual may be more sensitive to pain and other stimuli than usual. Nurses frequently see sensory deprivation in adult patients with bilateral eye patches or casts on various parts of their body. Perceptual deprivation is a common problem in critical care units in which the patient's environment is filled with various machines and supportive devices, each making its own unique hum, buzz, or beep. The monotonous environment is one without variation. This may be a nursing care problem for patients on bedrest; in casts; with burns over their face, hands, and chest; or in complete isolation, involving all the senses.

Lastly, prolonged fatigue and sleep deprivation are variables that alter the patient's response or sensitivity to pain. Hospitalized patients confronted with sleep deprivation are usually those in critical care units. Here the environment is noisy and patients are frequently awakened for various treatments or procedures. Fatigue has a tendency to slow down transmission of nerve impulses. The individual's reaction time is reduced and there is difficulty maintaining a normal train of thought. The fatigued patient has little energy remaining to cope with pain. Normal coping mechanisms of distraction or varying the stimuli are diminished.

In dealing with physiological pain, the nurse can have knowledge of the pain's physiological origin, purpose, and type; assess physiological manifestations of pain; and, finally, assess those variables or influencing factors that contribute to the physiological component of pain.

Psychological Component

Pain is an emotional, cognitive, and motivational experience. As an emotional experience, it is usually accompanied by anxiety, anger, resentment, depression, and other types of emotional feelings. The cognitive aspect of pain involves the communication of messages indicating that something is wrong. Until this message is recognized and heeded, the pain experience may continue unabated. As a motivator, pain moves one to take action that will reduce or prevent further damage (Bresler 1979).

Armstrong (1980) notes that pain perception refers to the physical sensation of pain and is sometimes referred to as the sensory discriminative component. This component involves sensory nerve pathways to the thalamus and does not require conscious awareness on the part of the affected individual. Therefore the psychological component of pain involves two types of perceptions. The first is perception of past experiences, such as early encounters with pain and the role significant others played in its alleviation. The second is perception of pain as a threat to the individual's physical or emotional integrity. In other words, the latter threat involves loss in varying degrees. Each individual varies in his perception of pain. As Melzack (1973) points out, the variation in perception may be due to a difference in pain threshold:

> That is, people are assumed to be physiologically different from one another so that one person may have a low threshold (and feel pain after slight injury), while another has a higher threshold (and feels pain only after intense injury). There is

now evidence that all people, regardless of cultural background, have a uniform sensation threshold—that is, the lowest stimulus value at which sensation is first reported. (P. 24)

Even though each individual has a low stimulus threshold at which he or she experiences pain, the perception of pain is nevertheless influenced by other factors.

A patient's current perception of pain takes into account early childhood experiences which were greatly influenced by his patients' perceptions and attitudes toward pain. Parents may have made an unrealistic fuss over a simple cut or bruise, or, on the other hand, may have demonstrated little sympathy toward a more serious injury. Therefore, earlier experiences with pain shape adulthood attitudes regarding it.

The second perception of pain involves a perceived threat. The threat may be a diffuse or specific feeling. The individual experiencing mental or nonbodily pain is aware of an uncomfortable feeling which he is unable to localize to any one part of his body. Mental pain causes the individual to realize that his psychological protective barrier has been broken. In this respect, the individual feels a loss or injury to his emotional wholeness. Psychological pain that is diffuse involves emotions such as grief, mourning, fear, anxiety, guilt, or painful ideas. These emotions are not confined to any one part of the body or particular experience. Consequently, this type of pain knows no boundary. The nurse can help a patient localize diffuse emotions by helping to identify those events that occurred prior to the anxiety or guilt state. When she does this, the nurse focuses the patient's emotions. Once he knows what contributed to the psychological pain, the patient can anticipate and cope with it.

The specific threat that is perceived may involve loss of all or part of a function. The myocardial infarction patient perceives the threat of pain involving loss of myocardial function and potential loss of life. The fear of pain focuses specifically on the heart whose function has been temporarily or permanently altered. Likewise, the renal patient perceives a threat of loss of independence and financial security. This is especially true if he must be totally dependent upon hemodialysis. The patient may suffer the pain of role changes which threaten his sense of personal integrity and self-esteem. Some patients, for their own reasons, may deny the existence of pain. Other patients may complain of severe pain, yet refuse therapy designed to alleviate the pain. These latter patients may feel the threat of pain due to curative procedures or treatments to be greater than the illness or injury itself.

A stimulus may be painful in one situation and not in another. The more anxious the patient, the less his ability to cope with pain or the threat of pain. In other words, the patient's stimulus threshold to pain is reduced. At another time, the same individual may not react to the same painful stimuli. Therefore, the nurse must be sensitive to those environmental factors which serve to lessen the patient's pain threshold. The patient's anxiety and fear regarding an illness and placement within a strange highly technical environment are examples of stimuli that reduce his pain threshold. Anxiety and fear are psychological variables that contribute to a high degree of variation between stimuli and its perception.

The psychological component of pain consists of past experiences and threats, diffuse or specific, to the individual. The patient's pain experience is a result of earlier encounters with pain. The adult patient is more cognizant of threats involving pain than are children. Each individual, regardless of his problem, is capable of manifesting pain on either a nonverbal or verbal communication level.

Besides obtaining a knowledge base regarding psychological pain, the nurse also assesses influencing factors. McCaffery (1973) believes that the factors influencing a patient's psychological response to pain include the degree of powerlessness experienced by the patient, the presence and attitudes of other people, the amount of information given the patient, the degree of threat the pain imposes on the life situation, personal and past experiences with pain, cognitive level, and the extent to which the patient has used pain for secondary gains. The last three variables are most important. Each patient is a product of past experiences, including those of childhood. Individuals unable to cope with emotional pain on a verbal basis may internalize conflicts, thus causing physical pain associated with gastritis, ulcerative colitis, or peptic ulcer. The nurse, through discussion with the patient and his family, assesses the significance of past pain experience as a variable in the patient's current pain experience. If the patient has been previously hospitalized, the nurse must assess whether or not it was a traumatic experience associated with intrusive procedures, complications, or threat of death.

The critically ill patient's cognitive ability is his understanding of the pain experience or events surrounding it. Of course, understanding is dependent upon knowledge input. The patient with indigestion who simultaneously experiences chest pain may think he is having a coronary, not realizing that the pain is not cardiac in origin but referred from the epigastric region. Furthermore, knowledge input gives the patient a sense of power. The patient understands what is happening internally to the biological systems and relates it to the various diagnostic procedures or supportive devices surrounding the bed. One patient may require a simple explanation of events whereas another might require more lengthy explanations. These factors are assessed by the nurse.

The last variable to be discussed briefly involves the extent to which pain provides secondary gains. Pain may become a way of gaining attention and/or recognition. The individual confronted with feelings of loneliness may temporarily have them alleviated during a pain experience. People in the immediate environment respond to the pain state and their response lessens the loneliness. Other individuals feel they can control people through their expression of pain. Whatever their reason, pain becomes a defense mechanism. As with all defense mechanisms, the nurse must assess its significance to the patient. Also, the nurse must assess the degree to which the patient depends upon pain for attention, when he seems to experience pain, and what effectively alleviates the pain. It is possible that visits from family members or staff members may reduce a patient's complaint of pain. If attention and freedom from loneliness is what the patient really desires, then the presence of significant others may alleviate the need to gain attention through pain.

NURSING ASSESSMENT OF PAIN

The nurse assesses pain through the patient's behavioral response. The responses can be categorized into regulatory behaviors and cognitive behaviors. The critical care nurse assesses patient behaviors in an attempt to predict pain. Predicting pain reaction is valuable in helping the nurse to understand the patient in relation to his pain behavior, and to assisting implementing interventions that are congruent with his cultural, socialized behaviors and previous experiences with pain (Ellis 1978).

Regulatory Behaviors

The regulator system involves inputs, processes, effectors, and feedback loops. It involves stimuli from the external environment and from changes in the internal state of dynamic equilibrium. The regulatory behaviors are physiological responses.

Physiological manifestations of pain involve assessment of visceral pain and the overall signs and symptoms of pain. As mentioned earlier visceral pain is the most difficult pain to assess. Physiological manifestation of pain in terms of signs and symptoms takes into account intensity, duration, and meaning of the pain experience.

Pain that is of low to moderate intensity and of superficial origin yields signs and symptoms that are of sympathetic origin. Pain that is very intense and of deep somatic or visceral origin yields its own regulatory behaviors. Depending on the type of pain, the following behaviors may be observed (Ellis 1978):

Regulatory Behaviors Related to Specific Types of Pain	
Low or Moderate Pain	Intense Somatic or Visceral Pain
Pallor	Pallor
Decreased blood pressure	Decreased blood pressure
Dilated pupils	Decreased heart rate
Skeletal muscular tension	Nausea and vomiting
Increased respiratory rate	Weakness and fainting
Increased heart rate	Possible loss of consciousness

There are also other regulatory behaviors which are·manifestations of pain (Ellis 1978):

Other Regulatory Behaviors
Posturing to minimize pain
Moaning or making other audible sounds
Blinking rapidly
Crying
Lying quiet and withdrawn
Grimacing and clinching teeth
Twitching of facial muscles
Diaphoresis

For the patient entering coronary care, cardiac pain originates from ischemia secondary to coronary ischemia. In assessing the pain's location, the nurse observes its origin in the base of the neck, over the shoulders, over the pectoral muscles, and down the arms. Furthermore, the nurse observes that the patient's pain is more frequently noted on the left side than the right. This occurs because the left side of the heart is more frequently involved in coronary disease. Guyton (1981) points out that when coronary ischemia is severe, such as after a coronary thrombosis, intense cardiac pain sometimes occurs directly underneath the sternum simultaneously with pain referred to other areas. It should be noted that skeletal nerve endings passing from the heart through the pericardial reflection around the great vessels conduct this direct pain. In addition, the nurse may assess other pain symptoms associated with coronary thrombosis. The cardiac patient complains of tightness in the chest. The exact mechanism behind the manifestations is unknown. However, it is believed that a reflex spasm of blood vessels, bronchioles, or muscles in the chest contribute to the pain. This may explain related symptoms of the cardiac patient such as shortness of breath and diaphoresis.

Esophageal and gastric pain can be easily confused with cardiac pain. Esophageal pain is usually referred to the pharynx, lower neck, or arms, or to midline chest regions beginning at the upper portion of the sternum and ending at the lower level of the heart. The nurse must realize that irritation of the gastric end of the esophagus may cause pain directly over the heart. The patient may believe this pain is cardiac in origin while in reality the pain is caused by spasm of the cardia. The cardia is the area where the esophagus empties into the stomach. Gastric pain, on the other hand, originates in the fundus of the stomach and is caused by gastritis. The patient complains of pain in the anterior surface of the chest or upper abdomen from below the heart to the xyphoid process. Patients describe the pain as a burning sensation. The health team who suspects peptic ulcer will assess the patient's pain to be located on either side of the pylorus in the stomach or in the duodemum. As with gastric pain, the patient complains of intense burning. The significant difference between gastric and ulcer pain lies in accurate assessment of the pain's location.

Acute to chronic pancreatitis causes pain in areas both anterior and posterior to the pancreas. The pain may be due to lesions in which pancreatic enzymes eat away the pancreas and surrounding structures. The nurse can recognize that the pancreas is located beneath the parietal peritoneum and that it receives many sensory fibers from the posterior abdominal wall. Such pain is localized behind the pancreas in the back and is described by the patient as a burning sensation. A skilled nurse is able to assist the patient in accurately locating a pain and assessing its significance.

The last visceral pain of clinical significance to the nurse consists of renal pain. Renal pain is better localized than those pains already discussed. Guyton (1981) points out that the kidney, kidney pelvis, and ureters are all retroperitineal structures and receive most of their pain fibers directly from the skeletal nerves. The patient usually experiences pain directly behind the ailing structure. Occasionally pain is referred via visceral afferent to the anterior abdominal wall below the umbilicus. Pain from the patient's bladder is localized directly over the bladder. Such localization helps the nurse in assessing bladder pain due to distention or cramp.

The critical care nurse needs to know how manifestations of pain are related to physiological origin in order to assess its location and true meaning. The nurse who does not have knowledge of the various visceral pains is unable to accurately assess the significance of a patient's pain. Furthermore, the nurse must be able to assess signs and symptoms of pain.

The nurse assesses various physiological parameters. The nature of physiological responses seems to be dependent upon two factors: the duration of pain experience and the degree of anxiety occurring with it. The regulatory behaviors are the result of increased sympathoadrenal activity. Each sign or symptom has clinical significance. For example, the patient in hypertensive crisis should not experience pain for a prolonged period since it could increase an already elevated blood pressure. Likewise, the patient in coronary care with supraventricular tachycardia does not need to have his pulse rate increased further. The list of examples could continue.

Physiological parameters may be the only means of assessing physiological pain in the patient who is unable to verbalize pain because of limited cognitive ability, comatose state, or speech impairment. The patient, regardless of age, may adapt to physiological pain. Adaptation takes place when the stimulus for activation is repeated frequently or over a long period of time. The adaptive response are compensatory, resulting from prolonged sympathetic responses. It is interesting to note that adaptation is the result of a decrease in sympathetic response. It can be assessed by only a slight increase in the pulse rate and blood pressure.

Cognitive Behaviors

The cognator system involves inputs from internal and external stimuli which include psychological and social factors. The specific aspects of the cognator mechanism consist of perceptual/information processing, learning, judgment, and emotion. The cognitive behaviors are psychological responses.

Factors influencing pain reaction include fear and anxiety, both of which tend to increase the subjective pain experience. Usually some degree of fear and/or anxiety accompanies pain. However, a high level of these feelings may cause the patient to perceive a greater sensation of pain which may lead to an intensifying of his usual behavioral response (Ellis 1978).

Patients experiencing pain exhibit varying cognitive behaviors due to the complexity of the pain phenomena. The following cognitive behaviors are associated with pain:

Cognitive Behaviors
Excitement
Irritability
Withdrawal
Hostility
Depression
Rigidity
Unusual posture
Knees drawn up to abdomen
Rubbing
Restlessness

The critically ill patient's cognitive behaviors can be categorized as nonverbal or verbal manifestations of pain.

Nonverbal response to pain is manifested as vocalization, facial expression, and body movements. The nonverbal clues are particularly significant for the patient who is unable to verbalize pain. Neurologically impaired, comatose, facial trauma, burned, and tracheal patients are unable to express themselves verbally. Likewise aphasia may limit the ability to accurately communicate pain. With other patients, a nonverbal response helps the nurse assess the validity of a patient's verbal denial of pain. Verbally the patient denies pain, while nonverbally giving clues indicating pain. Assessing nonverbal manifestations of pain can be a difficult task for the nurse, especially if she relies only on the patient's verbal denial or admission of pain.

Vocalization can be a nonverbal manifestation of pain. Vocalization consists of emitted sounds other than language and cannot be comprehended as verbal symbols. The critically ill patient vocalizes pain through screaming, groaning, grunting, or gasping. The patient who experiences a myocardial infarction or pulmonary embolism may vocalize pain before verbalizing its occurrence, location, duration, and intensity. These patients may make a sudden sharp gasp or groan. Other nonverbal responses follow shortly thereafter. The patient who experiences a painful intrusive procedure usually vocalizes a small scream or grunting noise. This vocalization occurs at the onset of the procedure (such as venipuncture or intravenous therapy) and then diminishes after the initial prick of the skin.

Like vocalization, facial expressions can provide significant nonverbal clues that the patient is in pain. Patients vary in their facial expressions. For example, a patient may have a very sober expression with opened eyes and no facial grimaces. Other facial expressions consist of clenched teeth, tightly shut lips and eyes, wrinkled forehead, or biting of the lower lip. Needless to say, the nurse may see many other facial contortions. If facial expressions are assessed as indicating pain, the nurse must validate whether or not the patient is really experiencing pain. Next, the nurse assesses those factors that contribute to the pain experience, with the aim of alleviating them. One patient may wrinkle the forehead in anticipation of a painful experience while others use facial expressions throughout the entire pain experience.

There are patients who use neither vocalizations or facial expressions to communicate their pain. Instead they communicate their pain with body movements. We have all witnessed the self-imposed immobility of postoperative surgical patients. They immobilize the part of their body altered through surgery. For example, the patient who experiences abdominal aneurysm may be observed holding the abdomen while gently trying to change position. Another individual with the same type of surgery may resist any type of movement in anticipation of pain. The patient with an injured arm or leg may request that the nurse immobilize that part of the body until he turns. The above patients immobilize primarily the surgical site or injured part. On the other hand, the patient who has sustained trauma or injuries may immobilize the entire body. Regardless of the reason, each individual is in essence using splinting as a means of protection against the threat of pain.

Besides immobility, the nurse may assess other body movements indicating pain. A patient in pain can be observed to have inappropriate or inaccurate body movements. The patient seems to thrash around the bed in a restless manner or frequently moves the legs or arms around in bed while tossing and turning. The patient is attempting to find relief from pain. It may take an observant nurse to assess what the patient's behavior signifies. Rather than scolding the patient for tearing apart the bed, pulling the tubes and wires, or sitting on the edge of the bed without assistance, the nurse verbally identifies such behaviors as nonverbal expressions of pain. The patient may then feel free to verbalize about the pain's location, duration, and intensity. Psychologically the patient feels relief in knowing that the health team is aware of the pain he has attempted to endure alone.

Other body movements include rubbing the affected body part. The nurse frequently sees an arthritic patient rubbing the tender joint prior to ambulation or while quietly sitting in the room. The patient with peripheral vascular insufficiency may rub his legs in an attempt to facilitate circulation and soothe pain. Even the cardiac patient may be observed rubbing his chest during or in anticipation of angina. Psychologically a rubbing body movement seems to soothe the affected site and possibly close the gate to pain.

The second major category of psychological manifestations consists of the patient's verbal response to pain. Verbalization involves certain cognitive abilities such as how the patient thinks and the manner in which thoughts are organized. The individual possesses the ability to communicate through language. There are times when the patient's cognitive ability is altered. The cognitive ability may be altered by drugs, brain damage, verbal ischemia, or hypoxia. Therefore the nurse must take into consideration a patient's physical problem and cognitive reliability when assessing pain.

Assessment of pain through verbalization involves both the nurse and patient. The nurse observes existence of pain, tolerance of pain, and factors affecting the pain. The patient, on the other hand, verbalizes location, quality, duration, intensity, rhythmicity, and meaning of the pain. The patient with reliable cognitive abilities locates a pain according to the body part involved and depth of involvement. Duration refers to the length of time spent in pain; intensity, to the perceived strength of the pain. One patient may experience pain of long duration and low intensity. Another patient experiences the same pain; however, his reduced tolerance makes the experience seem to be of greater intensity. Rhythmicity or patterning of pain is particularly significant to the obstetrical patient who may be at risk. Her verbalization of intensity and rhythmicity help the nurse time her contractions.

NURSING DIAGNOSIS OF PAIN

The nursing diagnosis of pain is dependent on the assessment of the type of injury, illness, or disease process. Regulatory and cognitive behaviors coupled with stressors causing the problem help the critical care nurse make the diagnosis. Stressors causing pain can be categorized as internal or external. Internal stressors consist of anxiety; fear; age; illness, disease, or injury; and medical or chemical alterations. External stressors can be attributed to the environmental noises associated with critical care, supportive devices, invasive procedures, and treatment modalities.

NURSING INTERVENTIONS TO RELIEVE PAIN

Pain is not only a sensory reaction to a stimulus. It is also a sensory discriminative experience affected by cognitive activities like anxiety, past experiences, and attention span (Locsin 1981).

The critical care team's goal is relief of pain. Total relief may not be possible for all patients. Nevertheless the nurse attempts to lessen the patient's pain as much as possible. This goal is accomplished by interventions in three categories, referred to by McCaffery (1973) as anticipation, presence, and aftermath of pain. For the purposes of discussion, these categories are labeled here as follows: prepain experience, actual pain experience, and postpain experience.

Prepain Experience

Whether or not the patient has previously experienced pain, the number of times he has had pain, and the associated circumstances will determine whether or not he is conditioned to expect pain, feel a pain sensation, and/or endure pain (Ellis 1978).

If the nurse has knowledge that a particular diagnostic study, surgical procedure, or other intrusive treatment will cause pain, she must prepare the patient for the pain experience. Part of preparation consists of assessing the absence or presence of anxiety. Because patients vary in their manifestation of anxiety, behaviors directly related to anxiety may be difficult to assess. The nurse can assume that the patient who faces diagnostic studies that might reveal a terminal illness, intrusive treatments involving needles, or a surgical procedure will experience a degree of anxiety. Studies show that a degree of anxiety is necessary to get the patient through a traumatic experience. McCaffery (1972) relates this principle directly to pain: "During the anticipation of pain, pain relief is enhanced if the patient experiences a moderate amount of anxiety and this anxiety is channeled into methods of coping with pain. When a pain sensation is felt, the reduction of anxiety associated with pain tends to decrease the perceived intensity of the sensation and/or increase the tolerance for pain" (p. 82). The nurse must assess whether or not the patient's anxiety state is related to prepain or postpain experience. The patient may be anxious regarding the outcome of the pain experience. The outcome may validate fears and fantasies. Therefore, the nurse intervenes by identifying the focus of the anxiety.

Another aspect of preparation in prepain experience includes providing the patient with information about what to expect. If pain will be a part of an experience, the patient must be told. The patient needs to know the intensity and duration of pain. In this respect, the patient knows what to expect and can even assist during the experience. It also gives the patient an opportunity to share with the nurse previous pain experience involving the same procedure. For example, a patient during a previous admission had a lumbar puncture. Due to arthritic changes in the spinal cord, multiple needle insertions were necessary before the procedure was successfully completed. For the patient, the experience was traumatic in that he sustained intense pain of long duration. The trauma was not anticipated by the health team or patient. With the current lumbar puncture, pain and difficulty are again anticipated. The patient may react with greater anxiety because of the previous experience. However, the health team's awareness of arthritic changes can lead to more precise insertion of the needle.

In a study by Voshall (1980), it was found that preoperative teaching about the type of postoperative pain that may be expected and the cause/control of pain will decrease the amount of pain and distress perceived by the patient. The findings indicated that postoperative patients who received information about postoperative pain ranked their sensation of pain lower, ranked their distress level lower, and received fewer analgesics than post-operative patients who did receive information about postoperative pain.

When the critically ill patient's reaction to pain appears inappropriate, it is important to examine the meaning the pain has for him. Memories of past pain experiences may be relevant. If an aspect of the present pain reminds him of a past experience, the memory will influence his total reaction to the current pain, decreasing or enhancing it (Armstrong 1980).

The nurse also plays a significant role in setting the stage for pain reduction. Prior to the pain experience, the nurse might decide to restrain the patient with hand restraints, posey belt, or another nurse. Such intervention only reinforces the expectation that the experience will be painful and causes the patient to interpret the procedure as punishment. If possible, restraining, as an alternative intervention, can be of low priority, reserved for the patient with an altered cognitive ability who must be restrained for his own protection.

Actual Pain Experience

During the actual pain experience, the nurse intervenes to facilitate meaningful sensory stimulation and reduce noxious stimulation. Meaningful sensory stimulation includes various methods of distraction. Distraction decreases intensity of pain and hopefully increases the patient's tolerance to it. Distraction can be accomplished through physical activity, or through auto-stimulation such as singing and visualization.

When possible, physical activity can be used as a distraction technique. Pain has a tendency to immobilize the patient, regardless of his physical problem. A patient with epigastric pain seems to find relief when ambulating. Patients on complete bedrest can still utilize physical activity as a means of distraction. For example, a patient with peripheral vascular insufficiency finds relief when exercising his legs in bed.

Another form of physical activity applies the principle involved in gate-control theory. The patient and/or nurse uses touch. Touch involves stroking, rubbing, or massaging. The nurse, while sitting at the patient's bedside can soothe an affected arm or leg by gently stroking it. Of course the nurse has assessed the origin of the patient's pain in order to further assess the appropriateness of the intervention. Rubbing an extremity with a thrombophlebitis would not be appropriate. Frequently stroking the forehead of an anxious patient in pain seems to lessen the pain by increasing the patient's tolerance. A backrub also has a soothing effect upon the patient and can be a meaningful form of sensory input. It also gives the patient and nurse an opportunity to get to know one another. Furthermore, the patient can be taught to rub the affected body part at the onset of pain. This becomes a type of autostimulation.

Autostimulation can involve such things as singing, listening to music if unable to sing, or visualization. The patient may feel embarrassed by singing alone; therefore, nurses can sing along. If the patient enjoys music, a tape recorder or radio can be available for autostimulation.

Verbalization, as a form of autostimulation, is possible through a variety of ways, such as reading stories or watching television or movies. For a short period of time the patient may be distracted from his pain. Patients may enjoy having their nurse read to them. Again, it provides a close interactional time in which the patient has the nurse's undivided attention. Such intervention may be most beneficial to the patient with facial burns or multiple fractures which necessitate total immobilization.

Television becomes a means of escape for all patients regardless of their physical problem. Television can be a companion to those who otherwise have limited autostimulation abilities. For example, the tracheostomy patient is unable to hum, sing, or talk. If he is hospitalized in respiratory care, the nurse may be unable to spend time reading to this patient. Therefore distraction becomes possible through television. Naturally, the appropriateness of its use must be assessed for each individual patient. Movies are often shown in chronic care facilities where patients are hospitalized for a long time. However, it is possible to show movies for patients in hemodialysis or respiratory critical care who need temporary distraction from pain.

The nurse helps to reduce pain by decreasing the amount of meaningless input. Meaningless sensory input can unintentionally occur from members of the health team. Therefore the nurse intervenes to control and/or eliminate unnecessary noise in the patient's environment. The nurse must carry out certain procedures that are necessary but painful. The nurse contributes to the patient's already existing painful state. The nurse can attempt to intervene in the least offensive manner possible.

The nurse, while intervening in the patient's actual pain experience, attempts to distract through another dimension. This dimension involves the use of waking-imagined analgesia (WIA) as a type of distraction. With this technique, according to Siegele (1974), "The person is taught to influence pain perception by imagining a pleasant situation involving the painful part and trying to recapture and relive the pleasurable sensation whenever he has pain" (p. 502). Unlike distraction, in which the patient uses objects or events in the immediate environment to lessen pain, WIA involves a pleasant experience. The patient is requested to recall the memory of a previous pleasant event like sailing into a beautiful sunset or a scenic vacation. If unable to recall a pleasant event, the patient can create one by using his imagination. Psychologically, the patient separates himself from the mind and body, utilizing all senses to recreate all the original sensations associated with the event while simultaneously experiencing a painful situation. WIA involves a degree of concentration and imagination. For the patient who has never used WIA, the nurse must intervene to stimulate the memory of previous pleasant sensations. The nurse helps the patient recall meaningful events in a general fashion. Depending upon the intensity and duration of the pain, the nurse helps the patient expand the memory from general to more specific. In other words if the actual pain experience will be prolonged, the patient can have sufficient pleasant details to mentally sustain him throughout the pain state.

The second major way in which the nurse intervenes during actual pain experience is to decrease noxious stimulation. Noxious stimulation is a result of internal physiological changes and external environmental conditions. Naturally, it is impossible to alleviate all pain resulting from both internal and external noxious stimulation. The nurse intervenes to make the patient as comfortable as possible. Those noxious stimuli resulting from internal physiological changes may be difficult to alter or reduce.

One source of noxious stimuli creating internal physiological change is surgical invasion. Surgical invasion results in trauma to tissues which is expressed by a physical sensation of pain. The response to pain includes the physiological, behavioral, and affective reactions to the stimuli. The quality, quantity, and duration of pain are related to the type of surgical procedure and techniques (McCauley and Polomano 1980). In order to fully appreciate the postoperative pain experienced by the coronary artery bypass patient, it is necessary to review the structures utilized during the procedure.

The superficial structures are composed of skin and soft tissue. Because nerve endings in the skin are numerous, incisional pain is one of the most distinguished types of postoperative pain. The pain is described as sharp and is well located to the traumatized area. The nerve endings in the subcutaneous tissue are sparse and less sensitive to pain. Pain in this area is described as producing a burning sensation. The deeper structures are not capable of producing the same sensations because they have fewer nerve endings. The pain here is more diffuse and radiates to the surrounding area. For the coronary artery bypass graft (CABG) patient, all structures described above are surgically altered. It should also be noted that parietal peritoneum and pleura and some visceral organs produce severe, sharp, referred pain or tenderness to cutaneous areas adjacent to the original site of trauma (McCauley and Polomano 1980).

The patient experiencing pain due to a muscle spasm finds temporary relief in medication, traction, or hot-wet packs. The nurse assesses which intervention is the best for the patient, basing her decision on evaluation of the reduction in pain and/or increased tolerance to pain. Such a patient experiences pain associated with movement. Pain of movement may be experienced by the severely disabled arthritic patient, the burned patient, or the postoperative patient with abdominal or chest surgery. The pain of each must be accurately assessed before movement begins. For example, the arthritic patient's pain is joint-related, and, therefore needs careful range-of-motion exercises to maintain what limited joint mobility remains.

The burn patient's pain is related to exposed or sensitive nerve endings. The nurse therefore changes the dressings as quickly as possible in an attempt to reduce pain associated with exposure to air. For patients with abdominal or chest injury, the nurse teaches them the less painful ways of turning. In addition, the nurse might teach them how to utilize accessory muscles for the purpose of coughing and deep breathing. Pain associated with internal physiological disease, injury, or illness is difficult to alleviate. The nurse's most effective intervention may be to help the patient cope with this pain.

Noxious stimulation can originate in the patient's immediate environment. The entire postoperative experience, including the critical care unit and the prospect of severe pain can be terrifying. When the patient is confronted with multiple sources of anxiety there is an increased need for coping mechanisms. The nurse who prepares the patient for the days following surgery can help reduce his anxiety and clarify misconceptions. For the highly anxious patient, only essential information is provided. The essential information consists of the location and length of incision or a description of the pain involved. During the postoperative period the nurse needs to discuss the patient's expectation of analgesics or other pain reduction measures (McCauley and Palomano 1980).

The critical care nurse keeps in mind that the CABG patient is totally motionless during the surgery and in the immediate postoperative period. The nurse helps the patient turn and begin active or passive range-of-motion exericses to the legs. The upper extremities remain immobilized because of intravenous lines, intraarterial lines, and Swan-Ganz line. When possible the nurse can tell patients how to move without accidently removing various supportive or monitoring devices.

As mentioned earlier, the critical care environment contains noxious stimuli. For example noise may originate from equipment, other patients, or the health team itself. Equipment and supportive devices, especially in critical care units, are sometimes distracting and noisy. The machines hum, beep, and buzz at varying levels of intensity, making sleep impossible for some patients. Sleep deprivation leads to reduction in the individual's tolerance to pain. The nurse needs to remove unnecessary supportive devices as soon as possible. Likewise the nurse may need to separate the noisy patient from other patients. In addition the health team members must be sensitive to the noxious stimulation created by their voices. Some critical care units are noisier than others.

Postpain Experience

The postpain experience comes in the period of time immediately after the pain experience. Normally once the pain experience or situation (that is, the pain-provoking procedure or treatment) has been completed, the nurse leaves the patient alone so she can complete other responsibilities. The patient remains with the fears and anxieties relating to the experience. The patient may think that the critical care team will return to complete the painful procedure, not understanding that the experience has been terminated. Consequently, the nurse must inform the patient when the situation is over. The nurse remains to alleviate the postpain fears and, if necessary, to discuss the actual pain state. When she does this, she helps the patient to learn from the experience so that the next time he will be able to cope more effectively.

Just as autostimulation such as music can be used during the actual pain experience, it can also be a significant postpain intervention. In a study by Locsin (1981), the effect of music on the pain of selected postoperative patient during a first 48-hour time period was investigated. Measurement of pain was achieved by using the Overt Pain Reaction Rating Scale (OPRRS). Analgesics received, arterial blood pressure, pulse rates, and respiratory rates were also used to test the hypothesis. Significant differences were found between the groups of postoperative patients in their musculoskeletal and verbal pain reactions during the first 48 hours. Therefore music seems to be a distraction stimulus which refocuses the attention given to pain to something pleasant. Furthermore, music occupies the patient's mind with something familiar, soothing, and preferred.

NURSING EVALUATION

Evaluation of the patient's problem and nursing care is an ongoing process. The critical care nurse assesses both regulatory and cognitive behaviors supporting the diagnosis of pain. The interventions designed to minimize pain are evaluated for their effectiveness. There are some patients whose pain will not be completely terminated. Nevertheless the nurse, together with other members of the critical care team, tries to provide alternative measures to assist the patient in coping with his pain.

SUMMARY

Pain affects all patients in critical care. A major variable is the patient's tolerance to pain based upon previous experience. The nurse assesses characteristics of pain such as intensity, location, duration, and type. From the assessment and observations of the patient's nonverbal and verbal behavioral responses, the nurse is able to formulate a plan of care designed to relieve pain. The nurse realizes that total relief is, in many instances, impossible. Therefore, the goal is to help the patient find the degree of relief that is possible. The effectiveness of the intervention is then based upon the attainment of relief. Nurses can and do creatively intervene to help the patient cope with pain.

REFERENCES

ARMSTRONG, D., "Pain-Producing Substance in Human Inflammatory Exudate and Plasma," *Journal Physiology*, 135 (1957), 135.

ARMSTRONG, MARGARET, "Current Concepts in Pain," *AORN Journal*, 32, no. 3 (September 1980), 383-390.

BOWERS, KENNETH, "Pain, Anxiety, and Perceived Control," *Journal of Consulting and Clinical Psychology*, 32, no. 3 (1968), 596-602.

BRESLER, DAVID, *Free Yourself From Pain*. New York: Simon & Schuster, 1979.

COPP, LAUREL ARCHER, "The Spectrum of Suffering," *American Journal of Nursing*, March 1974, pp. 491-495.

DRAKONTIDES, ANNA, "Drugs to Treat Pain," *American Journal of Nursing*, March 1974, pp. 508-513.

ELLIS, BETTY LOVE, "Predicting Postoperative Pain Behaviors," *Military Medicine*, 143, no. 12 (December 1978), 858-862.

GAUMER, WILLIAM, "Electrical Stimulation in Chronic Pain," *American Journal of Nursing*, March 1974, pp. 504-505.

GOLOSKOV, JOAN, "Use of the Dorsal Column Stimulator," *American Journal of Nursing*, March 1974, pp. 506-507.

GUYTON, ARTHUR, *Textbook of Medical Physiology*. Philadelphia: Saunders, 1981.

HACKETT, THOMAS, "Pain and Prejudice: Why Do We Doubt That the Patient is in Pain?" *Resident and Staff Physician*, May 1972, pp. 101-109.

KIM, SUSIE, "Pain: Theory, Research and Nursing Practice," *Advances in Nursing Science*, 2 (January 1980), 43-59.

LESHAN, LAWRENCE, "The World of the Patient in Severe Pain of Long Duration," *Journal of Chronic Disease*, 17 (February 1964), 121.

LESLE, KENNETH, "Pain: How It Varies from Person to Person," *Nursing Times*, July 20, 1972, p. 890.

LOCSIN, ROZZANO, "The Effect of Music on the Pain of Selected Postoperative Patients," *Journal of Advanced Nursing*, 6 (June 1981), 19-25.

MCCAULEY, KATHLEEN, and ROSEMARY POLOMANO, "Acute Pain: A Nursing Perspective with Cardiac Surgical Patients," *Topics in Clinical Nursing*, 2 (April 1980), 45-56.

MCCAFFERY, MARGO, *Nursing Management of the Patient with Pain*. Philadelphia: Lippincott, 1972.

——, "Patients in Pain," *Nursing '73* (November 1973), pp. 42-50.

MASTROVITO, RENE, "Psychogenic Pain," *American Journal of Nursing*, March 1974, pp. 514.

MELZACK, RONALD, *The Puzzle of Pain*. New York: Basic Books, 1973.

MENZEL, NANCY, and IDA MARTINSON, "Effects of Electrical Surface Stimulation on Control of Acute Postoperative Pain and Prevention of Atelectasis and Ileus in Patients Having Abdominal Surgery," *Communicating Nursing Research*, 8 (March 1977), 284-290.

SCHMIDEK, HENRY, "Pain: Current Physiologic and Surgical Concepts," *Hospital Formulary*, 12 (July 1977), 447-451.

SIEGELE, DOROTHY, "The Gate Control Theory," *American Journal of Nursing*, March 1974, p. 499.

VOSHALL, BARBARA, "The Effects of Preoperative Teaching on Postoperative Pain," *Topics in Clinical Nursing*, 2 (April 1980), 39-43.

WOLF, ZANE, "Pain Theories: An Overview," *Topics in Clinical Nursing*, 2 (April 1980), 9-18.

Index

Cardiac sounds, 33, 36
Cardiovascular system, 39, 44
Central venous pressure (CVP):
    about, 25
    status, 25, 27
Chest sounds, 33
Cognitive behaviors, 84, 112–14, 134–35

D

Denial:
    behavioral objectives, 197
    defensive reappraisal, denial, 211–14
    definition, 198–200
    direct-action tendency, avoidance,
        203–11
    nursing assessment, 214–15
    nursing diagnosis, 215–16
    nursing evaluation, 220
    nursing interventions, 216–20
Depersonalization:
    behavioral objectives, 276
    definitions, 277–79
    human design, humanization, 285
    nursing assessment, 287–88
    nursing diagnosis, 288
    nursing evaluation, 296
    nursing interventions, 288–96
    origin of depersonalization and
        dehumanization, 279–85
Depression:
    behavioral objectives, 457
    definition, 458
    nursing assessment, 468–70
    nursing diagnosis, 470
    nursing evaluation, 474
    nursing interventions, 470–74
    self-evaluation stage, 464–66
    self-monitoring stage, 459–64
    self-reinforcement stage, 466–68

E

Endocrine system, 52, 56

F

Family:
    behavioral objectives, 431

functions of family, 433–34
    nursing assessment, 447–48
    nursing diagnosis, 448
    nursing evaluation, 454
    nursing interventions, 448–54
    stress of illness, 436–43
    stress of social loss, 443–47

G

Gastrointestinal system, 56

H

Helplessness, 98–99
Hepatojugular reflex, 39
Hope, 97–98
Hopelessness:
    behavioral objectives, 95
    definitions, 97–101
    nursing assessment, 110–12
    nursing diagnosis, 112
    nursing evaluation, 117
    nursing interventions, 112–17
Hostility:
    behavioral objectives, 144
    definitions, 146–49
    externalization of hostility, 151–59
    internalization of hostility, 159–64
    nursing assessment, 164–65
    nursing diagnosis, 166
    nursing evaluation, 171
    nursing interventions, 166–71

L

Loneliness:
    behavorial objectives, 223
    definitions, 225–27
    existential loneliness, real experience,
        228–36
    loneliness anxiety, fear of aloneness,
        236–42
    nursing assessment, 242–43
    nursing diagnosis, 243
    nursing evaluation, 250
    nursing interventions, 243–49